Community Organizing and Community Building for Health and Social Equity

Community Organizing and Community Building for Health and Social Equity

Fourth Edition

EDITED BY
MEREDITH MINKLER
PATRICIA WAKIMOTO

RUTGERS UNIVERSITY PRESS

NEW BRUNSWICK, CAMDEN, AND NEWARK, NEW JERSEY, AND LONDON

Library of Congress Cataloging-in-Publication Data

Names: Minkler, Meredith, editor.
Title: Community organizing and community building for health and social equity /
edited by Meredith Minkler ; associate edited by Patricia Wakimoto.
Other titles: Community organizing and community building for health and welfare.
Description: Fourth edition. | New Brunswick, New Jersey : Rutgers University Press,
[2022] | Revision of: Community organizing and community building for health and
welfare. 3rd ed. 2012. | Includes bibliographical references and index.
Identifiers: LCCN 2021011296 | ISBN 9781978824744 (paperback) |
ISBN 9781978824751 (hardback) | ISBN 9781978824768 (epub) |
ISBN 9781978824775 (pdf)
Subjects: LCSH: Health promotion. | Community health services—Citizen
participation. | Community organization. | Community development.
Classification: LCC RA427.8 .C64 2022 | DDC 362.1—dc23
LC record available at https://lccn.loc.gov/2021011296

A British Cataloging-in-Publication record for this book is
available from the British Library.

References to internet websites (URLs) were accurate at the time of writing. Neither
the author nor Rutgers University Press is responsible for URLs that may have expired
or changed since the manuscript was prepared.

∞ The paper used in this publication meets the requirements of the American National
Standard for Information Sciences—Permanence of Paper for
Printed Library Materials, ANSI Z39.48-1992.

www.rutgersuniversitypress.org

Manufactured in the United States of America

CONTENTS

PART THREE

Building Effective Partnerships and Anticipating and Addressing Ethical Challenges

PART FOUR

Community Assessment and Issue Selection

PART FIVE

Community Organizing and Community Building within and across Diverse Groups and Cultures

PART EIGHT
Influencing Policy through Community Organizing and Media Advocacy

Appendixes

Note: In addition to the "Questions for Further Discussion" at the end of
each chapter and the following appendixes, supplementary materials for
instructors are available at rutgersuniversitypress.org/communityorganizing.

ILLUSTRATIONS

Figures

Tables

Boxes

FOREWORD

When I arrived in East Baltimore, Maryland, in the fall of 1985 to attend medical school, I was shocked by the living conditions that people were consigned to in the neighborhoods immediately adjacent to the medical school campus. As a young Black American who had been raised in Montreal, Canada, I had no context for what I was seeing. I had been inspired to come back to the United States by the soaring racial justice rhetoric of Martin Luther King Jr. and Malcolm X. I very much wanted to play a part in building a socially just society, but despite that motivation, what I encountered in East Baltimore was profoundly jarring. African Americans in East Baltimore were exposed to a seemingly endless constellation of injurious health privations, from dilapidated housing to poor-quality schools, a dearth of green space, failing infrastructure, high unemployment, mass incarceration, and aggressive, militarized policing. A few miles up the road I saw sprawling mansions nestled on the manicured lawns in Baltimore's Roland Park neighborhood. I would later come to learn of Baltimore's long and storied history of racial zoning, redlining, racially restrictive covenants, racial steering, and racial harassment, but as a naive and young Black man dropped into the midst of this inequity, I was left reeling and confused.

I also noticed a very peculiar thing. Many African American adults in East Baltimore would not make eye contact with me, and often had a faraway look in their eyes, while young African Americans, particularly adolescents, made direct eye contact, often with a look of frustration tinged with anger in their eyes. It was as if they had begun to internalize the devaluation that their desolate and resource-deprived environment was signaling. The cumulative emotional toll of years of dehumanizing conditions and treatment would begin to boil over. The look of frustration and anger often seemed to border on rage. Over time, that rage seemed to harden into a defeated resignation and what I perceived as a pervasive sense of futurelessness. It seemed to me as if people's spirits had been steadily broken by the indignity and chronic humiliation of living in conditions of relentless poverty and hopelessness. That crushing indignity was literally dimming the light in people's eyes.

While in medical school, I had the opportunity to travel to South Africa during apartheid to study the effects of that political system on the health of South African Blacks. I traveled on segregated buses and trains and visited Bantustans

throughout the country. But while working in clinics in Alexandra and the sprawling Baragwanath Hospital in Soweto, I saw a very different look in the eyes of Black
South Africans. Although they lived in materially far poorer circumstances than
what I saw in East Baltimore and suffered direct militarized and violent oppression by the minority White South African government, in their eyes I saw a strong
light. The Black South Africans I worked with in Alexandra and Soweto were organizing. They were coming together with political and community organizers to
strategize about building a new egalitarian and multiracial South Africa. In their
eyes I saw the bright light of hope and possibility. They had developed a powerful
sense of agency and had purpose in their lives. They had a vision for their future
and were set on achieving it.

My experience studying South Africa's apartheid gave me a much deeper
insight into East Baltimore and America's apartheid. I learned that at the core of
community health is hope. People who see a better future for themselves and their
communities will work toward it. Community organizers can help clarify that
vision and build the agency and sense of belonging that turn on the light in people's
eyes. So much of the skill set that I was acquiring in medical school was *technocratic*—
blood tests, cat scans, procedures—but I realized that much of what I needed to
learn to improve health in East Baltimore was instead *democratic*. And at the heart
of that democratic challenge lay community organizing.

Since those seminal experiences in East Baltimore and Soweto over thirty years
ago, I have committed my career to improving community health through community organizing. I have seen that in public health, as in social work, urban and
regional planning, and other fieldsthat interface with communities and social systems, practitioners must recognize the enduring consequences of deeply entrenched
structural and institutional racism and other forms of systemic injustice. I have
seen, too, that the only sustainable approach to eliminating health and social inequities employs policy and other means to facilitate intensive, multisectoral, place-
conscious interventions that are specifically designed to identify existing assets and
build social, political, and economic power among a critical mass of community
residents in historically under-resourced communities. Undoing racism and apartheid will require intensive work that creates and implements new policies, rebuilds
infrastructure, and heals and repairs human bonds damaged by generations of racism. Community organizing is the only proven tool that can deliver such results.

As the lead architect of Building Healthy Communities, the California Endowment's $1.8 billion, ten-year, statewide, place-conscious, community health
improvement initiative, I have taken the lessons of East Baltimore and South Africa
deeply to heart. Community organizing lives at the center of our work. The Minkler
and Wakimoto definition of *community organizing* as "a process by which communities identify their assets and concerns, prioritize and select issues, and intentionally build power and develop and implement action strategies for change"
guides the grant-making that fuels the initiative. In addition, the equity principle
dictates that the people most impacted by inequity must be directly engaged in

crafting the solutions. This must be foremost in the minds of practitioners in public health, social work, and regional planning, as well as of philanthropists, academics, and government officials, as they participate in this work. That requires ceding power, which is a difficult contortion for many of these institutional actors, particularly given America's long and continuing conflict with itself around two competing narratives: inclusion and exclusion.

As I write this foreword, an American president who has brutally mastered the narrative of exclusion refuses to concede his electoral loss to his opponent and instead sows division, ignites and fans conspiracy theories, and continues to demonize people of color and those who want to heal and rebuild this nation. Meanwhile, COVID-19 infects over 1 million Americans a week and is killing 1,000 people a day. Protests continue throughout the country seeking racial justice in the face of state-mediated murder through police violence.

Leaders and practitioners in fields like public health sit at the heart of these multiple epidemics and are often called upon to help communities navigate these fraught and dangerous times. In this context, and in the critical and uncharted territory ahead, the fourth and final edition of *Community Organizing and Community Building for Health and Social Equity* could not be more timely. For community organizing and community building are the port in the storm that we public health and other equity- and social change–focused practitioners must rededicate ourselves to in order to offer a way forward in this tumultuous period of our existence.

Threaded throughout this volume is the importance of working "with, rather than on communities," and using an equity lens to help promote impactful and multilevel change. A strong emphasis is placed as well on empowerment, or helping create the conditions in which people in exploited and disenfranchised communities can take the power they need to make changes now while also gaining a more permanent seat at the policymaking table.

The book also calls on practitioners to deeply and honestly confront the ethical challenges paramount in this work—from conflicting loyalties to engaging with hard questions like how to be a "White ally," and how to embed our work in a genuine commitment to authentic rather than tokenistic community leadership and engagement.

To address these and other issues, Minkler and Wakimoto have assembled a wide array of authors, from grassroots community organizers and community builders to their partners in academia, health departments, foundations, and the world of policymaking. They share conceptual frameworks for community organizing and community building, skills such as asset mapping, participatory evaluation, media advocacy, and policy analysis. Finally, the contributors share a wide range of case studies, from the building of a powerful People's Assembly in Jackson, Mississippi, to the creation in Seattle, Washington, of a unique health department/foundation/community collaborative that dramatically shifted power to communities while the health department worked internally to address structural racism and change its ways of doing business.

Despite the many challenges faced—especially when working to end such deeply entrenched and racialized problems as mass incarceration, the cases shared are also those of hope. And they brought me back to my own journey of discovery, from the dimly lit and troubled eyes of African Americans in a world devoid of hope or equity in the Baltimore of the 1980s to the eyes of impoverished people in Soweto working to end apartheid and showing the "bright light of hope and possibility," reflecting their powerful sense of agency, purpose, and a vision for the future.

In the words he wrote in the late 1980s as a young community organizer on the South Side of Chicago, in the essay that constitutes this book's second chapter, former president Barack Obama reminds us that "organizing teaches us, as nothing else does, the beauty and strength of everyday people." This book is built on the power of that belief.

Antony B. Iton, MD, JD, MPH

Community Organizing and Community Building for Health and Social Equity

PART ONE

Introduction

As this book goes to press, professionals and students in fields such as public health, social work, urban and regional planning, and community psychology are living through a time of almost unprecedented disjuncture. The worst pandemic in a century took well over half a million American lives in a single year as deep political divisions and conspiracy theories upended any hope of a broad national commitment to social distancing and wearing masks.

The depth and breadth of systemic racism and racial and social inequities were rarely as starkly in focus as in 2020. Whether in the brutal police killings of Black men and women and the unprecedented protests unleashed, or the fifty-year high in the Black–White gap in home ownership (Choi, 2020), racialized policies and practices were once again laid bare. We also saw stepped-up attacks on immigrants, women's reproductive rights, tribal sovereignty over rightfully owned land and water, and the rights of LGBTQ people, alongside the rolling back of environmental and worker protections as the existential threat of climate change looms ever larger. These threads are among many that form the tapestry within which public health professionals, social workers, community psychologists, and other social change professionals now find themselves working.

Yet, concurrently, that context includes positives: our unprecedented societal diversity, an electorate that voted in record numbers despite a raging pandemic, and the commitment and leadership of our youth and growing numbers of their elders on banning assault weapons and acknowledging the imperative of climate justice. We are also seeing bold new partnerships across differences, including countless collaboratives working for real and transformative change, with health departments and philanthropic funders increasingly playing key roles (Freudenberg et al., 2015; Iton & Ross, 2017; Plough & Ford, 2015; chapter 9).

Within this complex contextual tapestry, there is growing appreciation of the importance of community building and community organizing, and of working with, rather than on, communities (Minkler et al., 2019; Pastor et al., 2018).

The opening chapters of this book reflect the premise that for public health professionals, social workers, and other social change professionals, this aspect of our work has rarely been more important. In chapter 1, community organizing is defined as a process by which communities identify their assets and concerns, prioritize and select issues, and intentionally build power and develop and implement action strategies for change (Minkler et al., 2019, p. 10S). The related concept of community building is used not as a strategic framework or approach to fixing problems, but rather as an orientation to community practice, accenting building the capacities of complex and multidimensional communities (chapter 3).

The reality of the need for an even greater focus on such processes, however, and on such embedded concepts as high-level community participation and empowerment, has not begun to match the rhetoric (DeFilippis et al., 2010) nor, with few exceptions (Iton & Ross, 2017; chapter 9), is funding for such work as part of our professional practice even close to being adequate.

Yet, in the fight against some of our most intractable health and social problems, there are community-based organizations, a global health cities and communities movement, increasing use of tools such as coalitions and media advocacy, and partnerships between communities, academics, and health departments. Chapter 1 suggests that health educators, social workers, and other social change professionals can usefully adapt and apply community organizing and community building in their efforts to work with communities to combat HIV/AIDS, domestic violence, asthma, homelessness, and a host of other health and social problems. But it also makes a case for what it calls a "purer" approach to organizing, in which communities mobilize around the issues that they, not we as outsiders, identify and wish to collectively address. The role of the outside organizer in this latter approach is one of helping to create the conditions in which community groups can become empowered to determine their own health and social agenda and act effectively to help bring about the changes they wish to see.

Chapter 1 also introduces the concept of community building, which in recent years has achieved increasing currency in fields like health education, social work, community psychology, and urban planning (Blackwell & Colmenar, 2000; Corburn, 2013, 2017). As later described in chapter 3, however, an alternative perspective on community building views it not as a strategic framework or approach to fixing problems, but rather as an orientation to community practice, accenting building the capacities of complex and multidimensional communities, of which we as organizers and other practitioners are ideally a part.

The three major purposes of this book are highlighted in chapter 1:

1. To pull together recent and classic thinking about community organizing and community building theory and practice
2. To illustrate the concepts, principles, and methods explored through theory-driven case studies
3. To engage the reader in reflecting on many of the tough questions and ethical challenges that are often inherent in community practice

This first chapter highlights Tom Wolff et al.'s (2017) principles for collaborating for equity and justice designed to engage communities in collaborative action that can in turn lead to transformative changes in power, equity, and justice (p. 42). These principles range from explicitly addressing social and economic injustice and systemic racism to ensuring that the collaborative itself provides "basic facilitating structures that build member ownership and leadership" (p. 51). To this list, Minkler and Wakimoto add a seventh principle: "embodying cultural humility," with its commitment to critical self-reflection, an openness to others' cultures, redressing power imbalances, and developing authentic partnerships (Tervalon & Murray-Garcia, 1998), while also continually striving to be more culturally competent (Greene-Moton & Minkler, 2020). Although this list is far from exhaustive, the authors offer these principles as useful initial guidelines that are also thematic throughout the book.

Chapter 1 concludes with an overview of the various chapters and appendixes that make up this volume, illustrating in the process some of the central themes, such as empowerment and capacity building. We hope these offerings will provide the reader with an understanding of the theoretical bases, ethical challenges, and practical tools needed for engagement in this work, and with a new or renewed appreciation of community organizing and community building as potent approaches for improving the public's health and social well-being.

The first part of this book closes with former president Barack Obama's classic piece "Why Organize? Problems and Promise in the Inner City," which was originally published in 1988 as he reflected on his work as a young organizer on Chicago's South Side. Although some of the language (e.g., inner city) and key players (e.g., the Moral Majority) have changed, his message for organizers rings as true today as it did over thirty years ago. Obama has often commented that his experiences as a community organizer were the best preparation he had for the presidency. As he tells stories of his work with the Gamaliel Foundation (discussed in chapter 5) and all he has learned from ordinary folks who come together to make change, an uplifting view of what organizing can be unfolds. In Obama's words, "Organizing teaches, as nothing else does, the beauty and strength of everyday people" (1988, p. 40) and working collaboratively with everyday people can help us build healthy and strong communities.

REFERENCES

Blackwell, A. G., & Colmenar, R. (2000). Community-building: From local wisdom to public policy. *Public Health Rep, 115*(2–3), 161–166.

Choi, J. H. (2020, February 21). Breaking down the Black-White home ownership gap. The Urban Institute. https://www.urban.org/urban-wire/breaking-down-black-white-homeownership-gap.

Corburn, J. (2013). *Healthy City Planning: From Neighbourhood to National Health Equity.* Routledge.

Corburn, J. (2017). Equitable and healthy city planning: Towards healthy urban governance in the century of the city. In E. de Leeuw & J. Simons (Eds.), *Healthy Cities: The Theory, Policy, and Practice of Value-Based Urban Planning* (pp. 31–41). Springer.

DeFilippis, J., Fisher, R., & Shragge, E. (2010). *Contesting Community: The Limits and Potential of Local Organizing.* Rutgers University Press.

Freudenberg, N., Franzosa, E., Chisholm, J., & Libman, K. (2015). New approaches for moving upstream: How state and local health departments can transform practice to reduce health inequalities. *Health Educ Behav, 42*(1_suppl), 46S–56S.

Greene-Moton, E., & Minkler, M. (2020). Cultural competence or cultural humility? Moving beyond the debate. *Health Promot Pract, 21*(1), 142–145.

Iton, A., & Ross, R. K. (2017). Understanding how health happens: Your zip code is more important than your genetic code. In R. Callahan & D. Bhattacharya (Eds.), *Public Health Leadership* (pp. 83–99). Routledge.

Minkler, M., Rebanal, R. D., Pearce, R., & Acosta, M. (2019). Growing equity and health equity in perilous times: Lessons from community organizers. *Health Educ Behav, 46*(1_suppl), 9S–18S.

Obama, B. (1988). Why organize? Problems and promise in the inner city. *Illinois Issues* (42), 35–40.

Pastor, M., Terriquez, V., & Lin, M. (2018). How community organizing promotes health equity, and how health equity affects organizing. *Health Aff, 37*(3), 358–363.

Plough, A., & Ford, C. (2015). *From Vision to Action: A Framework and Measures to Mobilize a Culture of Health.* Robert Wood Johnson Foundation.

Tervalon, M., & Murray-Garcia, J. (1998). Cultural humility versus cultural competence: A critical distinction in defining physician training outcomes in multicultural education. *J Health Care Poor Underserved, 9*(2), 117–125.

Wolff, T., Minkler, M., Wolfe, S. M., Berkowitz, B., Bowen, L., Butterfoss, F. D., Christens, B. D., Francisco, V. T., Himmelman, A. T., & Lee, K. S. (2017). Collaborating for equity and justice: Moving beyond collective impact. *Nonprofit Q, 9*, 42–53.

1

Introduction to Community Organizing and Community Building in a New Era

MEREDITH MINKLER
PATRICIA WAKIMOTO

The second decade of the twenty-first century broke historic records, with 2020 alone bringing the worst global pandemic in over a hundred years. Within one year, COVID-19 has claimed 2.6 million lives worldwide and 529,000 lives in the United States alone. Deeply entrenched inequities in health and life chances by race and ethnicity in the United States were magnified by the pandemic, with Bassett and her colleagues' (2020) calculation of age-specific mortality rates revealing death rate ratios seven to nine times higher for Blacks, Hispanics, and Asian Pacific Islanders than for non-Hispanic Whites, reflecting the devastating toll COVID-19 has taken among communities of color.

The loss of over 20 million jobs in the first two months of the pandemic, and one in four American children being food insecure by late November (Feeding America, 2020), further highlight problems caused or exacerbated by the pandemic. So, too, does the dramatic increase in anti-Black and anti–Asian American Pacific Islander (AAPI) hate crimes linked to the pandemic (Ruiz et al., 2020). A study of police reports in sixteen of the nation's largest cities, for example, showed close to a 150 percent increase in anti-Asian hate crimes in 2020 alone, with racial slurs and taunts mimicking then president Donald J. Trump's frequent references to the "China virus" and other derogatory remarks (Center for the Study of Hate and Extremism, 2021).

Close on the heels of the pandemic's meteoric rise in early spring of 2020 were the Black Lives Matter (BLM)-led protests of the brutal police killing of George Floyd, an unarmed Black man. The protests were on a scale not seen since the civil rights demonstrations following the assassination of Martin Luther King Jr. over fifty years earlier. As many more names were added to the toll of tragic and unjustified deaths of Black people—among them Breonna Taylor, Ahmaud Arbery, Rayshard Brooks, Sandra Bland, Aura Rosser, and Jacob Blake—commentators began speaking of the twin viruses: COVID-19 and systematic racism. The latter is far more virulent, rooted in our history of genocide and displacement of Indigenous

7

people, the enslavement of Blacks, and "the continued racial ordering of humans and goods" (Hardeman et al., 2020, p. 2) underlying every aspect of our society. As discussed in chapter 4, this long-ignored racial ordering ranges from the civil legal system to finance, education, housing, employment, and health care, and manifests in the grave racial/ethnic health and social inequities in the United States (Blackwell & McAfee, 2020; Kendi, 2019; Reich, 2020).

In the context of these and other overlapping crises, however, there was reason for hope. In the words of acclaimed author Arundhati Roy (2020), "Historically, pandemics have forced humans to break with the past and imagine their world anew. This one is no different. It is a portal, a gateway between one world and the next. We can choose to walk through it, dragging the carcasses of our prejudice and hatred, our avarice, our data banks and dead ideas, our dead rivers and smoky skies behind us. Or we can walk through lightly, with little luggage, ready to imagine another world. And ready to fight for it." Although Roy was reflecting specifically on the coronavirus pandemic, her words apply equally to systemic racism and the future of racial justice, toward which the potentially transformative consequences of the protests and their aftermath have only begun to unfold. In summer 2020, a great national reckoning with race and systemic racism led 67 percent of Americans to express their support for BLM, although the percentage dropped to 55 percent by late autumn (Thomas & Horowitz, 2020). Numerous large corporations lined up with gestures of solidarity, albeit typically not with the bold changes in corporate culture and policies needed for real and sustainable change (Blackwell & McAfee, 2020; Hsu, 2020). Together with the pandemic, BLM protests and their aftermath cast into sharp relief the need for transforming policing, education, the economy, health care, the criminal legal system, immigration, and other broken systems that promote deep racial/ethnic, class, and other inequities (chapter 4). The need to boldly and firmly address growing online and virtual hate crimes, including expressions of homophobia, neo-Nazism, and White supremacy—sometimes with the tacit and vocal support of government leaders, including former president Trump—remain a bitter reminder of the long road ahead, both through and beyond the portal to racial equity and justice. Yet, as Kendi (2019) reminds us, racial discrimination is simply a more "immediate and visible manifestation" of a policy, whether written or unwritten, that sustains racial inequity (p. 19). Squarely facing the need to transform all such policies into those to support racial equity and justice must be a core commitment as we walk through Roy's portal toward a better future for all in our diverse society and world.

The COVID-19 pandemic's massive and escalating toll on morbidity, mortality, and national and global economies brought a small but measurable pause in carbon emissions. However, without dramatic reductions in emissions by 2030, we will be dangerously close to the threshold beyond which almost unimaginable human and planetary tolls will take place (Barone et al., 2020). Yet in the case of climate change, too, we have an opportunity to walk through Roy's portal "lightly, with little luggage, ready to imagine another world. And ready to fight for it." With the United States rejoining the Paris Accord early in 2021 and working to enact its own climate action plan, and with the commitment of the European Union and nations worldwide to rebuild economies differently and to transform how people live, work, and play (von der Leyen, 2020), the possibilities for real and sustainable change are heartening.

The social philosopher Cornel West (2017) found "grand signs of hope" captured by movements such as the 2017 women's mobilization that put class matters, gender matters, and LGBTQ matters at the center of race matters and empire matters; the historic protests at Standing Rock and others before it, in which Indigenous people came together in a struggle for sacred lands and self-respect; and the struggles in which military veterans, disabled people, and people of all races joined to stop oil pipeline companies from "invading and colonizing sacred land." West concludes that "the mounting coalition—or solidarity work—of mobilizations of peoples of color here and around the world is a beacon of hope" (p. xxiii).

In each of these movements and struggles, people of all races, ethnicities, and identities have used community building and organizing, as well as movement building, to try to undo centuries-old power imbalances, to right wrongs, and to aspire to a society in which equity and justice are centric. Some of us engage in such work as separate from our day jobs, while others of us are fortunate enough to work in fields or with organizations in which community building and organizing for equity and justice are recognized as among the most important parts of our professional lives. As Iton and Shrimali (2016) remind us, "Attempts to address health disparities will fail unless we acknowledge that changing our practice is inherently political and controversial," and unless we act now to change power inequities, share power with those we serve, and design new programs and policies "to build collective power for change" (p. 1757).

Community Organizing, Community Building, and Equity: Definitions and Intersections

In this time of reimagining our world while confronting extraordinary challenges, including historic imbalances in privilege and power, renewed attacks on women's reproductive health, and immigrant and LGBTQ rights, the importance of community organizing and community building has seldom been clearer. As Manuel Pastor and colleagues (2018) note, a growing evidence base "recognizes community organizing as a vehicle for unleashing the collective power necessary to uproot the socioeconomic inequities at the core of health disparities" (p. 358). Further, the language of equity or fairness that is increasingly central in fields including public health, social work, urban and regional planning, and community psychology enables practitioners as community builders and organizers to work *with*, rather than *on* communities, through an equity lens to help support multilevel change (Minkler et al., 2019). Central to this work, moreover, is creating the conditions necessary for the empowerment of marginalized populations that have been historically exploited and neglected by the economically and racially privileged and powerful (Blackwell & McAfee, 2020; Corburn, 2017; Kleba et al., 2021; Pastor et al., 2018).

We define *community organizing* as "a process by which communities identify their assets and concerns, prioritize and select issues, and intentionally build power and develop and implement action strategies for change" (Minkler et al., 2019, p. 10S). Reflected in this definition, core tenets of organizing frequently include building community power and empowerment, starting with issues that matter to the people, and *praxis*, defined by Brazilian adult educator, Paulo Freire (1970) as "action based on critical reflection." As discussed in chapter 3, however, no single set of tenets captures the complexity of community organizing, nor the breadth and depth of thinking and approaches encompassed by this term.

In health education and public health more broadly, growing interest in community organizing approaches to equity and health equity have stressed the importance of systems change with a focus on the Social Determinants of Health (SDOH). Indeed, as Paula Braveman and her colleagues (2017) note, getting to health equity "*requires* removing obstacles to health such as poverty, discrimination and their consequences, including powerlessness, lack of access to good jobs with fair pay, quality education and housing, safe environments, and health care" (p. 2; emphasis added). Helping to remove such barriers to equity is often a major part of the raison d'être of community organizers and community builders, and of public health professionals, social workers, city and regional planners, and other practitioners embracing these roles.

The Bidirectionality of Community Organizing and Equity

In a seminal article, Pastor and colleagues (2018) point out that not only has community organizing gained traction in fields like public health that are increasingly concerned with health and social equity, but conversely, the health equity frame has become a useful and important one for effective community organizing. The value of framing community issues through a health lens was one of five core themes to emerge from convenings of community organizers from throughout the United States as part of the Robert Wood Johnson Foundation's efforts to inform its thinking about a broad "Culture of Health." As discussed later in this book, a Culture of Health is a society in which "every person has a fair and equal opportunity to live as healthy a life as possible" (Plough & Gandhi, 2019, p. 490). The Foundation's recognition that grassroots community organizers have much to teach the funders and public health professionals was encouraging. And so was the organizers' clear articulation of the strategic value of partnering with public health departments and professionals and leveraging public health's expertise to gain credibility with stakeholders, while receiving their assistance with data collection and advocacy efforts (Minkler et al., 2019).

As discussed in chapter 10, the increasing adoption of a Health in All Policies approach on the municipal through the global health levels is helping stakeholders and leaders in areas from urban and regional planning to consider the potential health impacts of their education, transportation, and financial policies (Iton & Ross, 2017; Rudolph et al., 2013). The impact of such efforts on the local level is well illustrated in the work of fourteen communities, plagued by health inequities, but whose residents, as part of The California Endowment's Building Healthy Communities initiative, have helped craft, advocate for, and secure the adoption of over one hundred policies in a range of municipal sectors that, in turn, have fostered access to fresh food, clean water, parks, and more walkable communities (Iton & Ross, 2017).

Community Building

Closely related to community organizing and deeply concerned with equity, are the approaches collectively known as *community building*. Although several views of community building are used in this book, it is conceptualized most often as an orientation to practice focused on community, rather than a strategic framework or approach used by outside professionals in their efforts to support community economic development and other goals. As Walter and Hyde (2012) point out, the former view of community building conceptualizes community as "an inclusive, multidimensional, and dynamic system" of which the practitioner ideally is a part (p. 85).

Identifying and building individual and community capacities, as well as the broader notion of community capitals, such as social capital and the built environment (Beaulieu, 2014; Flora & Flora, 2008), is a key part of community building and mapping (chapters 3, 11), which then can be used to help effect change.

A second view of community building, also reflected in this volume, is more deliberately focused on action for change. As defined by PolicyLink founder Angela Glover Blackwell (Blackwell & Colmenar, 2000), community building in this view involves "continuous, self-renewing efforts by residents and professionals to engage in collective action, aimed at problem solving and enrichment, that creates new or strengthened social networks, new capacities for group action and support, and new standards and expectations for the life of the community" (p. ii). The basic tenets of this view of community building, as summarized by Blackwell and Colmenar (2000, p. 162), include

- "strengthening communities holistically," rather than addressing "bits and pieces," such as housing or transportation;
- building local capacity for problem solving, and building relationships between communities and resource institutions;
- fostering community participation in the policymaking process;

- dealing up front with "race," and ethnicity and their pervasive ties to systemic health and social inequities;
- breaking down the isolation of poor communities, linking neighborhoods to the larger context of regional development;
- tailoring programs to local conditions and engaging the community in the local problem solving as the most effective solutions come from within the community; and
- building mechanisms for accountability, enabling communities to "maintain improvements and monitor [progress] toward achieving a better quality of life."

The book's focus on community building, and not merely community organizing, is well justified from the perspectives of public health, social welfare, urban and regional planning, community psychology, and other fields. We confront daily the fraying social fabric of our information (and disinformation) age society, in which individuals often lack secure embeddedness in a family, a workplace, a neighborhood, or a community of common interest (Moore & Kawachi, 2017; Putnam, 2000). This lack of connectedness and, on the community level, the different forms of social capital it represents, are not only a social hazard but also a public health one, as alienation and lack of a sense of connection are associated with an epidemic of "deaths of despair" from suicides, alcoholism, and drug overdoses. Sehgal (2020) calculated for 2018 that children had a lifetime risk of 1 in 70 for deaths from drug overdoses alone, a figure that increased still further during the pandemic. Heart disease, depression, risky health behaviors, and difficulty healing from trauma are among the numerous health outcomes also associated with social isolation and lack of embeddedness in the social fabric (Iton & Ross, 2017; Nurius et al., 2013).

Cross-Sector and Community-Engaged Collaboration for Equity

As discussed throughout this book, the sheer complexity of many health and social problems and inequities in the United States and globally has long highlighted the importance of community-engaged, cross-sector approaches better able to understand and address such concerns than more siloed and top-down approaches (Baciu et al., 2017; Schultz et al., 2020; Towe et al., 2016). Numerous governmental and global health bodies, including the Centers for Disease Control and Prevention (CDC), the National Institutes of Health (NIH), the Pan American Health Organization, and the World Health Organization, have called for and supported cross-sector collaboration, high-level community engagement, and increasingly, community-led partnerships in public health practice (Kleba et al., 2021; Pan American Health Organization, 2020; World Health Organization, 2017; chapter 3). Similarly, large and small philanthropic entities, prominently including the W.K. Kellogg Foundation, The California Endowment, and the Robert Wood Johnson

Foundation in the United States, have long emphasized cross-sector collaborations that include communities as major actors, in efforts to study and address health inequities (Baciu et al., 2017; Iton & Shrimali, 2016; Wallerstein et al., 2018; chapters 3, 9, 20).

Support for community engagement and cross-sector collaboration has taken on still greater significance during the COVID-19 pandemic and the profound economic recession and other national and global transformations in its wake. The rapidly changing contexts in which we live and work further underscore the need for developing new theoretical models and testing the relevance and effectiveness of existing ones to better guide and assess such collaborative endeavors. Such models must be grounded in, or supplemented by, a principles-focused approach to ensure that we measure our work against the criteria of equity and justice (Butterfoss & Kegler, 2009; Wolfe et al., 2020; Wolff et al., 2017; chapters 18, 19).

The many common threads that link the aforementioned approaches to community building and community organizing and the need for both cross-sector collaboration and high-level community engagement are explored in more detail in chapter 3 and subsequent parts of this volume. Yet these and other commonalities across approaches are also well captured in the six principles for collaborating for equity and justice developed by Wolff et al. (2017) and a seventh added by Greene-Moton & Minkler (2020). These themes are introduced here, and are thematic throughout the book.

Collaborating for Equity and Justice: Seven Principles

In 2016, against the backdrop of growing racial ethnic and income inequities and the increasing popularity of simplistic and largely top-down approaches to deeply entrenched problems, Tom Wolff and his colleagues developed a set of principles to guide alternative, community-driven social change approaches (Wolff et al., 2017). Grounded in decades of experience and research and practice in and with communities, the original six principles for "collaborating for equity and justice" (CEJ) were explicitly designed to facilitate impactful cross-sector collaboration for social change "in a way that explicitly lifts up equity and justice for all and creates measurable change" (Wolff et al., 2017, p. 42). As the authors point out, "No single model or methodology can thoroughly address the inequity and injustice facing communities that have historically experienced powerlessness" (p. 42). They therefore offer CEJ principles that can enhance the development of authentic, community-led collaborations more likely to promote equity and justice in both the processes and the outcomes of the work for systemic change (see box 1.1).

The third CEJ principle focuses specifically on the imperative of community organizing *as an intentional strategy and as part of the process*, and one that includes a strong emphasis on building local leadership and power. Yet each of the other principles, from the first (*explicitly address issues of social and economic injustice and structural racism*) to the sixth (*emphasize approaches that facilitate member*

BOX 1.1

Seven Principles for Collaborating for Equity and Justice

1. Explicitly address issues of social and economic injustice and structural racism.

2. Employ a community development approach in which residents have equal power in determining the coalition or collaborative's agenda and resource allocation.

3. Employ community organizing as an intentional strategy and as part of the process. Work to build resident leadership and power.

4. Focus on policy, systems, and structural change.

5. Build on the extensive community-engaged scholarship and research over the last four decades that show what works, that acknowledge the complexities, and that evaluate appropriately.

6. Construct core functions for the collaborative based on equity and justice that provide basic facilitating structures and build member ownership and leadership.

7. Embody cultural humility by critically reflecting on our own values and biases, working to understand others' cultures and beliefs, committing to authentic partnership and redressing power imbalances, while continually striving to become more culturally competent.

Sources: Principles 1–6 are from Wolff et al. (2017); principle 7 is adapted from Tervalon & Murray-Garcia (1998) and Greene-Moton & Minkler (2020).

---

ownership and leadership), relate directly to the diverse approaches to community building and community organizing explored in this book (Wolff et al., 2017).

Added to this list is a seventh principle (*embody cultural humility, while continually striving to become more culturally competent*), which we believe to be as foundational as the other six to successful work in CEJ. The concept of cultural humility was first described almost twenty-five years ago by physician Melanie Tervalon and health educator and community clinic director Jane Murray-Garcia, who saw it as an alternative to the popular notion of cultural competence, viewed narrowly as an end point that a health or other professional either attains or fails to achieve (Tervalon & Murray-Garcia, 1998). They defined *cultural humility* as "a lifelong commitment to self-evaluation and critique, to redressing power imbalances . . . and to developing mutually beneficial and non-paternalistic partnerships with communities on behalf of individuals and defined populations" (p. 117).

More recently, some of us have sought a road around the choice between cultural competence and cultural humility, arguing that both concepts are useful, particularly when a more nuanced view of cultural competence is embraced. Such an approach recognizes cultural humility as part of the process of cultural competence, which has been shown to increase individual and community control over and participation in decisionmaking (Danso, 2018; Greene-Moton & Minkler, 2020). In adopting the embodiment of cultural humility and striving to improve our cultural competence as a seventh principle to guide collaborating for equity and justice, we recognize the imperative of both, particularly in our diverse nation, in which systemic racism and other isms lie at the base of so many of the challenges and inequities that we face.

We hope that the seven principles, both individually and in their totality, provide readers with a useful set of guidelines in their own reflection on, and collaborative work with, communities and other partners committed to the quest for equity and social justice

Purpose and Organization of the Book

This volume is designed for professionals and students in fields like public health, social work, community psychology, and urban and regional planning, which lie at the interface of health, broadly defined, and social systems and communities. Like its predecessors, this fourth edition has three major purposes. First, it attempts to put together in one place much of the critical thinking in community organizing and community building theory and practice. These contributions address both long-valued aspects of community building and organizing and newer approaches that are playing transformative roles in organizing and building healthy communities today.

Second, the book attempts to demonstrate, through a series of case studies, the concrete application of many of the concepts and methods discussed in real-world organizing and community building settings. The frequent use of such analytical case studies and illustrations is designed to help bridge the still sizable gap between theory and practice in community organizing and community building.

A third purpose of the book is to make explicit the kinds of hard questions and ethical challenges on which those of us who engage in community organizing or community building as part of our professional practice should continually reflect. Such questions include the following: How can we foster true power sharing in our work with communities? What are the appropriate roles of "White allies" in work with communities of color? And how can we effectively build bridges across differences based on race and ethnicity, but also social class, gender and gender identity, nativity, ability/disability, and so many more? How do we address conflicting priorities between our agency or funder and the communities we serve? How do we anticipate and address the potential unanticipated consequences of an intervention or organizing campaign? And how do we develop empowering, rather than disempowering, approaches to community health assessment and the evaluation of community health initiatives or organizing projects? By raising such questions rather than providing simplistic answers, the book attempts to foster an approach to community organizing and community building that is, above all, self-critical, reflective, and respectful of the diverse communities with which we are engaged.

Before providing a chapter-by-chapter overview of what this third edition includes, we must state up front what it does not. First, it does not provide a step-by-step approach to community organizing or community building, which can be found elsewhere (Bobo et al., 2010; Homan, 2016; Sen, 2003; Staples, 2016). Second, the book is not a comprehensive casebook, and consequently cannot begin to do justice to the myriad exciting community building and organizing efforts taking place among and with different racial/ethnic communities in both urban and rural areas, or among the disability, LGBTQ, and other communities based on shared interests or identity both locally and globally. Third, this book does not attempt to cover the growing literature on social movements for health and social justice, which themselves are the topics of other comprehensive volumes and substantive reviews (Brown & Fee, 2014; Brown et al., 2011; Della Porta & Diani, 2006; Pastor et al., 2015).

This book is focused primarily on community organizing and community building efforts in the United States. Although globalization is a frequent backdrop for the perspectives offered, and while we believe many of the principles and case studies shared will have relevance beyond our borders, the importance of adequately taking context into account, coupled with space limitations, precluded a broader geographic focus.

Despite these limitations, we hope that this book will enable you, the reader, to think critically about community organizing and community building for health and social equity, asking hard questions and exploring their relevance in practice settings.

Following this introduction to the book is chapter 2, an early writing by former president Barack Obama, in which he eloquently asks and answers the bedrock question, "Why organize?" Although originally published in 1988 when a young Obama reflected on his work as an organizer on Chicago's South Side, the piece provides a compelling introduction to the thinking of one of the most important figures of our times. While some of the players and language have changed, the lessons of this chapter about core principles and approaches in community organizing practice have stood the test of time.

The four chapters in Part Two provide several approaches to practice and conceptual frameworks within which community organizing and community building for health and social equity can be better understood. In chapter 3, Meredith Minkler, Nina Wallerstein, and Cheryl A. Hyde provide an expanded theoretical and historical introduction to community organizing and community building, highlighting the key themes of power, empowerment, and community capacity to set the stage for their more detailed examination in later chapters. As the authors note, the strengths-based philosophy and principles of relevance and participation inherent in both community building and organizing, and their emphasis on creating environments in which communities can become empowered, take on special relevance in today's rapidly changing cultural and sociopolitical context.

Well before the national reckoning with systemic racism catalyzed by the Black Lives Matter protests over the police murder of George Floyd and other Black people, scholars such as Heather Came and Derek Griffith (2018), Ibram X. Kendi (2019), and Cornel West (2017) had provided critical conceptual and historical framing for our understanding of systemic racism its impacts. In chapter 4, Derek M. Griffith and Heather Came present these and other insights into racism, systemic racism, and "anti-racism practice," with particular attention to their utility for community organizing as an approach to health and social equity. Drawing on strategies shared by Kendi (2019) in his landmark book *How to be an Antiracist*, chapter 4 reminds us to view racial inequity as a problem not of people, but of policy, and to strive for broad structural change as a key foci of our organizing and community building work.

In chapter 5, Marty Martinson, Celina Su, and Meredith Minkler provide an in-depth comparison of the philosophy and methods of Saul D. Alinsky, who is known as the "father of social action organizing," and Paulo Freire, who is considered one of the most influential adult educators of modern times and whose methods were subsequently adapted and used in community organizing, These two giants in the field provided different yet seminal contributions (Alinsky, 1971; Friere, 1970) that continue to influence much of the more recent thinking and work in the field today. Contemporary examples of both approaches are provided and demonstrate some of the growing complementarity of these organizing traditions in practice.

We conclude Part Two with chapter 6, activist and writer Makani Themba's moving piece about the genesis and evolution of the Jackson People's Assembly in Mississippi, and its successful efforts to build a Black-led, multiracial, working-class resident organization that became a major force in the city's government. Grounding her analysis in a long tradition of southern organizing, Themba explores how history and contemporary challenges, including the pandemic, have shaped the work. She describes important lessons learned about the value and relevance of the People's Assembly approach for communities well beyond Jackson, and poses some tough questions going forward.

In Part Three, we turn our attention to the challenging and often difficult roles of health educators, social workers, and other social change professionals as community builders and organizers. Canadian scholar and activist Ronald Labonté begins chapter 7 by questioning prevailing views about community and raising cautions for health workers who engage in community organizing (termed community development in Canada) toward the aim of building authentic partnerships. Stressing the difference between *community-based* and true *community organizing* approaches, he provides criteria to be met if authentic partnerships between health agencies and communities are to be realized.

Several of the hard questions and issues raised by Labonté are examined in greater detail in chapter 8. Meredith Minkler, Cheri A. Pies, Patricia Wakimoto, and Cheryl A. Hyde provide theoretical perspectives and case examples that shed light on the ethical and practical challenges frequently faced by health educators, social workers, community psychologists, and others in their roles as community organizers. They explore problems such as conflicting priorities, the potential for negative unanticipated consequences, and the role of the isms (racism, sexism, ableism, homophobia, etc.) in our work. Additional questions are posed for practitioners and social change professionals to ask themselves and each other, in an effort to make more explicit the difficult ethical terrain in which we operate.

We conclude Part Three with a look at how genuine partnerships can be built between health departments and communities when racism, capacity building, and cultural humility are seriously addressed. In chapter 9, Roxana Chen, Kirsten Wysen, Blishda Lacet, Whitney Johnson, and Stephanie A. Farquhar use two Seattle case studies to highlight the work of the Transgender Economic Empowerment Coalition and the Seattle Urban Native Nonprofits, a leadership roundtable that aims to unite Native-led organizations' efforts. The authors apply a successful model that works on internal change in a health department and not merely changing the community. Their examples illustrate how community-agency partners and promising practices build on the issues raised in the chapters in Part Two.

In Part Four, chapter 10, Trevor Hancock and Meredith Minkler challenge the reader to move away from the traditional needs assessments, or even community health assessments, to *healthy community assessments*, using a range of tools to broaden the lens through which we view and help conduct such processes—ideally in partnership with community members themselves (appendixes 2 and 4). From Community Health Indicators to PolicyLink's Racial Equity Index (Langstron, 2020) and unique indicators only community members would know to include, we are provided a wide range of resources as we gather information for both change and empowerment.

In chapter 11, the traditional community assessment process is further scrutinized as John L. McKnight, John P. Kretzmann, and Lionel J. Beaulieu present and update the classic piece, "Mapping Community Capacity," adding both a focus on its utility for rural areas and the value of seven *community capitals* (Flora & Flora, 2008), which can further broaden our vision of the building blocks available in mapping strengths and assets that can be called upon in building healthier communities.

We conclude Part Four by turning our attention to the related area of issue selection with communities in chapter 12. Social work leader and scholar Lee Staples and feminist organizer and writer Rinku Sen lay out the criteria for a "good issue," as well as the factors to be considered in developing and framing the issue as part of a strategic analysis. With useful tools and examples, they illuminate the ways in which outside professionals can help ensure that the issue selected comes from the community and is developed in ways that help the community achieve its goals.

A major theme running through much of this book involves the role of community organizing and community building in and across diverse groups. In Part Five chapter 13, social work leaders and scholars Lorraine M. Gutiérrez and Edith A. Lewis describe their classic approach to organizing with women of color through the application of an empowerment framework stressing principles of education, participation, and capacity building. Arguing that traditional models of community organizing fail to adequately address the strengths, needs, and concerns of women of color, they present a feminist perspective on organizing that specifically addresses organizing by and with this critical population.

In chapter 14, Laura A. Linnan, Stephen B. Thomas, and Susan R. Passmore offer a unique approach to health education and community building to address health disparities, using as a base Black beauty salons and barber shops. These small businesses were among the first that were Black owned and run. They have served as important community meeting places and are facing new challenges in the COVID-19 pandemic. The historical significance of these cultural sites of meanings is provided as a critical backdrop to two exemplary case studies of their contemporary use in addressing health problems while building on community strengths. Although not community organizing in the traditional sense, this chapter demonstrates the utility and importance of respecting, and partnering with, valued cultural institutions in the fight against health disparities.

We conclude Part Five with chapter 15's presentation of a case study that demonstrates how popular education, community organizing, and community-based participatory research were a potent mix for helping a low-income community of immigrant Chinatown restaurant workers build capacity while addressing wage theft and other key concerns. Charlotte Chang, Alicia L. Salvatore, Pam Tau Lee, Shaw San Liu, and Meredith Minkler emphasize the engagement of all partners throughout this process as well as its outcomes in both community building and the repayment of millions of dollars in back wages resulting from their action research. The use of participatory evaluation throughout this project, and a ten-year retrospective look at later community, policy, and research outcomes to which it contributed, are also discussed.

Although community building and organizing often conjure up images of community meetings and door-to-door canvassing, the COVID-19 pandemic with its stay-at-home and other social distancing guidelines, was an important reminder of the essential role of online approaches in this work. In Part Six, chapter 16, public health trainers and practitioners Nickie Bazell and Evan vanDommelen-Gonzalez consider the powerful roles of the internet and social media in community building, organizing, and advocacy. But they intentionally do not include a long list of currently popular web links and other resources since given the rapidity of change in the online universe, many of these would likely be extinct by the time this book is published. Instead, they focus on the bigger issues and questions, and remind us that such tools are effective only when embedded in a broader and carefully designed strategy that includes real-world engagement as well as cyberactivism.

While discussing the ever-evolving opportunities for our online capacity to support community building and organizing, and offering the inspiring example of Enterprise for Youth, the authors also remind us of the challenges faced, from a shrinking, but still important digital divide, to cyber security, and the trauma that users may experience as graphic images of horrific events become part of our daily (if not hourly) lives.

In chapter 17, Caricia Catalini, Anne Bluethenthal, Dierdre Visser, María Elena Torre, and Meredith Minkler explore how a wide range of art forms have been used to promote community building and organizing around community-driven issues and social movements both historically and in today's rapidly changing world. The goodness of fit between the arts and health promotion is highlighted, and the theoretical bases for using the arts in organizing explored, through a wealth of illustrative examples. The chapter then provides a more detailed look at three diverse efforts to use the arts for community building and social change: a videovoice project in the aftermath of Hurricane Katrina in New Orleans; poetry, music, and other modalities in an economically impoverished but culturally historic neighborhood in San Francisco; and painting and other powerful visuals to bring alive the findings of a participatory action research project on police harassment of Black and Brown people in the Bronx, New York. The authors conclude by reminding us that as we work to address often unprecedented health and social inequities, the arts can be a valuable ally.

Building and maintaining effective coalitions have increasingly been recognized as often vital components of effective community organizing and community building. In Part Seven, chapter 18, health education leaders and scholars Frances D. Butterfoss and Michelle C. Kegler offer their Community Coalition Action Theory (CCAT) as a conceptual model that emerged in large part from years of practice in the field (Butterfoss & Kegler, 2009). They provide a set of constructs and practice-proven propositions for understanding coalition development, maintenance and effective functioning of the tasks associated with each stage, and such key issues as coalition context, leadership and staffing, dealing with conflict, and documenting both short-term successes and longer-term impacts to further improve practice.

In chapter 19, Patricia Wakimoto, Susana Hennessey Lavery, Meredith Minkler, and Jessica Estrada illustrate the utility and challenges of using CCAT in their assessment of a community coalition in San Francisco's Tenderloin neighborhood and its efforts to address food insecurity and tobacco control in this heavily impacted community. They describe the coalition's three stages of development and implementation and its adherence to such CCAT propositions as attention to context and the utility of multilevel interventions for change. But the authors also draw on Wolff et al.'s (2017) principles for Collaborating for Equity and Justice (CEJ) and Wolfe et al.'s (2020) questions for incorporating these principles in CCAT evaluations to ensure that our assessments explicitly use an equity lens.

In chapter 20, R. David Rebanal offers a lively look at a topic typically overlooked in books and articles on community organizing, namely the importance of fundraising as a critical part of the work itself. As he notes, although most funders still tend to support primarily direct service, and many are hesitant to embrace controversial causes, growing numbers of foundations and other donors *are* supporting community organizing and related strategies that can help promote health equity and address the SDOH. The many tips and examples in this chapter, from how to find and reach out to prospective donors to how to build a diversified funding strategy, while also increasing funders' interest in putting more of their resources into support for community organizing, provide important take homes for those of us interested in both doing, and building sustainable support for, equity-focused community organizing.

Although also rarely included in academic books on community building and community organizing, a central dilemma faced by professionals as organizers is how to facilitate the evaluation of community organizing and community building efforts in ways that do not *disempower* communities in the process. In chapter 21, Chris M. Coombe, Patricia Wakimoto, and Zachary Rowe describe how the process of evaluation can be used as a capacity building tool in organizing, as well as a source of knowledge for project improvement through a systematic and collaborative approach known as participatory or empowerment evaluation. Limitations of traditional approaches to evaluation are discussed, the theoretical underpinnings of participatory evaluation described, along with an eight-step process for applying this approach in the messy and complex world of community organizing and coalition building.

In Part Eight, the book's final part, we address the truth behind a popular saying among politicians and community organizers: "If you're not at the table, you're on the menu." In chapter 22, Lisa Cacari Stone, Manuel Pastor, Joseph Griffin, Rachel Morello-Frosch, and Meredith Minkler stress the importance of using an equity lens and bringing the lived experiences of communities most burdened by health and social inequities into the policymaking process. A conceptual framework is offered for bridging evidence, community organizing, and equity policy, including a look at the key steps or streams involved in this process. A case study of the Los Angeles Collaborative for Environmental Health and Justice is used to demonstrate the utility of the conceptual model in terms of both processes and outcomes. The authors conclude that high-level community engagement is essential if we are to achieve equity policy, and that community building should itself become a central consideration in how policies are shaped and what they look like.

In chapter 23, Amber Akemi Piatt, Christine Mitchell, Wayland "X" Coleman, and Meredith Minkler explore how two coalitions, led by currently and formerly incarcerated people and their families, used the window of opportunity provided by COVID-19 to advance the struggle for ending mass incarceration and related abolitionist change. The work of Decarcerate Alameda County is in part explored using Kingdon's model (2011; chapter 22) of the policymaking process to illustrate how coalition leaders and allies, including health educators at the nonprofit Human Impact Partners, brought attention to the urgent need for decarceration, helped craft policy solutions, and presented them to decisionmakers, achieving some (albeit far too limited) policy wins, through the process. The authors then turn to the very different approach of the #DeeperThanWater Coalition in Massachusetts, including its intentional decision *not* to collaborate with elected officials for policy change, but instead to focus on exposing environmental and other abuses and building broad public momentum for abolishing the criminal legal system. Finally, and far too infrequently in books of this kind, we hear firsthand from Wayland "X" Coleman, an incarcerated organizer with #DeeperThanWater, whose insights and experiences behind prison walls, and whose determination to share those realities with those of us outside, even at great personal cost, help convey, as little else can, the urgency of the work.

We conclude Part Eight with chapter 24, a detailed look at media advocacy, or the strategic use of mass media to promote policy initiatives (Wallack et al., 1993). Authors Lori Dorfman, Prisila Gonzalez, and Shaddai Martinez Cuestas walk us through the layers of strategy that must take place if we are to compete for the media's attention by replacing individually focused "portrait" stories of adverse health outcomes with "landscape" stories that center instead on how the systems and structures surrounding individuals contribute to their health status. The potent role of media advocacy in enabling community groups and advocates to reframe local and national problems from gun violence to housing to sugary beverages, and change the ways in which they are presented and viewed is highlighted, as is its role as a critical tool for building healthier communities through advocacy for healthy public policy.

The book concludes with appendixes designed to provide the reader with concrete tools and applications that correspond to the themes and issues raised in the chapters. We start with Cheryl A. Hyde's thoughtful reflection about the need to challenge ourselves to explore and deal with our own cultural identity to more effectively work in communities. Another appendix describes an exercise called River of Life, which is grounded in part in Indigenous tradition and presented as one way to engage coalition or community organization members in developing a historical timeline. Other appendixes offer valuable resources to employ digital technology and community mapping, Human Impact Partners' Community Health Indicators, as well as a Ladder of Community Participation, which never outlives its usefulness as a guide for understanding effective participation and power dynamics. The authors of the appendixes provide practical tips and useful tools for community assessment; coalition membership and process assessment; and measurement of perception of control at individual, organizational, and neighborhood levels. Together, the twelve appendixes will help trainees and established health and social change professionals put into practice messages central to community organizing and community building.

Although this book is written primarily for students and practitioners in fields such as community health education, social work, community psychology, and urban and regional planning, we hope it will be of interest, as well, to a wide range of social justice activists and professionals across a wide range of disciplines concerned with the many hard questions and realities that surround community building and organizing in the early twenty-first century. As in earlier editions, the contributors to this volume have attempted to write provocatively and critically, challenging readers to ask hard questions and rethink some of our most basic assumptions. We ask you, the reader, to join us in this process of critical questioning and dialogue as you seek to apply theory to practice, and practice to the rethinking of theory, toward the end of helping build health and social equity and more caring and humane communities and societies.

REFERENCES

Alinsky, S. D. (1971). *Rules for Radicals: A Practical Primer for Realistic Radicals.* Random House.

Baciu, A., Negussie, Y., Geller, A., Weinstein, J. N., & National Academies of Sciences, Engineering, and Medicine (2017). The root causes of health inequity. In *Communities in Action: Pathways to Health Equity* (pp. 99–184). National Academies Press.

Barone, E., Tweeten, L., Wilson, C., & Law, T. (2020, July 9). The coronavirus pandemic has caused carbon emissions to drop. *Time.* https://time.com/5864374/coronavirus-carbon-emissions/.

Bassett, M. T., Chen, J. T., & Krieger, N. (2020). Variation in racial/ethnic disparities in COVID-19 mortality by age in the United States: A cross-sectional study. *PLoS Medicine, 17*(10), e1003402.

Beaulieu, L. J. (2014, October). Promoting community vitality and sustainability: The Community Capitals Framework. Purdue University Center for Regional Development. https://docplayer.net/48294421-Community-vitality-sustainability-the-community-capitals-framework.html.

Blackwell, A. G., & Colmenar, R. (2000). Community-building: From local wisdom to public policy. *Public Health Rep, 115*(2–3), 161.

Blackwell, A. G., & McAfee, M. (2020, June 26). Banks should face history and pay reparations. *New York Times.* https://www.nytimes.com/2020/06/26/opinion/sunday/banks-reparations-racism-inequality.html.

Bobo, K., Kendall, J., & Max, S. (2010). *Organizing for Social Change* (4th ed.). The Forum Press.

Braveman, P., Arkin, E., Orleans, T., Proctor, D., & Plough, A. (2017). *What Is Health Equity? And What Difference Does a Definition Make?* Robert Wood Johnson Foundation.

Brown, P., Morello-Frosch, R., & Zavestoski, S. (2011). *Contested Illnesses: Citizens, Science, and Health Social Movements.* University of California Press.

Brown, T. M., & Fee, E. (2014). Social movements in health. *Annu Rev Public Health, 35*, 385–398.

Butterfoss, F. D., & Kegler, M. C. (2009). Community coalition action theory. In R. DiClemente, L. Crosby, & M. C. Kegler (Eds.), *Emerging Theories in Health Promotion Practice and Research* (2nd ed., pp. 236–276). Jossey-Bass.

Came, H., & Griffith, D. (2018). Tackling racism as a "wicked" public health problem: Enabling allies in anti-racism praxis. *Soc Sci Med, 199*, 181–188.

Center for the Study of Hate and Extremism. (2021). *Report to the Nation on Anti-Asian Prejudice and Hate Crime.* California State University at San Bernadino; CSHE. https://www.csusb.edu/sites/default/files/Report%20to%20the%20Nation%20-%20Anti-Asian%20Hate%202020%20Final%20Draft%20-%20As%20of%20Apr%2030%202021%206%20PM%20corrected.pdf.

Corburn, J. (2017). Urban place and health equity: Critical issues and practices. *Int J Environ Res, 14*(2), 117.

Danso, R. (2018). Cultural competence and cultural humility: A critical reflection on key cultural diversity concepts. *J Soc Work, 18*(4), 410–430.

Della Porta, D., & Diani, M. (2006). *Social Movements: An Introduction.* Blackwell Publishers.

Feeding America. (2020, October). The impact of the coronavirus on food insecurity in 2020. Feeding America. https://www.feedingamerica.org/sites/default/files/2020-10/Brief_Local%20Impact_10.2020_0.pdf.

Flora, C. B., & Flora, J. L. (2008). *Rural Communities: Legacy and Change* (3rd ed.). Westview Press.

Freire, P. (1970). *Pedagogy of the Oppressed.* Translated by M. B. Ramos. Seabury Press.

Greene-Moton, E., & Minkler, M. (2020). Cultural competence or cultural humility? Moving beyond the debate. *Health Promot Pract, 21*(1), 142–145.

Hardeman, R. R., Medina, E. M., & Boyd, R. W. (2020). Stolen breaths. *N Engl J Med, 383*(3), 197–199.

Homan, M. S. (2016). *Promoting Community Change: Making It Happen in the Real World* (6th ed.). Cengage Learning.

Hsu, T. (2020, May 3). Corporate voices get behind "Black Lives Matter" cause. Updated June 10. *New York Times.* https://www.nytimes.com/2020/05/31/business/media/companies-marketing-black-lives-matter-george-floyd.html.

Iton, A., & Ross, R. K. (2017). Understanding how health happens: Your zip code is more important than your genetic code. In R. Callahan & D. Bhattacharya (Eds.), *Public Health Leadership* (pp. 83–99). Routledge.

Iton, A., & Shrimali, B. P. (2016). Power, politics, and health: A new public health practice targeting the root causes of health equity. *Matern Child Health J, 20*(8), 1753–1758.

Kendi, I. X. (2019). *How to Be an Antiracist.* One World.

Kingdon, J. W. (2011). *Agendas, Alternatives, and Public Policies.* Longman.

Kleba, M. E., Wallerstein, N., Belon, A. P., van der Donk, C., Gastaldo, D., Avery, H., & Wright, M. (2021). Empowerment and participatory health research. Position Paper 4. International Collaboration for Participatory Health Research.

Langstron, A. (2020). Introducing the National Equity Index. PolicyLink/USC Equity Research Institute, National Equity Atlas. www.nationalequityatlas.org.

Minkler, M., Rebanal, R. D., Pearce, R., & Acosta, M. (2019). Growing equity and health equity in perilous times: Lessons from community organizers. *Health Educ Behav, 46*(1_suppl), 9S–18S.

Moore, S., & Kawachi, I. J. (2017). Twenty years of social capital and health research: A glossary. *J Epidemiol Community Health, 71*, 513–517.

Nurius, P. S., Uehara, E., & Zatzick, D. F. (2013). Intersection of stress, social disadvantage, and life course processes: Reframing trauma and mental health. *Am J Psychiatr Rehabil, 16*(2), 91–114.

Pan American Health Organization. (2020). Strategic plan of the Pan American Health Organization 2020–2025: Equity at the heart of health (Official Document, 359). Pan American Health Organization. License: CC BY-NC-SA 3.0 IGO. https://iris.paho.org/handle/10665.2/52473.

Pastor, M., Benner, C., & Matsuoka, M. (2015). *This Could Be the Start of Something Big: How Social Movements for Regional Equity Are Reshaping Metropolitan America.* Cornell University Press.

Pastor, M., Terriquez, V., & Lin, M. (2018). How community organizing promotes health equity, and how health equity affects organizing. *Health Aff, 37*(3), 358–363.

Plough, A. L., & Gandhi, P. (2019). Promoting social justice through public health practice. In B. S. Levy & H. L. McStowe (Eds.), *Social Injustice and Public Health* (pp. 481–494). Oxford University Press.

Putnam, R. (2000). *Bowling Alone: The Collapse and Revival of American Community.* Simon and Schuster.

Reich, R. B. (2020). *The System: Who Rigged It, How We Fix It*. Alfred A. Knopf.

Roy, A. (2020, April 3). The pandemic is a portal. *Financial Times*. https://www.ft.com/content /10d8f5e8-74eb-11ea-95fe-fcd274e920ca.

Rudolph, L., Caplan, J., Ben-Moshe, K., & Dillon, L. (2013). *Health in All Policies: A Guide for State and Local Governments*. American Public Health Association and Public Health Institute.

Ruiz, N. G., Horowitz, J. M., & Tamir, C. (2020, July 1). Many Black and Asian Americans say they have experienced discrimination amid the COVID-19 outbreak. Pew Research Center.

Schultz, J., Fawcett, S., Holt, C., & Watson-Thompson, J. (2020). Strengthening collaborative action for community health and development. *Am J Health Stud, 35*(2), 152–163.

Sehgal, A. R. (2020). Lifetime risk of death from firearm injuries, drug overdoses, and motor vehicle accidents in the United States. *Am J Med, 133*, 1162–1167.

Sen, R. (2003). *Stir It Up: Lessons in Community Organizing and Advocacy*. Jossey-Bass.

Staples, L. (2016). *Roots to Power* (3rd ed.). Praeger.

Tervalon, M., & Murray-Garcia, J. (1998). Cultural humility vs. cultural competence: A critical distinction in defining physician training outcomes in medical education. *J Health Care Poor Underserved, 9*(2), 117–125.

Thomas, D., & Horowitz, J. M. (2020). Support for Black Lives Matter has decreased since June but remains strong among Black Americans. Pew Research Center. https://www.pew research.org/fact-tank/2020/09/16/support-for-black-lives-matter-has-decreased-since -june-but-remains-strong-among-black-americans/.

Towe, V. L., Leviton, L., Chandra, A., Sloan, J. C., Tait, M., & Orleans, T. (2016). Cross-sector collaborations and partnerships: Essential ingredients to help shape health and well-being. *Health Aff, 35*(11), 1964–1969.

von der Leyen, E. (2020, May 27). Proposal for Recovery Plan, Next Generation European Union. European Commission. https://ec.europa.eu/commission/presscorner/detail/en/speech _20_941.

Wallack, L., Dorfman, L., Jernigan, D., & Themba, M. (1993). *Media Advocacy and Public Health: Power for Prevention*. Sage.

Wallerstein, N., Duran, B., Oetzel, J. G., & Minkler, M. (2018). On community-based participatory research. In N. Wallerstein, B. Duran, J. G. Oetzel, & M. Minkler (Eds.), *Community-Based Participatory Research for Health: Advancing Social and Health Equity* (3rd ed., pp. 3–16). Jossey-Bass.

Walter, C. L., & Hyde, C. A. (2012). Community building and practice: An expanded conceptual framework. In M. Minkler (Ed.), *Community Organizing and Community Building for Health and Welfare* (3rd ed., pp. 78–94). Rutgers University Press.

West, C. (2017). *Race Matters, 25th Anniversary: With a New Introduction*. Beacon Press.

Wolfe, S. M., Long, P. D., & Brown, K. K. (2020). Using a principles-focused evaluation approach to evaluate coalitions and collaboratives working toward equity and social justice. *New Dir Eval, 2020*(165), 45–65.

Wolff, T., Minkler, M., Wolfe, S. M., Berkowitz, B., Bowen, L., Butterfoss, F. D., Christens, B. D., Francisco, V. T., Himmelman, A. T., & Lee, K. S. (2017). Collaborating for equity and justice: Moving beyond collective impact. *Nonprofit Q, 9*, 42–53.

World Health Organization. (2017). WHO community engagement framework for quality, people-centered and resilient health services. World Health Organization (WHO/HIS/ SDS/2017.15). License: CC BY-NC-SA 3.0 IGO. https://apps.who.int/iris/handle/10665/259280.

2

Why Organize?

Problems and Promise in the Inner City

BARACK OBAMA

First published in 1988

Over the past five years, I've often had a difficult time explaining my profession to folks. Typical is a remark a public school administrative aide made to me one bleak January morning, while I waited to deliver some flyers to a group of confused and angry parents who had discovered the presence of asbestos in their school.

"Listen, Obama," she began. "You're a bright young man, Obama. You went to college, didn't you?"

I nodded.

"I just cannot understand why a bright young man like you would go to college, get that degree and become a community organizer."

"Why's that?"

"Cause the pay is low, the hours is long, and don't nobody appreciate you." She shook her head in puzzlement as she wandered back to attend to her duties.

I've thought back on that conversation more than once during the time I've organized with the Developing Communities Project, based in Chicago's far south side. Unfortunately, the answers that come to mind haven't been as simple as her question. Probably the shortest one is this: It needs to be done, and not enough folks are doing it.

The debate as to how black and other dispossessed people can forward their lot in America is not new. From W. E. B. Du Bois to Booker T. Washington to Marcus Garvey to Malcolm X to Martin Luther King Jr., this internal debate has raged between integration and nationalism, between accommodation and militancy, between sit-down strikes and boardroom negotiations. The lines between these strategies have never been simply drawn, and the most successful black leadership has recognized the need to bridge these seemingly divergent approaches. During the early years of the Civil Rights movement, many of these issues became submerged in the face of the clear oppression of segregation. The debate was no longer whether to protest, but how militant must that protest be to win full citizenship for blacks.

Twenty years later, the tensions between strategies have reemerged, in part due to the recognition that for all the accomplishments of the 1960s, the majority of blacks continue to suffer from second-class citizenship. Related to this are the failures—real, perceived and fabricated—of the Great Society programs initiated by Lyndon Johnson. Facing these realities, at least three major strands of earlier movements are apparent.

First, and most publicized, has been the surge of political empowerment around the country. Harold Washington and Jesse Jackson are but two striking examples of how the energy and passion of the Civil Rights movement have been channeled into bids for more traditional political power. Second, there has been a resurgence in attempts to foster economic development in the black community, whether through local entrepreneurial efforts, increased hiring of black contractors and corporate managers, or Buy Black campaigns. Third, and perhaps least publicized, has been grass-roots community organizing, which builds on indigenous leadership and direct action.

Proponents of electoral politics and economic development strategies can point to substantial accomplishments in the past 10 years. An increase in the number of black public officials offers at least the hope that government will be more responsive to inner-city constituents. Economic development programs can provide structural improvements and jobs to blighted communities.

In my view, however, neither approach offers lasting hope of real change for the inner city unless undergirded by a systematic approach to community organization. This is because the issues of the inner city are more complex and deeply rooted than ever before. Blatant discrimination has been replaced by institutional racism; problems like teen pregnancy, gang involvement and drug abuse cannot be solved by money alone. At the same time, as Professor William Julius Wilson of the University of Chicago has pointed out, the inner city's economy and its government support have declined, and middle-class blacks are leaving the neighborhoods they once helped to sustain.

Neither electoral politics nor a strategy of economic self-help and internal development can by themselves respond to these new challenges. The elections of Harold Washington in Chicago or of Richard Hatcher in Gary were not enough to bring jobs to inner-city neighborhoods or cut a 50 percent drop-out rate in the schools, although they did achieve an important symbolic effect. In fact, much-needed black achievement in prominent city positions has put us in the awkward position of administering underfunded systems neither equipped nor eager to address the needs of the urban poor and being forced to compromise their interests to more powerful demands from other sectors.

Self-help strategies show similar limitations. Although both laudable and necessary, they too often ignore the fact that without a stable community, a well-educated population, an adequate infrastructure and an informed and employed market, neither new nor well-established companies will be willing to base themselves in the inner city and still compete in the international marketplace.

Moreover, such approaches can and have become thinly veiled excuses for cutting back on social programs, which are anathema to a conservative agenda. In theory, community organizing provides a way to merge various strategies for neighborhood empowerment. Organizing begins with the premise that (1) the problems facing inner-city communities do not result from a lack of effective solutions, but from a lack of power to implement these solutions; (2) the only way for communities to build long-term power is by organizing people and money around a common vision; and (3) a viable organization can only be achieved if a broadly based indigenous leadership—and not one or two charismatic leaders—can knit together the diverse interests of their local institutions.

This means bringing together churches, block clubs, parent groups and any other institutions in a given community to pay dues, hire organizers, conduct research, develop leadership, hold rallies and education campaigns, and begin drawing up plans on a whole range of issues-jobs, education, crime, etc. Once such a vehicle is formed, it holds the power to make politicians, agencies and corporations more responsive to community needs. Equally important, it enables people to break their crippling isolation from each other, to reshape their mutual values and expectations and rediscover the possibilities of acting collaboratively—the prerequisites of any successful self-help initiative.

By using this approach, the Developing Communities Project and other organizations in Chicago's inner city have achieved some impressive results. Schools have been made more accountable; job training programs have been established; housing has been renovated and built; city services have been provided; parks have been refurbished; and crime and drug problems have been curtailed. Additionally, plain folk have been able to access the levers of power, and a sophisticated pool of local civic leadership has been developed.

But organizing the black community faces enormous problems as well. One problem is the not entirely undeserved skepticism organizers face in many communities. To a large degree, Chicago was the birthplace of community organizing, and the urban landscape is littered with the skeletons of previous efforts. Many of the best-intentioned members of the community have bitter memories of such failures and are reluctant to muster up renewed faith in the process.

A related problem involves the aforementioned exodus from the inner city of financial resources, institutions, role models and jobs. Even in areas that have not been completely devastated, most households now stay afloat with two incomes. Traditionally, community organizing has drawn support from women, who due to tradition and social discrimination had the time and the inclination to participate in what remains an essentially voluntary activity. Today the majority of women in the black community work full time, many are the sole parent, and all have to split themselves between work, raising children, running a household and maintaining some semblance of a personal life—all of which makes voluntary activities lower on the priority list. Additionally, the slow exodus of the black middle class into the suburbs means that people shop in one neighborhood, work in another, send their child to a school across town and go to church someplace other than the place where they live. Such geographical dispersion creates real problems in building a sense of investment and common purpose in any particular neighborhood.

Finally, community organizations and organizers are hampered by their own dogmas about the style and substance of organizing. Most still practice what Professor John McKnight of Northwestern University calls a "consumer advocacy" approach, with a focus on wrestling services and resources from the outside powers that be. Few are thinking of harnessing the internal productive capacities, both in terms of money and people, that already exist in communities.

Our thinking about media and public relations is equally stunted when compared to the high-powered direct mail and video approaches successfully used by conservative organizations like the Moral Majority. Most importantly, low salaries, the lack of quality training and ill-defined possibilities for advancement discourage the most talented young blacks from viewing organizing as a legitimate career option. As long as our best and brightest youth see more opportunity in climbing the corporate ladder than in building the communities from which they came, organizing will remain decidedly handicapped.

None of these problems is insurmountable. In Chicago, the Developing Communities Project and other community organizations have pooled resources to form cooperative think tanks like the Gamaliel Foundation. These provide both a formal setting where experienced organizers can rework old models to fit new realities and a healthy environment for the recruitment and training of new organizers. At the same time the leadership vacuum and disillusionment following the death of Harold Washington have made both the media and people in the neighborhoods more responsive to the new approaches community organizing can provide. Nowhere is the promise of organizing more apparent than in the traditional black churches. Possessing tremendous financial resources, membership and—most importantly—values and biblical traditions that call for empowerment and liberation, the black church is clearly a slumbering giant in the political and economic landscape of cities like Chicago. A fierce independence among black pastors and a preference for more traditional approaches to social involvement (supporting candidates for office, providing shelters for the homeless) have prevented the black church from bringing its full weight to bear on the political, social and economic arenas of the city.

Over the past few years, however, more and more young and forward-thinking pastors have begun to look at community organizations such as the Developing Communities Project in the far south side and GREAT in the Grand Boulevard area as a powerful tool for living the social gospel, one which can educate and empower entire congregations and not just serve as a platform for a few prophetic leaders. Should a mere 50 prominent black churches, out of the thousands that exist in cities like Chicago, decide to collaborate with a trained organizing staff, enormous positive changes could be wrought in the education, housing, employment and spirit of inner-city black communities, changes that would send powerful ripples throughout the city.

In the meantime, organizers will continue to build on local successes, learn from their numerous failures and recruit and train their small but growing core of leadership—mothers on welfare, postal workers, CTA drivers and school teachers, all of whom have a vision and memories of what communities can be. In fact, the answer to the original question—why organize?—resides in these people. In helping a group of housewives sit across the negotiating table with the mayor of America's third largest city and hold their own, or a retired steelworker stand before a TV camera and give voice to the dreams he has for his grandchild's future, one discovers the most significant and satisfying contribution organizing can make.

In return, organizing teaches as nothing else does the beauty and strength of everyday people. Through the songs of the church and the talk on the stoops, through the hundreds of individual stories of coming up from the South and finding any job that would pay, of raising families on threadbare budgets, of losing some children to drugs and watching others earn degrees and land jobs their parents could never aspire to—it is through these stories and songs of dashed hopes and powers of endurance, of ugliness and strife, subtlety and laughter, that organizers can shape a sense of community not only for others, but for themselves.

Acknowledgments

"Why Organize? Problems and Promise in the Inner City" was first published in the August/September 1988 *Illinois Issues* (published by then Sangamon State University, now the University of Illinois at Springfield). Reprinted with permission of the publisher of *Illinois Issues* at NPR Illinois.

PART TWO

Contextual Frameworks
and Approaches

Over thirty years ago, political scientist Richard Couto (1990) pointed out that "because Americans have so little sense of community, we pay a great deal of attention to it." He suggested that "our rose-tainted view of community and the processes we describe as empowerment, community development, and community organizing" have led to considerable conceptual confusion, with groups from political progressives to far right conservatives using terms like *grass roots* and *populist* "as if [they] were herbal medicine for current public problems and to renew American social health" (p. 144).

The contributors to this part of the book attempt to move us beyond the prevailing confusion by offering conceptual frameworks and models within which community, community organizing, and community building can be better understood. Although additional perspectives on these concepts are offered throughout the book, this section seeks to lay a foundation for their subsequent exploration.

In chapter 3, Meredith Minkler, Nina Wallerstein, and Cheryl A. Hyde offer initial definitions of community organizing and community building and underscore the centrality of the notion of empowerment to both of these processes. Following a brief historical review, they then introduce the best-known typology of community organizing, developed by social work leader and scholar Jack Rothman (2007), emphasizing three primary modalities: community capacity development, social planning and policy, and social advocacy. Alternative and complementary models are explored, including community building and feminist organizing (Hyde, 2018). The latter is explored more deeply in chapter 13, with special attention to feminist organizing with women of color.

Chapter 3 also considers several key concepts in community organizing and community building central to effecting change on the community level: power, empowerment, and community capacity. Although this chapter covers a wide terrain, it does so primarily as a prelude to more in-depth discussion of these concepts in subsequent chapters.

One of the most critical–and overlooked–conceptual frameworks for our work in public health, social work, and other fields in the twenty-first century involves understanding race, systemic racism, and the essential role of anti-racist practice in our work for health and social equity. In chapter 4, Derek M. Griffith and Heather Came ground the need for such understanding in the fact that "The problem in America is not race . . . the problem is racism" (Jenkins et al., 2019, p. 35). They describe anti-racism as both an educational and an organizing framework designed to face, address, and ultimately end racism and "unearned white privilege" (Came & Griffith, 2018; appendix 1). Building on the authors' own earlier work and the insights of scholars including Ibram X. Kendi (2019), chapter 4 offers a range of strategies for infusing anti-racism into community organizing and community building practice to enhance our effectiveness in working for equity and social justice.

In chapter 5, Marty Martinson, Celina Su, and Meredith Minkler begin by introducing the philosophy and approach of two of the individuals whose contributions to our thinking and practice in community organizing have been among the most profound. Saul D. Alinsky (1971), the father of social action organizing from the 1930s into the 1960s, is best known for his controversial ethics, confrontational style, and building of often faith-based "organizations of organizations" that wield considerable power and continue to win many campaigns against well-funded corporate and other interests (Schulz & Miller, 2015). In contrast, adult educator Paulo Freire (1973), whose "education for critical consciousness" is seminal for many community builders and organizers in fields like health education and social work, emphasized problem-posing dialogue to unearth the root causes of problems as a basis for "action based on critical reflection" as part of transformative change processes (Freire, 1973; Su, 2009). After situating the thinking and actions of these key figures in their personal biographies, Martinson, Su, and Minkler illustrate their contrasting approaches using powerful contemporary case examples from faith-based organizing through ISAIAH Minnesota and youth organizing through Sistas and Brothas United in the northwest Bronx, New York, respectively. But they also show how groups like ISAIAH have gone beyond Alinsky's insistence on winnable, local issues to instead confront systemic racism and build broad social movements more in keeping with the realities of the twenty-first century (Fisher et al., 2018; Kotz, 2019; Schulz & Miller, 2015), and with Freirian organizing's long appreciation of the need to move from local organizing to transformative systems change (Carroll & Minkler, 2000; Freire, 2000; Su, 2009).

In a provocative recent essay, feminist organizer and writer Rinku Sen (2020) suggests that "the combined disruption of an ongoing deadly pandemic, record unemployment and multiracial uprisings to defend Black lives will soon make many of our existing models irrelevant" (p. 2). Chapter 6 concludes this part with a case study by organizer and movement builder Makani Themba, who both illustrates this thinking and hearkens back to some of the earliest community building and organizing traditions. Themba shares the genesis and evolution of the Jackson People's Assembly in Mississippi, and its successful efforts to build a Black-led, multiracial, working-class resident organization that then became a major force in the city's government. She explores how some of the history of the long tradition of southern organizing, as well as contemporary challenges, including the pandemic, have shaped the work. Themba highlights lessons learned about the value and relevance of the People's Assembly approach for communities well beyond Jackson, and poses some tough questions going forward.

REFERENCES

Alinsky, S. D. (1971). *Rules for Radicals: A Practical Primer for Realistic Radicals.* Random House.
Came, H., & Griffith, D. (2018). Tackling racism as a "wicked" public health problem: Enabling allies in anti-racism praxis. *Soc Sci Med, 199,* 181–188. doi:http://dx.doi.org/10.1016/j.socscimed.2017.03.028.
Carroll, J., & Minkler, M. (2000). Freire's message for social workers: Looking back, looking ahead. *J Community Pract, 8*(1), 21–36.
Couto, R. A. (1990). Promoting health at the grass roots. *Health Affairs, 9*(2), 144–151.
Fisher, R., DeFilippis, J., & Shragge, E. (2018). Contested community: A selected and critical history of community organizing. In R. A. Cnaan & C. Milofsky (Eds.), *Handbook of Community Movements and Local Organizations in the 21st Century* (pp. 281–297). Springer.
Freire, P. (1973). *Education for Critical Consciousness.* Seabury Press.
Freire, P. (2000). *Cultural Action for Freedom.* Harvard Educational Press.

Hyde, C. A. (2018). Charisma, collectives, and commitment: Hybrid authority in radical feminist social movement organizations. *Soc Mov Stud, 17*(4), 424–436.

Jenkins, W. C., Schoenbach, V. J., Rowley, D. L., & Ford, C. L. (2019). 2. Overcoming the impact of racism on the health of communities: What we have learned and what we have not. In C. L. Ford, D. M. Griffith, M. A. Bruce, & K. L. Gilbert (Eds.), *Racism: Science & Tools for the Public Health Professional* (pp. 15–45).Washington, DC: APHA Press.

Kendi, I. M. (2019). *How to Be an Antiracist.* One World.

Kotz, P. (2019, March 6). The kindness revolt: A not-so-secret plot to make a better Minnesota. *CityPages.* http://www.citypages.com/news/the-kindness-revolt-a-not-so-secret-plot-to-make-a-better-minnesota/506724471.

Rothman, J. (2007). Multi modes of intervention at the macro level. *J Community Pract, 15*(4), 11–40.

Schutz, A., & Miller, M. (2015). *People Power: The Community Organizing Tradition of Saul Alinsky.* Vanderbilt University Press.

Sen, R. (2020, July 1). Why today's social revolutions include kale, medical care and help with rent. Zócalo Public Square. https://www.zocalopublicsquare.org/2020/07/01/mutual-aid-societies-self-determination-pandemic-community-organizing/ideas/essay/.

Su, C. (2009). *Streetwise for Book Smarts: Grassroots Organizing and Education Reform in the Bronx.* Cornell University Press.

3

Improving Health through Community Organizing and Community Building

Perspectives from Health Education and Social Work

MEREDITH MINKLER

NINA WALLERSTEIN

CHERYL A. HYDE

Although community organizing has long been a central method of practice in both health education and social work, it has achieved even greater prominence in recent decades as both fields have increasingly focused on collaborating for health and social equity to redress the deep inequities underlying so many of the health and social problems we face. The pivotal role of community building and organizing in such efforts is well documented (Minkler et al., 2019; Pastor et al., 2018; Staples, 2016), and both the Society for Public Health Education (SOPHE) and the National Association of Social Workers (NASW) have adopted position statements on the importance of community organizing in their fields.

As defined in chapter 1, community organizing is "a process by which communities identify their assets and concerns, prioritize and select issues, and intentionally build power and develop and implement action strategies for change" (Minkler et al., 2019, p. 10S). The newer and related concept of community building may be seen not so much as a method as an approach for people who identify as members of a shared community to engage together in identifying and building on their strengths, developing leadership and power, and working together for community change (Walter & Hyde, 2012).

Implicit in both of these definitions is the concept of empowerment, classically defined by Rappaport (1984) as an enabling process through which individuals or communities take control over their lives and environments. Indeed, we argue that without empowerment, reflected in enhanced community capacity or problem-solving ability, community organizing is not taking place. Further, and while a public health or social work professional may help mobilize a community around climate justice or improved access to mental health services, he or she can't be said to be doing community organizing in the pure sense unless the community itself has identified the issue around which their work together will take place (chapters 8, 12). There is another important reason for emphasizing community issue selection, however. The public health educator, social worker, or other professional who adheres to the bedrock principle of *starting with the community's felt need or concern*, will be more likely to foster true community ownership of programs and actions, which, in turn, can increase the likelihood of success (Pastor et al., 2018; Minkler et al., 2019; Wolff et al., 2017).

In addition to helping promote changes in health or social conditions or specific community change targets, community organizing and community building are also important in light of the substantial evidence that civic and related forms of social participation can themselves significantly improve perceived control, psychological empowerment, individual coping capacity, health behaviors, and both physical and mental health status (Coombe et al., 2017; Kleba et al., 2021; Rivkin, 2014; Wallerstein, 2006). Further, as noted in chapter 1, the growing accent on community partnerships, coalitions, and community-engaged research, supported by government agencies, philanthropic organizations, and community-based organizations has spurred even greater attention to the concepts of community building and organizing often central to this work (Pastor et al., 2018; Wolff et al., 2017).

Following an introduction to the concept of community, we provide a brief historical grounding of community organizing and community building, and we offer conceptual models of these approaches in practice. We then discuss three concepts at the core of community organizing and community building—power, empowerment, and community capacity—and conclude by underscoring the pivotal strategies both community building and organizing offer for improving the public's health and welfare in the deeply challenging yet potentially promising times ahead.

The Concept of Community

Integral to a discussion of community organization and community building is an examination of the concept of community. While typically thought of in geographic terms, communities may also be based on shared interests, norms, or identity characteristics, such as race/ethnicity, sexual orientation, gender identity, disability status, or occupation (Rothman, 2008). Historically, communities have been defined as (1) *functional spatial units* meeting basic needs for sustenance, (2) *units of patterned social interaction*, or (3) *symbolic units of collective identity* (Hunter, 1975). Eng and Parker (1994) added a fourth definition of communities *as social units* where people come together politically to make change.

Multiple theories are relevant to understanding the concept of community. The *ecological systems perspective* is useful in the study of autonomous geographic communities, focusing on population characteristics, such as size, density and heterogeneity, the physical environment, the social organization of the community, and the technological forces that have an impact on it (chapters 10, 11). In contrast, the *social systems perspective*, classically articulated by Warren (1963) focuses primarily on formal and informal organizations, exploring the interactions of community subsystems (economic, political, etc.), both horizontally within the community and vertically as they relate to other systems of power (Fisher & DeFilippis, 2015). Political communities, such as tribal sovereign nations or municipalities, combine elements of both of these definitions.

Clearly, a person's perspective on community influences his or her view of the appropriate domains and functions of the community organization process. Community development specialists (e.g., agricultural extension workers and Peace Corps volunteers), have focused on *geographic communities*. In contrast, proponents of a broader social action approach (Schutz & Miller, 2015) have organized around *issues* such as affordable health care, housing, and a living wage in recognition of the profound impact of such bedrock concerns on local communities. Finally, as Chávez et al. (2010) and others (chapters 4, 13) have suggested, an appreciation of the history of particular societal oppressions and modes of survival within communities of color should be a key consideration. In Black communities, market exploitation thus led to a shattering of religious and civic organizations that had previously buffered these communities from hopelessness and nihilism (Blackwell & McAfee, 2020; West, 2017). The Black Lives Matter protests of 2020 shined a harsh and much needed light on how our long history of racialized police brutality and mass incarceration has contributed to devastating race-based inequities in health and life chances (Khan-Cullors & Bandele, 2017; Minkler et al., 2020; chapters 4, 23).

These perspectives suggest another definition of communities as created by the *actions and practices* of their members, whether in person or through social media, which cultivate actions together as well as a sense of belonging and identity (Cnaan & Milofsky, 2018). These include communities defined by *sociopolitical actions*, such as Black Lives Matter and the Me Too movement; *communities of practice* that exchange learnings within a knowledge base (Wenger-Trayner & Wenger-Trayner, 2015); and *multisector communities*, such as the World Health Organization Healthy Cities and Communities program (https://www.who.int/healthpromotion /healthy-cities/en/). But they also increasingly include *academic-community research communities*, such as longtime community-based participatory research (CBPR) partnerships that have cultivated projects, actions, and connectedness over time (Coombe et al., 2020; Wallerstein et al., 2018).

Reflecting on such realities, scholar and activist Cornel West (2017) called for community change through re-creating a sense of agency and political resistance based on "subversive memory—the best of one's past without romantic nostalgia." Likewise, in Indigenous communities in the United States and globally, robust cultural renewal movements and collaborations with academic partners in recent decades embrace organizing and healing from historical traumas that have been wrought over centuries by the dominant society (Corntassel, 2012; Smith, 2012; Walters et al., 2020).

A view of community that incorporates such perspectives would be grounded in an understanding of historical trauma across generations, and oppressions based on race/ethnicity, class, geography and nativity, gender identity, and disability and LGBTQ status. Violation of treaties and sovereign nation status has been a particular oppression for Indigenous peoples. But it would also build on community strengths. Included here are community self-determination, power, and empowerment, as these have been used by oppressed and disenfranchised groups to critically reflect on their realities and engage in praxis to address historical trauma and promote change on the local through the national and global policy levels (Chávez et al., 2010; Hyde, 2018; Minkler et al., 2019; chapter 13).

Community Organizing and Community Building in Historical Perspective

The term *community organization* was coined by American social workers in the late 1800s in reference to their efforts to coordinate services for newly arrived immigrants and the poor. Yet, as Garvin and Cox (2001) pointed out, although community organization is often seen as the offspring of the settlement house movement, several important milestones well outside that movement should by rights be included in any history. The following are prominent among these:

1. African American efforts in the post-Reconstruction period to salvage newly won rights that were rapidly slipping away
2. The populist movement, which began as an agrarian revolution and became a multisectoral coalition and a major political force
3. The labor movement of the 1930s and 1940s, which taught the value of forming coalitions around issues, the importance of full-time professional organizers, and the use of conflict as a means of bringing about change

Within the field of social work, early approaches to community organizing stressed collaboration, consensus, and mutual aid as communities were helped to self-identify and increase their problem-solving ability (DeFilippis et al., 2010; Hyde, 2018; Sen, 2020; chapter 13). By the 1950s, however, a new, increasingly popular brand of community organizing stressed confrontation and conflict strategies for social change and put its greatest emphasis on getting and effectively using power (Schutz & Miller, 2015; Staples, 2016; chapter 5). Most closely identified with Saul Alinsky (1971), social action organizing emphasized redressing power imbalances by creating dissatisfaction with the status quo among the disenfranchised, building community-wide identification, and helping members devise winnable goals and nonviolent conflict strategies as a means to bring about change (Phulwani, 2016; Schutz & Miller, 2015; chapter 5).

From the late 1950s on, strategies and tactics of community organizing were increasingly applied to broader social change objectives, through the civil rights movement, followed by the women's movement, LGBTQ organizing, disability rights, the antiwar movement, and, more recently, immigrants' rights, Black Lives Matter, and environmental and climate justice movements. Many of these movements illustrate a hybrid or post-Alinsky tradition in organizing (Phulwani, 2016; Stall & Stoecker, 2005; Stoecker, 2018; chapter 5). In such approaches, Alinsky's reticence to tackle issues like racism is replaced by embracing the need to do so (Phulwani, 2016; Schutz & Miller, 2015), and more attention is paid to the importance of mutual aid and building community capacity and leadership (chapters 5, 6).

Finally, both Alinsky and post-Alinsky organizing owe a large and generally unacknowledged debt to radical feminist organizing, and the "collective charisma" at its core. Hyde (2018) describes the latter as "a hybrid form of authority and a touchstone for movement commitment and action" (p. 431). Collective charisma thus laid the groundwork for the development of oppositional consciousness, defined as "an empowering mental state that prepares members of an oppressed group to act to undermine, reform, or overthrow a system of human domination" in which they experience grave injustices (Mansbridge, 2001, p. 4).

In often stark contrast to the Alinsky tradition, and more in keeping with the radical feminist organizing highlighted earlier, the Freirian approach to organizing grew out of the philosophy and approach to adult literacy for transformative social change developed by Brazilian adult educator Paulo Freire in the 1950s and 1960s (Freire, 1973, 2016). As described in chapter 5, with its accent on popular education, critical consciousness, and action based on critical reflection, Freire's approach quickly gained traction in both the Global South and the United States and other Global North nations as a potent new approach to community organizing (Carroll & Minkler, 2000; Wallerstein & Auerbach, 2004/2020). Through praxis, or ongoing cycles of reflection and action, Freirian emancipatory educational processes of listening/dialogue/action engage community members in identifying and listening to their own issues, engaging in critical dialogues to prioritize their actions, which they then evaluate and restart the next cycle of reflection and action. In the United States, many have used his approach in adult education, grassroots organizing, leadership, and public health programs with community health workers, community members, or leaders to promote community empowerment and transformation (Wiggins, 2012; Wiggins et al., 2018).

Alongside these developments, an appreciation of *community building* has grown, conceptualized in this chapter as an orientation that emphasizes community assets and shared identity, whether or not task-oriented organizing takes place (Chávez et al., 2010; Rothman, 2008; Walter & Hyde, 2012). Such community building projects are strength based and often borrow, from feminist organizing, an accent on the integration, through dialogue, of personal and political experiences (Frisby et al., 2009; Hyde, 2005, 2018; Reger, 2017; Sen, 2020; Whittier, 2017). Yet even absent an accent on integrating the personal and political, community building can play a critical role for both individuals and the groups with which they identify.

A potent example may be found in gay-straight alliances (GSAs), school-based clubs that can help create a more health promoting school environment for lesbian, gay, bisexual, transgender, and questioning (LGBTQ) youth, with positive impacts on their physical and mental health and well-being (Poteat et al., 2012; Toomey et al., 2011). In a qualitative study of LGBTQ youth participating in GSAs in several parts of the United States and Canada, the clubs were described by youth as enabling them to be part of a community and providing a sense of connection, belonging, and social support, as well as safety. But participants also described the clubs as serving as "a gateway to resources outside of the GSA, such as supportive adults and informal social locations" (Porta et al., 2017, p. 489). Although for some youth, the opportunity provided by their GSA to develop as leaders and connect to the larger LGBTQ community did include developing skills in advocacy, for most, the accent on potential political dimensions of community building was not stressed (Porta et al., 2017).

The different models of community organization and community building described in this and subsequent chapters and appendixes illustrate how alternative assumptions about the nature and meaning of community heavily shape our conceptualization and practice.

Models of Community Organizing and Community Building Practice

While community organizing is frequently treated as though it were a single model of practice, several different typologies of organizing have been developed. The best known was first developed by social work and community organization theorist Jack Rothman (2008) and consists of three distinct but overlapping models of practice; originally described as locality development, social planning, and social action, the language and sophistication of these concepts were later broadened (Rothman, 2008). *Community capacity development* stresses consensus and cooperation as an organizing approach and building group identity and problem-solving ability as key goals. This revised nomenclature avoids a narrower geographic focus implied by "locality development" and strongly incorporates the community building notion. *Social planning and policy* stresses the use of data and rational-empirical problem solving, while also making room for new approaches, including participatory planning and policy development, more in keeping with the spirit of true community organizing than the earlier term *social planning*.

Finally, the third category, *social advocacy*, like its predecessor, social action, emphasizes the use of pressure tactics, including confrontation, to help bring about concrete changes to redress power imbalances, and is more in keeping with social change tactics and strategies used in the early twenty-first century (Minkler et al., 2019; Pastor et al., 2018). As discussed in subsequent chapters, these include both neighborhood actions and far larger efforts, often aided by online organizing, to foster national and even global change efforts. Such efforts are diverse in focus and include immigrant and refugee rights, climate change, or actions involving identity based on race/ethnicity, sexual orientation or gender identity (e.g., efforts to reclaim and protect the rights of transgender people), or status as a disabled person (the disability rights movement). But they share a commitment to working for social change through myriad social action strategies and tactics—and where appropriate, combining these with other, quite different, approaches discussed in this chapter.

Rothman's (2008) three models are often mixed, for example, with community capacity development combined with social advocacy to stress identity activism. Feminist community organizing, for example, may combine the goals and assumptions of social advocacy organizing with methods that are often consistent with community capacity development (Hyde, 2008, 2018). Similarly, the Healthy Heartlands Initiative across five midwestern states (https://www.heartlandalliance .org/heartland-alliance/research-and-policy/initiatives/health-healing-initiatives/) combines faith-based community capacity development, planning and policy (or "setting the table with technical experts"), and social advocacy aimed at legislators and other key players to promote racial and health equity.

Alternative models of community capacity development have also been proposed, including Himmelman's (2001) "collaborative empowerment," Kretzmann and McKnight's asset-based community development (chapter 10) and Walter and Hyde's (2012) community-building approach. Such models emphasize collaboration but also stress *community-driven development*, wherein community concerns lead the organizing in a process that creates healthy and more equal power relations (García, 2020; Walter & Hyde, 2012; chapters 7, 15, 19).

Community building models emphasize community strengths, not as nostalgia for the good old days but as a diversity of groups and systems that identify and nurture shared values and goals. Himmelman's (2001) "collaborative empowerment model" and Wolff et al.'s (2017) *principles for collaborating for equity and justice*, for example, include facets of traditional organizing (e.g., building a community's power base), but put their heaviest accent on enabling communities to take the lead so that real power and empowerment are achieved rather than merely "community betterment." Cultural renewal initiatives, whether in Indigenous or in other identity-based communities, also emphasize centering organizing within cultural traditions, knowledge, and values for empowered future generations (Walters et al., 2020).

Along similar lines, Walter and Hyde's (2012) community building approach describes community building practice as "a way of orienting one's self in community" that places community "at the center of practice" (p. 84), rather than having the professional organizer as the center. Their concept of community building attempts to balance and blend such elements of community as history, identity, and autonomy with the dimensions of community development, community planning, community action, community consciousness, and "the commons." While placing a similarly strong emphasis on identifying and promoting community strengths, a macroconceptualization of community building also emphasizes regional economic development and federal and state policy-level reinvestment in local communities as critical (Blackwell & Colmenar, 2000; Blackwell & McAfee, 2020). Finally, approaches such as "feminist organizing" incorporate elements of both community building and organizing (Hyde, 2018; Stout, 2010; chapter 13). As Hyde (2005, p. 361) points out, feminist organizing need not address "quintessentially feminist issues," such as gender-based violence or pay equity; "rather, it is the empowering aspects of such endeavors that render them feminist." In Stall and Stoecker's (2005) view, in a "women-centered" model, "power begins in the private sphere of social relationships," but once again, the goal is empowerment, or "the cultivation of individual and collective skills and resources for social and political action" (p. 302).

The Community Coalition Action Theory (Butterfoss & Kegler, 2009; chapter 18) and related collaborative approaches (Wolff et al., 2017) are alternately defined as examples of community organizing practice or as strategies used across models. Coalitions and regional collaboratives are increasingly popular in diverse areas of health, social work, and urban and regional planning, from asthma prevention to gender-based violence, food insecurity, and health-focused land-use planning (chapters 19, 22; appendix 2).

Finally, and while not organizing per se, CBPR approaches often use community organizing strategies and gauged their success on the ability of partnerships to achieve policy or systems transformations that promote greater equity (Cacari Stone et al., 2018; Minkler, 2010; chapter 22). Using a mix of Rothman's social planning (with the inclusion of data), locality development (with often place-based projects), and social action (understanding that advocacy is critical for translation of data into action), many CBPR initiatives have sought to enhance racial and class equity (Cacari Stone et al., 2018; Devia et al., 2017; Minkler, 2010; chapters 15, 22).

In sum, as suggested earlier, although no single model of community organizing or community building exists, three concepts in particular—power, empowerment, and community capacity—are emphasized in each. They are discussed and illustrated in more detail in later chapters; we introduce them here to underscore their importance to this work, particularly during the complex and troubling era in which we live and practice and the uncharted territory ahead.

Core Concepts in Community Building and Community Organizing

Power and Empowerment

Power has always been a central concept within community organizing, community building, and the processes and outcomes of community empowerment. A starting point for empowerment has been the recognition of inequities in power among different groups in society (e.g., communities of color, lower socioeconomic-status groups, disabled people etc.), which then suffer from disenfranchisement and poorer health outcomes.

"Power over," as an oppressive force, resides in multiple systems that affect these communities on a daily basis, from histories of social exclusion and racist policies to the current maintenance of economic, political, or ideological power inequities (Blackwell & McAffee, 2020; Gaventa & Cornwall, 2015; Stoeffler, 2018). These systems can then become internalized within cultures and individuals, creating feelings of powerlessness, potentially leading to inaction. While oppressive power can be seen as monolithic, Foucault (1977) upends these ideas by discussing power as a productive and inherently unstable resource within institutional practices and webs of social relations that can be challenged and resisted.

Empowerment and organizing strategies therefore mean confronting the multiple mechanisms of control, whether structural, cultural, or internalized. The perspectives of *power with others* and *power to act* support advocacy and resistance against oppression have been threaded throughout the empowerment literature, as well as the feminist notion of *power within ourselves* (Stoeffler, 2018).

While the term *empowerment* has been justifiably criticized as a catch-all phrase in social science (Rappaport, 1984), it represents a central tenet of community organizing and community building practice. Classically, empowerment has been defined as having three levels, psychological, organizational, and community (Zimmerman, 2000). Although these are all important, we focus here on community empowerment as "a group-based, participatory, developmental process through which marginalized or oppressed individuals and groups gain greater control over their lives and environment, acquire valued resources and basic rights, and achieve important life goals and reduced societal marginalization" (Maton, 2008, p. 5). This definition recognizes the power of the collective in organizing, the potential continuum and developmental nature of empowering processes for people in gaining control over their lives, and outcomes of enhanced resources and improved conditions. Israel and her colleagues' "Scale for measuring perceptions of control at the individual, organizational, neighborhood, and beyond-the-neighborhood levels" (appendix 12), has proven a particularly useful tool for capturing the degree to which individuals believe they and their organizations and communities can have an impact on decisions affecting their lives and their organizations and communities. Additionally, however, it can help assess people's perceptions of the degree to which their neighborhood members work together to influence decisions on the city, state, or national level, and the extent to which they have connections to people in positions of power who can help influence decisionmaking (appendix 12).

Community empowerment also helps to address such key public health concerns as achieving equity (Marmot et al., 2008) as well as people having the capacity to identify problems and solutions (Goodman et al., 1999; chapters 10, 11) and to influence and hold accountable the institutions that impact their lives (chapter 22). Ultimately, community empowerment is an integrated social action process by which individuals, communities, and organizations gain mastery over their lives in the context of changing their social and political environment to improve equity and quality of life (Kleba et al., 2021; Wallerstein, 2006).

From these perspectives, community empowerment is an action-oriented concept with a focus on transforming power relations between communities, institutions, and broader social-political forces. It assumes that communities have the cultural and organizing strengths to take actions against inequitable conditions. The dialogical process of Paulo Freire (1973, 2016), with its accent on critical consciousness and praxis, or cycles of listening, dialogue, and action, adds to our understanding of the interaction between the multiple levels of empowerment. Praxis engages individuals with others to claim their personal power through political and collective action (Douglas et al., 2016; Laverack, 2006; Su, 2009; chapters 5, 15).

As a theory and methodology, community empowerment is multilayered, representing both processes and outcomes of change for individuals, the organizations of which they are a part, and the community social structure itself (Zimmerman, 2000). "Psychological empowerment" includes people's perceived control in their lives, their critical awareness of their social context, and their political efficacy and participation in change. Empowerment challenges the perceived or real "powerlessness" resulting from the injuries of poverty, chronic stressors, lack of control, and insufficient resources to meet demands. Social epidemiology founder S. Leonard Syme (Syme & Ritterman, 2009), describes this simply as "control over destiny." Organizational empowerment incorporates both *processes* of organizations (e.g., whether they are acting to influence societal change) and *outcomes*, such as their effectiveness in gaining new resources (Hughey et al., 2008). At the community level, community empowerment outcomes can include increased sense of community, greater perceived control on multiple levels (appendix 12), more civic engagement, and actual changes in policies, transformed conditions, or increased resources that may reduce inequities (Kleba et al., 2021; Minkler 2010; Wallerstein, 2006).

Community-based participatory research (CBPR) also supports these multiple levels of empowerment and of confronting power inequities as key to its practice. Defined by Wallerstein et al. (2018) as multisector collaboration that uses data and information to advocate for goals of social and health equity, the learnings about power within CBPR can contribute to community organizing and community building strategies. CBPR theory and practice have identified the importance of seeking power sharing among partners in addition to redressing power inequities in communities (Coombe et al., 2020; Muhammad et al., 2015; Wallerstein et al., 2020; chapter 15). This consideration may be even more important when outside organizers are brought into a community organizing effort, elevating the importance of cultural humility, for example, being reflexive about their positions of power, whether on the basis of race-ethnicity, education, or other status, in order to improve power-sharing within the organizing group (Greene-Moton & Minkler, 2020).

The concept of commitment to "collective empowerment," based on the Engage for Equity CBPR study of 179 academic-community partnerships across the United States, incorporates ideas of actions based on their fit within a community or culture, and people perceiving that they have influence on decisions, adopting ongoing collective reflection, and sharing values (Wallerstein et al., 2020). This concept supports Freirian praxis of reflection and action by people themselves within their own communities, and mirrors classic empowerment literature regarding people participating collectively, with core principles for change, and critical reflection and influence within their community to improve their living conditions.

As communities become empowered and better able to engage in collective problem solving, key health and social indicators may reflect this, such as increased voter participation, increased representation of women and people of color in positions of power, and governmental budgets allocated to community priorities (Kleba et al., 2021; Rivkin, 2014; chapters 15, 22). Participatory approaches to evaluation can also lead to enhanced community capacity building and empowerment at the local level (Fetterman et al., 2012; Wiggins et al., 2018; chapters 15, 21). Moreover, and even prior to the coronavirus pandemic, empowered communities were helping to address some of the deeply entrenched social determinants of health (SDOH) that contribute to ill health in the first place (chapters 15, 22; Minkler et al., 2019; Pastor et al., 2018; Schultz et al., 2020; Wolff et al., 2017).

Community Capacity

Closely related to the concept of empowerment is the notion of community capacity, classically defined by Goodman et al. (1999) as "the characteristics of communities that affect their ability to identify, mobilize, and address social and public health problems" (p. 259). As these scholars further note, community capacity has multiple dimensions: active participation, leadership, rich support networks, skills and resources, critical reflection, sense of community, understanding of history, articulation of values, and access to power.

Complementing the above, and widely adopted in public health, social work, and numerous other fields, is political scientist Robert Putman's (2000) concept of social capital or the features of social organization that facilitate coordination and cooperation for mutual benefit. Social capital is operationalized both as a *horizontal relationship* between community members, with variables of trust, reciprocity, and civic engagement (Cockerham, 2013; Kawachi et al., 2008) and as a vertical linking relationship with external communities and people in positions of power (Moore & Kawachi, 2017; Rubin, 2016; chapter 11). Within epidemiology, low social capital has been correlated with poor health status (Kawachi et al., 2008; Rodgers et al., 2019). Yet, while an important descriptor of community well-being, social capital itself is not a strategy, and requires community organizing and capacity building approaches in order to strengthen the health and social outcomes with which it is concerned.

Social networks (the relationships in which people are embedded) and the social support people give and receive through these networks are important to consider within the context of community capacity building (Berkman, 2000). Social network mapping techniques, for example, may be employed to help identify natural helpers or leaders within a community. They may help these natural leaders in turn identify both their own networks and high-risk groups within the community. Further, such techniques may involve network members in undertaking their own community assessments and actions necessary to strengthen networks within the community (Eng et al., 2009; Hindhede & Aagaard-Hansen, 2017; chapters 10, 11; appendix 2). Finally, leadership development represents a key aspect of fostering community capacity. In particular, it is critical to develop leaders who can stimulate people to be self-reflective, to think critically and across differences, identifying problems and potential solutions outside their comfort zones (Brown & Mazza, 2005; Jones et al., 2010; Lasker & Guidry, 2009).

As Gutiérrez and Lewis suggest in chapter 13, an emphasis on leadership development may be especially important in communities of color where "a unidirectional outreach approach" often treats such communities as "targets of change rather than active participants and collaborators." Further, and in the diverse communities in which many of us live, work, play, and age, leadership requires "reclaiming courage," embodied in the "strong early voices" that are often silenced in polite adult society (Browne & Mazza, 2005, pp. 62, 63).

Lay health worker strategies have been key to promoting community empowerment, capacity, competence, social capital, and leadership, especially if they emphasize transformations in the lay health workers themselves, and changes in clinical and community practices, instead of only their impact on clients (Bracho et al., 2016; Eng et al., 2009; Wiggins et al., 2018). Sometimes, moreover, empowered lay health workers have gone on to run for and attain political office, serve on municipal or regional task forces, or in other ways serve their communities on the policy level (chapter 10).

Summary

The continued pivotal role of community organizing in health education and social work practice reflects both this approach's time-tested efficacy and its fit with the most fundamental principles of these fields. Community organizing thus stresses strengths-based approaches, the principle of relevance or starting where the people are, the principle of participatory issue selection and choice of actions, and the importance of creating environments in which individuals and communities can become empowered as they increase their community capacity or problem-solving ability.

Similarly, newer conceptualizations of community building stress many of the same principles, within an overall approach that focuses on community growth and change from the inside, through increased group identification; discovery, nurturing, and mapping of community assets; and creation of "critical conscious-ness," all toward the end of building stronger and more caring communities. Finally, new tools and approaches, including the power of the internet for facili-tating community organizing and community building (chapter 16), have greatly increased the reach of these methods over the last decade.

Whether engaged in "pure" community-driven organizing around issues the community identifies, or borrowing skills from community organizing and com-munity building practice, professionals in fields like public health, social work, and urban and regional planning can challenge themselves to examine their own dynamic of power. Such reflection should include dynamics of power with their professional colleagues and community members, to understand the com-plexities of working in partnership toward the goals of community ownership and empowerment (Wallerstein, 1999; appendixes 1, 5). In sum, both community organizing and community building practice bring essential strategies in a wide variety of community and organizational settings and may hold particular rele-vance in the changing cultural and sociopolitical climate of the twenty-first century.

Questions for Further Discussion

1. The authors argue that health and social work professionals cannot empower communities, but they can help create the conditions in which people and their communities can become empowered. As a professional in one of these or a related field, what actions might you or your agency take to help create such conditions?

2. As a newly hired social worker or health educator, you are charged with help-ing organize a largely Black community with high rates of diabetes and heart disease around these serious health problems. But when you raise this issue at a community meeting, residents make clear that they are much more inter-ested in organizing around police harassment, particularly that directed toward Black men and youth. You are committed to doing genuine commu-nity organizing, but you also understand your agency's position and the fact that they have funding for organizing communities around diabetes and heart disease prevention. How might you proceed?

REFERENCES

Alinsky, S. D. (1971). *Rules for Radicals: A Pragmatic Primer for Realistic Radicals.* Random House.

Berkman, L. F. (2000). Social integration, social networks, and health. In N. B. Anderson (Ed.), *Encyclopedia of Health and Behavior* (Vol. 2, pp. 754–759). Sage.

Blackwell, A. G., & Colmenar, R. (2000). Community-building: From local wisdom to public policy. *Public Health Rep, 115*(2–3), 161–166.

Blackwell, A. G., & McAfee, M. (2020, June 26). Banks should face history and pay reparations. *New York Times.* https://www.nytimes.com/2020/06/26/opinion/sunday/banks-reparations-racism-inequality.html.

Bracho, A., Lee, G., Giraldo, G. P., De Prado, R. M., & Latino Health Access. (2016). *Recruiting the Heart, Training the Brain: The Work of Latino Health Access*. Hesperian Health Guides.

Brown, C. R., & Mazza, G. J. (2005). *Leading Diverse Communities: A How-to Guide for Moving from Healing into Action*. Jossey-Bass.

Butterfoss, F., & Kegler, M. (2009). A community coalition action theory. In R. Di Clemente, R. A. Crosby, & M. C. Kegler (Eds.), *Emerging Theories in Health Promotion Practice & Research* (2nd ed, pp. 237–276). Jossey-Bass.

Cacari Stone, L., Themba-Nixon, M., Freudenberg, N., & Minkler, M. (2018). The role of community-based participatory research in policy advocacy. In N. Wallerstein, B. Duran, J. G. Oetzel, & M. Minkler (Eds.), *Community-Based Participatory Research for Health: Advancing Social and Health Equity* (3rd ed., pp. 277–292). Jossey-Bass.

Carroll, J., & Minkler, M. (2000). Freire's message for social workers: Looking back, looking ahead. *J Community Pract, 8*(1), 21–36.

Chávez, V., Minkler, M., Wallerstein, N., & Spencer, M. S. (2010). Community organizing for health and social justice. In L. Cohen, V. Chávez, & S. Chehimi (Eds.), *Prevention Is Primary: Strategies for Community Well-Being* (2nd ed., pp. 87–112). Jossey-Bass.

Cnaan, R. A., & Milofsky, C. (2018). *Handbook of Community Movements and Local Organizations in the 21st Century*. Springer International.

Cockerham, W. (2013). *Social Causes of Health and Disease* (2nd ed.). Polity Press.

Coombe, C. M., Chandanabhumma, P., Brush, B. L., Jensen, M., Lachance, L., Lee, S. Y. D., Meisenheimer, M., Minkler, M., Greene-Moton, E., Muhammed, M., Reyes, A. G., Rowe, Z., Wilson-Powers, E., & Israel, B. A. (2020, August). A participatory, mixed methods approach to define and measure partnership synergy in long-standing equity-focused CBPR partnerships. *Am J Community Psychol, 66*(3–4), 427–438. DOI:10.1002/ajcp.12447.

Coombe, C. M., Israel, B. A., Reyes, A. G., Clement, J., Grant, S., Lichtenstein, R., Schulz, A. J., & Smith, S. (2017). Strengthening community capacity in Detroit to influence policy change for health equity. *Michigan Journal of Community Service Learning, 23*(2). https://doi.org/10.3998/mjcsloa.3239521.0023.208.

Corntassel, J. (2012). Re-envisioning resurgence: Indigenous pathways to decolonization and sustainable self-determination. *Decolonization, Indigeneity, Education, and Society, 1*(1), 86–101.

DeFilippis, J., Fisher, R., & Shragge, E. (2010). *Contesting Community: The Limits and Potential of Local Organizing*. Rutgers University Press.

Devia, C., Baker, E., Sanchez-Youngman, S., Barnidge, E., Golub, M., Motton, F., Muhammad, M., Ruddock, C., Vicuña, B., & Wallerstein, N. (2017). Advancing system and policy changes for social and racial justice: Comparing a rural and urban community-based participatory research partnership in the U.S. *Int J Equity Health, 16*, 17.

Douglas, J. A., Grills, C. T., Villanueva, S., & Subica, A. M. (2016). Empowerment praxis: Community organizing to redress systemic health disparities. *Am J Community Psychol, 58*(3–4), 488–498.

Eng, E., & Parker, E. (1994). Measuring community competence in the Mississippi Delta: The interface between program evaluation and empowerment. *Health Educ Q, 21*(2), 199–220.

Eng, E., Rhodes, S., & Parker, E. A. (2009). Natural helper models to enhance a community's health and competence. In R. J. DiClemente, R. A. Crosby, & M. C. Kegler (Eds.), *Emerging Theories in Health Promotion Practice and Research* (2nd ed., pp. 303–330). Jossey-Bass.

Fetterman, D., Kaftarian, S. J., & Wandersman, A. (2012). *Empowerment Evaluation Knowledge and Tools for Self-Assessment, Evaluation Capacity Building, and Accountability* (2nd ed.). Sage.

Fisher, R., & DeFilippis, J. (2015). Community organizing in the United States. *Community Dev J, 50*(3), 363–379.

Foucault, M. (1977). *Power/Knowledge: Selected Interviews and Other Writings, 1972–1977.* C. Gordon (Ed.). Pantheon Books.

Freire, P. (1973). *Education for Critical Consciousness.* Seabury Press.

Freire, P. (2016). *Pedagogy of the Heart.* Bloomsbury.

Frisby, W., Maguire, P., & Reid, C. (2009). The "f" word has everything to do with it: How feminist theories inform action research. *Action Res, 7*(1), 13–29.

García, I. (2020). Asset-Based Community Development (ABCD): Core principles. In R. Phillips, E. Trevan, & P. Kraeger (Eds.), *Research Handbook on Community Development* (pp. 67–75). Edward Elgar.

Garvin, C. D., & Cox, F. M. (2001). A history of community organizing since the Civil War with special reference to oppressed communities. In J. Rothman, J. Erlich, & J. E. Tropman (Eds.), *Strategies of Community Intervention* (6th ed., pp. 65–100). Peacock Publishers.

Gaventa, J., & Cornwall, A. (2015). Power and knowledge. In H. Bradbury (Ed.), *The SAGE Handbook of Action Research: Participative Inquiry and Practice* (3rd ed., pp. 465–471). Sage.

Goodman, R. M., Speers, M., McLeroy, K., Fawcett, S., Kegler, M., Parker, E. S., Smith, R., Sterling, T. D., & Wallerstein, N. (1999). Identifying and defining the dimensions of community capacity to provide a basis for measurement. *Health Educ Behav, 25*(3), 258–278.

Greene-Moton, E., & Minkler, M. (2020). Cultural competence or cultural humility? Moving beyond the debate. *Health Promot Pract, 21*(1), 142–145.

Himmelman, A. (2001). On coalitions and the transformation of power relations: Collaborative betterment and collaborative empowerment. *Am J Community Psychol, 29*(2), 277–284.

Hindhede, A. L., & Aagaard-Hansen, J. (2017). Using social network analysis as a method to assess and strengthen participation in health promotion programs in vulnerable areas. *Health Promot Pract, 18*(2), 175–183.

Hughey, J., Peterson, N. A., Lowe J. B., & Oprescu, F. (2008). Empowerment and sense of community: Clarifying their relationship in community organizations. *Health Educ Behav, 35*(5), 651–663.

Hunter, A. (1975). The loss of community: An empirical test through replication. *Am Sociol Rev, 40*(5), 537–552.

Hyde, C. A. (2005). Feminist community practice. In M. Weil (Ed.), *Handbook of Community Practice* (pp. 360–371). Sage.

Hyde, C. A. (2008). Feminist social work practice. In T. Mizrahi & L. Davis (Eds.), *Encyclopedia of Social Work* (20th ed., pp. 216–221). Oxford University Press.

Hyde, C. A. (2018). Charisma, collectives, and commitment: Hybrid authority in radical feminist social movement organizations. *Soc Mov Stud, 17*(4), 424–436.

Jones, M., Rae, R., Frazier, S., Maltrud, K., Varela, F., Percy, C., & Wallerstein, N. (2010, December). Healthy Native Communities Fellowship: Advancing leadership for community changes in health. *Indian Health Service Provider, 35*(12), 279–284.

Kawachi, I., Subramanian, S. V., & Kim, D. (2008). *Social Capital and Health.* Springer.

Khan-Cullors, P., & Bandele, A. (2017). *When They Call You a Terrorist: A Black Lives Matter Memoir.* St Martin's Griffin.

Kleba, M. E., Wallerstein, N., Belon, A. P., van der Donk, C., Gastaldo, D., Avery, H., & Wright, M. (2021). Empowerment and participatory health research. Position Paper 4. International Collaboration for Participatory Health Research.

Lasker, R. D., & Guidry, J. A. (2009). *Engaging the Community in Decision Making.* McFarland.

Laverack, G. (2006). Improving health outcomes through community empowerment: A review of the literature. *Health Popular Nutr, 24*(1), 113–120.

Mansbridge, J. (2001). The making of oppositional consciousness. In J. Mansbridge & A. Morris (Eds.), *Oppositional Consciousness: The Subjective Roots of Social Protest* (pp. 1–19). University of Chicago Press.

Marmot, M., Friel, S., Bell, R., Houweling, T. A. J., & Taylor, S. (2008). Closing the gap in a generation: Health equity through action on the social determinants of health. *Lancet, 372* (9650), 1661–1669.

Maton, K. I. (2008). Empowering community settings: Agents of individual development, community betterment, and positive social change. *Am J Community Psychol, 41*(1), 4–21.

Minkler, M. (2010). Linking science and policy through community-based participatory research to study and address health disparities. *Am J Public Health, 100*(1_suppl), S81–S87.

Minkler, M., Griffin, J., & Wakimoto, P. (2020). Seizing the moment: Policy advocacy to end mass incarceration in the time of COVID-19. *Health Educ Behav, 47*(4), 514–518.

Minkler, M., Rebanal, R. D., Pearce, R., & Acosta, M. (2019). Growing equity and health equity in perilous times: Lessons from community organizers. *Health Educ Behav, 46*(1_suppl), 9S–18S.

Moore, S., & Kawachi, I. (2017). Twenty years of social capital and health research: A glossary. *J Epidemiol Community Health, 71*(5), 513–517.

Muhammad, M., Wallerstein, N., Sussman, A., Avila, M., & Belone, L. (2015). Reflections on researcher identity and power: The impact of positionality on community based participatory research (CBPR) processes and outcomes. *Crit Sociol, 41*(7–9), 1045–1063.

Pastor, M., Terriquez, V., & Lin, M. (2018). How community organizing promotes health equity, and how health equity affects organizing. *Health Affairs, 37*(3), 358–363.

Phulwani, V. (2016). The poor man's Machiavelli: Saul Alinsky and the morality of power. *Am Polit Sci Rev, 110*(4), 863–975.

Porta, C., Sane, A., Singer, E., Mehus, C. J., Gower, A. L., Saewyc, E., Fredkove, W., & Eisenberg, M. E. (2017). LGBTQ youth's views on gay-straight alliances: Building community, providing gateways, and representing safety and support. *J School Health, 87*(7), 489–497.

Poteat, V. P., Sinclair, K. O., DiGiovanni, C. D., Koenig, B. W., & Russell, S. T. (2012). Gay-straight alliances are associated with student health: A multischool comparison of LGBTQ and heterosexual youth. *J Res Adolesc, 23*(2), 319–330.

Putnam, R. (2000). *Bowling Alone: The Collapse and Revival of American Community.* Simon and Schuster.

Rappaport, J. (1984). Studies in empowerment: Introduction to the issue. *Prev in Human Services, 3*(2–3), 1–7.

Reger, J. (2017). Finding a place in history: The discursive legacy of the wave metaphor and contemporary feminism. *Fem Stud, 43*(1), 193–221.

Rivkin, S. (2014). Examining the links between community participation and health outcomes: A review of the literature. *Health Policy Plan, 29*(suppl_2), ii98–ii106.

Rodgers, J., Valuev, A. V., Hswen, Y., & Subramanian, S. V. (2019). Social capital and physical health: An updated review of the literature for 2007–2018. *Soc Sci Med, 236*, 112360.

Rothman, J. (2008). Multi modes of community intervention. In J. Rothman, J. L. Erlich, & J. E. Tropman (Eds.), *Strategies of Community Intervention* (7th ed., pp. 141–170). Eddie Bowers Publishing.

Rubin, O. (2016). The political dimension of "linking social capital": Current analytical practices and the case for recalibration. *Theory Soc, 45*(5), 429–449.

Schultz, J., Fawcett, S., Holt, C., & Watson-Thompson, J. (2020). Strengthening collaborative action for community health and development. *Am J Health Stud, 35*(2), 152–163.

Schutz, A. & Miller, M. (2015). *People Power: The Community Organizing Tradition of Saul Alinsky.* Vanderbilt University Press.

Sen, R. (2020, July 1). Why today's social revolutions include kale, medical care and help with rent. Zócalo Public Squre. https://www.zocalopublicsquare.org/2020/07/01/mutual-aid -societies-self-determination-pandemic-community-organizing/ideas/essay/.

Smith, L. T. (2012). *Decolonizing Methodologies: Research and Indigenous Peoples* (2nd ed.). Zed Books.

Stall, S., & Stoecker, R. (2005). Toward a gender analysis of community organizing models: Liminality and the intersection of spheres. In M. Minkler (Ed.), *Community Organizing and Community Building for Health* (2nd ed., pp. 296–317). Rutgers University Press.

Staples, L. (2016). *Roots to Power: A Manual for Grassroots Organizing* (3rd ed.). Praeger.

Stoecker, R. (2018). About the localized social movement. In R. Cnaan & C. Milofsky (Eds.), *Handbook of Community Movements and Local Organizations in the 21st Century* (pp. 211–227). Springer.

Stoeffler, S. W. (2018). Community empowerment. In R. Cnaan & C. Milofsky (Eds.), *Handbook of Community Movements and Local Organizations in the 21st Century* (pp. 265–280). Springer.

Stout, J. (2010). *Blessed Are the Organized: Grassroots Democracy in America.* Princeton University Press.

Su, C. (2009). *Streetwise for Book Smarts: Grassroots Organizing and Education Reform in the Bronx.* Cornell University Press.

Syme, S. L., & Ritterman, M. L. (2009). The importance of community development for health and well-being. *Community Dev Invest Rev, 5*(3), 1–13.

Toomey, R. B., Ryan, C., Diaz, R. M., & Russell, S. T. (2011). High school gay-straight alliances (GSAs) and young adult well-being: An examination of GSA presence, participation, and perceived effectiveness. *Appl Dev Sci, 15*(4), 175–185.

Wallerstein, N. (1999). Power between evaluator and community: Research relationships within New Mexico's healthier communities. *Soc Sci Med, 49*, 39–53.

Wallerstein, N. (2006). What is the evidence on effectiveness of empowerment to improve health? Health Evidence Network Report. WHO Regional Office for Europe. http://www.euro.who.int/Document/E88086.pdf.

Wallerstein, N., & Auerbach, E. (2004/2020). *Problem-Posing at Work: English for Action* (2nd ed.). Grass Roots Press (re-issued in e-book, 2020).

Wallerstein, N., Duran, B., Oetzel, J. G., & Minkler, M. (2018). *Community-Based Participatory Research for Health* (3rd ed.). Jossey-Bass.

Wallerstein, N., Oetzel, J. G., Sanchez-Youngman, S., Boursaw, B., Dickson, E., Kastelic, S., Koegel, P., Lucero, J. E., Magarati, M., Ortiz, K., & Parker, M. (2020). Engage for equity: A long-term study of community-based participatory research and community-engaged research practices and outcomes. *Health Educ Behav, 47*(3), 380–390.

Walter, C. L., & Hyde, C. A. (2012). Community building and practice: An expanded conceptual framework. In M. Minkler (Ed.), *Community Organizing and Community Building for Health and Welfare* (3rd ed, pp. 78–94). Rutgers University Press.

Walters, K. L., Johnson-Jennings, M., Stroud, S., Rasmus, S., Charles, B., John, S., Allen, J., Kaholokula, J. K. A., Look, M. A., de Silva, M., & Lowe, J. (2020). Growing from our roots: Strategies for developing culturally grounded health promotion interventions in American Indian, Alaska Native, and Native Hawaiian communities. *Prev Sci, 21*(1), 54–64.

Warren, R. (1963). *The Community in America.* Rand McNally.

Wenger-Trayner, E., & Wenger-Trayner, B. (2015). Introduction to communities of practice: A brief overview of the concept and its uses. https://wenger-trayner.com/introduction-to-communities-of-practice/.

West, C. (2017). *Race Matters, 25th Anniversary: With a New Introduction.* Beacon Press.

Whittier, N. (2017). *Identity Politics, Consciousness-Raising, and Visibility Politics.* Oxford University Press.

Wiggins, N. (2012). Popular education for health promotion and community empowerment: A review of the literature. *Health Promot Int, 272*, 356–371.

Wiggins, N., Parajon, L. C., Coombe, C., Duldulao, A., Garcia, L., & Wang, P. (2018). Participatory evaluation as a process of empowerment: Experiences with community health workers in the United States and Latin America. In N. Wallerstein, B. Duran, J. G. Oetzel, & M. Minkler (Eds.), *Community-Based Participatory Research for Health: Advancing Social and Health Equity* (3rd ed., pp. 251–264). Jossey-Bass.

Wolff, T., Minkler, M., Wolfe, S. M., Berkowitz, B., Bowen, L., Butterfoss, F. D., Christens, B. D., Francisco, V. T., Himmelman, A. T., & Lee, K. S. (2017). Collaborating for equity and justice: Moving beyond collective impact. *Nonprofit Q, 9*, 42–53.

Zimmerman, M. (2000). Empowerment theory: Psychological, organizational and community levels of analysis. In J. Rappaport & E. Seidman (Eds.), *Handbook of Community Psychology* (pp. 43–63). Kluwer Academic Publishers/Plenum.

4

Anti-racism Praxis

A Community Organizing Approach for Achieving Health and Social Equity

DEREK M. GRIFFITH

HEATHER CAME

It was courage. It was Black people standing up saying . . . "I'm a human being. I have a right to go and to be treated like a human being," even more so than the jobs. . . . I heard . . . that the leadership didn't want to use the children . . . but as soon as the idea got around among the kids . . . we moved on it. [O]ther folk had already gone to jail and we knew what to expect. I think that we have never been powerless since that day.

–Washington Booker III, fourteen years old in 1963

On Thursday, May 2, 1963, more than 1,000 Black elementary, middle, and high school students participated in a nonviolent protest in Birmingham, Alabama. The next day, when hundreds more gathered for another march, ardent segregationist and commissioner of public safety Theophilus Eugene "Bull" Connor directed the local police and fire departments to use high-pressure fire hoses, police clubs, police dogs, and other tools to stop the demonstration. The television and newspaper coverage of these events, now known as the Children's Crusade, triggered global outrage and led to the eventual passage of the Civil Rights Act of 1964 ("The Children's Crusade," 2021). Washington Booker III was among the children who participated in this protest. For the next fifty years, Mr. Booker was a "foot soldier," community organizer, and activist until his death in 2016 (Stein, 2016). This is the power of anti-racism praxis and community organizing. But let us first define racism.

Racism and Racialization

The problem in America is not race. The problem is not that people look different from each other. The problem is that people are treated differently because of the way they look. The problem is racism. (Jenkins et al., 2019, p. 35)

53

Historically, public health, medicine, and the social sciences have focused on defining and addressing race, not racism. "In so doing, it has helped to reify the notion of race and obscure the underlying role of racism in producing the patterns of health inequities that persist in our society" (Jenkins, et al., 2019). Racism is real. In public health, considerable attention, resources, and effort are dedicated to documenting and measuring the health effects of racism and other forms of discrimination (Ford et al., 2019).

It is only through activism, community organizing, and community building that scholars have been able to use the term *racism* to describe the root cause of racial differences in health equity and well-being (Jenkins et al., 2019; Williams & Griffith, 2019). Whether racism can be eliminated or simply mitigated remains a matter of contention, debate, and disagreement (Came & Griffith, 2018; Ford et al., 2019). Until the last few decades, scholars, activists, and advocates were unable to use the term *racism* to describe the focus of their efforts, and initiatives to achieve health equity were hampered by the lack of any sustained institutional presence (Jenkins, 2019). The establishment of policies, organizations, offices, centers, and institutes dedicated to addressing racial inequities in health and social conditions have provided a foundation to support efforts to achieve health equity (Jenkins et al., 2019).

Racism is an analytic tool that can be used to explain power systems, patterns, and outcomes that vary by population groups and that are broader than the explicit decisions and practices of individuals, organizations, or institutions. Racism is a useful frame for characterizing the policies and practices that create underlying social conditions that lead to disease concentration, clustering, and interaction (Poteat et al., 2020). Racism is a system, not an individual characteristic or a personal moral failing. Racism is *a system of power* whose mechanisms are in the structures, policies, practices, norms, and values of our decisionmaking (Jones, 2019). Focusing on prejudicial attitudes and discriminatory behavior ignores the historical, social, and political aspects of the system of oppression and focuses the issue on race-contingent behavior or actions ("disparate treatment"), rather than identifying how decisions not seemingly affected by race can still produce differential outcomes ("disparate impact") (Came & Griffith, 2018). Racism unfairly disadvantages some individuals and communities, unfairly advantages others, and saps the strength of the whole society through the waste of human resources (Jones, 2019).

Structural racism is a useful frame for these factors because it reflects the totality of ways that ideologies of inherent racial inferiority of socially defined groups (i.e., races) create ranking or a caste system that differentially allocates societal resources and advantage (Bailey et al., 2017). Structural racism illustrates how these ideologies (i.e., cultural racism) (Cogburn, 2019; Griffith et al., 2010) operate through mutually reinforcing sectors of society (e.g., health care, housing, education, criminal justice) in ways that determine population-level patterns of health and well-being (i.e., the experience of health, happiness, and prosperity) (Bailey et al., 2017).

While cultural narratives and media coverage often present it as reflecting aberrant views of a minority of people, racism is often aligned with the normative culture of particular eras, geographic contexts, and locales (Came & Griffith, 2018).

Although historically, racism has been used to describe discrimination based on race, *racialization* provides a framework for understanding how the social and historical context makes ethnic groups, religious minorities, and others subject to racism and xenophobia similar to racial groups (LeBrón & Viruell-Fuentes, 2019; Samari et al., 2019). In contrast to groups being able to define themselves, racialization describes a process by which others define a group and ascribe to it characteristics associated with where the group comes from, what it believes in, or how it organizes itself socially and culturally (Samari et al., 2019). In addition to these external definitions, groups can elect to racialize themselves as a political strategy, an act of resistance, and a demonstration of power rooted in a positive racialized identity.

Why Anti-racism Organizing?

In the very act of working for the impersonal cause of racial freedom, a man experiences, almost like grace, a large measure of private freedom. Or call it a new comprehension of his own identity, an intuition of the expanding boundaries of his self, which, if not the same thing as freedom, is its radical source.

–James Farmer Jr., cofounder of what became the
Congress of Racial Equality (CORE)

The art and science of devising and implementing strategies to address racism and racialization is called *anti-racism*. Anti-racism is not a status or event; it is a process (Griffith & Semlow, 2020). Jones (1997) defines anti-racism as "the rejection of the racist ideology, practices, and behavior in oneself: the active opposition of all forms of racism in individuals and institutions; and the advocacy of individual conduct, institutional practices, and cultural expressions that promote inclusiveness and interdependence and acknowledge and respect racial differences" (p. 517). But well-meaning and committed people define and practice anti-racism differently (Friedersdorf, 2020). There have always been differences in the strategic visions of various leaders, institutions, and social-protest organizations about what practical steps should be taken to improve the material conditions of people (Marable, 1995).

Anti-racism praxis seeks to help individuals and communities create a vision of the goals and objectives, not simply the problem (i.e., racism) (Came & Griffith, 2018). An anti-racism approach often includes a structural analysis that recognizes that the world is controlled by systems, with traceable historical roots, that batter some and benefit others. Anti-racism presumes, accepts, and embraces different views as essential ingredients to facilitate new ways of thinking (Eliasson, 2016). There is no strategy known to these authors to effectively engage and change those who are not at least open to new ideas and principles. However, for those who are even somewhat open to considering new ideas, concepts, and strategies to achieve health equity, we offer some tools for anti-racism praxis (see table 4.1).

Because the task of *pursuing health equity* is not simply one of science but of translating science into narratives, beliefs, practices, and policies, we have to recognize that efforts to make a moral or social justice case for eliminating health disparities and achieving health equity have been largely ineffective (Williams, 2012). Reviews of *anti-racism interventions* (Clarke et al., 2013; Rankine, 2014; Shapiro, 2002) have found that the objective of the majority of interventions is to heal, organize, and empower those who are the targets of racism by helping them see how the world is shaped by systems, with traceable historical roots, that advantage some and disadvantage others. And yet, one of the fundamental challenges of *anti-racism organizing* is to increase individual and collective capacity to look at the world as if it could be otherwise (Allsup, 2003), and to identify and remember why it is important for each person to participate. People who organize and build community often do so around "gut issues" that motivate members to get involved and remain involved (Kieffer, 1984). *Spirituality* has been a fundamental source of motivation for many efforts to organize and create social change. Spirituality has been the foundation that facilitates hope and optimism and mitigates discouragement, disillusionment, and pessimism (Watts et al., 1999).

Successful interventions need to be targeted, context specific, and focused on changing behavior rather than deeply held attitudes or beliefs (Pederson et al., 2005). Many anti-racism programs and initiatives seek to change awareness of cultural differences, reducing prejudice, and increasing individual growth, transformation, and activism (Came & Griffith, 2018; Shapiro, 2002). The problem is that even the most well intentioned people bring with them entrenched beliefs, attitudes, and experiences that shape how they learn and critically unlearn and apply new information (Came & Griffith, 2018). Even with these new tools, however, there are often questions about what one can do (see table 4.2 for a list of potential actions).

The actions in this list, culled from Dr. Ibram X. Kendi's (2019) landmark book *How to Be an Antiracist*, include a wide range of steps we can take to eliminate racial inequity in the spaces we inhabit. These steps include viewing racial inequity "as a problem of policy, not people," though digging deep to identify its myriad "intersections and manifestations." But it also moves into action, from finding various anti-racist policy options, to identifying diverse actors with the power to make the desired policy changes, and mobilizing driving forces for change, including "like-minded policymakers" and community and other players that can effectively fight for the enactment of the desired policy focused on racial equity. Finally, as also discussed in chapter 22, Kendi (2019) further emphasizes the importance of carefully monitoring "politics, policies, and practices" to both evaluate their efficacy in expanding (or reducing) racial inequities, and the extent to which they are likely to do so in the future.

TABLE 4.1

Five Key Elements of Anti-racism Praxis

Element	Description
Reflexive relational practice	• Anti-racism work is relational; it involves listening, respect, understanding, relationship building, nurturing relationships, addressing mistrust and distrust, and demonstrating trustworthiness.
	• Beneficiaries of privilege and those targeted by oppression need to first critically analyze and commit to a process of self-awareness and self-actualization.
Structural power analysis	• Understand sources of formal and informal power.
	• Conduct an analysis of the organization, institution, or setting to examine how racism is operating, whose voices are privileged, and whose voices are silenced or unheard.
	• Examine three faces of power by asking three questions: a. Who frames the issue(s), and how are the issues framed? b. Who controls and sets the agenda (i.e., what is considered a relevant or priority issue to be included and discussed)? c. Who controls the actual decisions made and who benefits from the decisions?
Systems change theory	• Consider the organization or institution's external context, organizational culture and climate, and values, attitudes, beliefs, and behaviors of individuals.
	• Critically examine five elements of a system: (1) core values and assumptions, (2) social and organizational context and consequences, (3) the relationship among monitoring and evaluation methods, (4) the relationship among explanations of the problem, and (5) actions to achieve health and social equity.
Sociopolitical education	A. Decolonize one's mind by (re)engaging with traditional knowledge, problematizing and unlearning myths/misinformation, and (re)learning accurate information.
	B. Devise new ways of thinking that address the limitations or errors in the way a problem has been conceptualized, examined, or addressed.
	C. Create new ways of thinking for the purpose of action. Recognize that insights from action will help to refine how we think about the problem and potential solutions in ways that increase hope, confidence, and motivation to act.
Monitoring progress	• Use process, impact, and outcome evaluation data to monitor policies and practices, measure racism, and guide where and how to intervene.
	• Use health impact assessment tools (e.g., indigenous impact assessment tool, *Health Equity Assessment Tool*) to evaluate the impact of existing or planned policy and investment decisions.

Source: Adapted from Came and Griffith (2018), with permission of the publisher.

TABLE 4.2

Actions to Eliminate Racial Inequity

1. View racial inequity as a problem of policy, not people.

2. Identify racial inequity in all its intersections and manifestations.

3. Investigate and uncover the racist policies causing racial inequity.

4. Develop or identify anti-racist policy options that may help to achieve racial equity.

5. Identify what individuals or groups have the power to institute.

6. Teach others about policies that cause or perpetuate racial inequity and strategies to mitigate or eliminate these policies.

7. Work with like-minded policymakers to institute policies to achieve and sustain racial equity.

8. Identify sources of power that can help to mobilize power to achieve and sustain racial equity, and sources of power that remove or reduce the power of policymakers and stakeholders that do not share these goals.

9. Closely monitor politics, practices, and policies to evaluate the extent to which policies are expanding or reducing racial inequities.

10. Closely monitor politics, practices, and policies to evaluate the extent to which new policies are likely to expand or reduce racial inequities.

Source: This selected list is adapted from Kendi's (2019) steps we can take to eliminate racial inequity in our spaces.

Conclusion

Echoing public health activist and scholar Bill Jenkins (Jenkins et al., 2019), this chapter has emphasized that "The problem in America is not that people look different from each other. The problem is that people are treated differently because of how they look."

Anti-racism is an educational and organizing framework that seeks to confront, ameliorate, and eradicate racism and unearned White privilege (Came & Griffith, 2018). Anti-racist community organizing builds on the core components and principles of community organizing and infuses anti-racism as core values and ethical beliefs. As such, anti-racist organizing is based on two premises: (1) racism is the defining form of oppression in the United States (and elsewhere), and (2) racism is among the most critical and largest obstacles to social equity and community organizing for social change (Shapiro, 2002). Anti-racism praxis seeks to enable equity, social justice, and peace and move toward a world where racism is nonexistent or its health effects are negligible. While sometimes labeled differently, these efforts build on long-standing traditions of Indigenous public health practices that center Indigenous wisdom and ways of knowing and the experiences, traditions, and strengths of racialized groups in the United States and across the globe (Baumhofer & Yamane, 2019; Came et al., 2020; Marable, 1995; Million & Pete, 2019).

Organizing and activism are often rooted in moral and ethical values, and efforts to create a better world, not for oneself, but for others who may or may not have yet been born. Organizations and collective efforts are important in providing a vehicle for collective action, and for honing one's sociopolitical awareness and insight. A key ingredient of organizing and other community mobilization strategies is the relationships that create the foundation for solidarity and collective action. These relationships can be the foundation and fuel to inspire and sustain people like Washington Booker III to fight racism alongside other "foot soldiers" throughout their lives. We should all be so lucky to find such a noble cause and legacy.

Questions for Further Discussion

1. As defined by Ibram X. Kendi and discussed in this chapter, an *anti-racist* is someone who supports an anti-racist policy through their actions or by expressing anti-racist ideas. These ideas include that racial groups are equals and do not need "developing," and supporting policies that reduce racial inequity. Reflecting on this definition and on the chapter more broadly, describe how you personally might have defined an "anti-racist" before becoming familiar with these perspectives. What surprised you most in the above definition and/or other ideas expressed in the chapter? Why? If a fellow student or colleague not in this class asked your advice on concrete ways of being an anti-racist, what two to three suggestions would you offer?

2. The authors suggest that community organizing is a valuable avenue for moving from naming problems (e.g., a racist policy) to helping mobilize and take action for policy change. Identify a policy, in any area, that you believe must be changed to live up to anti-racist praxis. Why did you choose that policy, and how does it promote or reinforce racism and/or race-based inequities? Building, in part, on the messages of this and other readings, what steps or strategies would you recommend to professionals wishing to engage with communities in organizing to change the policy you identified? List and discuss at least three such steps or approaches and why you selected them.

REFERENCES

Allsup, R. E. (2003). Praxis and the possible: Thoughts on the writings of Maxine Greene and Paulo Freire. *Philos of Music Educ Rev, 11*(2), 157–169.

Bailey, Z. D., Krieger, N., Agénor, M., Graves, J., Linos, N., & Bassett, M. T. (2017). Structural racism and health inequities in the USA: Evidence and interventions. *Lancet, 389*(10077), 1453–1463. doi:https://doi.org/10.1016/S0140-6736(17)30569-X.

Baumhofer, N. K., & Yamane, C. (2019). Multilevel racism and Native Hawaiian health. In C. L. Ford, D. M. Griffith, M. A. Bruce, & K. L. Gilbert (Eds.), *Racism: Science & Tools for the Public Health Professional* (pp. 375–391). APHA Press.

Came, H., & Griffith, D. (2018). Tackling racism as a "wicked" public health problem: Enabling allies in anti-racism praxis. *Soc Sci Med, 199*, 181–188. doi:http://dx.doi.org/10.1016/j.socscimed.2017.03.028.

Came, H., Warbrick, I., McCreanor, T., & Baker, M. (2020). From gorse to ngahere: An emerging allegory for decolonising the New Zealand health system. *N Z Med J, 133*(1524), 102–110.

The Children's Crusade. (2021). National Museum of African American History & Culture. https://nmaahc.si.edu/blog/childrens-crusade.

Clarke, A. R., Goddu, A. P., Nocon, R. S., Stock, N. W., Chyr, L. C., Akuoko, J. A., & Chin, M. H. (2013). Thirty years of disparities intervention research: What are we doing to close racial and ethnic gaps in health care? *Med Care, 51*(11), 1020–1026.

Cogburn, C. D. (2019). Culture, race, and health: Implications for racial inequities and population health. *Milbank Q, 97*(3), 736–761.

Eliasson, O. (2016, January 18). Why art has the power to change the world. World Economic Forum. https://www.weforum.org/agenda/2016/01/why-art-has-the-power-to-change-the-world/.

Ford, C. L., Griffith, D. M., Bruce, M. A., & Gilbert, K. L. (2019). Introduction. In C. L. Ford, D. M. Griffith, M. A. Bruce, & K. L. Gilbert (Eds.), *Racism: Science & Tools for the Public Health Professional* (pp. 1–8). APHA Press.

Friedersdorf, C. (2020, August 20). Anti-racist arguments are tearing people apart. *The Atlantic.* https://www.theatlantic.com/ideas/archive/2020/08/meta-arguments-about-anti-racism/615424/.

Griffith, D. M., Johnson, J., Ellis, K. R., & Schulz, A. J. (2010). Cultural context and a critical approach to eliminating health disparities. *Ethn Dis, 20*(1), 71–76.

Griffith, D. M., & Semlow, A. R. (2020). Art, anti-racism and health equity: "Don't ask me why, ask me how!" *Ethn Dis, 30*(3), 373–380. doi:10.18865/ed.30.3.373.

Jenkins, W. C., Schoenbach, V. J., Rowley, D. L., & Ford, C. L. (2019). Overcoming the impact of racism on the health of communities: What we have learned and what we have not. In C. L. Ford, D. M. Griffith, M. A. Bruce, & K. L. Gilbert (Eds.), *Racism: Science & Tools for the Public Health Professional* (pp. 15–45). APHA Press.

Jones, C. P. (2019). Action and allegories. In C. L. Ford, D. M. Griffith, M. A. Bruce, & K. L. Gilbert (Eds.), *Racism: Science & Tools for the Public Health Professional* (pp. 223–241). APHA Press.

Jones, J. M. (1997). *Prejudice and Racism* (2nd ed.). McGraw-Hill.

Kendi, I. X. (2019). *How to Be an Antiracist.* One World.

Kieffer, C. H. (1984). Citizen empowerment: A developmental perspective. *Prevention in Hum Services, 3*(2–3), 9–36.

LeBrón, A. M. W., & Viruell-Fuentes, E. A. (2019). Racism and the health of Latina/Latino communities. In C. L. Ford, D. M. Griffith, M. A. Bruce, & K. L. Gilbert (Eds.), *Racism: Science & Tools for the Public Health Professional* (pp. 414–428). APHA Press.

Marable, M. (1995). *Beyond Black and White: Transforming African-American Politics.* London: Verso.

Million, D., & Pete, D. (2019). "We are peoples": Reclaiming Native health. In C. L. Ford, D. M. Griffith, M. A. Bruce, & K. L. Gilbert (Eds.), *Racism: Science & Tools for the Public Health Professional* (pp. 363–374). APHA Press.

Pederson, A., Walker, I., & Wise, M. (2005). "Talk does not cook rice": Beyond anti-racism rhetoric to strategies for social action. *Aust Psychol, 40*(1), 20–30. doi:10.1080/00050060512 33131729.

Poteat, T., Millett, G. A., Nelson, L. E., & Beyrer, C. (2020). Understanding COVID-19 risks and vulnerabilities among Black communities in America: The lethal force of syndemics. *Ann of Epidemiol, 47*, 1–3. doi:https://doi.org/10.1016/j.annepidem.2020.05.004.

Rankine, J. (2014). *Creating Effective Anti-racism Campaigns: Report for Race Relations Commissioner.* Words and Pictures.

Samari, G., Alcalá, H. E., & Sharif, M. Z. (2019). Racialization of religious minorities. In C. L. Ford, D. M. Griffith, M. A. Bruce, & K. L. Gilbert (Eds.), *Racism: Science & Tools for the Public Health Professional* (pp. 445–463). APHA Press.

Shapiro, I. (2002). *Training for Racial Equity and Inclusion: A Guide to Selected Programs.* Aspen Institute, Roundtable on Comprehensive Community Initiatives for Children and Families.

Stein, K. (2016, January 20). Washington Booker: Vigil planned to honor civil rights foot soldier, veteran, political activist. *Birmingham Real-Time News.* https://www.al.com/news/birmingham/2016/01/vigil_planned_to_honor_civil_r.html.

Watts, R. J., Griffith, D. M., & Abdul-Adil, J. (1999). Sociopolitical development as an antidote for oppression. *Am J Community Psychol, 27*(2), 255–271.

Williams, D. R. (2012). Miles to go before we sleep: Racial inequities in health. *J Health Soc Behav, 53*(3), 279–295. doi:10.1177/0022146512455804.

Williams, D. R., & Griffith, D. M. (2019). "We just haven't put our minds to it": An interview with David Williams describing the trajectory of his career studying racism. In C. L. Ford, D. M. Griffith, M. A. Bruce, & K. L. Gilbert (Eds.), *Racism: Science & Tools for the Public Health Professional* (pp. 73–95). APHA Press.

5

Contrasting Organizing Approaches

The "Alinsky Tradition" and Freirian Organizing Approaches

MARTY MARTINSON

CELINA SU

MEREDITH MINKLER

Community organizing efforts across the country and the globe reflect a range of models with different philosophies and strategies for systematically bringing people together to bring about social change. This chapter explores two such models of community organizing—the Alinsky tradition and Freirian approaches. Here, we examine the key components of each model, contrast the basic assumptions and strategies embedded in each, and identify the ways in which these models might complement or inform each other. Community organizing in practice, of course, rarely reflects an ideal model in its pure form, as each effort requires strategies and tactics that are specific to the given situation (Rothman, 2008; Sen, 2003). Nevertheless, the influence of the ideas and practices of Saul Alinsky and Paulo Freire over the past several decades have been significant and thereby warrant more detailed examination.

Saul Alinsky (1909–1972)

Born into a middle-class Jewish immigrant household in Chicago, Alinsky worked as an early labor organizer with the Congress of Industrial Organizations. He emerged in the 1930s as a formidable community organizer when he worked with the Back of the Yards neighborhood in Chicago. There, he built an "organization of organizations" that brought together churches, labor, and service organizations to successfully fight for expanded social services, education, and other community needs in the meatpacking and stockyards section of Chicago. As community organizer Miller (2009) notes, Alinsky "borrowed from the tough approach of the industrial union movement, grafted its strategy and tactics onto the poor, working-class communities that surrounded the great industrial stockyards of the Midwest, and found in the local traditions and values that supported organizing." Alinsky's efforts succeeded in achieving his goal of using "people power" to counter the "money power" of the Chicago political machine and to gain seats at the decision-making tables (Schutz & Miller, 2015).

Alinsky went on to cofound the Industrial Areas Foundation in 1940 to expand his pragmatic and conflict-oriented style of organizing to other parts of the country. In his words, "The first step in community organizing is community disorganization," achieved by identifying the controversial issues on which people feel most compelled to act (Alinsky, 1971, p. 116). While Alinsky himself said that there is no such thing as a step-by-step prescription for organizing because each effort is situation specific, the ideas, tactics, and strategies he described in his books *Reveille for Radicals* (1946) and *Rules for Radicals* (1971) suggest the general principles that make up an Alinsky style of community organizing.

The Alinsky Tradition of Community Organizing

According to Alinsky, the organizer's role is that of an outsider who agitates, listens to the concerns of the people, and then mobilizes them to act on those concerns. He believed that no action should be taken until the "mass power base" has been built, for without that base, the organizer "has nothing with which to confront anything" (Alinsky, 1971, p. 113). Alinsky's organizing efforts focus on recruitment of large numbers of people. Once these numbers are obtained, the organizer helps the people identify specific, concrete actions in which to use that "people power" and concurrently assesses the power base of the opposition (Alinsky, 1971).

As Alinsky (1971) noted, to build people power, the organizer needs to first "get a license to operate" (p. 98) within a community by establishing legitimacy. The organizer describes their prior organizing successes as "credentials of competency" (p. 101) to gain trust and agitates within the community so that people will voice their concerns. The organizer must agitate to "rub raw the resentments of the people" and "fan the latent hostilities" so the community members will see and hear their own frustrations (p. 116). The organizer then helps the people to move from this generalized discontent to a focus on specific issues around which they can organize campaigns and create change. The organizer must persuade the people that they are not powerless, and that they *can* do something about those issues *if* they mobilize to create a mass-based organization. The organizer makes it clear that the organization will give them the power, the ability, the strength, and the force to be able to do something about these specific problems. "The organization is born out of the issues and the issues are born out of the organization" (p. 120).

Issue selection is key to organizing, and according to Alinsky (1971), a "good issue" is one that is simple, specific, and winnable (Schutz & Miller, 2015; Staples, 2016; chapter 12). Notably, this stands in contrast to other organizing strategies that integrate or focus on broader social justice issues, such as anti-racism or antiviolence campaigns (Came & Griffith, 2018; Sen, 2020; Su, 2009). Alinsky steered away from such campaigns as ideological and divisive, and instead chose specific battles that could be won quickly through targeted actions to give the community a sense of confidence and achievement.

Alinsky also asserted the importance of choosing a campaign *target*—a specific individual or organization that has the power to make decisions and therefore make change (Schutz & Miller, 2015; Sen, 2003). In Alinsky's (1971) words, "Pick the target, freeze it, personalize it, and polarize it" (p. 130). For example, when organizing with the low-income Black community in Rochester, New York, he identified Eastman Kodak, the antilabor industrial giant of Rochester, as being largely responsible for the economic plight of the community. After picking this target, he "froze" it with provocative comments to the media and personalized and polarized it by deliberately confusing the identity of one of Eastman Kodak's directors with a known segregationist and racist. That director, W. Allen Wallis, had a tense relationship with Black students in his position as president of the local university. Alabama governor George Wallace was nationally known for racist policies and he famously stood in the doorway of the University of Alabama to stop two Black students from entering. When the media asked Alinsky about Wallis, Alinsky responded, "Wallis? Which one are you talking about—Wallace of Alabama, or Wallis of Rochester—but I guess there isn't any difference" (p. 137). Alinsky's quip was widely quoted and served as a means for personalizing and polarizing Eastman Kodak as the enemy of the people, and Black communities in particular.

Alinsky was well known for his controversial "ethics of means and ends," which he detailed in *Rules for Radicals* (1971). His list of ten rules pertaining to these ethics is summed up well in his tenth rule, "You do what you can with what you have and clothe it with moral garments" (p. 26). In general, Alinsky believed that the ends justify the means, and they depend on whose side you are on, how passionate you feel about the issue, or how close you are to defeat.

Overall, as noted by Minkler (2005), organizing in the Alinsky tradition "emphasize(s) redressing power imbalances by creating dissatisfaction with the status quo among the disenfranchised, building community-wide identification, and helping members devise winnable goals and nonviolent conflict strategies to bring about change" (p. 28). In the end, this kind of social action organizing serves to shift power from being concentrated among elite power brokers to being shared with previously marginalized communities. Through their organizing into a mass power base, these communities gain access to the decisionmaking table. Alinsky organizing thus moves individuals from a place of invisibility and voicelessness to that of visibility and influence. Community organizer Rinku Sen (2013) asserted that while Alinsky described himself as a radical, "he was not in the business of overthrowing existing structures but, rather, of making them more responsive" (p. 251).

Alinsky-Tradition Organizing and Its Evolution

A number of powerful Alinsky-based organizations remain strong, including the expansive and long-standing Industrial Areas Foundation (IAF), which he cofounded. IAF's strategy of building "organizations of organizations" grew into a vast network of local and faith-based organizations that in 2020 operated in sixty-five cities in the United States, Canada, Germany, the United Kingdom, and Australia. While Alinsky's successor at IAF, Ed Chambers, modified the approach to create more sustainable structures with formal leadership training and diversified leadership, IAF remains grounded in the Alinsky tradition (Kleidman, 2004; Schutz & Miller, 2015) as reflected in its mission to build "organizations and relationships that equip families and communities to participate with power in the public decisions that impact their lives" (www.industrialareasfoundation.org).

An example of IAF's attention to Alinsky's foundations of self-interest, shared values, and specific winnable goals is its organizing around census participation in Texas. Deeply concerned about immigrant communities' already deep disenfranchisement, IAF joined forces with local religious leaders and organizations to educate undocumented and mixed-status Latinx families in Texas about the importance of being counted in the 2020 census, the role it plays in their political power, and the need to ignore fear-inducing misinformation about risks to their safety (https://www.industrialareasfoundation.org/updates).

Other notable examples of Alinsky-tradition organizing include the Association of Community Organizations for Reform Now (ACORN), a formidable antipoverty organizing group that disbanded in 2010 after forty years, but whose members went on to form new organizations. The Direct Action Training and Research Center (DART) trains leaders and organizers "to build power and take direct action on problems facing their communities" (thedartcenter.org). Gamaliel is another Alinsky-style network of powerful faith-based and community organizations. Based in Chicago with regional and nationwide affiliates in seventeen states, Gamaliel trains local leaders to build strong organizational bases through member recruitment, with the broad aim being "to empower ordinary people to effectively participate in the political, environmental, social and economic decisions affecting their lives" (http://www.gamaliel.org).

Faith in Action (formerly known as the Oakland Training Institute in California), the Pacific Institute for Community Organization (PICO), and the PICO National Network are examples of organizing networks that adheres to many of Alinsky's key precepts while also evolving to address head on some issues that Alinsky avoided, such as systemic racism. As discussed earlier, while he frequently worked with Black congregations and communities, Alinsky cautioned against dealing directly with race and systemic racism, which he described as "ideological" and divisive. Faith in Action, however, concerns itself explicitly with "how anti-blackness, White Supremacy, and patriarchy have shaped our society," as their organizing "bring[s] people together across race, class, religion, urban/suburban/rural, and region to make progress on racial and economic justice" (https://faithinaction.org/). ISAIAH Minnesota, which is one of Faith in Action's affiliates, demonstrates well this commitment to justice-focused organizing.

ISAIAH Minnesota: Shifting Alinsky Organizing toward Racial and Economic Justice

ISAIAH Minnesota, which is a coalition of over 200 congregations, 38 mosques, a dozen Black barbershops, and other partners, has mobilized to address community concerns, including toxic waste, transportation, health care and childcare, and, especially in recent years, racial and economic justice. In the Alinsky tradition that strives to bring together diverse groups to "struggle together to realize their common interests" and "[build] relationships that cut across historic lines of antagonism" (Miller, 2009, p. 12), ISAIAH Minnesota provides "a vehicle for congregations, clergy, and people of faith" across diverse religious communities "to act collectively and powerfully towards racial and economic equity" (https://isaiahmn.org/).

ISAIAH Minnesota has had numerous successes, including leveraging $68 million in state funds to clean up 3,000 acres of toxic "brownfields" in Minneapolis and St. Paul, and obtaining land and funding for affordable senior housing. It played a key role in helping to restore three light rail stops in predominantly low-income communities of color, which were also home to many people with disabilities (Blackwell et al., 2012), and worked with coalition partners to restore $1.5 million in funding for shelters and services for women and children experiencing domestic violence.

In the wake of the 2016 election of Donald J. Trump as president, many ISAIAH Minnesota members were deeply concerned that rural Minnesotans had voted overwhelmingly for a person whose values they saw as directly contradicting those of people of faith. Over the next twelve months, ISAIAH responded by holding hundreds of house meetings across the state "to simply listen, to press beyond the tribal discourse of winning and losing to matters of the heart" (Kotz, 2019). In the words of organizer Alexa Horwart, among the key questions asked were, "What keeps you up at night?" and "Where are you and your family struggling?"

In many rural areas, economic hardships were blamed on the arrival of growing numbers of Latinx and East African immigrants—immigrants that President Trump viciously described as criminals, moochers, and the source of (read White) hard-working Americans' struggles. Race-based distrust had grown, but ISAIAH Minnesota's house meetings provided a chance to look more deeply, which helped residents see that "the Somali next door had no say in the tripling price of insulin, the poverty wages of poultry plants, or the economics driving the little guy from the farm" (Kotz, 2019). Their conversations revealed that the real causes of their struggles lay in the corridors of corporate and political power, not in each other (chapter 4). ISAIAH Minnesota organizers brought people together to "speak their fears," which led to open discussions of race, religion, shared concerns, and how to mobilize for change. Out of this came campaigns to address those shared concerns, such as the very low (13 percent) rate of paid sick leave in their state. Many in the campaign had never been activists before, but they now saw that they could make change.

The specific concerns of immigrants were also addressed. Residents of Northfield supported the first municipal ID law in the state, allowing undocumented residents to open bank accounts. In Rochester, an immigrant defense fund was established, and in St. Cloud, ISAIAH members worked with the city to hammer out an agreement "on what policing should look like" (Kotz, 2019).

Faith in Minnesota, the organization's separate political arm, built and diversified ISAIAH's power base even further. They made hundreds of thousands of phone calls, did extensive door knocking, and organized a phone bank that called 14,000 Muslim voters—efforts that engaged many more residents in political participation, sometimes for the first time (Kotz, 2019).

Against this backdrop, when the brutal police killing of George Floyd took place in their own state capitol, ISAIAH quickly joined the Black Lives Matter protests that followed and continued their work to promote racial justice in policing (https://isaiahmn.org/). ISAIAH joined close to a hundred other organizations to support a set of police accountability reforms put forward by Minnesota's People of Color and Indigenous (POCI) Caucus. They kept the pressure on the House, which eventually passed a bill that included several important reforms, such as a ban on chokeholds and a mandatory duty to intervene and report officer use of force). ISAIAH also called out the omission of important additional measures and the Senate majority leader's stoking of fear, division, and misinformation through the false claim that the House bill would literally "defund the police." Ultimately, ISAIAH committed to continuing to work for police reform through 2021 and beyond, "until all Minnesotans, especially Black, Brown, Asian, and Indigenous Minnesotans, are safe from police brutality" (Bates, 2020).

Critiques of the Alinsky Approach

The foregoing case study of ISAIAH Minnesota illustrates how some notable organizers have revised the Alinsky model over time to better align with social justice movements. While organizations like ISAIAH maintain key Alinsky tenets, such as building "an organization of organizations" with a strong power base, they have also moved beyond Alinsky's model by working toward broader systems change, challenging systemic racism and anti-immigrant practices. Such shifts in the Alinsky model, often led by organizers of color, came through critique of the Alinsky model for its unwillingness to attend to analysis of racial and gender hierarchies, the predominance of White staff and leadership in Alinsky organizations, and inflexibility in the rules and tactics of Alinsky organizing that did not always fit well with the values and experiences of communities of color (Delgado, 1986; Fisher et al., 2018; Sen, 2003, 2013).

The original Alinsky model has also been criticized for failing to build local capacity and leadership, and for focusing on local targets in an increasingly interconnected and multinational world (Chávez et al., 2010; Fisher et al., 2018; Phulwani, 2016; Schutz & Miller, 2015). Finally, Sen (2020) and Stall and Stoecker (2005) underscore the feminist critique of the Alinsky tradition, with key concerns including the emphasis on "public sphere" interventions, the lack of work/life balance for organizers, the use of narrow self-interest as a primary motivation, and the reliance on conflict and confrontational tactics.

While organizations such as IAF, Gamaliel, and Faith in Action have notably modified the Alinsky model to better address the limitations of the original approach, many community organizations instead use alternative approaches to frame their organizing efforts in ways that better match their philosophical and cultural values. The "woman-centered organizing" model described by Stall and Stoecker (2005), feminist approaches to organizing explored by Hyde (2018) and others, as well as the classic approach of Gutierrez and Lewis (1999; chapter 13) to organizing with women of color, are illustrative. We turn now to an approach that has become increasingly recognized across geographic, gender, and cultural lines as an approach that significantly differs from Alinsky's community organizing, namely Paulo Freire's (1970) model of liberation or popular education for critical consciousness and structural transformation and its use in community organizing and community building.

Paulo Freire (1921–1997)

Paulo Freire grew up in northwest Brazil in a middle-class family that then endured hunger and poverty during the Great Depression. Although Freire was trained as a lawyer, his passion was adult education. After working as a teacher, he began to study and critique the Brazilian education system for its perpetuation of the oppression, exploitation, and powerlessness of poor people. Freire promoted an alternative model of education that supports human liberation and makes people the subjects of their own learning (Chávez et al., 2010; Freire, 1970). He argued that to build a stronger democracy, education must be rooted in the lived experiences of the people and in the development of critical consciousness.

Freire first employed his liberation education ideas in the early 1960s, in a successful pilot literacy program with 300 sugarcane sharecroppers. He then developed broader literacy campaigns for the poor in Brazil through which people learned to read, while they also learned to "'read' the political and social situation in which they lived" in order to transform it (Carroll & Minkler, 2000, p. 23).

When a coup d'état in 1964 led to Freire's imprisonment and forced exile in Chile, he used this time to further develop his ideas about education and human liberation from oppression, wrote his landmark book, *Pedagogy of the Oppressed* (1970), and saw his "liberation education" approach increasingly being used in other parts of Central and South America and beyond. Freire returned to Brazil in 1980. After the country's military dictatorship ended in 1985, Freire became head of São Paulo's vast public education system, while continuing to write, teach, and inspire students in many parts of the world (Freire, 2000).

Popular Education as Liberation Education

At the heart of Freire's approach is popular, or liberation, education, which starts with people's own experiences and provides them the tools to analyze their situation and take action to transform both themselves and their conditions.

Although we focus here on Freire's use of popular education, the approach itself preceded him. The Highlander Folk School (now the Highlander Research and Education Center), founded by Myles Horton and others in Appalachian Tennessee in the 1932, has used popular education and literacy since its inception as a means of promoting civic participation and social action organizing (Horton, 1998; Horton & Freire, 1990; chapter 15).

A Freirian approach to liberation education involves a facilitated social action process in which groups come together in "culture circles" to listen to each other, engage in dialogue about the struggles in their lives and the social and historical roots of those struggles, envision and employ collective actions to create change, and reflect upon those actions as they develop further actions for change (Carroll & Minkler, 2000; Wallerstein et al., 2005). Teachers act as facilitators in helping students (or "learner-teachers") think through issues and put forward their own analyses. This methodology of listening–dialogue–action–reflection represents a participatory model of learning that promotes the development of *conscientization*, or critical consciousness, that leads to action. As such, the process is transformative for both the individual and the community (Chávez et al., 2010; Freire, 1970; Wallerstein et al., 2005).

Freire believed that social change can happen only through the development of critical consciousness, because people must understand the root causes of their daily life conditions before they can work toward addressing and transforming those root causes.

Liberation Education as a Community Organizing Approach

As theories of action for structural transformation, popular or liberation education has long been adopted by people outside the field of education—including community organizers and public health activists—as essential strategies for mobilizing communities to work for health equity and social change. As Sen (2003) notes, community organizers thus have adopted Freirian premises that people learn best when learning is connected to their day-to-day lives, and when there is shared power. She further suggests that when organizers use popular education approaches, and particularly in leadership development, there is "greater engagement of participants in the material [skills of organizing], more opportunities to build community among members, and . . . to raise participants' confidence by stressing internal knowledge" (p. 105). Further, using liberation education methods can also advance two critical dimensions of the work in changing the reality of people's lives and moving toward social justice as they "democratize the learning process and produce new knowledge for all involved" (Sen, 2003, p. 106).

We turn now to an example of a Freirian approach to organizing with youth that illustrates these and other core concepts.

Using a Freirian Approach to Organizing: Sistas and Brothas United

Founded in 1999, Sistas and Brothas United (SBU) is a student activist organization that began as the youth arm of a large, Alinsky-style organization—the Northwest Bronx Clergy Community Coalition (https://www.northwestbronx.org/sbu). Yet, while both organizations engaged poor to low-income, predominantly Black and Latinx residents in this neighborhood, and began with a focus on education, SBU's organizing model has, since the beginning, been far more in line with a Frieiran approach to organizing (Su, 2009). We look at three areas in which its Freirian approach differed sharply from Alinsky organizing: organizational activities that focus on support services and community building, an emphasis on individual development, and a model of leadership development where the organizer acts as partner-mentor.

EMPHASIS OF ORGANIZATIONAL ACTIVITIES: RECRUITMENT AND CAMPAIGNS. In contrast to a more traditional Alinsky focus on campaigns and recruitment, SBU's Freirian approach is generally more holistic and less immediately pragmatic, with activities like soul food events, hip-hop workshops, "sister-bonding" and rap sessions, tutoring, and yoga. Dozens of teenagers from local public schools show up to discuss local education politics, orient new members, carry out research, chair meetings, and strategize campaigns. But as Su describes, the close attention to the emotional and social needs of members has also helped create conditions for their empowerment (Su, 2009).

Further, many of the socializing, consciousness-raising, and political educa-tion activities of SBU serve as foundational components of its community organ-izing strategies. In addition to providing informal opportunities for the development of relationships and trust between members, these activities allow participants to engage in dialogue about the issues that concern them and to identify the root causes of those issues. Shiller (2012) thus describes how after "one-on-ones" with an adult leader-guide and other relationship building exercises, an "isms" train-ing was offered to help youth look more deeply at the meaning of racism, sexism, and homophobia, and "through the process, explore their own identities and expe-riences with oppression" in a deeply personal way, followed by sharing their feel-ings with another group member (p. 79).

Freire's emphasis on the importance of engaging in critical reflection and dia-logue before deciding on a course of action is also routinely integrated into SBU's organizational activities. To encourage critical reflection, adult leader-guides in this example encouraged youth to think about their neighborhood by taking walk-ing tours, during which they focused on things they previously may not have noticed: the quality and forms of housing and schools, the location and types of stores, transportation, noise, and the general feel of the blocks they walked (Shiller, 2012; appendix 3). Shiller thus noted youths' subsequent discussion of the juxtaposition of run-down and well-resourced schools, the overcrowding, but also large, unused spaces that could be transformed into schools.

In classic Freirian tradition, the youths' observations in this case example led to deeper questions and reflections on why things were the way they were, and how they might be changed (Shiller, 2012). The leader-guides also asked questions enabling the youth to reflect on and dialogue more concretely about things they could do to help change the situation. The youth discussed, for example, whether they could get an old and dilapidated armory converted into a new school, and they began studying and working to make this goal a reality. As SBU members began attending community meetings, developing "talking points," and working with other groups who shared their interest in this idea, they became increasingly confident in their ability to help effect change, and in the process build their collective and political efficacy (Bandura, 2004, 2018). Although they were not able to convert the armory into a school, they were able to form a coalition with other community groups to defeat a private developer's plan to turn the armory into a market, convincing local elected officials that the armory should be used in a way that would contribute to social good. They went on to win a community benefits agreement for subsequent proposals (Dolnick, 2009; Fullerton & Arterian Chang, 2015).

EMPHASIS ON INDIVIDUAL DEVELOPMENT. Dovetailing with the wide range of activities that took place as part of SBU, and consistent with a Freirian approach, an emphasis on individual development alongside organizational campaigns was evident. Organizers often blurred the line between "traditional" community organizing and social services (Sen, 2020). The organization thus paid careful attention to individual development through peer tutoring, spoken word workshops, college application workshops and mentoring, and informal socializing. One organizer described this essential component of developing emerging leaders when he noted, "I spend quality time hanging out with leaders. . . . We talk about how they're doing in schools. We get into family business. . . . Building them as individuals is as important as campaign work. . . . We need to build the skills and inner confidence so that they can maintain a certain level of conversation amongst themselves" (Su 2009, p. 87).

Through these opportunities for individual development, SBU leaders and members experienced personal transformation that often led them to a greater commitment to each other, to the work of the organization, and in some cases, to major leadership roles. Yorman Nuñez, for instance, went from being an active participant in SBU to the program manager for the Bronx Cooperative Development Initiative, working with small businesses and residents to build economic power, and the director of Just Urban Economies at the MIT Co-Lab (Fullerton & Arterian Chang, 2015).

NATURE OF LEADERSHIP DEVELOPMENT: ORGANIZER AS PARTNER. In keeping with Freire's notions of a liberatory, rather than a banking, mode of pedagogy (Freire, 1970), organizers at SBU also worked hard to engage member-leaders as partners. Leaders repeatedly stated that friendship and solidarity, not just overlapping self-interests per se, underlaid their decision to join the organization.

Further, and rather than building interchangeable leaders, organizers encouraged individual members to pursue tailored interests and build expertise in the policy issues, research methods, or organizing activities they found most compelling. Thus SBU meetings were more likely than those at traditional Alinsky organizations to include leaders taking turns reporting back findings from research, or presenting ideas for an ongoing campaign. They were also more likely to insist on active consensus at meetings, whereby each attendee explicitly approved or questioned an agenda item before votes occurred. Ultimately, and consistent with Freire's (1970) approach, organizers aimed to engage in dialogue, as essential to "generating critical thinking" (p. 81).

Limitations of Freirian Organizing

Partly because the Freire-inspired model of organizing is participatory and focused on building both trust and relationships, it is also more labor intensive than traditional Alinsky approaches. With less emphasis on large numbers, and more on individual transformation and building deep, sustainable foundations of support based on relationships, Freirian groups struggle to achieve the large scale of those in the Alinsky tradition. Further, Freirian organizations emphasize the importance of looking at root causes, not just winnable issues, making it much more difficult to capture the "clincher" of a decisive campaign victory. As Schultz (2007) argued, Freirian approaches do not always help marginalized constituencies move beyond social critique and build concrete political power. Ideally, however, this sort of deep-seated commitment helps to build sustainable, meaningful participation and lifetime activists for social change overall, not just for the specific campaigns or organizations.

Implications for Policymaking

The Alinsky- and Freire-inspired organizational approaches illustrated in this chapter suggest different political strategies for policy reform. Overall, and despite some recent and important changes discussed following here, Alinsky-type groups aim to "pursue strategies that help constituents to win referenda of existing policy proposals or elections, engage in confrontational strategies, and build broad-based coalitions in the name of 'color-blind' equality" (Su, 2009, p. 3). In contrast, Freirian-style organizations like SBU primarily work to construct and implement new policy proposals, engage in mostly collaborative strategies (rather than confrontational ones), and address issues of race, ethnicity, and racism directly and adeptly (rather than taking a "color-blind" approach).

Sistas and Brothas United and other classically Freirian organizations emphasize means as much as ends, and they deliberately blur the two, such that critical dialogue is interwoven throughout the organizing and policymaking processes. In contrast, Alinsky organizations typically call for "policy after power" (Alinsky, 1971, p. 104), so that actions are not taken until the mass organization has been mobilized. In Alinsky's words, "Change comes from power and power comes from the organization" (p. 113). Overall, the impression, when looking at these different policymaking strategies in terms of the case studies, is that "the Alinsky-informed [organization] ultimately tries to help its constituents obtain a larger slice of the social, political, and economic pie while the Freirian organization tried to [create] a whole new kind of bigger, better pie altogether" (Su, 2009, p. 3).

Despite their differences, however, Alinsky and Freirian organizations not infrequently have worked together to achieve important policy wins. A joint campaign by SBU and its Alinsky-style parent organization, the Northwest Bronx Clergy and Community Coalition, for example, succeeded in reducing public school overcrowding, increasing community engagement, and modifying zero-tolerance policies in local schools to reduce the frequency of suspensions and expulsions of local youth of color. By holding politicians accountable for things such as deteriorating school conditions, youth members of SBU further send a powerful message about the dangers of "investing" in incarceration and police surveillance instead of education (Goddard et al., 2015). In 2004, SBU cofounded the citywide Urban Youth Collaborative (UYC) to argue that police violence in New York City schools was not about "a few bad apples," but about systemic violence baked into the system. In 2010, SBU and its partners successfully pressured the New York State Legislature and Mass Transit Authority to restore $25 million in financing to keep student Metrocards free, and as part of a years-long effort with other organizations, they helped get an act passed requiring the NYCPD to publicly report the number of arrests and suspensions in public schools. In 2015, they also helped get amendments passed to strengthening reporting and transparency within this act (Urban Youth Collaborative & Center for Popular Democracy, 2017).

Since then, most of SBU's work has been in coordination with other groups in UYC and national Dignity in Schools campaigns. Throughout, they have worked to grapple with complex conceptualizations of "public safety" in schools, acknowledging that some students might seek protection by authorities from bullies, and articulating an anti-racist vision of "restorative justice" (chapter 17) of what good schools and safe communities would look like for citywide and national campaigns (Brennan, 2020; Moise, 2020). SBU also continued to build on its early and continuing efforts to help youth gain a deeper understanding of the meaning of racism, sexism, and homophobia while exploring their own identities and experiences with oppression. The organization's recent campaigns now incorporate queer, global, and intersectional analyses beyond their earlier work. For instance, in their work as part of the alliance Communities United for Police Reform (CPR), SBU has collaborated with Desis Rising Up & Moving to examine how the global War on

Terror has impacted local policing of Muslim communities. Similarly, SBU's work with FIERCE, an advocacy group for LGBTQ youth, has highlighted the ways in which queer youth of color are mistreated by police in rapidly gentrifying, historically queer-friendly neighborhoods like Chelsea. In 2013, CPR helped to pass the Community Safety Act, which aims to end racial profiling and discriminatory policing in New York (Goodman, 2013). This evolution in SBU's work dovetails well with the growth of the Black Lives Matter and abolitionist movements (chapter 23).

Conclusion: Learning from Both Models

While the Alinsky and Freirian approaches to community organizing differ in their philosophies, strategies, and end goals, each offers a useful and relevant framework for creating social and structural change to improve the public's health and welfare and advance social justice. Alinsky-type groups, for example, play an important role in helping to mobilize popular support for specific legislative bills, such as for a living wage and affordable health care. In contrast, a Freirian model may be more useful in helping urban communities address complex, seemingly intractable, problems like geographical concentrations of respiratory illness, where no single problem source or "target" exists (Solomon et al., 2016).

Much can be learned from the respective strengths and limitations of each of these models in terms of how they might complement each other to create a stronger model overall. Freirian groups, for example, can learn to achieve greater scale and clinch campaign wins from Alinsky-type groups, while organizations in the Alinsky tradition can help prevent organizer and member-leader burnout, sustain policy formulation strategies, and tackle seemingly (but not inherently) divisive issues by learning from Freirian groups. As Sen (2003) notes, "The beauty of innovation in organizing emerges from the marriage of [the two approaches]: political education creates the reflection and growth opportunities that motivate action, and action provides the expression of newly clarified values" (p. 182). Finally, by using a combination of Alinsky and Freirian approaches, community organizing efforts can attain the "people power" necessary to gain influence in the policymaking process, while also facilitating transformative experiences focused on critical consciousness and praxis and helping people gain a greater sense of control over their lives.

Questions for Further Discussion

1. Name three or four key tenets of Alinsky-type organizing. Name three or four key tenets of Freirian organizing. What do they have in common? How do they differ?
2. Grassroots groups tackling public health issues, such as environmental injustice and local pollution, police brutality, or food deserts, face enormous challenges. The deleterious health effects they wish to address and avert often

take years, if not decades, to document and prove. The policies they wish to implement instead can take a long time as well, and involve a complex network of allies and policymakers. Are some issues or campaigns better suited for Alinsky-type organizing? For Freirian organizing? What are the strengths and weaknesses of Alinsky-type organizing in helping grassroots groups to sustain campaigns over long timelines, and to build coalitions in their work? What are the strengths and weaknesses of Freirian organizing on these challenges?

Acknowledgments

Portions of this chapter were adapted from Celina Su's, *Streetwise for Book Smarts: Grassroots Organizing and Education Reform in the Bronx.* Copyright 2009. Used by permission of the publisher, Cornell University Press. The authors offer our deepest gratitude to Doran Schrantz and the staff and volunteers at ISAIAH and Crystal Reyes and the other present and former leaders at SBU for their inspiring work and contributions to equity and social justice.

REFERENCES

Alinsky, S. D. (1946). *Reveille for Radicals.* University of Chicago Press.

Alinsky, S. D. (1971). *Rules for Radicals: A Pragmatic Primer for Realistic Radicals.* Random House.

Bandura, A. (2004). Swimming against the mainstream: The early years from chilly tributary to transformative mainstream. *Behav Res Ther, 42*, 613–630.

Bandura, A. (2018). Toward a psychology of human agency: Pathways and reflections. *Perspect Psychol Sci, 13*(2), 130–136.

Bates, J. (2020, July 21). ISAIAH Statement on MN Legislature Police Accountability Legislation. Citizen Justice Democracy. https://isaiahmn.org/2020/07/21/isaiah-statement-on-mn-legislature-police-accountability-legislation/.

Blackwell, A. G., Thompson, M., Freudenberg, N., Ayers, J., Schrantz, D., & Minkler, M. (2012). Using community organizing and community building to influence public policy. In M. Minkler (Ed.), *Community Organizing and Community Building for Health and Welfare* (3rd ed., pp. 371–385). Rutgers University Press.

Brennan, R. (2020, August 30). To protect and serve—far away from the classroom. The Riverdale Press. https://riverdalepress.com/stories/to-protect-and-serve-far-away-from-the-classroom,72379.

Came, H., & Griffith, D. (2018). Tackling racism as a "wicked" public health problem: Enabling allies in anti-racism praxis. *Soc Sci Med, 199*, 181–188.

Carroll, J., & Minkler, M. (2000). Freire's message for social workers: Looking back and looking ahead. *J Community Pract, 8*, 21–36.

Chávez, V., Minkler, M., Wallerstein, N., and Spencer, M. S. (2010). Community organizing for health and social justice. In L. Cohen, S. Chehimi, & V. Chávez (Eds.), *Prevention Is Primary* (2nd ed., pp. 87–112). Jossey-Bass.

Delgado, G. (1986). *Organizing the Movement: The Roots and Growth of Acorn.* Temple University Press.

Dolnick, S. (2009, December 14). Voting 45–1, council rejects $310 million plan for mall at Bronx Armory. *New York Times.* https://www.nytimes.com/2009/12/15/nyregion/15armory.html.

Fisher, R., DeFilippis, J., & Shragge, E. (2018). Contested community: A selected and critical history of community organizing. In R. A. Cnaan & C. Milofsky (Eds.), *Handbook of Community Movements and Local Organizations in the 21st Century* (pp. 281–297). Springer International.

Freire, P. (1970). *Pedagogy of the Oppressed.* Translated by M. B. Ramos. Seabury Press.

Freire, P. (2000). *Cultural Action for Freedom.* Harvard Educational Review.

Fullerton, J., and Arterian Chang, S. (2015). The Bronx Cooperative Development Initiative continues its regenerative journey. In *Capital Institute Field Guide to a Regenerative Economy.* http://fieldguide.capitalinstitute.org/bcdi.html.

Goddard, T., Myers, R. R., & Robison, K. (2015). Potential partnerships: Progressive criminology, grassroots organizations and social justice. *Int J Crime, Justice Soc Democr, 4*(4), 76–90.

Goodman, J. D. (2013, June 27). City council votes to increase oversight of New York police. *New York Times.* https://www.nytimes.com/2013/06/27/nyregion/new-york-city-council -votes-to-increase-oversight-of-police-dept.html.

Gutiérrez, L. M., & Lewis, E. A. (1999). *Empowering Women of Color.* Columbia University Press.

Horton, M. (1998). *The Long Haul: An Autobiography.* Doubleday.

Horton, M., & Freire, P. (1990). *We Make the Road by Walking: Conversations on Education and Social Change.* Temple University Press.

Hyde, C. A. (2018). Charisma, collectives and commitment: Hybrid authority in radical feminist social movement organizations. *Soc Mov Stud, 17*(4), 424–436.

Kleidman, R. (2004). Community organizing and regionalism. *City and Community, 3*(4), 430–421.

Kotz, P. (2019, March 6). The Kindness Revolt: A not-so-secret plot to make a better Minnesota. *CityPages.* http://www.citypages.com/news/the-kindness-revolt-a-not-so-secret-plot -to-make-a-better-minnesota/506724471.

Miller, M. (2009). *A Community Organizer's Tale: People and Power in San Francisco.* Heyday Books.

Minkler, M. (2005). Community organizing with the elderly poor in San Francisco's Tenderloin District. In M. Minkler (Ed)., *Community Organizing and Community Building for Health and Welfare* (3rd ed., pp. 272–287). Rutgers University Press.

Moise, L. (2020, September 8). Why we organize for police-free schools. City Limits. https:// citylimits.org/2020/09/08/opinion-why-we-organize-for-police-free-school/.

Phulwani, V. (2016). The poor man's Machiavelli: Saul Alinsky and the morality of power. *Am Polit Sci Rev, 110*(4), 863–875.

Rothman, J. (2008). Multi modes of community intervention. In J. Rothman, J. L. Erlich, & J. E. Tropman (Eds.), *Strategies of Community Intervention* (7th ed., pp. 141–170). Eddie Bowers.

Schutz, A. (2007). Education scholars have much to learn about social action: An essay review of learning power. *Educ Rev Online, 10*(3). http://edrev.asu.edu/essays/VI0n3index.html.

Schutz, A., & Miller, M. (2015). *People Power: The Community Organizing Tradition of Saul Alinsky.* Vanderbilt University Press.

Sen, R. (2003). *Stir It Up: Lessons in Community Organizing and Advocacy.* Jossey-Bass.

Sen, R. (2013). New theory for new constituencies: Contemporary organizing in communities of color. In M. Weil, M. Reisch, & M. L. Ohmer (Eds.), *The Handbook of Community Practice* (2nd ed., pp. 249–264). Sage.

Sen, R. (2020, July 1). Why today's social revolutions include kale, medical care, and help with the rent. Zócalo Public Square. https://www.zocalopublicsquare.org/2020/07/01/mutual -aid-societies-self-determination-pandemic-community-organizing/ideas/essay/.

Shiller, J. T. (2012). Preparing for democracy: How community-based organizations build civic engagement among urban youth. *Urban Educ, 48*(1), 69–91.

Solomon, G. M., Morello-Frosch, R., Zeise, L., & Faust, J. B. (2016). Cumulative environmental impacts: Science and policy to protect communities. *Annu Rev Public Health, 37*, 83–96.

Stall, S., & Stoecker, R. (2005). Toward a gender analysis of community organizing models: Liminality and the intersection of spheres. In M. Minkler (Ed.), *Community Organizing and Community Building for Health and Welfare* (3rd ed., pp. 196–217). Rutgers University Press.

Staples, L. (2016). *Roots to Power: A Manual for Grassroots Organizing* (2nd ed.). Praeger.

Su, C. (2009). *Streetwise for Book Smarts: Grassroots Organizing and Education Reform in the Bronx.* Cornell University Press.

Urban Youth Collaborative and the Center for Popular Democracy. (2017). *The $746 Million a Year School-to-Prison Pipeline: The Ineffective, Discriminatory, and Costly Process of Criminalizing New York City Students.* Urban Youth Collaborative and the Center for Popular Democracy.

Wallerstein, N., Sanchez, V., & Velarde, L. (2005). Freirian praxis in health education and community organizing: A case study of an adolescent prevention program. In M. Minkler (Ed.), *Community Organizing and Community Building for Health* (2nd ed., pp. 218–236). Rutgers University Press.

6

It's All Organizing, It's All Love

Building People's Power in Jackson, Mississippi

MAKANI THEMBA

Love is the basic quality that we need. If you do not love, if you do not love
the people, sooner or later you are going to betray them.

—Chokwe Lumumba, late mayor of Jackson, Mississippi,
in his inaugural speech, July 1, 2013

These words by Chokwe Lumumba challenge us to adjust our idea of organizing
work. Yet, the idea of love as a compass for organizing flies in the face of what is
often considered "traditional" transactional organizing—epitomized in the Alinsky approach (Alinsky, 1971; chapter 5). Transactional organizing focuses on people
as a set of interests and the process of organizing as coming together to pressure
decisionmakers to achieve "wins" that, hopefully, improve conditions. In this
framework, efforts like feeding people and providing medical care are considered
"direct services" and therefore outside of organizing. However, this principle of
loving "the people," of tending to community needs as a critical component of
organizing and building power, calls on organizers to let go of the false dichotomy
between community care and community organizing (Sen, 2020). This idea that
building authentic communities of care is part of building power is not new. It is
practiced on a global scale and is rooted in love for the people and the places in
which we live.

People's assemblies are part of a long democratic tradition in progressive
movements worldwide that draw on this more expansive approach to organizing
(Themba-Nixon, 2017). They are essentially a forum for mass engagement to address
the issues that affect a community's life. Assemblies can focus on issues or projects that are independent of government action, and they can act as advocates to
influence and make demands on government in their interests. This chapter looks
at the developing People's Assembly in Jackson, which endeavors to do both.

Organizing Rooted in Resistance as Love

To understand organizing in Jackson, one must understand what it means to have a sense of place, of home, of nation; to feel that unalterable sense of homeland that no matter what happens, this place belongs to you and you to it. Mississippi is one such place, where there are Black people with that kind of fierce love for their land. It is often said to those from the North, "We are the ones that didn't run. We stayed. We fought. We ain't giving up no ground without a fight."

The 2018 movie *Black Panther* sparked new conversations about safety, nationhood, and sanctuary. Wakanda, the fictional nation that is home to the Black Panther king and super hero character, captured the imagination of millions. Black people went to see the film six times and more, just so they could spend more time in the fictional Wakanda. Amid persistent racism, terror, and marginalization, here was a place where Black people ruled; where we had the resources that we needed, and where our brilliance and beauty were recognized. It was a nation of our own, if only in our minds.

Countries are political constructions forged by boundaries and governments, but what makes a nation is a matter of the heart. You can't have democracy without nationhood—that sense of real belonging. Authentic democracy at its core is an act of faith—and love. It is much deeper than voting, more potent than politics. It is the sense that it is up to you to participate because the place you call home is "yours" to govern.

Mississippi—and Jackson in particular—has a history of people's governance in a variety of forms. The area around Natchez was an Indigenous metropolis known for its democratic systems and vibrant trade prior to its violent invasion by European "settlers." In the early twentieth century, Mound Bayou was an international showcase of Black self-governance and cooperative economics. The storied Mississippi Freedom Democratic Party, famously cofounded by Fannie Lou Hamer, centered the practice of people's assembly-like organizing in the building of the party. In fact, they even held their own elections—a critically important strategy as Black residents faced such violent voter suppression—where residents practiced collective decisionmaking.

The first Jackson People's Assembly was launched and coordinated by Malcolm X Grassroots Movement (MXGM) (Themba-Nixon, 2017). It was organized in Ward 2, the home ward of Chokwe Lumumba, in 2006. Based in North Jackson, Ward 2 is a mix of homeowners, stable working class renters, as well as Tougaloo College. Although students played an important role in the development of the Assembly (they volunteered to do outreach and other forms of support), much of the organizing was done by senior leadership with Lumumba playing a primary role. Lumumba's charisma, wit, and sharp systemic analysis was an important factor in engaging residents, as was the trust and respect people felt for him and his decades of work in the community. Faith communities also played a critical role. For example, collaborators New Hope Baptist and Anderson South United Methodist were among the key spaces where assemblies were convened. Churches not only hosted assemblies, they also helped to promote them, with both church members and their leadership participating. These partnerships were important because they helped to extend the volunteer infrastructure of MXGM and helped more strongly root the process with local leadership.

Moving into Electoral Politics

Although originally conceived as an "outside" strategy to provide a space for resident engagement in building alternative, community-serving forms of governance, the People's Assembly quickly became a force to reckon with on city government issues as well. The Ward 2 Assembly was gaining momentum and residents from other wards expressed an interest in taking the People's Assembly citywide. In the meantime, Lumumba's active leadership in the Assembly as well as his extensive knowledge of municipal functions were increasingly in the spotlight. Residents made it known that they wanted a progressive leader like Lumumba on Jackson's city council and the base built through Assembly outreach turned to work on trying to elect one of their own (Lartey, 2017).

When Lumumba was successfully elected to represent Ward 2 in 2009, MXGM refocused efforts on building the People's Assembly as a platform for resident voice and reshaping municipal policy. With a strong ally on the city council, the Assembly kicked off its "Deepening Democracy" campaign to organize low- and moderate-income Black communities. The goal was to develop progressive policy initiatives "around community/economic development, food security and health issues"—priorities identified in assemblies. By 2010, the People's Assembly was the fastest-growing organizing force in Jackson, with more than 300 members citywide (Themba-Nixon, 2017).

Training and political education were important to this process, both in terms of building hope and belief in people's own ability to govern and make decisions together and in terms of residents' understanding of the issues and what can be done to address them. Political education took place during the large assemblies, in the task forces (smaller groups charged with developing strategies for implementing priorities surfaced in the assemblies), and even during outreach efforts. Perhaps the most ambitious effort of the People's Assemblies was the engagement of residents in a participatory budget process (Su, 2017) in which a number of residents would collectively identify budget priorities, in this case for the city of Jackson.

The process was modeled on best practices from the growing participatory budget movement (Su, 2017) in which resident leaders were working with MXGM organizers to develop the process. Lumumba participated in the political education process providing participants with information on city mechanisms and potential targets for change. Budget priorities were identified and delivered to the council. Lumumba played a leadership role in advancing the issues on the coun-cil, leveraging the fact that it was the only policy agenda developed directly by residents.

Over time, resident energies were increasingly split between independent, "self-determination" projects, such as its cooperative garden projects, its "reform" work to change municipal policy, and its "solidarity economy" work as part of a movement to build a just and sustainable economy in which people are front and center and in the driver's seat in creating history. Local policy work was drawing more of the Assembly's resources, and while residents were encouraged by the real and potential impact of policy work, they also knew that they were going to have to build more power if they were going to win their policies on council.

By 2011, Assembly leaders were starting to focus on the next mayoral election and organized to elect then councilmember Lumumba as mayor. By 2012, the Assembly network was in full swing working to build the citywide infrastructure necessary to support Lumumba in a mayoral run. Lumumba was elected in 2013 receiving 90 percent of the vote. The People's Assembly agenda had moved from an outside campaign to the official platform of the mayor.

As the People's Assembly and the Lumumba administration infrastructure became increasingly interlinked, the work of the Assembly focused on moving its policy agenda at city council. A critical challenge was funding. Jackson did not have the kind of tax base to provide the kind of resourcing that the People's Assembly agenda required. It was decided that Jackson should hold a referendum to raise the sales tax by 1 percent to generate additional revenues for infrastructure and other public improvements.

The People's Assembly played a pivotal role in the successful referendum in 2014, holding educational forums and mobilizing people to get involved in the cam-paign. It also helped organize residents to push the state legislature to grant Jack-son permission to hold the January 2014 referendum, and it continues to defend the tax increase and focus resources on the priorities that surfaced in the People's Assembly participatory budgeting process.

Chokwe Lumumba died suddenly after just eight months in office. In a rocky special election, his son, Chokwe Antar Lumumba, was a leading contender but the late mayor was "replaced" by Tony Yarber, a councilmember who did not share Lumumba's vision. However, Yarber's lackluster performance as mayor helped pave the way for Chokwe Antar Lumumba's massive victory in 2017, where he garnered 94 percent of the vote in the final election and breezed past a crowded field of eight candidates in the Democratic primary.

Lumumba's campaign slogan, "When I become mayor, you become mayor" (a riff off of Newark, New Jersey mayor Ras Baraka's "When I become mayor, we all become mayor") was inspiring to Jackson residents who felt locked out of govern-ment with little say. The campaign itself reflected a diverse representation of Jack-sonians, including gender-nonconforming individuals, elders, youth, and the city's small but growing immigrant community. At the emotionally charged victory party celebrating Lumumba's decisive win, people were weeping, laughing, and hugging one another saying, "We're mayor now!"

The inauguration in July 2017 emphasized this point as participants were asked to stand and swear to a "people's oath" of participation and co-governance. People's Assemblies were also reinstated as a central vehicle for achieving that vision. However, despite Jackson's rich organizing history, the city had limited civic infrastructure and resources. There were few advisory groups or resident oversight structures—places in the *decisionmaking* process that provide roles for residents. "We're all becoming mayor" meant more formal mechanisms for listening and engagement. Another reason for developing formal infrastructure for participation is that to achieve real change, Jackson needed to mobilize residents as volunteers, donors, and more. People's Assemblies and neighborhood associations play a critical role in mobilizing resident engagement in city initiatives.

Strengthening civic engagement also meant ensuring open access to information so that residents could provide informed input. People's Assembly organizers worked with the city to disseminate information about upcoming city council agenda items and answer questions on the budget and other key facets of city business. Assembly representatives attend council meetings and city leaders attended People's Assemblies on a regular basis. Yet, with all of these efforts in place, more work was required to increase the participation of those who are often marginalized from decisionmaking. People's Assembly organizers used a variety of popular education strategies, including a daylong LoveFest with music and games to increase resident engagement. They also always include a significant amount of the small group discussion and collective visioning that are critical to popular education (Friere, 1994). The city of Jackson's chief administrative officer, Dr. Robert Blaine, even developed a Monopoly-like board game to provide an accessible, practical, and fun way for residents to learn about budgets.

Contributions and Continued Challenges

The assemblies are significant in at least five ways:

1. *They provide clear, formal venues for listening to the local residents' issues.* This is particularly important given the significant number of organizers who were not Mississippi natives.
2. *They serve as a training ground and leadership pipeline.* Everything from outreach to meeting logistics provides opportunities to test new leadership, mentor new members, and build skills. The assemblies are also intergenerational, engaging a significant number of youth and elders and providing yet another opportunity for learning and skills exchange.
3. *They provide a vehicle for coalition building around a broad agenda.* As a vehicle for mass organizing, the assemblies allow for engagement around a much broader set of issues and, as a result, attract a diverse set of partners. As assemblies

(pushed by residents) take on critical bread and butter issues like wages, land use, and budgeting, they also evolve their own political life.

4. *The focus on public policy pushes members into deeper engagement with governance structures—at the local and state level.* Residents are trained on local budgeting and tax policy and the role of state agencies, the legislature, and the governor in the decisions that affected Jacksonians' quality of life. This focus is also building a cadre of activated residents who learn how to conduct research on policy issues and make independent proposals to policymakers.

5. *Assemblies have also taken on independent projects to improve quality of life that serve as concrete examples of the power of self-determination and collective action.* Assembly projects include the establishment of food gardens and cleanup and beautification efforts.

But the People's Assemblies are also a constant reminder that, while Jackson is nearly 90 percent Black, the city still has a great deal of political diversity. In fact, the People's Assemblies invariably uncover the need for deeper political discussion and education, if Jackson is to build a truly radical city from the ground up. Of course, there are a lot of progressive values that many residents already share around economics, shared prosperity, and caring for one another as neighbors and as a city. And there are others—including gender justice and community safety—that require a lot more conversation before values are more widely shared.

Policing and public safety are great examples of how residents have strong, divergent views. Although Mayor Chokwe Antar Lumumba ran on a platform of alternatives to prison and prevention, abolition is still a difficult (though not impossible) topic for many Jacksonians (see chapter 23). Jackson has one of the highest per capita murder rates in the nation (Vicory 2020), most of it related to poverty and interpersonal violence. These tensions played out in the People's Assemblies, as many residents tied safety to policing, while more progressive groups are working toward defunding and de-emphasizing police in safety. However, the media attention generated by a rash of police-involved shootings in spring 2019 was helping to drive a public conversation about accountability—specifically in regard to pushing the city to change its policy and release the names of officers involved in shootings.

National allies and police accountability activists on the ground expected that the mayor would use his executive authority to repeal the policy and release the names. For them, the mayor's condemnation of the shootings was not enough; they wanted more decisive action. Some even accused him of collaborating with police. The police were advocating to keep the city policy in place, framing it as a workers' rights issue for this predominantly Black force. Consistent with a core precept of media advocacy (see chapter 24), both sides were attempting to frame their arguments from a human dignity standpoint.

The mayor decided to convene a commission to review the policy and propose changes that included several members of the People's Assemblies. The commission was consistent with the Lumumba administration's people's governance frame-work in giving the public an opportunity to weigh in. The process took just short of three months—laser speed for bureaucracy but an eternity for grieving family members seeking justice. Tensions ran high. In the end, the commission released compromise guidelines that required the police department to release the names of officers involved in shootings, as long as they were not operating undercover. Other important reforms followed, including the establishment of independent oversight, bans on excessive force, and mandating officers to intervene to stop the use of excessive force.

However, and as is so often the case in municipal politics, the political pen-dulum has swung in the other direction as a recent spike in homicides, exacer-bated by pandemic pressures, has at this writing put 2020 on course to be Jackson's deadliest on record. Residents and the media pushed hard for more of Jackson's resources to be spent on police. And answering this call, the city budget passed in September 2020 featured increases for police salaries as well as an expanded force even as many cities are rolling back police budgets.

Concluding Thoughts and Hard Questions Ahead

Governing in a state like Mississippi, in a country like the United States, has many constrictions that progressives may find difficult to navigate. What does it mean to espouse justice and fair wages in a time of austerity? What does co-governance look like when people don't share key values? To what extent do you engage in dom-inant culture institutions—like public schools or the Democratic Party—because it is where many residents are engaged? These questions are important because centering love and care in our organizing is about engaging people right where they are. That is why People's Assembly organizers will stand out in the Mississippi sun handing out food and toilet paper, and testing residents for COVID-19; or build broad coalitions that include service providers, faith communities, businesses, and radical students (Themba 2020). This is organizing that blurs the lines between direct services and so-called traditional organizing because ensuring that people have what they need and investing time in building their capacity to govern them-selves gives people a sense of what is possible when we look out for one another.

Questions for Further Discussion

1. The author states that "Centering love and care in our organizing is about engaging people right where they are." What are some examples of the ways members of the People's Assembly did this in Jackson, Mississippi? Think about a community group you know or are a part of, and whether or how they are "engaging people where they are." How else might they do this, or do it better?

2. The author notes that people's assemblies are important in five key ways (e.g., providing a venue for listening to residents' concerns, creating a training ground and pipeline for leadership development, etc.). Thinking about a grass-roots organization you know of or have been involved in, does one of these in particular stand out as an area in which the organization is doing well or in which it needs to focus more of its time and energy? Please share concrete examples to illustrate.

REFERENCES

Alinsky, S. D. (1971). *Rules for Radicals: A Practical Primer for Realistic Radicals.* Random House.

Freire, P. (1994). *Pedagogy of Hope: Reliving Pedagogy of the Oppressed.* Continuum.

Lartey, J. (2017, September 11). A revolutionary, not a liberal: Can a radical black mayor bring change to Mississippi? *The Guardian.* https://www.theguardian.com/us-news/2017/sep/11/revolutionary-not-a-liberal-radical-black-mayor-mississippi-chokwe-lumumba.

Sen, R. (2020, July 1). Why today's social revolutions include kale, medical care, and help with the rent. Zócalo Public Square. https://www.zocalopublicsquare.org/2020/07/01/mutual-aid-societies-self-determination-pandemic-community-organizing/ideas/essay/.

Su, C. (2017). Beyond inclusion: Critical race theory and participatory budgeting. *New Polit Sci, 39*(1), 126–142.

Themba, M. (2020, July 8). An island amid Mississippi's COVID madness. *The Nation.* https://www.thenation.com/article/society/coronavirus-racism-america/.

Themba-Nixon, M. (2017). The city as liberated zone: The promise of Jackson People's Assemblies. In *Jackson Rising.* PressBooks. https://jacksonrising.pressbooks.com/chapter/the-city-as-liberated-zone-the-promise-of-jacksons-peoples-assemblies/.

Vicory, J. (2020, January 6). "It puts a dark cloud over the city": Can Jackson get a handle on gun violence, homicides? *Mississippi Clarion Ledger.* https://www.clarionledger.com/story/news/local/2020/01/06/gun-violence-jackson-mississippi-how-many-homicides-2019/2794601001/.

PART THREE

Building Effective Partnerships and Anticipating and Addressing Ethical Challenges

One of the most important parts of the professional's role in community organizing and other aspects of community practice involves building and maintaining effective partnerships that enable working with, not on, communities. But before we can talk seriously about community partnerships, we should take a good look at our own and others' understandings of what "community" really means. As Fisher and his colleagues (2018) point out, the very notion of community is, and should be, contested, particularly in light of its increasing co-optation by government bodies and others in ways that support the current political economy "and those who have the most to gain from the status quo."

This part begins with just such a critique, as Canadian scholar and activist Ronald Labonté (chapter 7) looks more deeply at some of the assumptions that underlie our notions of community and our related approaches to community organizing. Drawing on both his extensive work as a health promotion consultant nationally and globally, and his in-depth study of the Toronto health department, Labonté begins by asking professionals to free themselves from their often uncritical and romanticized notions of community. In a similar vein, he reminds us that community involvement and decentralized decision making, although wonderful concepts in theory, may translate into tokenism, both sapping a community's limited energy and inadvertently supporting government cutbacks (Fisher et al., 2018; Raphael et al., 2019).

Labonté then applies this attitude of critical rethinking to the whole domain of community organizing (which, in Canada, has roughly the same meaning as *community development*). Central to this discussion is the distinction he draws between *community-based* efforts and true *community organizing*. In the former, Labonté suggests, health professionals or their agencies define and name the problem, develop strategies for dealing with it, and involve community members to varying degrees in the problem-solving process. In contrast, community organizing supports community groups as they identify problems or issues and plan strategies for confronting them. Building on these and related distinctions, Labonté suggests that community organizing approaches are far more conducive to the building of authentic partnerships. The latter require, among other things, that "all partners [establish] their own power and legitimacy" (Butterfoss & Kegler, 2009; Wolff et al., 2017; chapter 18). Further, they underscore the need for health educators, social workers, and other community-engaged practitioners to support community group partners, whether or not the latter buy into the concerns and mandates of the professional or agency (Minkler et al., 2019).

In chapter 8, Meredith Minkler, Cheri A. Pies, Patricia Wakimoto, and Cheryl A. Hyde revisit many of the issues and challenges raised in the preceding chapter, focusing special attention on the ethical dimensions of these issues. Six areas are explored: the problem of conflicting priorities; the difficulties involved in eliciting genuine rather than tokenistic community participation; cross-cultural misunderstanding and problems of real and perceived racism and other isms in organizing; the dilemmas posed by funding sources; problematic, unanticipated consequences of our organizing efforts; and questions of whose "common good" is being addressed by the organizing effort.

Drawing on both theoretical literature and relevant case studies, the authors highlight the ethical challenges raised in each of these areas and pose hard questions for professionals as organizers regarding their assumptions, appropriate roles, and potential courses of action. Several tools are provided, such as the classic DARE criteria for measuring empowerment: Who determines the goals of the project? Who acts to achieve the goals? Who receives the benefits? Who evaluates the project? (Rubin and Rubin, 2007), and the "publicity test of ethics" for helping communities decide whether to accept money from a controversial source (chapter 20). The real purpose of the chapter, however, is to raise questions, rather than answer them. A key message of chapter 8, and indeed of this whole part of the book, is that thoughtful and sometimes difficult questioning of our assumptions and values, and careful exploration of the ethical dimensions of our work, must be both preliminary and ongoing aspects of our work with communities.

The importance of taking this message seriously is well illustrated in chapter 9, as Roxanna Chen and her colleagues at Public Health–Seattle & King County, the Seattle Foundation, and community leaders share their experiences with a bold new "Communities of Opportunity" (COO) initiative. The COO was designed to enable the awarding of grants and other support to community-driven partnerships in King County wishing to address issues within the broad umbrella of housing, health, and equity. From the beginning, the health department looked inward, at its own processes and practices that might effectively exclude from participation the very communities it most hoped to reach—and made the necessary changes. Having ten community leaders as part of the COO's fourteen-member governing body, for example, was a critical way to shift power. So, too, was developing a simple, four-page request for proposals, which specified, in turn, that the proposals were also to be just four pages in length. This leveled the playing field, giving low-resource community organizations a much better chance of getting funded than had been the case with complicated proposal processes, which had favored the larger and better-resourced competitors. Community demands, for example, that an asset-based approach, rather than a deficit mentality (Kretzmann & McKnight, 1993) be used in characterizing them, were taken seriously, and this, too, helped build the trust essential to effective partnerships.

Lessons learned from and with the two grantees highlighted in this chapter, the Transgender Economic Empowerment Coalition and the Seattle Urban Native Nonprofits (SUNN), were illuminating, especially as neither was a traditional "place-based" grantee. The case study is a powerful example of what initiatives supported by health departments or funders can help catalyze when they take seriously the need for cultural humility, addressing their own isms, sharing power and creating systems through which communities can take the lead (Freudenberg et al., 2015; Iton & Ross, 2017; Wolff et al., 2017). As one community partner put it, you need to "Go slow to go fast" in this work, and COO is an exemplary case in point.

REFERENCES

Butterfoss, F. D., & Kegler, M. C. (2009). The Community Coalition Action Theory. In R. DiClemente, R. A. Crosby, & M. C. Kegler (Eds.), *Emerging Theories in Health Promotion Practice and Research* (2nd ed., pp. 238–274). Jossey-Bass.

Fisher, R., DeFilippis, J., & Shragge, E. (2018). Contested community: A selected and critical history of community organizing. In R. Cnaan & C. Milofsky (Eds.), *Handbook of Community Movements and Local Organizations in the 21st Century* (pp. 281–297). Springer.

Freudenberg, N., Franzosa, E., Chisholm, J., & Libman, K. (2015). New approaches for moving upstream: How state and local health departments can transform practice to reduce health inequalities. *Health Educ Behav, 42*(1_suppl), 46S–56S.

Iton, A. B., & Ross, R. K. (2017). Understanding how health happens: Your zip code is more important than your genetic code. In R. Callahan and D. Bhattachara (Eds.), *Public Health Leadership* (pp. 83–99). Routledge.

Kretzmann, J. P., & McKnight, J. L. (1993). *Building Communities from Inside Out: A Path Toward Finding and Mobilizing a Community's Assets.* Center for Urban Affairs and Policy Research.

Minkler, M., Rebanal, R. D., Pearce, R., & Acosta, M. (2019). Growing equity and health equity in perilous times: Lessons from community organizers. *Health Educ Behav, 46*(1_suppl), 9S–18S.

Raphael, D., Bryant, T., & Rioux, M. (2019). *Staying Alive: Critical Perspectives on Health, Illness, and Health Care* (3rd ed.). Canadian Scholars Press.

Rubin, H., & Rubin, I. (2007). *Community Organizing and Development* (4th ed.). Macmillan.

Wolff, T., Minkler, M., Wolfe, S. M., Berkowitz, B., Bowen, L., Butterfoss, F. D., Christens, B. D., Francisco, V. T., Himmelman, A. T., & Lee, K. S. (2017). Collaborating for equity and justice: Moving beyond collective impact. *Nonprofit Q, 9*, 42–53.

7

Community, Community Organizing, and the Forming of Authentic Partnerships

Looking Back, Looking Ahead

RONALD LABONTÉ

Note from the author: Much of this chapter is based on my insights into some of the challenges of an "empowering" public health practice, something I had spent the first twenty years of my working life grappling with. The practice was inherently political (since anything dealing with policy is by definition political), and explicitly directed at reducing inequities in health embedded within societal structures. It was good practice then and is even more critical today, given the unprecedented pace of change in the contexts in which we work and the need to evaluate and take local action in light of increasingly dynamic national and global changes and what they may portend.

IT IS HARD TO BE critical of community when one spends most of the day working in the stuffy cubicles of a government building or in the isolated offices of universities. Community represents something more positive and affirming than the bureaucratic rigidities or academic competitiveness of one's daily working experience. It is difficult to question community's importance when the main positive comments about frontline workers' efforts tend to come from small groups gathered in church basements or cluttered storefront meeting rooms. Yet questioning and critiquing the notion of community are precisely what I do in this chapter. My concern is that an uncritical adoption of community rhetoric can, paradoxically, work against the empowerment ideals that lie at the heart of many health practitioners' intent.

Let me clarify the meaning of a few key terms before proceeding. Several concepts bearing a community label are now common in the health sector, notably community organization, community mobilization, and community development. But different people use different terms to mean the same thing. In Canada, for example, *community development* is often used to describe what in the United States is called *community organizing*. For the purposes of my argument, *community organizing* refers to efforts to create a new group or organization, often with the assistance of an outsider, such as a health educator or social worker (Rothman, 2008). *Community mobilization* describes attempts to draw together a number of such groups or organizations into concerted actions around a specific topic, issue, or event. *Community development* (or community organizing in the United States) incorporates both but describes a particular practice in which both practitioner and agency are committed to broad changes in the structure of power relations in society through the support they give community groups (Freudenberg et al., 2015; Labonté, 1995, 1996; Schutz & Miller, 2015). Hereafter, and to avoid confusion, I use the term *community organizing* to encompass both community organizing and community development. Finally, I make a distinction in vantage point, though not in underlying values or goals, between my definition of community organizing and that of the book's editors. In chapter 1, borrowing from Minkler and her colleagues (2019), the authors thus define community organizing as "a process by which communities identify their assets and concerns, prioritize and select issues, and intentionally build power and develop and implement action strategies for change" (p. 9S). Our definitions are, in reality, quite similar in their accents on community capacity and agency in determining issues, building power, and working collectively for change. Where they differ is in my focus, as well, on the role of the health educator, social worker, or other practitioner or agency in working with and supporting the community in its organizing efforts. For although most community organizing takes place in and by communities of geography or identity, without the help or involvement of outsiders, for those of us in fields like public health and social welfare who *do* wish to help support communities in their efforts, reflecting more deeply on our roles in this process, and their attendant promise and challenges, is a discussion well worth having (chapters 1, 8, 9, 13; appendix 6).

I begin by examining the conceptual confusion that continues to surround the term *community* and offer five cautions about its uncritical invocation in health and social practice. Drawing in part on insights gained through my in-depth study of the Toronto Department of Public Health in the 1990s (Labonté, 1996), and more recent observations, I argue that while the *concept* of "community organizing" continues some of this confusion, the *practice* of community organizing has demonstrated considerable potential for fostering self-reliance and the creation of authentic partnerships with communities. I conclude by presenting nine characteristics of authentic partnerships that health educators and other social change professionals are encouraged to strive for in our practice.

The Contested Meaning of Community

Numerous historical developments contributed to the conceptual prominence of community in health work. Although a detailed discussion is beyond the scope of this chapter, the surrounding boundaries have expanded in relation to a wide range of developments. Among these are growing appreciation of the role of the

Social Determinants of Health (SDOH) and of both individuals and the places in which they live, work, and recreate (Braveman et al., 2017; Iton & Ross, 2017; Marmot et al., 2008). New and escalating health and social problems, including the COVID-19 pandemic and the global recession in its wake, together with rising health care costs amid loss of coverage, have also broadened the boundaries of community in this work and contributed to the growing focus on community factors in both disease causation and prevention (Cockerham, 2006, 2015; Fawcett et al., 2011, 2016; Iton & Ross, 2017).

As noted in earlier chapters, the centrality of community and the importance of community organizing for health were reflected in such influential documents as the Ottawa Charter for Health Promotion (World Health Organization, 1986), which regarded "the empowerment of communities, their ownership and control of their own endeavors and destinies" as the heart of the "new" health promotion. Many commentators view community as the venue for, if not the very definition of, the new health promotion practice (Fawcett et al., 2011; Robertson & Minkler, 1994; chapter 3), a view commonly expressed by practitioners themselves (Diers, 2006; Rupp et al., 2020). Indeed, as Walter and Hyde (2012) suggest, a general weakness of professional and institutional discourses on community has been the largely atheoretical and uncritical way in which the term has entered common usage.

Initially in the health field, *community* was simply a reflexive adjective. In Canada, hospitals became community health centers, nurses became community health workers, state health departments became community health departments, and health promotion and health education programs became community-based efforts. In the syntax of everyday language, "community" ceased being a subject, a group of people acting with their own intent, and became an object (community as a "target" for health programs) or an adjective to the real subjects, which remained health institutions, which had become, by linguistic sleight of hand, community modified. The problem was not that community-enamored practitioners and their agencies did not know their grammar well. The problem was the way in which community became objectified as fact and posited as a solution to most all health problems rather than treated as a definitional conundrum whose development is inherently problematic.

When community is defined at all, it is usually in the static vocabulary of data, creating categories based on identity (the low-income community, the women's community, the disabled community), geography (the neighborhood, the small town, a particular housing project), or issue (the environmental community, the heart health community, the social justice community). Often, community is simply *assumed* to be those persons using the services of an institution and living within administratively drawn catchment boundaries (the hospital community, the school community, the university community).

Community has all of these elements of identity, geography, shared issue of concern, even institutional relations, but it is also more. *Community* derives from the Latin *communitas*, meaning "common or shared," and the *ty* suffix, meaning "to have the quality of." Sharing is not some demographic datum; it is the dynamic act of people being together. Community is, in effect, organization. There is no "low income community" outside of poor people coming together to share their experience and act to transform it. There is no "women's community" outside of two or more women sharing their reality, and empowering themselves to act more effectively upon it. As defined by the Toronto Department of Public Health (1994b) over twenty-five years ago, a community is "a group of individuals with a common interest, and an identity of themselves as a group. We all belong to multiple communities at any given time. The essence of being a community is that there is something that is 'shared.' We cannot really say that a community exists until a group with a shared identity" exists (n.p.). Even recognition of the active, organizational nature of community, however, does not fully clarify the term.

Romanticization

Community, as implied in the landmark Ottawa Charter (Epp, 1986), and critiqued in more recent writings (DeFilippis et al., 2010; Fisher et al., 2018), can do no wrong. The building of stronger communities, for example, is often regarded as an elemental strategy for strengthening community health (Fawcett et al., 2016; Iton & Ross, 2017; chapter 9). Though it is important to accept community self-determination in principle, it is also vital to recognize that what communities do for their own health may be inimical to a broader public health. Nazi Germany was a classic example of a strong community, as is the small but growing neo-Nazi group in that country today. So, too, are many radical fringe groups, such as QAnon, among the growing number of White supremacist organizations and militias. Similarly, one could define as a community lobbyists against stricter pollution controls and people who work together to block supportive housing for homeless persons, or those with mental disabilities. Neighborhoods, towns, cities, and states comprise myriad communities, as often in conflict with one another as seeking consensus and understanding. Under conditions of conflict, which community should be supported, and why? Unless linked to a political theory of social organization and change and an analysis of social power relations, this question cannot be answered, and the notion of "community" becomes somewhat fatuous. Worse, it becomes romanticized in a way that can obscure very real and important power inequities between different communities that may subtly imperil the health and well-being of less powerful groups, for example, the community of urban land developers versus the community of the unhoused.

Bureaucratization

Whose interests are most served by increasing community involvement in health? And what is it, exactly, that health workers are asking communities to become involved in? Apart from concerns over tokenism (participation without authority), community involvement in health programs may not always "strengthen" the community. Health professionals may bureaucratize thriving community initiatives if they are insensitive to the fact that a community organizing approach to issues is intrinsically unmanageable by conventional planning standards, which rigidly specify goals, objectives, and outcomes before action can begin. Even when health agencies engender new initiatives, they may unintentionally sap the political vitality of community group leaders. The health educator or social worker who gets "permission" from her senior managers to include local activists on a housing and health committee will likely see little progress if these community advocates are simply involved in the agency's bureaucratic process of committee meetings, reports, and senior management approvals. In contrast, if that same practitioner assists these activists in educating, advocating, and collaborating with decision-makers in a partnership for social change, the likelihood of change may be substantially increased. While the former, tokenistic engagement (Arnstein, 2019; chapter 8) may effectively, if unintentionally, have silenced the political voice of some of the strongest community leaders, the latter, more empowering process, would instead help amplify it (chapters 8, 9; appendix 6).

Antiprofessionalism

Just as health authorities can risk elitism in their desire to demonstrate health promotion "leadership," community groups and some of their health worker supporters can undermine effective collaborations through a festering antiprofessionalism. Professional is not the antithesis of community. Indeed, the Latin root of the word *professional* means to "profess" or "vow," a reference to the medieval practice of surrendering personal gain to the larger community of a religious order or workers' guild. It is true that health professionals, like others in the "poverty industry," can increase the victimization of people living in socially disadvantaged conditions through their attitudes and exercise of power over their "clients." But to imply, as some have, that most past public health practice has been wrong or that, as McKnight (1987) has argued, "resources empower; services do not" denigrates the community of health and social workers. It reinforces a we/they polarity and ignores the formative role that respectfully delivered useful, and usable services have often played in developing new community organizations and overcoming the isolation of society's most marginalized or oppressed (Hyatt, 2008; Mathie et al., 2017; Sen, 2020).

Many health professionals are also community activists. If they respect the leadership prerogative of community groups and are seen as valued and trusted parts of the community, there is no reason for them to be self-deprecatory or to disparage the value of their own "professional" efforts. Indeed, community groups supported by health workers not infrequently cite the professional status, legitimacy, and influence such workers bring to the relationship, which community groups can then use to enhance their own social change efforts (Minkler et al., 2019; chapter 15). I liken the process of policy change, for example, to a nutcracker. One arm is the data-rich reports, policy documents, charters, and frameworks produced by health professionals primarily for internal consumption and bureaucratic legitimacy. The other arm, exerting the greatest force, is a community group able to put pressure on politicians, "cracking" the issue against the more conservative arm of professional validation. Both arms are necessary, if different in their strategic placement and use in creating healthy social change.

Decentralization

The decentralization of decisionmaking over public programs, another oft-cited tenet of community organizing, allows for programs unique to community groups and their perceived needs. But the concept must be tempered with the recognition that most economic and social policy is national and transnational in nature. Local decisionmaking, by definition, can take place only within narrow parameters at best and is unlikely to include substantial control over economic resources (DeFilippis et al., 2010; Fisher & DeFilippis, 2015).

The rhetoric of decentralized local control may also inadvertently support growing health and social inequities by failing to defend social programs against austerity cutbacks or regressive tax reform by more senior government levels. Indeed, part of the appeal of community, especially to neoliberals and neoconservatives, is that it can readily justify dramatic social service cutbacks in the name of increasing community control (Fisher et al., 2018; Hyatt, 2008). In Canada, decentralized community decisionmaking in health care became a fact only as public funding for health care began shrinking, hospitals closing, and thousands of health care workers losing their jobs (Bryant et al., 2010). Similarly, during the crucial early weeks and months of the COVID-19 pandemic, the Trump administration's reluctance to serve as a "shipping clerk," procuring and distributing needed personal protective equipment and other assistance to local and state governments, was couched in the language of decentralization—that it was up to local and state entities to figure out how to do this. In this instance, "decentralized decisionmaking," without adequate resources, both resulted in states and municipalities negotiating on their own (and sometimes in conflict with each other) and provided former president Trump a rationale for shifting the blame for the rapidly escalating number of cases and fatalities to the local and state levels.

Self-Help

The promotion of self-help and mutual aid groups parallels the call for decentralized decisionmaking. Professional coordination of self-help networks is sometimes advanced as a means of "humanizing" the welfare system and of coping with program cutbacks driven by neoliberal economic policies. The first rationale is sound;

the second accepts reprivatization of social policy, better known as charity. That self-help and mutual aid groups can be empowering and health enhancing is undeniable (chapter 5; Sen, 2020). But there is typically little recognition in government policies on health promotion and community organizing that self-help primarily taps the volunteer energies of women, society's "traditional" care providers. Will government support and professional coordination of self-help simply increase voluntarism at the economic expense of women? Moreover, the type of self-help usually being promoted is what is sometimes called "defensive"—groups of people with a common problem or disease providing peer support.

There is also a history of "offensive" self-help, those groups concerned with meso- and macrolevel social change strategies. These groups are less likely to receive government or other outside support because they are regarded as too political, self-interested, or advocacy oriented. Yet, unless the right of groups to advocate for changes in government policy is recognized and supported in health promotion funding policy, the self-help ethos restricts to a personal level problems that have both personal and political dimensions. Further, and with the active support of many of the nation's large philanthropic funders, local health departments and other sectors are increasingly joining coalitions, typically led by grassroots, community-based organizations, to work for the "transformative change" needed if we are to truly address the social determinants of health (Freudenberg et al., 2015; Iton & Ross, 2017; Minkler et al., 2019; chapter 9).

Community Organizing: Assumptions, Cautions, and Potential

Many of the cautions just raised cut to the quick of community organizing as a specific health practice. There is no theory of community organizing any more than there is a singular theory of or approach to health promotion. Rather, the term describes a range of practices in which it has existed historically, such as international development, literacy, economic development, housing, and social work / social services.

Community organizing involves assumptions about the nature of society, social change, and the relationship among community, organizers, state agencies, and community groups. These assumptions are sometimes made explicit in community organization and development literature and models (e.g., Fisher et al., 2018; Rothman, 2008; Walter & Hyde, 2012; chapter 10). But with some important exceptions (Iton & Ross, 2017; Plough & Gandhi, 2019; Rudolph et al., 2013; chapter 9), they are rarely explicitly present in government or other health agency policy statements on community organizing and often remain unexplored among practitioners themselves (Labonté, 1996; Minkler et al., 2019). One early and succinct statement of these assumptions was that of the Toronto Department of Public Health (1994a), which defined community organizing as "the process of supporting community groups in identifying their health issues, planning and acting upon their strategies for social action / social change, and gaining increased self-reliance and decision-making power as a result of their activities" (n.p.). There are five important components to this definition.

1. *Community organizing describes a relationship between outside institutions and community groups.* In fields like public health and social work, the "doer" of community organizing has traditionally been seen as a professional in a health department or nonprofit health agency or organization. Yet increasingly, health departments and other outside entities from the United States and Canada to South Africa, New Zealand, and Australia are seeing their role as that of supporting *community-driven* organizing (Freudenberg et al., 2015; Iton & Ross, 2017; Kleba et al., 2021; chapters 3, 9, 15), in which outside professionals are ideally valued partners but are not running the show. Instead, their role is one of nurturing relations with and among institutions and community groups, with a focus on equity, community leadership, and power-shifting (Iton & Ross, 2017; chapter 9).

A helpful tool in this regard is the "ladder of community participation" developed by health educators at the Contra Costa County Department of Health Services in California (Morgan & Lifshay, 2006; appendix 6). Using this simple tool, health or other organizations can better see the level of control that they and their community partners actually possess in any given project or partnership (e.g., from "health department leads" at the bottom rung through "limited input and consultation" near the middle to "power sharing" and "community leads" at the top (appendix 6). Such tools can be useful for organizations and their community partners seeking more equitable relationships (Arnstein, 2019; Morgan & Lifshay, 2006; appendix 4).

But playing this role effectively requires that practitioners acknowledge the differences in power (status, authority, resources, legitimacy) that exist among themselves, their agency, and community groups. Further, as Wallerstein (1999) classically pointed out, failing to recognize the power and authority conferred by our own sources of unearned power and privilege can disrupt or prevent real and authentic partnerships with communities.

If practitioners presume without questioning that they are "equals" with community groups, they risk making invisible the types of power that they do hold "over" groups, thereby increasing the risk of abusing that power or of failing to recognize the potential for making it available to groups for their own use (Wallerstein, 1999; chapters 8, 9; appendix 6).

There has been a long history of anti-racist, critical gender, and now nonbinary forms of training in Canada and the United States. And in and beyond North America, the MeToo and Black Lives Matter movements have brought renewed scrutiny to the intersectionality of these power differences and the need for more critical reflective practices that are actively anti-racist, pro-feminist, and acutely sensitive to the institutionalized forms of discrimination and exclusion (Carter & Snyder, 2020; appendix 1). Increasingly, moreover, local health departments, university departments in fields like health and social welfare, and other outside entities that interface with communities are recognizing the importance of holding "dismantling racism" and intersectionality trainings (Came & Griffin, 2018; Carter & Snyder, 2020; Kendi, 2019; chapter 9; appendix 1) for their own staff or member organizations.

2. *Community organizing is always a matter of choosing some groups over others.* Accepting a professional interest in community organizing compels practitioners to define which groups we are actually interested in, and why. The choices made by health and social workers and their agencies are rarely made explicit or include only those groups that might agree to mobilize around particular health or social issues, such as heart health, homelessness, or anti-tobacco advocacy. This renders choice a matter of personal preference or institutional convenience. There is an ethical concern in the first instance: public agencies should be publicly accountable. Favoritism in choice should be informed by an explicit analysis of the SDOH, theories of social change, and power relations, not simply by ideologies kept from organizational or public view and debate. Second, both ethical and practical issues emerge when the majority of health and social workers' time is spent with groups (e.g., youth with mental health problems but living with caring parents who earn a good wage versus unhoused, hard-core drug abusers). To the extent that community organizing is a public resource that can help affect a redistribution in material resources (DeFilippis et al., 2010; Freudenberg et al., 2015), a high ratio of middle-class clients or groups represents an upward redistribution of resources that contradicts the social justice rhetoric of documents, such as the Ottawa Charter for health promotion (World Health Organization, 1986).

3. *Community organizing involves "making private troubles public issues."* Community organizing work is not support group work. We can distinguish a "support group" from a "community group" based on whether its members look primarily inward to their immediate psychosocial needs or outward to the socioenvironmental context that creates those needs in the first place. To paraphrase C. Wright Mills (1956), community groups transform the private troubles of support groups into public issues for policy remediation. Support group work, or *defensive self-help*, is central to what many public health nurses, educators, social workers, and some community organizers do. It is fundamentally important work and necessary to community organizing, for without the support of a group, many historically marginalized people will lack the confidence to look outward to the harder-to-change sociopolitical conditions that created their marginality in the first place.

But whereas support group work concerns the creation of healthy (equitable) power relations within groups, community organizing concerns the creation of healthy (equitable) power relations among community groups and institutions, or *offensive self-help.* The reason for making this distinction is twofold. It prevents community organizing or development from becoming a term so large in practice that it no longer serves any useful conceptual purpose (DeFilippis et al., 2010), a critique aptly, made years ago of health promotion (Robertson & Minkler, 1994). It also

TABLE 7.1

Community-Based and Community Organizing Programming

Community-Based Programming	*Community Organizing Programming*
The process in which health professionals or health agencies define the health problem, develop strategies to remedy the problem, involve local community members and groups to assist in problem solving, and work to transfer major responsibility for an ongoing program to local community members and groups.	The process of organizing or supporting community groups in their identification of important concerns and issues and their ability to plan and implement strategies to mitigate their concerns and resolve their issues.
Example:	*Example:*
Nobody's Perfect or heart health programs	Healthy Communities projects
Characteristics:	*Characteristics:*
The problem name is given.	The problem name starts with that of the community group, and then is negotiated strategically, that is, to a problem naming that advances the shared interest of the group and the institution.
There are defined program time lines.	
Changes in specific behaviors or knowledge levels are the desired outcome.	Work is longer term, requiring many hours.
Decisionmaking power rests principally with the institution.	A general increase in the group's capacities is the desired outcome.
	Power relationships are constantly negotiated.

requires that health professionals, social workers, and their agencies grapple with power relations at a higher level of social organization and not restrict themselves to the necessary but insufficient work of support group organizing.

4. *Community organizing is not simply bringing institutional programs into "community" settings.* We can distinguish between community-based and community organizing approaches to our work. The distinction lies in who sets the agenda and who names the issue or problem (table 7.1). In the community-based approach, the agency finds existing individuals or groups and links up its programs with them. It is an important approach to public health and social work, but it is not community organizing, which attempts to support community groups in resolving concerns as group members define them (Minkler et al., 2019; Morgan & Lifshay, 2006; Pastor et al., 2018; appendix 6). Of course, as already noted, not all groups or group

concerns will or should be supported. Community organizing requires making choices that, in turn, require explicit analyses of social power relations and agency/staff commitments to shifting these relations toward greater equity. But despite important steps forward (Freudenberg et al., 2015; Iton & Ross, 2017; chapter 9) much community organizing and community mobilizing work in health continues to concern itself primarily with specific diseases, lifestyle behaviors, and those public policies that influence their risks (Alvaro et al., 2011; Labonté & Robertson, 1996; Raphael, 2010). These issues may not always be of concern to lower income groups or localities. To the extent that institutional support and financial resources for community work are streamed through these "set agendas," the more political empowerment work of groups or localities can actually be undermined (chapter 8).

Community organizing, however, can emerge from a community-based program, just as community-based programs can arise in the context of a larger community organizing effort (Bell & Standish, 2005; Iton & Ross, 2017; Labonté & Robertson, 1996; Minkler et al., 2019). In the first instance, the practice issue becomes one of health and social workers and their agencies accepting as legitimate and finding ways to support action on more structurally defined health problems (e.g., unemployment, violence, food insecurity, or environmental racism) that participants in community-based programs (e.g., asthma prevention) might raise as concerns. In the second instance, the practice issue becomes one that health or social workers and their agencies negotiate with local residents, to ensure that the content and timing of community-based programs fit within the context of community residents' other political mobilizations.

5. *Community organizing promotes self-reliance, not self-sufficiency.* In defining community organizing as a process of creating more equitable relationships among groups and institutions, we can bury the myth of community self-sufficiency. According to that myth, the community group can mobilize and/or provide its own resources and the skills to enable it to function autonomously from others. This is often assumed to be the goal of community organizing or a measure of maximum community participation (Bjaras et al., 1991; Rifkin, 2012). However, the health sector's rhetorical acceptance of such terms as partnerships and intersectoralism should lead practitioners and their agencies to foster equitable and effective interdependencies rather than to promote the autonomy of localities. The goal of community organizing is not self-sufficiency, it is the ability of the group to negotiate its own terms of relationship with those institutions or other agencies that support it.

Community Organizing and the Creation of Effective and Authentic Partnerships

An equitably negotiated arrangement among different groups is often referred to by the shorthand notion of "partnership." Whether practitioners and their agencies rally behind the ideas of community organizing, community mobilization, or community development, they are essentially entering a partnership with a variety of different groups or organizations.

Effective Partnerships and Conflict

Community organizing may strive for inclusivity in community building, for agreement among as broad a collection of community groups as possible. The reality, however, is that powerless groups usually seek to shift skewed social relations by limiting the power that other groups have over them. Powerless individuals often create their identity as a community group only in opposition to or conflict with groups that are more powerful than themselves. This dynamic has been at the base of the confrontational approach to community organizing favored by Saul Alinsky and his adherents (Alinsky, 1971; Schutz & Miller, 2015; chapter 5) and has been used successfully to create communities from seemingly intractable conditions of isolation and apathy (Labonté, 1995; Schutz & Miller, 2015; chapter 5). More generally, research in social identity theory finds that group identities often require conflictual forms of "who's in / who's out" boundary setting (Abrams & Hogg, 1990), and a large body of sociological theory argues that intergroup conflict is the norm rather than the exception and provides the necessary "fuel" for social change.

In a landmark piece, Barbara Gray (1989), whose work on collaboration theory remains seminal to an understanding of partnerships, acknowledges that collaboration usually requires a period when less powerful groups establish their legitimacy through conflictual relations with more powerful groups. But conflict may also be necessary during collaboration. One reason that environmental groups now participate in collaborative policy bodies with industry and government is that they have demonstrated their ability, through direct conflictual actions, to prevent unilateral decisions by the other parties. Those environmental groups that participate in collaboration generally no longer engage in direct action. But if all environmental groups ceased conflict relations with industry or government, what would prevent a return to unilateral decisionmaking by either of the two more powerful stakeholders?

The Striving for Collaboration

That intergroup conflict is healthy and perhaps essential to social change should not lead health workers to shun the necessity of uniting diverse, conflicting groups at some higher level of community. Community-as-ideal, the moral resonance of the term, is what gives it power and appeal (Lyon, 1989) even if this ideal must be approached with an analytical caution about how it can be used for anti-community right-wing political agendas (Berlet & Sunshine, 2019; Defilippis et al., 2010). Nonetheless, as Gardner (1991) classically remarked, pluralism without commitment to the common good is pluralism gone berserk. Pragmatically, the community born in conflict or struggle rarely survives the eventual peace "unless those involved create the institutional arrangements and non-crisis bonding experiences that carry them through the year-in-year-out tests of community functioning" (p. 14).

Gray (1989) provides a comprehensive partnership model for promoting those functions, which she describes as "collaboration" and "a mutual search for information and solution." There are five features that characterize the process-as-outcome. First, recognition of stakeholder interdependence is enhanced. Second, differences are handled constructively. Third, joint ownership of decisions is developed. Fourth, stakeholders assume collective responsibility for "managing the problem domain" through formal and informal agreements. Fifth, the process is accepted as continually emergent.

There are several steps in effective collaboration, the first and most important being problem setting. This requires a "common definition of the problem," a "commitment to collaborate," and "identification of the stakeholders." This stage subsumes a pre-negotiation stage, the goal of which is to arrive at a common definition of problem and intent broad enough to get stakeholders to the table. This differentiates collaboration from the all-too-frequent form of government or other health agency consultation, in which the issue and desired outcome are already defined (appendix 6; Arnstein, 2019; chapter 8).

Effective collaboration requires the efforts of persons Gray refers to as "midwives," the community developers of organizations-as-communities. They are functionally distant from all of the stakeholders and work with them before they come to the table, seeking to find the "superordinate goal" that Sherif (1966) famously argued was the basis for initiating any reduction in intergroup conflict. This goal must be "compelling for the groups involved, but unattainable by [any] one group, singly; hence it is not identical with 'common goal.' . . . [It must also] supersede all other goals each group may have" (Sherif, 1966, p. 88).

Whatever the initiating superordinate goal, the conditions for authentic collaboration allow a sharper delineation of the differences among consultation, involvement, and participation (collaboration). Briefly, *consultation* involves the seeking of information from citizens, but with no ongoing dialogue. *Involvement* does involve dialogue, but such dialogue is typically controlled by the government or outside agency. Citizen involvement tends to be advisory only, around a problem or issue that the government or outside agency has predetermined or named (Arnstein, 2019; Morgan & Lifshay, 2006; appendix 6). There is no agreement on power sharing. In contrast, true *participation* involves negotiated relationships with citizens, who are treated as constituencies and take part in "naming the problem" or selecting the issue. All affected groups participate, and resources are made available to enable the full participation of less powerful groups (Arnstein, 2019; Labonté, 1993; Morgan & Lifshay, 2006; chapter 9; appendix 6).

What makes for the effective and authentic partnerships that community organizing creates? Building on the foregoing and drawing on Panet-Raymond's (1992) insights gleaned from attempts to forge relations between community health and social service centers and neighborhood volunteer centers in Quebec, and on Butterfoss and Kegler's (2009) Community Coalition Action Theory (chapter 18), we might say that partnerships exist only when the following are true:

1. All partners have established their own power and legitimacy. This often requires a period of conflict and some enduring strain between powerful and powerless groups. The provision of resources to these groups is one facet of community organizing work, provided such resources remain in the autonomous control of the groups.
2. All partners have well-defined mission statements. They have a clear sense of their purpose and organizational goals.
3. All partners respect one another's organizational autonomy by finding a visionary goal that is larger than any one of their independent goals. This requires extensive midwifing work to set the shared agenda. The achievement of this shared agenda is another facet of community organizing work.
4. Community group partners are well rooted in the locality. They have a constituency to which they are accountable.
5. Institutional partners have a commitment to partnership approaches in work with community groups.
6. Clear objectives and expectations of the partners are developed. The partners create a commitment among themselves to jointly "manage the problem domain."
7. Written agreements are made that clarify objectives, responsibilities, means, and norms. Regular evaluation allows adjustments to these agreements.
8. Outside agency or organization partners have clear mandates to support community group partners without attempting to get them to "buy into" the institutional partner's mandate and goal. This distinguishes community organizing from community-based approaches to work.
9. All partners strive for and nurture the human qualities of open-mindedness, patience, respect, and sensitivity to the experiences of persons in all partnering organizations.

Concluding Thoughts: Looking Back, Looking Ahead

Community is a potent idea, but its reality is the more modest process of people organizing themselves, or being helped to organize, into identity-forging, issue-solving groups. The multiplicity of people's group (community) experiences requires health and social work practitioners and their agencies to specify clearly whom they mean when they invoke the term. Romantic notions of community are more likely to support neoliberal political agendas, the dismantling of social welfare programs, and the upward redistribution of wealth and power than to empower localities in any significant way. As health practitioners attempt to support community groups and help them organize, they must be wary of "colonizing" these groups with institutional, often disease-based ways of defining health and social issues. Moreover, they must locate their choice of issues and groups to support within some analytical framework of society and social change. This framework needs to take account of the many forms of power that partly constitute the relationship among institutions, health professionals, and community groups, for the essence of community (organizing) is the transformation of these power relations such that there is more equity within and between institutions and groups.

At base, community organizing opposes those inequalities between people that are created by people and their economic and political practices. For, as French philosopher Raymond Aron once commented, "When inequalities become too great, the idea of community becomes impossible."

Parts of this chapter were first written more than thirty years ago. Over the intervening decades, the ability of local actions to "empower" became increasingly constrained by a neoliberal form of globalization. New economic rules were crafted that began reshaping the distribution of wealth and power within and between nations. Liberalized trade and financial markets created global tax competition and new ways for the rich to avoid or evade contributing to public revenues and the public good. The "local" is where all of us in some sense still and must reside, and often vibrantly so. But its capacity to leverage progressive change at the policy levels that conditions what we now call the "social determinants of health" became more difficult. The contradictions of an economy predicated on ever increasing levels of production and consumption in the midst of climate change and ecosystem collapse had become, for many, too palpable to ignore. Environmental justice joined with social justice as the new imperatives for human health, vastly increasing the space in which community partnerships must be developed. Both forms of justice continue to demand local attention and action, but neither can be assured or sustained in the absence of global agreements and international cooperation. One need only remember that one of Trump's first acts in office in 2016 was to abandon America's participation in the historic Paris Agreement on climate change, even as the great majority of Americans in poll after poll expressed their belief that climate change was a real and existential threat.

The local is now global, and the global is now local. Poorer countries have been experiencing this truism for decades. The first global taste of it came with the 2008 financial crisis. Many of us thought the moment had come for a reversion from an economics of pathology to one of health. We were wrong. Wealth and power continued to accrue to an ever smaller proportion of the world's population. Even as the health conditions continued to improve for many who were extremely poor and low income (and most of the rest of us), we were simply drawing down irreplaceable environmental capital at a rate that would soon (and quite literally) drown many of us.

Our second taste has come with the COVID-19 pandemic, still in dislocating play as this book goes to press, with millions dead and case and hospitalization rates again surging in much of the world. The *communitas* of what we hold in common and share, and which has long been at the heart of the human condition, is being strained by lockdowns even as it is being transformed by technologies. The disruptions the pandemic has wreaked on a global political and economic order already in disarray are ones that could herald a fundamental shift toward a more equitable and environmentally healthy future. They could as easily lead to new nationalisms, exaggerated xenophobia, and autocratic diktats that imperil war. Or they could simply be followed by a slow return to a pre-COVID-19 "normal" that was already killing us, albeit slowly and unequally.

Can the ideals of community partnerships conveyed in this chapter help tilt us in one direction over another? I believe they can. There is nothing inherent in good local-scale praxis that does not also apply at more global scales. Nor do the rules of partnership engagement alter. "Community" takes on an enlarged geographic meaning, although it still demands localized efforts to avoid becoming an empty abstraction. The ethos of having to choose sides and accept, albeit not embrace, the necessity of conflict as a bridge to collaboration is all the more important as civil and social rights become seen by antidemocratic rulers as pandemic collateral damage.

Questions for Further Discussion

1. "Community" is a contested concept with multiple meanings. As a health or social work professional and community activist, and someone who works for a health system, you have an interest in and have also been asked to join a community group advocating for changes in local health policies affecting the community. What criteria would you use in choosing to join and engage in their organizing efforts, and why?

2. Community organizing is often seen as a geographically local activity. Although localities are often the level at which citizen participation is most directly experienced and empowering, their influence over the deeper structural determinants of health is often limited. Should community organizing focus primarily on issues that are within the power or authority of local decisionmaking? If not, what other actions or strategies can community organizers use to affect equitable health positive changes in such determinants?

Acknowledgments

Portions of this chapter are based on Labonté, R. (1989). Community empowerment: The need for political analysis. *Can J Public Health, 80*(2), 87–88; and Labonté, R. (1993). Community development and partnership. *Can J Public Health, 84*(4), 237–240, adapted and reprinted by permission of the Canadian Public Health Association.

REFERENCES

Abrams, D., & Hogg, M. (1990). *Social Identity Theory: Constructive and Critical Advances.* Springer-Verlag.

Alinsky, S. D. (1971). *Rules for Radicals: A Pragmatic Primer for Realistic Radicals.* Random House.

Alvaro, C., Jackson, L. A., Kirk, S., McHugh, T. L., Hughes, J., Chircop, A., & Lyons, R. F. (2011). Moving Canadian governmental policies beyond a focus on individual lifestyle: Some insights from complexity and critical theories. *Health Promot Int, 26*(1), 91–99.

Arnstein, S. R. (2019). A ladder of citizen participation. *J Am Plann Assoc, 85*(1), 24–34.

Bell, J., & Standish, M. (2005). Communities and health policy: A pathway for change. *Health Aff, 24*(2), 339–342.

Berlet, C., & Sunshine, S. (2019). Rural rage: The roots of right-wing populism in the United States. *J Peasant Stud, 46*(3), 480–513.

Bjaras, G., Haglund, B. J. A., & Rifkin, S. (1991). A new approach to community participation assessment. *Health Promot Int, 6*(3), 199–206.

Braveman, P., Arkin, E., Orleans, T., Proctor, D., & Plough, A. (2017, May 1). What is health equity? And what difference does a definition make? Robert Wood Johnson Foundation. https://www.rwjf.org/en/library/research/2017/05/what-is-health-equity-.html.

Bryant, T., Raphael, D., & Rioux, M. (2010). *Staying Alive: Critical Perspectives on Health, Illness and Health Care* (2nd ed.). Canadian Scholars' Press.

Butterfoss, F. D., & Kegler, M. C. (2009). Community coalition action theory. In R. DiClemente, L. Crosby, & M. C. Kegler (Eds.), *Emerging Theories in Health Promotion Practice and Research* (2nd ed., pp. 236–276). Jossey-Bass.

Came, H., & Griffith, D. (2018). Tackling racism as a "wicked" public health problem: Enabling allies in anti-racism praxis. *Soc Sci Med, 199*, 181–188.

Carter, J. C., & Snyder, I. (2020). A beginner's guide to intersectionality. National League of Cities. https://www.nlc.org/article/2020/09/03/a-beginners-guide-to-intersectionality/.

Cockerham, W. C. (2006). *Social Causes of Health and Disease.* Polity Press.

Cockerham, W. C. (2015). *Medical Sociology on the Move: New Directions in Theory.* Springer.

DeFilippis, J., Fisher, R., & Shragge, E. (2010). *Contesting Community: The Limits and Potential of Local Organizing.* Rutgers University Press.

Diers, J. (2004). *Neighborhood Power: Building Community the Seattle Way.* University of Washington Press.

Epp, J. (1986). *Achieving Health for All: A Framework for Health Promotion.* Health and Welfare Canada.

Fawcett, S., Abeykoon, P., Arora, M., Dobe, M., Galloway-Gilliam, L., Liburd, L., & Munodawafa, D. (2011). Constructing an action agenda for community empowerment at the 7th Global Conference on Health Promotion in Nairobi. *Glob Health Promot, 17*(4), 52–56.

Fawcett, S. B., Schultz, J., Collie-Akers, V., Holt, C., & Watson-Thompson, J. (2016). Community development for population health and health equity. In P. Erwin & R. Brownson (Eds.), *Scutchfield and Keck's Principles of Public Health Practice* (4th ed., pp. 443–460). Cengage Learning.

Fisher, R., & DeFilippis, J. (2015). Community organizing in the United States. *Community Dev J, 50*(3), 363–379.

Fisher, R., DeFilippis, J., & Shragge, E. (2018). Contested community: A selected and critical history of community organizing. In R. A. Cnaan & C. Milofsky (Eds), *Handbook of Community Movements and Local Organizations in the 21st Century* (pp. 281–297). Springer.

Freudenberg, N., Franzosa, E., Chisholm, J., & Libman, K. (2015). New approaches for moving upstream: How state and local health departments can transform practice to reduce health inequalities. *Health Educ Behav, 42*(1_suppl), 46S–56S.

Gardner, J. W. (1991). *Building Communities*. John Gardner Papers (SC0908), Department of Special Collections and University Archives, Stanford University Libraries, Stanford, CA.

Gray, B. (1989). *Collaborating: Finding Common Ground for Multiparty Problems*. Jossey-Bass.

Hyatt, S. (2008). The Obama victory, asset-based development and the re-politicization of community organizing. *North American Dialogue, 11*(2), 17–26.

Iton, A., & Ross, R. K. (2017). Understanding how health happens: Your zip code is more important than your genetic code. In R. Callahan & D. Bhattachara (Eds.), *Public Health Leadership* (pp. 83–99). Routledge.

Kendi, I. X. (2019). *How to Be an Antiracist*. One World.

Kleba, M. E., Wallerstein, N., Belon, A. P., van der Donk, C., Gastaldo, D., Avery, H., & Wright, M. (2021). Empowerment and participatory health research. Position Paper 4. International Collaboration for Participatory Health Research.

Labonté, R. (1993). *Health Promotion and Empowerment: Practice Frameworks*. Centre for Health Promotion/Participation.

Labonté, R. (1995). Population health and health promotion: What do they have to say to each other? *Can J Public Health, 86*(3), 165–168.

Labonté, R. (1996). *Community Development in the Public Health Sector: The Possibilities of an Empowering Relationship between State and Civil Society* [Ph.D. dissertation, York University].

Labonté, R., & Robertson, A. (1996). Health promotion research and practice: The case for the constructivist paradigm. *Health Edu Q, 23*(4), 431–447.

Lyon, L. (1989). *The Community in Urban Society*. Lexington Books.

Marmot, M., Friel, S., Bell, R., Houweling, T. A., Taylor, S., & Commission on Social Determinants of Health (2008). Closing the gap in a generation: Health equity through action on the social determinants of health. *Lancet, 372*(9650), 1661–1669.

Mathie, A., Cameron, J., & Gibson, K. (2017). Asset-based and citizen-led development: Using a diffracted power lens to analyze the possibilities and challenges. *Prog Dev Stud, 17*(1), 54–66.

McKnight, J. (1987). Comments at Prevention Congress III. Waterloo, ON.

Mills, C. W. (1956). *The Power Elites*. Oxford University Press.

Minkler, M. (1994). Challenges for health promotion in the 1990s: Social inequities, empowerment, negative consequences, and the public good. *Am J of Health Promot, 8*(6), 403–413.

Minkler, M., Rebanal, R. D., Pearce, R., & Acosta, M. (2019). Growing equity and health equity in perilous times: Lessons from community organizers. *Health Educ Behav, 46*(1_suppl), 9S–18S.

Morgan, M. A., & Lifshay, J. (2006). Community engagement in public health. Contra Costa Department of Health Services, Public Health Division. http://www.barhii.org/resources/downloads/community_engagement.pdf.

Panet-Raymond, J. (1992). Partnership: Myth or reality? *Community Dev J, 27*(2), 156–165.

Pastor, M., Terriquez, V., & Lin, M. (2018). How community organizing promotes health equity, and how health equity affects organizing. *Health Aff, 37*(3), 358–363.

Raphael, D. (2010). Setting the stage: Why quality of life? Why health promotion? In D. Raphael (Ed.), *Health Promotion and Quality of Life in Canada: Essential Readings* (pp. 1–14). Canadian Scholars' Press.

Rifkin, S. B. (2012). Translating rhetoric to reality: A review of community participation in health policy over the last 60 years. In *Conference: WZB Social Science Center Berlin*. https://www.researchgate.net/publication/280386846_Rhetoric_to_Reality_a_review_of_community_participation_and_health_policy.

Robertson, A., & Minkler, M. (1994). New health promotion movement: A critical perspective. *Health Educ Q, 21*(3), 295–312.

Rothman, J. (2008). Multi modes of community intervention. In J. Rothman, J. L. Erlich, & J. E. Tropman (Eds.), *Strategies of Community Intervention* (7th ed., pp. 141–170). Eddie Bowers Publishing.

Rudolph, L., Caplan, J., Mitchell, C., Ben-Moshe, K., & Dillon, L. (2013). Health in all policies: Improving health through intersectoral collaboration. *NAM Perspectives*. Discussion Paper, National Academy of Medicine, Washington, DC. https://doi.org/10.31478/201309a.

Rupp, L. A., Zimmerman, M. A., Sly, K. W., Reischl, T. M., Thulin, E. J., Wyatt, T. A., & Stock, J. J. P. (2020). Community-engaged neighborhood revitalization and empowerment: Busy streets theory in action. *Am J of Community Psychol, 65*(1–2), 90–106.

Schutz, A., & Miller, M. (2015). *People Power: The Community Organizing Tradition of Saul Alinsky*. Vanderbilt University Press.

Sen, R. (2020, July 1). Why today's social revolutions include kale, medical care, and help with rent. Zócalo Public Square. https://www.zocalopublicsquare.org/2020/07/01/mutual-aid -societies-self-determination-pandemic-community-organizing/ideas/essay/.

Sherif, M. (1966). *Group Conflict and Cooperation*. Routledge and Kegan Paul.

Toronto Department of Public Health. (1994a). *Making Choices*. Toronto: Toronto Department of Public Health.

Toronto Department of Public Health. (1994b). *Making Communities*. Toronto: Toronto Department of Public Health.

Wallerstein, N. (1999). Power between evaluator and community: Research relationships within New Mexico's healthier communities. *Soc Sci Med, 49*(1), 39–53.

Walter, C., & Hyde, C. (2012). Community building practice: An expanded conceptual framework. In M. Minkler (Ed.), *Community Organizing and Community Building for Health and Welfare* (3rd ed., pp. 78–90). Rutgers University Press.

World Health Organization. (1986). *Ottawa Charter for Health Promotion*. WHO Europe.

8

Ethical Issues in Community Organizing and Capacity Building

MEREDITH MINKLER

CHERI A. PIES

PATRICIA WAKIMOTO

CHERYL A. HYDE

Fields such as public health and social work may be described as inescapably moral enterprises (Petrini, 2010), concerned as they are with determining what we as societies and communities ought to do to pursue the public's health and well-being. These social change professions are governed by codes of ethics that serve as primarily prescriptive guidelines for appropriate conduct; for example, see the Coalition of National Health Education Organizations (2020) and the National Association of Social Workers. Central to these codes are the core values of social justice, empowerment, participation, wellness, self-determination, dignity, and respect.

Ethical dilemmas can arise when core values come into conflict and as solutions are sought or an intervention is implemented (Harrington & Dolgoff, 2008; Long, 2018). Recognizing and resolving dilemmas are essential skills for practitioners, including community organizers, health educators, and capacity builders. And while there are numerous frameworks for ethical decision making, the process boils down to three essential elements: the means, the circumstances, and the ends being sought (Childress, 2020). In this chapter, we present some common ethical dilemmas in community practice.

When community organizer Saul Alinsky asserted "the ends justify the means," he essentially placed a higher value on what is accomplished than on how it is accomplished (Alinsky, 1971; chapter 5). This approach presents ethical questions and risks downplaying core values. We argue that community determination and participation are critical. Active involvement of people, beginning with their identification of their needs and goals, can result in improved communal ownership of an initiative, community capacity development, and reduced vulnerability to outside manipulation (Barsky, 2019; chapter 3; Hardina et al., 2015; Smith & Blumenthal, 2012; chapter 3). When community organizing is conceptualized as placing equal importance on means and ends, it can be clearly distinguished from other approaches, such as consultation and outside expert–driven planning (Arnstein, 2019).

The significant emphasis in organizing on fostering community self-determination may at first suggest that health and social work professionals may not need to engage in extensive ethical reflection. Despite lofty ambitions and guiding principles, the practice of community organization is in reality one of the most ethically problematic arenas in which practitioners work.

Those of us who are practitioners must first identify the circumstances that inform a community organizing effort. Such circumstances are the political, economic, cultural, and social contexts of an organizing campaign or intervention and may include the reasons why community mobilization is necessary in the first place. Second, we must work closely with community members and emphasize the importance of their lived experience as community experts, while helping them develop the skills to understand and respond to relevant opportunities or obstacles, as needed to be successful. Sometimes, conflicting circumstances generate ethical conflicts. Social factors, such as strong community networks that might support an organizing effort may be undermined by economic realities, which in turn may lead to competition among community subgroups for scarce resources. Important questions routinely arise, and whether and how we think about them can have critical implications for the process. For example, in the interest of authentic community participation and empowerment, how do we facilitate dialogue rather than direct it? How do we tease apart our own agenda from that of the community? And what happens when there are multiple, and often conflicting, community agendas?

This chapter explores six areas in which health educators, social workers, and other practitioners frequently experience tough ethical dilemmas in relation to community organizing and community building: (1) the eliciting of real, rather than symbolic, participation; (2) the challenges of conflicting priorities; (3) the dilemmas posed by funding sources, rules and regulatory organizations; (4) the perils of cultural conflict, including challenging the isms (racism, sexism, etc.); (5) the unanticipated consequences of organizing; and (6) the matter of whose "common good" is being addressed. We present case examples to illustrate factors that contribute to community-related ethical dilemmas, as well as possible strategies for resolution.

Community Participation: Real or Symbolic?

Community participation has historically been recognized as a central value in public health, social work, education, urban and regional planning, and other areas that emphasize organizing and capacity building (Corburn, 2009; Reisch & Garvin, 2016; Rivkin, 2014; appendix 6). In the 1970s, calls for "maximum feasible participation" coincided with the birth of the neighborhood health center movement

(DeBuono et al., 2007). Community or public participation, together with the concept of empowerment, emerged as the defining feature of the health promotion movement (Robertson & Minkler, 1994; chapter 3) and community capacity building efforts in fields such as public health, social work, community psychology, and urban and regional planning (Corburn, 2009, 2020; Wallerstein, 2006; chapter 11).

However, despite increased rhetoric of participation, acting on calls for high-level community involvement has proved difficult. As Siler-Wells (1989) pointed out, "Behind the euphemisms of participation and empowerment lay the realities of power, control and ownership" (p. 142). Even as we attempt to blur hierarchical distinctions by talking in the health field about health care "providers" and "consumers" and calling for partnerships between health professionals and communities, power imbalances remain.

In an attempt to bring clarity to issues of control and ownership, Arnstein (2019) developed a "ladder of participation." At the bottom rungs of the ladder are forms of "nonparticipation" (e.g., therapy and manipulation). In the middle, are several "degrees of tokenism" (e.g., placation, consultation, and informing), through which community members are heard and might have a voice, but their input is not necessarily heeded. Finally, the top rungs of the ladder are degrees of "citizen power" (e.g., partnership, delegated power, and finally, true power).

Morgan and Lifshay (2006; appendix 6) developed a "ladder of community participation in public health" specifically related to local health departments and the communities they serve. They acknowledged that in some circumstances (e.g., a sudden health emergency), the health department must call the shots. Even so, outcomes are more likely to be effective if top-down directives are built on a high degree of authentic prior partnership and trust between the health department and the community (appendix 6). Similarly, *not* attending to basic relationship building prior to the start of an initiative often leads to poorly realized outcomes once an effort is underway (Hyde et al., 2012).

Realistically, authentic community participation and determination are easier said than done, and it is in the gap between ideal and real that ethical dilemmas reside. Practice in the health promotion field often uses the rhetoric of high-level community participation. However, there is a tendency to operate at the lower rungs of the participation ladder, even as professionals "attempt to get people in the community to take ownership of a professionally defined health agenda" (Robertson & Minkler, 1994, p. 305; chapter 7).

Special challenges may arise when there are certain limiting conditions. In one example, the community was adolescent youth engaged in a school-based or after-school community organizing or youth participatory action research (YPAR) project. School district restrictions or parental concerns limited the extent to which youth could fully determine the agenda for action or the methods to be used (Ozer, 2017; Wilson et al., 2007). Psychologist and YPAR founder Emily Ozer and her colleagues borrowed the term *bounded empowerment* from organizational theory to capture the realities when goals and activities take place within limiting conditions, such as participants' legal status as minors and school districts' regulations (Ozer et al., 2013).

In other instances, a community's input may be sought and then discounted, further reinforcing unequal power relationships. As true partners in decisionmaking, community advisory boards (CABs) can make a real difference in the ways that practitioners approach community-based programs, initiatives, or research (Switzer et al., 2020). CABs can provide valuable input on community needs and strengths, the likely effectiveness of strategies, and cultural nuances and sensitivities that need to be respected and addressed. Increasingly, CABs are being established in response to a funding mandate or similar inducement, rather than out of a sincere concern for eliciting and acting on community input. In such instances, CABs often perceive that they are expected to rubber-stamp decisions that the outside professionals have already made.

Even programs committed to community participation through advisory boards and other means may occasionally find themselves ignoring input that conflicts with predetermined projects and plans. This can come at a considerable cost to earned trust and credibility in the community. An unfortunate example occurred in what was, in most respects, a national and global model for effective health promotion on multiple levels, and it underscores that even the best programs can slip into paternalistic ways of doing things on occasion, with negative results. The California Tobacco Control Program (CTCP) was created when a successful 1992 ballot initiative put a 25 cent tax on cigarettes and allocated a quarter of the money generated to anti-tobacco health education and advocacy. CTCP is extremely successful and has been a major contributor to the state's decline in cigarette smoking by nearly 60 percent since 1989 (California Department of Public Health, 2016, p. 6). When CTCP professionals designed a billboard aimed at the Black community, they showed it to their African American community advisory group. The billboard depicted a young Black man smoking a cigarette under the caption "Eric Jones just put a contract out on his family for $2.65. Secondhand smoke kills." Advisory group members perceived the ad as extremely racist and strongly urged against using it. Rather than heed the advice, CTCP ran the ad, only to receive the same kind of negative reaction from community members. The story is a poignant reminder that it is not enough to talk the talk of community competence and community participation. We must indeed be willing to walk the walk; in this case, trust in the CAB was needed to teach the outside experts how to avoid stigmatizing their community in the name of health promotion.

Evident in the "lessons learned" literature are the challenges to real community participation when community members are used in a tokenistic advisory or lip service capacity, leading to mistrust of outsiders and exclusion of essential perspectives (Hyde et al., 2012; Katz-Wise et al., 2019; Switzer et al., 2020). As professionals in public health, social work, and other fields, without a strong commitment to authentic community participation we risk undermining our future efforts and dissipating the often fragile trust that communities invest in us (chapter 9). Instead, genuine commitment to the concept of true partnership must serve as a guiding principle for ensuring meaningful community participation (Switzer et al., 2020).

Community organizers Herbert Rubin and Irene Rubin (1992, p. 77) offered a useful tool for applying guiding principles in the form of the "DARE" criteria of empowerment:

Who *Determines* the goals of the project?

Who *Acts* to achieve them?

Who *Receives* the benefits of the actions?

Who *Evaluates* the actions?

The more often we answer these questions by responding "the community," the more likely our efforts contribute to real community empowerment and high-level participation.

Conflicting Priorities

Conflicting priorities may arise when practitioners are responsible to a health or social service agency employer, the community being served by that agency, and a supporting funding source or program, and as they serve to both facilitate consumer participation in the agency and act as community advocates. From an agency perspective, the practitioner's role may be viewed as helping people choose from a narrow range of options that fit within the organization's or funder's predetermined goals. However, if agency agendas fail to adequately respond to community needs and desires, practitioners may face difficult ethical dilemmas deciding the degree to which they feel comfortable complying with agency expectations and directives.

Community self-determination and justice are two ethical precepts that lie at the heart of community organizing and building, and keeping them at the forefront in practice can help address dilemmas. Both precepts reflect an inherent faith in people's ability to accurately assess their strengths and needs and their right to act on these insights to set goals and determine strategies. They are reflected in the early reminder to "start where the people are" (Nyswander, 1956), a guiding principle in both health education and social work. But beginning with an issue that matters to the community, and using methods and approaches that reflect community wisdom and lived experience, may be easier said than done.

Consider an HIV/AIDS prevention program that has the goal of mobilizing a community around safer sex, medication adherence, and early diagnosis. If the program is embedded in a community that is more concerned about homophobia or the increasing rate of drug overdose deaths among young people, should the health professional put the agency's formal agenda on the back burner and truly start where the people are? Within the bounds of certain limiting conditions (as discussed later), our response is affirmative, since in choosing to start with the people's concerns, the practitioner asserts a commitment to the principles of self-determination and liberty, and the rights of individuals and communities to affirm and act on their own values.

Yet there is also a practical rationale for starting where the people are. When this ethical principle is followed, when trust in the community has been demonstrated, and when the immediate concerns of people have received primary attention, the organizer's original concerns are frequently seen by community members as relevant to their lives. Through active listening and thoughtful and probing questioning, the organizer may learn how the community perceives the agency's issues versus their own, and whether bridges or links can be formed when there are seemingly disparate agendas.

Conflicting priorities may surface when there are multiple communities or community factions that have different or competing agendas. For example, a community committed to preventing and addressing homelessness may be deeply torn over an effort to organize around a needle exchange program. A mixed-use residential community near a proposed site for a new "big box" store, such as Walmart or Home Depot, may be divided between residents who organize against this perceived threat to local businesses and traffic flow, and residents who prioritize a source of needed employment. Efforts to organize could generate more conflict and confrontation than consensus among community members. The question of whether a practitioner should intervene, and if so on what level and with what ethical precepts, takes on added importance.

Dilemmas Posed by Funding Sources, Rules, and Regulations

The restrictions that funders or other key stakeholders impose on community-based organizations are among the most frequently mentioned sources of ethical conflict (Fisher et al., 2018; chapter 20). Practitioners report that the rules of a resource provider or state regulatory agency may severely limit the type of and access to programs and activities. This requires community-based practitioners to continually assess and balance compliance at the possible risk of program accessibility and innovation.

In times of severe economic constraints, realities of scarce funding and the nature and source of the funding can severely limit the practice of starting where the people are. Decreased availability of government and foundation funding has sometimes resulted in community-based organizations and community coalitions having to accept financial support from controversial sources. When strings are attached to that funding, it can create real or perceived conflicts of interest for the community, and problems may intensify.

A well-known cautionary tale of risks that can come with funding from an ethically questionable source is associated with Mothers Against Drunk Driving (MADD). Founded nearly forty years ago, MADD has been identified as "one of the most successful public health grassroots citizen advocacy organizations in the

United States in the past century" (Fell and Voas, 2006, p. 195) and it remains the most powerful and prominent force behind DUI laws (Yu et al., 2020). When MADD accepted a $180,000 donation from Anheuser-Busch, the nation's largest beer manufacturer, affiliation with the alcohol industry was widely viewed as having compromised MADD's ability to take a strong stand on the liquor industry's role in the nation's alcohol problem (Marshall and Oleson 1994). In defense of MADD, Dejong and Russell (1995) pointed out the organization's leadership role in pushing for a national minimum drinking age and other policy changes opposed by the alcohol industry. Yet MADD did not significantly strengthen its position on alcohol advertising until some years later. After cutting the ties, it belatedly concluded that it "was truly not interested in solving problems due to the misuse of alcohol," despite its propaganda to the contrary (p. 234).

Even when money comes without apparent strings, conflicts between an agency or group's values and those of a potential financial sponsor may raise difficult ethical questions. For example, HIV/AIDS prevention organizations have been offered substantial financial support from alcohol and tobacco companies to underwrite events such as awareness walks and media campaigns. Similarly, communities fundraising for cash-strapped schools or community centers may benefit from corporate efforts to "give something back" to local communities via support for their sports activities (Bragg 2018; Coburn & McCafferty 2016). The support in turn provides opportunities to promote industries' interests in profiting through branding or advertising of less healthy options.

Nowhere is the influence of corporations on the community good more visible than during the Olympics. Coca-Cola has been a top corporate sponsor of the Olympics since 1928, and it recently extended its contract through 2032. The campaign aims to make the Olympics more approachable to children, teens, and millennials, portraying athletes as young people who enjoy having fun with friends. Digital platforms are used for targeting ads of Coke products in Coca-Cola's "Taste the Feeling" campaign to promote Olympic events. For the 2016 Olympics in Rio de Janeiro, Coca-Cola built a hangout space where teens could take photos with the Olympic Torch (Bragg et al., 2018).

Health professionals aware of the harmful health effects of sugary beverages (Malik & Hu, 2019) and of "lethal but legal" products, such as tobacco (Freudenberg, 2014), may view acceptance of certain corporate donations as morally or ethically untenable. Yet community-based groups may argue that all money is tainted, or they may agree with Saul Alinsky (1971) that the ends justify the means. When community coalitions are conflicted about whether to accept funding from a controversial source, practitioners may help by suggesting application of "the publicity test of ethics." This test involves having a group ask, "If the funding source for the project became known, would the group's integrity or reputation be damaged?" (chapter 20).

For donations from Big Tobacco and alcohol industries, "alternative sponsorship projects" have helped link health and social programs and organizing efforts with alternative corporate or other sources of financial assistance, and in the process deal a public relations blow to the companies. Although such programs are far less available today, some alternatives have emerged. For example, with a solid evidence base on the contributions of sodas and other sugary beverages to problems such as heart disease and diabetes (Malik & Hu, 2019), alternative funding has sometimes been secured through mechanisms like city soda tax revenues. Albeit still in their early stages, soda taxes typically place a one- to two-cent-per-ounce tax on sugar-sweetened beverages, with some of the revenue generated designated for community grants to groups supporting healthy food access and physical activity (Falbe et al., 2018). To date, few cities have passed such taxes, and funds distributed are often earmarked for new programs. A San Francisco soda tax measure failed in 2014, in part due to the immense fiscal resources and lobbying of the American Beverage Association (ABA), its monetary gifts to cash-strapped departments (e.g., sports and recreation), and a popular city supervisor (appendix II). These realities created conflicts of interest for actors who might otherwise have been strong supporters of the measure. Further, and while a revised measure did pass in San Francisco two years later, the ABA spent a total of $28 million to defeat three measures in nearby municipalities in 2016 alone (https://cspinet.org.resources /big-sodas-spending-spree-fight public-health-measures; appendix II).

Alternative funding strategies are important, especially in times of a recession, fiscal retrenchment in health and social services, and declining support for a whole host of worthy organizing endeavors, but they cannot solve the long-term funding needs. When needs are great, where should the line be drawn? And when community participation and empowerment are a value, who draws the line? When community members are offered a financial offer of assistance from a source that may pose ethical implications, practitioners are frequently confronted with the reaction, "We need the money so go for it!" Are we truly promoting community participation and empowerment if we disregard the community's desire to accept needed resources from a source that we consider problematic? Or will the community's long-run agenda be undermined if taking the money may at some point put constraints on decisionmaking, priority setting, or program direction? If we aim for promotion of the common good, how do we accomplish this in a climate of declining public funding and the concurrent pull of likely support from potentially problematic sources? These are important questions that health educators and other social change professionals encounter and need to address.

Where government or philanthropic funding has been received for a public health or social welfare project accenting community participation, dilemmas may arise in the face of change. The community's priorities may shift over time, or members' interest may wane before project completion. Should practitioners urge community groups to continue working on what is now a low priority to fulfill a funding mandate? Do they propose returning remaining money to the funders? We propose a third way, namely, approach the funding source about accepting the community's change in direction and continue to provide overall project support, particularly if the new direction is compatible with the funder's broader goals (e.g., to build healthy communities). Writing grants that emphasize community capacity building outcomes and processes is often a key role of the practitioner. Working with the community and funders, whenever shifts in the areas of concern to participants arise, is a critical means (albeit, not foolproof) of helping ensure funding continuity while still honoring community priorities.

Another set of ethical challenges may arise for community organizers working with nonprofit organizations in the United States that have tax-exempt 501(c)3 (nonprofit) status, and therefore are limited in the amount of lobbying activity in which they may engage (chapter 20). The California Senior Leaders Alliance (CSLA), a grassroots organization of older volunteer organizers and activists largely from underserved communities, wanted to move from general public and policymaker education to advocacy for bills benefiting low income elders. Its philanthropic funder was sympathetic but did not feel it could support the new activity, and when a newspaper cover story highlighted the work of the senior leaders at the state capitol as "lobbying," the group had to cease such work until alternative funding could be found. By raising individual donations for unrestricted use, and seeking an additional grant from a second foundation that was willing and able to support policy measure advocacy more directly, CSLA maintained its original funding while moving, with a new funding base, into advocacy arenas not previously sanctioned (Martinson et al., 2013; chapter 20).

Cultural Conflicts and the Isms

Professionals engaged in community organizing and capacity building frequently differ from the community members or constituent groups that they serve racially, ethnically, or culturally. With communities more diverse than ever, opportunities for misunderstandings, real or perceived racism, sexism, homophobia, or other problems arising between practitioners and the community or within communities, are plentiful. Practitioners must be willing to deal openly with their own isms as well as cross-cultural misunderstandings by employing critical organizing and capacity building skills of self-reflection (appendix 1), listening and dialoguing, and participatory engagement (chapters 5, 21). This requires juggling cultural norms and values of the community with broader ethical values grounded in egalitarianism or justice (Defilippis et al., 2010; Fisher et al., 2018; chapter 7) to avoid misunderstandings and loss of community trust.

Further, practitioners may need to address intragroup cultural conflicts because communities are rarely free of the isms (chapter 7). Discriminatory or culturally offensive statements and actions can emerge at any time in a community campaign, requiring practitioner dexterity in respecting the community's opinions or customs while creating a space for education or development. For one of us (Hyde), a fairly routine community meeting was made difficult when the group's leader began to make homophobic comments. Not wanting to confront the leader publicly, the practitioner chose to have a private, one-on-one conversation with this individual after the meeting to explain how hurtful those comments were. Because these two had already developed a solid working relationship, they were able to have an honest discussion and reach an agreement on how to proceed, which included the leader not offering her personal opinions that were so upsetting. Even though the practitioner lost an initial opportunity to address this with the group, the leader appreciated not being called out publicly in front of her members. Maintaining that relationship proved important in enabling the outside practitioner to later return to the group for a workshop on how to deal with various isms, including homophobic remarks. Building trust was prioritized over immediately addressing discriminatory comments, though they were examined within an educational and safe context.

When contentious public political discourse is frequent, a practitioner may need to assist a community or constituency group in dealing with hate speech directed their way. This requires the need to be adept at guiding community members toward ethical practices, especially when the initial tendency might be to return vitriol with more of the same. Practitioners who work with low-income people often contend with mean-spirited stereotypes directed toward that group, stereotypes that are typically laden with classist, racist, or sexist meaning.

Dealing with cultural conflict and isms cannot be fully or effectively done in communities unless agency staff and practitioners are also willing and able to deal with their own isms (Iton, 2006; Iton & Ross, 2017; chapter 9). Anti-racism trainings are not new. An excellent early example in 1997 involved building community–university–health agency partnerships in Greensboro, North Carolina, and Pittsburgh, Pennsylvania, which were grounded in anti-racism training and committed to addressing race-based disparities in cancer care (Eng et al., 2018). In the wake of widespread Black Lives Matter (BLM)-led protests of police brutality in 2020, increasing numbers of health departments, social service agencies, and university departments are holding mandatory anti-racist or dismantling/undoing racism trainings for their staffs (Came & Griffin, 2018; Iton & Ross, 2017; chapter 9). This is recognition that systemic interventions to dismantle racism and foster deep, internal changes in one's *own* attitudes, beliefs, and behaviors, in this case, among agency staff members, are prerequisites to effectively working within communities to address racial/ethnic health inequities (Iton & Ross, 2017; chapter 9; appendix 1).

Tools like McIntosh's (1989) classic (albeit sometimes criticized) "White Privilege" checklist and Hyde's framework for critical self-reflection on power and privilege (appendix 1), are useful to community practitioners attempting to better explore their own isms. DiAngelo's *White Fragility* (2018), Kendi's *How to Be an Antiracist* (2019), Came and Griffith's (2018; chapter 4) approach to "anti-racism praxis," and resources on cultivating cultural humility (Chávez, 2018; Greene-Moton &

Minkler, 2020; Judkis, 2020) are often considered integral to effective and culturally sensitive practice. The work is not easy, but current movements have opened new opportunities to educate and increase awareness and sensitivity.

Of all the isms, systemic racism is the most insidious, and it makes our attention to its many manifestations all the more critical. The 2020 resurgence of the BLM movement, brought on by a series of violent and often deadly police actions against Black people, thus raised critical ethical issues for White supporters. Too often, White activists and practitioners focus on their intentions without seeing how some aims can result in practices that inadvertently uphold White supremacy. This can be seen in instances of White paternalism and saviorism, the need to do good but in the process making the story about White experiences and benefits (Flaherty, 2016). Such developments can do significant harm to collective mobilizations like BLM because they divert attention away from actual racial injustices and the work done by people of color to combat injustices. Yet, because of the claim of good intentions, the self-serving aspect of White interests are difficult to confront as they appear to be and to some extent are supporters of causes such as racial justice and ending police brutality against Black and Brown people. This is one of the insidious ways in which white supremacy gets reproduced.

What, then, does it mean to be an ethical "White ally" (Minkler et al., 2019; Woods, 2014)? This is, in part, a call to decenter what is usually recognized as movement leadership from White individuals to Black activists. White supporters and proponents of BLM and related racial justice initiatives need to step back and redirect those who continue to prioritize a White lens, so that issues, experiences, and voices of Black people guide and ground change efforts. To do so necessitates cultural humility and mindfulness of White activists and willingness to hold other Whites accountable (Burghardt, 2014). It requires a hard look at one's own racial privilege (not just reading about how to do it) and how often this, even unknowingly, results in the views and actions of Whites receiving preferential attention that needs to be countered. Much of this work entails acknowledging the defensiveness and denial of self and other Whites regarding Black and Brown people's experiences with and responses to racism, along with intentionally challenging racist actions and sentiments of others. Yet, without doing this work of self-education and self-accountability, and without adopting a stance of supporting, rather than leading, multiracial coalitions and partnerships at the grassroots level will not flourish (Carruthers, 2018). Becoming a White ally means undertaking a deeply ethical commitment to engage in the challenging work of becoming an authentic anti-racist practitioner. In Kendi's (2019) words, "Being an antiracist requires persistent self-awareness, constant self-criticism, and regular self-examination."

The "Wall of Moms" in Portland, Oregon, learned this lesson the hard way. What began as a way of bringing mothers in this largely White city together to fight racism and other isms devolved into a "problematic but predictable place" when the group was called out for having far too many non-Black administrators, and a leader seen as using the group to further her own personal goals and visibility. As Cineas (2020) noted, "critics were quick to point out how the women managed to gain international acclaim *because* of the very privilege they were able to exercise while out on the front lines: whiteness. While whiteness was part of the tactic of getting noticed as many of the mothers were aware that their white bodies would yield attention and were intentional about their positioning at the protests, Black mothers, who have been losing their children to police violence at an alarming rate for decades, have received little attention for their activism." Although the White administrators resigned their posts to make room for Black and Indigenous women, the hurt felt by Black community members could have been avoided. Not surprisingly, many former Wall of Mom members abandoned it for a new group, Moms United for Black Lives, with 12,000 members by late July. The original Wall of Moms, meanwhile, used its Facebook page to urge White activists to "consider what skills you have to give, think about how you can participate without seeking rank or power, and welcome our new leadership."

Unanticipated Consequences

The guiding principles of fostering self-determination and meaningful participation can go a long way toward avoiding problems that can plague the community organizing process. Yet, even when these principles are followed, organizing efforts may result in unanticipated outcomes or by-products with negative consequences. Two examples are illustrative, one that focused on injury prevention campaigns and one that involved leadership and community organizing training of health workers.

Many recent prevention and health promotion campaigns have done an excellent job involving youth, people of color, LGBTQ groups, and other traditionally neglected communities in the design and pretesting of programs and materials aimed at better reaching these populations. However, health promotion and community organizing efforts often inadvertently reproduce and transmit problematic aspects of the dominant culture. A poignant example was observed by Caroline Wang (1992), in the stigmatization of people with disabilities that is often communicated through well-meaning injury-prevention campaigns. One in a series of billboards featured a teenager in a wheelchair with the caption, "If you think fourth period English is endless, try sitting in a wheelchair for the rest of your life!" Another that was captioned, "One for the road," showed a man on crutches with his leg partially amputated. As Wang points out, the implicit message in such ads is, "Don't let this happen to you!" or, in the words of a disabled person viewing these injury prevention ads, "I feel like I should be preventing myself" (Wang 1992).

The problem of inadvertent stigmatization in the name of public health also may be found as part of the "war on childhood obesity," which a former surgeon general likened to the war on terror following the 9/11 attacks. Author and self-described "fat person" Aubrey Gordon shares the example of a children's hospital in Atlanta, which took a cue from an earlier campaign against methamphetamines in crafting its anti–childhood obesity efforts (Gordon, 2020). The hospital's campaign used billboards with black and white pictures of sad-appearing overweight children and the captions, "WARNING: My fat may be funny to you, but it's killing me," and "WARNING: Fat prevention begins at home. And in the buffet line" (p. SR6). As someone first shamed by a pediatrician as a young child, and many times subsequently, and who frequently experienced depression and low self-esteem as a result, Gordon stated that even a popular and well-financed national campaign like Let's Move! "wasn't a campaign against foods with little nutritional value, or against the unchecked poverty that called for such low-cost, shelf-stable foods. *It was a campaign against a body type.*" In fields like public health, with a solid evidence base on the adverse consequences of obesity in children (Malik & Hu, 2019), the importance of educational campaigns and messaging that target the *social determinants of health* and not the overweight child, are essential to addressing the root causes of the problem without victim blaming in the process.

In some instances, the very nature of the processes involved in community organizing can have negative unanticipated consequences. The training of health promoters in low-resource communities provides a case in point. From a health education and a community organizing standpoint, the activities make eminent sense, as they typically identify and build on the strengths of natural helpers in a community and practice homophily, the idea that people learn best and prefer to receive services from people who are like themselves in race, social class, and other qualities. Many excellent models for community health worker training emphasize empowerment (Bracho et al., 2016; Eng et al., 2009) and employ methods such as Paulo Freire's "education for critical consciousness" (Freire, 1970; chapter 5). However, as Freire cautioned, leadership training can alienate community members by making them strangers in their own communities. Once trained and, in a sense, "indoctrinated" into the culture of the public health or social welfare organization or department, they may find it difficult to relate to or interact with peers as they had previously. In the case of an environmental health coalition in a Latino community, impressive local women were hired and trained as *promotoras* (lay health workers and organizers), but once hired, they were frequently referred to as *chismosas*, or gossips, by some older women. Some husbands were suspicious of their wives' new role in the community (Minkler et al., 2010). Is it the training they receive that gives them a new vocabulary and consequently a different way of addressing identified problems? Is it the fact that they feel unstated pressure to "fit in" to the agency that hired them, where most people are professionally trained and where the culture of the office environment is different from that of the community? Or is it that once they are identified as a community leader who tries to mobilize peers around an issue recognized as important, they are distrusted as being on the other side? How should we proceed when we are committed to involving indigenous community workers in education and organizing, yet aware that such efforts may alienate individuals and limit their credibility in the community?

In the environmental health coalition, the coalition head, a White male, began by going out for beer with local men to dispel suspicion about their wives and partners' involvement as *promotoras*. Additional outreach to other community members and establishment of a tutoring and training program for children dissipated initial suspicion of the *promotoras* and resulted in heavy community turnout at city council and other meetings, which in turn contributed to the achieved policy changes (Minkler et al., 2010).

Thoughts on the Common Good

Acknowledging and confronting ethical dilemmas may help enhance community capacity building and ultimately greater empowerment of community groups. When we start where the people are, we make every attempt to be responsive to the needs, concerns, and agendas of the community. We affirm a commitment to self-determination and liberty and promote the rights of individuals to act on their own values. But important questions remain: Do we have an ultimate end in our efforts of promoting and preserving the common good of the communities with which we work? If so, whose common good is being addressed, and who is determining what constitutes the common good? Finally, should we also be concerned with notions of common good that transcend local communities?

Alinsky (1971) long argued that a cardinal rule in effective community organizing is to appeal to self-interest; people will not organize unless they see what's in it for them. In the United States, which is characterized by a heavy accent on rugged individualism, stressing only self-interest may feed into an already impoverished notion of the common good. Contemporary thought leaders with left or right political leanings are largely in agreement that America has lost its sense of a common good, something that our dominant systems of capitalism and individualism make difficult at best. As Larry Churchill (1987) noted over thirty years ago, our very notions of justice are based on "a moral heritage in which answers to the questions 'what is good?' and 'what is right?' are lodged definitively in a powerful image of the individual as the only meaningful level of moral analysis" (p. 21). He argued that "a more realistic sense of community is one in which there are shared perceptions of the value of individual lives and a social commitment to protect them all equitably" (p. 101).

Lack of a genuine sense of community and a well-developed notion of the common good may be especially troubling for practitioners for whom a strong sense of social justice often lies at the base of their personal and professional values (chapter 1). Although an appeal to self-interest may be pragmatic in helping to mobilize a community for achievement of its self-interested goals, there are dangers associated with this limited approach. Key among these is the possibility that a local community group may fail to see or reflect on the connection between its goals and concerns and the broader need for social justice in a democratic society (Defilippis et al., 2010; Fisher et al., 2018; chapter 7).

Even though a focus on self-interest may be necessary from an organizing perspective, we argue that it is too narrow to be sufficient. Therefore, we advocate against an overly simplistic utilitarian notion of the common good that focuses solely on achieving the greatest good for the greatest number, because it may not truly reflect the ends that those engaged in community organizing are attempting to realize. Instead, we look to a definition of common or collective good that speaks both to local organizing efforts and to a broader vision of society.

The new era that began in 2020 included a COVID-19 pandemic, almost unprecedented economic losses, historic and continuing BLM protests over police killings of Black people, and a deeply contentious presidential election with deep distrust and sometimes violence between those who identified as "red" and "blue" rather than simply as Americans. The breaching of the Capitol on January 6, 2021, by an angry mob spurred on by then president Trump, designed to disrupt the certification of the election results he and his followers refused to accept, was the ultimate manifestation of this profound distrust. Immense pain occurred on multiple levels, is continuing, and will likely continue well into the future. But as discussed in chapter 1, this era has also seen renewed moral and ethical reflection. Practitioners who engage in organizing and other community-based work must be part of this discussion, reflection, and debate, both to understand the issues and to bring their perspectives to a dialogue that will be critical to the future of communities, community organizing, and community participation. Through such discussions, we can help demonstrate how community organizing can serve as a bridge to thinking more deeply about the collective good not only of this or that community but also of the broader society.

Conclusion

Throughout this chapter, we asked hard questions about values and ethics that go to the core of our practice as community organizers. However, all too often in practice, such reflection has been an afterthought, occurring when we are met with unanticipated dilemmas and painful ethical challenges. By making such reflection and dialogue an early and continuing part of our organizing efforts, we can enhance our ability to ensure that the actions we take in working with communities meet the criteria of ethically sound practice.

We have tried to address specific ethical dilemmas in this chapter but recognize that many others cannot be anticipated. We must commit ourselves to articulating the dilemmas we face in our practice, with special attention to recognizing contradictions with which we must cope and understanding where our responsibilities lie. But we must also identify and articulate the underlying values that drive our work. How do we communicate the importance of the values of community participation and empowerment when conflicting priorities present us with the task of meeting different needs and sometimes different and conflicting agendas? When our agencies or funders propose what is really only symbolic or lip service community participation and capacity building, how do we formulate effective values-based arguments to reinforce the importance of not only bringing community members to the table but ensuring that their input is both heard and heavily reflected in the final product? What role can we play in helping community groups reflect on their own values as a means of grappling with difficult dilemmas over issue selection or whether to accept funding from a potentially ethically problematic source? When systemic racism underlies so much of what takes place in the organizations for which we work, how are we to stand up for the need to get our own house in order, through anti-racist trainings and the like, before we can effectively partner with communities of color? Finally, what role can we play in helping communities to explore the connections between their perceptions of their own common good and a broader vision of society?

Although we cannot anticipate the possible consequences of all our actions, we can be confident that some consequences of our community organizing efforts will be different from what was expected. We must expect the unexpected and recognize that in the process, we are likely to find ourselves in ethically challenging situations that require discussion, dialogue, and difficult choices.

Questions for Further Discussion

1. Identify an ethical challenge that you had to contend with as a practitioner, or one a friend or colleague had to deal with. Did this dilemma get resolved in a satisfactory or unsatisfactory way, and why? What would you have done differently? What lessons might be learned?

2. Your health agency secured funding for you and a local public school to develop an afterschool empowerment program for diverse high school youth where they would learn and practice skills in community organizing. The project starts out beautifully, but when the majority of group members, including Latinx, select anti-immigrant bias as the area they want to organize around, things get tricky. A small group of Latinx students and the only two students from Muslim countries are worried that organizing around this issue could call attention to them and their parents, some of whom are undocumented. What steps might you take to help the students think through this dilemma? What ethical issues or precepts might guide you (and the group) as you think more deeply about it? And who else might you consult for guidance?

REFERENCES

Alinsky, S. D. (1971). *Rules for Radicals: A Practical Primer for Realistic Radicals.* Random House.

Arnstein, S. R. (2019). A ladder of citizen participation. *J Am Plann Assoc, 85*(1), 24–34.

Barsky, A. E. (2019). Practice, values, and ethics—social work with communities. In *Ethics and Values in Social Work* (2nd ed., pp. 214–243). Oxford University Press.

Bracho, A., Lee, G., Giraldo, G. P., De Prado, R. M., & Latino Health Access. (2016). *Recruiting the Heart, Training the Brain: The Work of Latino Health Access.* Hesperian Health Guides.

Bragg, M. A., Roberto, C. A., Harris, J. L., Brownell, K. D., & Elbel, B. (2018). Marketing food and beverages to youth through sports. *J Adolesc Health, 62*(1), 5–13.

Burghardt, S. (2014). *Macro Practice in Social work for the 21st Century* (2nd ed.). Sage.

California Department of Public Health. Tobacco Control Program. (2016). *Tobacco Facts and Figures 2016.* California Department of Public Health.

Came, H., & Griffith, D. (2018). Tackling racism as a "wicked" public health problem: Enabling allies in anti-racism praxis. *Soc Sci Med, 199,* 181–188.

Carruthers, C. (2018). *Unapologetic: A Black, Queer, and Feminist Mandate for Radical Movements.* Beacon Press.

Chávez, V. (2018). Cultural humility: Reflections and relevance for CBPR. In N. Wallerstein, B. Duran, J. G. Oetzel, & M. Minkler (Eds.), *Community-Based Participatory Research for Health: Advancing Social and Health Equity* (3rd ed., pp. 357–362). Jossey-Bass.

Childress, J. F. (2020). *Public Bioethics: Principles and Problems.* Oxford University Press.

Churchill, L. (1987). *Rationing Health Care in America: Perceptions and Principles of Justice.* University of Notre Dame Press.

Cineas, F. (2020, July 19). How Portland's Wall of Moms collapsed—and was reborn under Black leadership. Vox. https://www.vox.com/21353939/portland-wall-of-moms-collapses-to-form -moms-united-for-black-lives.

Coalition of National Health Education Organizations. (2020). *Code of Ethics for the Health Education Profession.* Coalition of National Health Education Organizations. http://cnheo .org/ethics-of-the-profession.html.

Coburn, A., and McCafferty, P. (2016). The real Olympic Games: Sponsorship, schools, and the Olympics—the case of Coca-Cola. *Taboo: J Culture Educ, 15*(1), 5.

Corburn, J. (2009). *Toward the Healthy City: People, Places, and the Politics of Urban Planning.* MIT Press.

Corburn, J. (2020). Street science: Community knowledge for global health equity. In *Oxford Research Encyclopedia of Global Public Health.* Oxford University Press. https://oxfordre.com /publichealth/view/10.1093/acrefore/9780190632366.001.0001/acrefore-9780190632366 -e-265.

DeBuono, B., Gonzalez, A. R., & Rosenbaum, S. (2007). *Moments in Leadership: Case Studies in Public Health Policy and Practice.* Pfizer.

DeFilippis, J., Fisher, R., & Shragge, E. (2010). *Contesting Community: The Limits and Potential of Local Organizing.* Rutgers University Press.

Dejong, W., & Russell, A. (1995). MADD's position on alcohol advertising: A response to Marshal and Oleson. *J Public Health Policy, 16*(2), 231–238.

DiAngelo, R. (2018). *White Fragility: Why It's So Hard for White People to Talk about Racism.* Beacon Press.

Eng, E., Rhodes, S., & Parker, E. A. (2009). Natural helper models to enhance a community's health and competence. In R. J. DiClemente, R. A. Crosby, & M. C. Kegler (Eds.), *Emerging Theories in Health Promotion Practice and Research* (2nd ed., pp. 303–330). Jossey-Bass.

Eng, E., Schaal, J., Baker, S., Black, K. Cykert, S., Jones, N., Lightfoot, A., Robertson, L., Samuel, C., Smith, B., & Thatcher, K. (2018). Partnership, transparency, and accountability: Changing systems to enhance racial equity in cancer care and outcomes. In N. Wallerstein, B. Duran, J. G. Oetzel, & M. Minkler (Eds.), *Community-Based Participatory Research for Health: Advancing Social and Health Equity* (3rd ed., pp. 107–121). Jossey-Bass.

Falbe, J., Minkler, M., Dean, R., & Cordeiero, J. (2018). Power mapping: A useful tool for understanding the policy environment and its application to a local soda tax initiative. In N. Wallerstein, B. Duran, J. G. Oetzel, & M. Minkler (Eds.), *Community-Based Participatory Research for Health: Advancing Social and Health Equity* (3rd ed., pp. 405–410). Jossey-Bass.

Fell, J. C., & Voas, R. B. (2006). Mothers against Drunk Driving (MADD): The first 25 years. *Traffic Inj Prev, 7*(3), 195–212.

Fisher, R., DeFilippis, J., & Shragge, E. (2018). Contested community: A selected and critical history of community organizing. In R. Cnaan & C. Milofsky (Eds.), *Handbook of Community Movements and Local Organizations in the 21st Century* (pp. 281–297). Springer.

Flaherty, J. (2016). *No More Heroes: Grassroots Challenges to the Savior Mentality.* AK Press.

Freire, P. (1970). *Pedagogy of the Oppressed.* Translated by M. B. Ramos. Seabury Press.

Freudenberg, N. (2014). *Lethal but Legal: Corporations, Consumption, and Protecting Public Health.* Oxford University Press.

Gordon, A. (2020, November 13). Leave fat kids alone. *New York Times Sunday Review.* https://www.nytimes.com/2020/11/13/opinion/sunday/childhood-obesity-health.html.

Greene-Moton, E., & Minkler, M. (2020). Cultural competence or cultural humility? Moving beyond the debate. *Health Promot Pract, 21*(1), 142–145.

Hardina, D., Jendian, M., & White, C. (2015). Tactical decision-making: Community organizers describe ethical considerations in social action campaigns. *J Sociol Soc Welf, 42*(1), 73–94.

Harrington, D., & Dolgoff, R. (2008). Hierarchies of ethical principles for ethical decision making in social work. *Ethics Social Welfare, 2*(2), 183–196.

Hyde, C. A., Hopkins, K., and Meyer, M. (2012). Pre-capacity building in loosely-coupled collaborations: Setting the stage for future initiatives. *Gateways: International Journal of Community Research and Engagement, 5*, 76–97.

Iton, A. (2006). Tackling the root causes of health disparities through community capacity building. In R. Hofrichter (Ed.), *Tackling Health Inequities through Public Health Practice: A Handbook for Action* (pp. 115–136). National Association of County and City Health Officials.

Iton, A., & Ross, R. K. (2017). Understanding how health happens: Your zip code is more important than your genetic code. In R. Callahan & D. Bhattachara (Eds.), *Public Health Leadership* (pp. 83–99). Routledge.

Judkis, M. (2020, July 8). Anti-racism trainers were ready for the moment. Is everyone else? *Washington Post.* https://www.washingtonpost.com/lifestyle/style/anti-racism-trainers-were-ready-for-this-moment-is-everyone-else/2020/07/07/df2d39ea-b582-11ea-a510-55bf26485c93_story.html.

Katz-Wise, S. L., Pullen Sansfaçon, A., Bogart, L. M., Rosal, M. C., Ehrensaft, D., Goldman, R. E., & Bryn Austin, S. (2019). Lessons from a community-based participatory research study with transgender and gender nonconforming youth and their families. *Action Res, 17*(2), 186–207.

Kendi, I. X. (2019). *How to Be an Antiracist.* One World.

Long, D. D. (2018). Practice-informed research: Contemporary challenges and ethical decision-making. *J Soc Work Pract, 15*(2).

Malik, V. S., & Hu, F. B. (2019). Sugar-sweetened beverages and cardiometabolic health: An update of the evidence. *Nutrients, 11*(8), 1840.

Marshall, M., & Oleson, A. (1994). In the pink: MADD and public health policy in the 1990s. *J Public Health Policy, 15*(1), 54–68.

Martinson, M., Minkler, M., & Garcia, A. (2013). Honoring, training, and building a statewide network of elder activists: The California Senior Leaders Program (2002–2012). *J Commun Pract, 21*(4), 327–355.

McIntosh, P. (1989, July–August). White privilege: Unpacking the invisible knapsack. *Peace and Freedom,* 10–12. https://www.racialequitytools.org/resourcefiles/mcintosh.pdf.

Minkler, M., Garcia, A. P., Williams, J., LoPresti, T., & Lilly, J. (2010). Sí se puede: Using participatory research to promote environmental justice in a Latino community in San Diego, California. *J Urban Health, 87*(5), 796–812.

Minkler, M., Rebanal, R. D., Pearce, R., & Acosta, M. (2019). Growing equity and health equity in perilous times: Lessons from community organizers. *Health Educ Behav, 46*(1_suppl), 9S–18S.

Morgan, M. A., & Lifshay, J. (2006). *Community Engagement in Public Health.* Contra Costa Department of Health Services, Public Health Division.

Nyswander, D. (1956, November). Education for health: Some principles and their application. *California Health, 14,* 65–70.

Ozer, E. J. (2017). Youth-led participatory action research: Overview and potential for enhancing adolescent development. *Child Dev Perspect, 11*(3), 173–177.

Ozer, E. J., Newlan, S., Douglas, L., & Hubbard, E. (2013). "Bounded" empowerment: Analyzing tensions in the practice of youth-led participatory research in urban public schools. *Am J Community Psychol, 52*(1–2), 13–26.

Petrini, C. (2010). Ethics-based public health policy? *Am J Public Health, 100*(2), 197–198.

Reisch, M., & Garvin, C. D. (2016). *Social Work and Social Justice: Concepts, Challenges, and Strategies.* Oxford University Press.

Rivkin, S. (2014). Examining the links between community participation and health outcomes: A review of the literature. *Health Policy Plann, 29* (suppl_2), ii98–ii106.

Robertson, A., & Minkler, M. (1994). New health promotion movement: A critical perspective. *Health Educ Q, 21*(3), 295–312.

Rubin, H., & Rubin, I. (1992). *Community Organizing and Development* (2nd ed.). Macmillan.

Siler-Wells, G. L. (1989). Challenges of the Gordian Knot: Community health in Canada. In *International Symposium on Community Participation and Empowerment Strategies in Health Promotion* (pp. 42–55). Center for Interdisciplinary Studies, University of Bielefeld.

Smith, S., & Blumenthal, D. (2012). Community health workers support community based participatory research ethics: Lessons learned along the research-to-practice-to-community continuum. *J Health Care Poor Underserved, 23,* 77–87.

Switzer, S., Carusone, S. C., Guta, A., & Strike, C. (2020). *Lessons Learned for Designing a Flexible, Activity-Based Community Advisory Committee for People Living with HIV Who Use Drugs.* Sage.

Wallerstein, N. (2006, February). *What Is the Evidence on Effectiveness of Empowerment to Improve Health?* Health Evidence Network Report. WHO Regional Office for Europe. https://www.euro.who.int/__data/assets/pdf_file/0010/74656/E88086.pdf.

Wang, C. (1992). Culture, meaning, and disability: Injury prevention campaigns in the production of stigma. *Soc Sci Med, 35*(9), 1093–1102.

Wilson, N., Dasho, S., Martin, A., Wallerstein, N., Wang, C., & Minkler, M. (2007). Engaging young adolescents in social action through Photovoice: The youth empowerment strategies (YES!) project. *J Early Adolesc, 27*(2), 241–261.

Woods, J. (2014, August 19). 12 ways to be a white ally to Black people. *The Root.* https://www.theroot.com/12-ways-to-be-a-white-ally-to-black-people-1790876784.

Yu, J., Jennings, E. T., & Butler, J. S. (2020). Lobbying, learning and policy reinvention: An examination of the American states' drunk driving laws. *J Public Policy, 40*(2), 259–279.

9

Communities Driving Change

A Case Study from King County's Communities of Opportunity

ROXANA CHEN

KIRSTEN WYSEN

BLISHDA LACET

WHITNEY JOHNSON

STEPHANIE A. FARQUHAR

The past two decades have seen growing calls for community health department partnerships to study and address health equity, while in the process building community power and capacity (Butterfoss & Kegler, 2012; Wolff et al., 2017). Yet the call for community partnerships coming from health departments and funders has been met, in many communities, with the response that before authentic partnerships can be formed, local health departments and funding agencies must look inward, examining their own personal and professional beliefs, behavior, and assumptions. Particularly important, and in a spirit of cultural humility, these potential partners must acknowledge and address structural racism and demonstrate a genuine commitment to power sharing as prerequisites to success in partnering with low income communities of color and other often disenfranchised communities they serve (Iton & Ross, 2017; Minkler et al., 2019; Wolff et al., 2017).

In 2014, this recognition led community leaders, staff, and leadership from Public Health—Seattle & King County (PHSKC) and the Seattle Foundation to come together to create Communities of Opportunity (COO), investing in community partnerships and community-driven strategies that aimed to increase housing, health, and economic equity in King County, Washington.

From the beginning, the COO initiative aimed to promote equity by shifting power to community leaders. As noted elsewhere in the literature, these types of initiatives must prioritize leadership by those most affected by injustice and inequity in order to effect structural and systemic changes (Freudenberg et al., 2015; Iton & Ross, 2017; Wolff et al., 2017). As part of this process, the community-led partnership demanded new roles, skills, capacities, and relationships from the local health department. The PHSKC partner has contributed to this process by making changes in the health department's decisionmaking, grant contracts, evaluation and performance monitoring, staffing, and capacity building processes. In this chapter, we provide a case study that describes COO's launch and evolution, and the experiences of two COO-funded projects: the Transgender Economic Equity Coalition and Seattle Urban Native Nonprofits (SUNN). We share our successes, the challenges faced, and lessons learned in hopes of accelerating the shift among other local health departments to community-driven practice.

Communities of Opportunity: Genesis and Evolution

Since its inception in 2014, staff from the local health department (PHSKC) have worked with community and philanthropic leaders to invest in community partnerships and community-driven strategies that aim to increase housing, health, and economic equity in King County, Washington. With an initial investment of $2.5 million funded by philanthropy and local government, COO expanded to include support from a local property tax levy, "Best Starts for Kids" (BSK), passed in November 2015. Its initial focus was on geographic areas where COO's index of health and well-being were in the lowest fortieth percentile (index indicators included obesity, adverse childhood experiences, poor housing, smoking, diabetes, 200% poverty rate, frequent mental distress, life expectancy, and unemployment). Community leaders were adamant that asset-based framing be used and that their neighborhoods not be known by their deficits. Consequently, and consistent with Kretzmann & McKnight's (1993) "asset-based community development" approach (chapter 11) the phrase "Communities of Opportunity" was coined.

COO was governed by a fourteen-member decisionmaking group with community leaders in the majority (ten community representatives and four funder representatives from the Seattle Foundation and the health department). This composition of the leadership group provided an opportunity to rethink cultural humility as including the entrenched culture of the public health professional, which, when done well, requires humility in partnering with families and communities (Tervalon & Murray-Garcia, 1998). The health department and the Seattle Foundation representatives were required to wake up to the realities of groups with whom they were working to allow the partnership to flourish (Greene-Moton & Minkler, 2020).

Since 2014, COO has awarded over $15 million to nine place-based and cultural community partnerships, which included sixty-eight organizational partners, and over a hundred organizations through its systems and policy change funding. The funds were allocated through competitive request for proposal (RFP) processes, and four new Learning Community programs. A Learning Community, or community of shared practice, creates spaces for communities and organizations to share their work and gain skills to advance their impact across the region.

Challenging Institutional Racism: Best Starts for Kids (BSK)

Communities of Opportunity leads with racial equity, openly naming past and current governmental structural racism. This chapter provides examples of corrective actions taken by the health department. The COO team at the health department worked to counteract these systems by changing internal institutional processes. Community leaders and the Seattle Foundation saw a willingness within county government to shift away from practices such as typical contracting rules, which created advantages for larger organizations and did little to close racial and geographic gaps. New grant-making processes offered technical assistance (TA) for applicants as they prepared proposals, simplified contract monitoring procedures, worked with funded partners to identify data and evaluation measures, and offered post-award coaching, thereby "increasing community capacity to shape outcomes" (Best Starts for Kids Blog, 2017a, 2017b).

Co-creating Strategies and Outcome Measures

Similar to informing the grant review and contracting processes, the COO Governance Group helped to shape COO's outcome measures that guide the initiative goals (see box 9.1). In 2014, before the first COO grants were made, a small group of community leaders who were from and worked with Seattle communities partnered with PHSKC to develop a new kind of RFP. Monthly meetings took place at a community development association building half an hour south of Seattle, a location central for community partners, and called for centering racial equity and recognizing community power. One community leader asked government and philanthropy staff to listen and be ready to shift.

To avoid a familiar pattern from past rounds of health department and foundation funding, the group of community leaders urged the county and the Seattle Foundation to release short RFPs (four pages), ask for short proposals (four pages),

---

BOX 9.1

Communities of Opportunity Goals

Thrive economically—Workforce development that included local hires, support of new local businesses, and inclusion of youth

Have quality affordable housing—Preservation and development of affordable housing close to transit, jobs, and education

Are connected to community—Increased civic participation and engagement, cultural preservation, and access to safe public spaces

Are healthy—Access to healthy, affordable food and safe places outside to be physically active, especially for youth offer site visits to finalists, and give several weeks to respond so that applicants had time to coordinate with other organizations. The group strongly recommended that funder staff conduct site visits with finalists to ensure that an authentic local partnership was in place. They had seen too many grants and contracts in the past go to larger organizations able to hire talented grant writers but unable to engage in real partnerships with community members. As Freudenberg et al. (2015) note, "Redistributing the power and wealth that shape health will require health departments and universities to provide . . . more autonomy to engage key players without political interference" (p. 51S). COO funding supported many community organizations whose leaders in turn helped county and foundation staff navigate complex local political situations (Communities of Opportunity, 2015). As constituents, the community members often had better access to elected leaders than did staff from county departments. When the county's BSK levy was developed in 2015 to improve well-being for children, families, and the communities they live in, community leaders helped get out the vote and were credited with helping secure its passage. Ten percent of these new revenues went toward supporting and expanding COO—$6.5 million each year for the six years of the levy. COO received an additional $600,000 each year from the Seattle Foundation to support its systems and policy change efforts (Communities of Opportunity, 2015).

Early Grantees

Tony To, the executive director of Community Organization, HomeSight Washington, was stunned when he read a new RFP from the COO partnership between Seattle Foundation and King County government in June 2014. The announcement was focused on communities in South Seattle and South King County, which he knew experienced significant social, racial, and economic inequities, and would fund strategies *devised and led by the people affected.* Tony had worked in the Rainier Valley in Southeast Seattle for twenty years, pulling together grants from the city, federal government, and private foundations to improve the neighborhood. HomeSight and organizational partners in the Rainier Valley went on to be funded as one of COO's original place-based community partnerships.

Michael Woo, a founder of Got Green, a local nonprofit working on food access, youth leadership development, and climate justice noted that "the Communities of Opportunity funding approach is a game changer. Communities have well-defined priorities and need the resources to act on them" (King County Press Release, 2015). Got Green received funding to develop paid internship programs for youth to advance the goal of diversifying the workforce in the environmental sector.

A third grantee, the Somali Health Board, was also able to navigate a streamlined granting process and received COO funding. The Somali Health Board had been working with PHSKC since 2012 to foster two-way communication between local Somali residents, the health department, and the health care system. With

COO funding, the Somali Health Board was able to lead a coalition of ten racial and ethnic health boards to create a joint policy agenda to improve health equity. Partners included health boards sponsored by Latinx, Ethiopian, Eritrean, Vietnamese, Iraqi/Arab, African American, Cambodian, Cham, Congolese, and Pacific Islander health advocates. In the words of one community health board member, "We believe the Community Health Board model will cultivate broad participation, advocacy and input [because they are] led by health professionals representing communities of color. It is our communities, after all, that experience a disproportionate share of inequities in health, housing and economic opportunity. It is imperative that our voices are represented at policy making tables" (Somali Health Board, 2018).

The next section highlights two COO-funded projects. The case studies were selected because they highlight the role of the health department in supporting community-driven work as well as the special considerations of these types of partnerships.

Case Study I: Transgender Economic Empowerment Coalition (TEEC)

Although COO started with a focus on place-based partnerships, PHSKC and the Seattle Foundation recognized that displacement was adversely impacting the ability of cultural communities to maintain geographic cohesion. With that in mind, COO released an RFP that included supporting cultural community partnerships not bound by geography. The application defined cultural communities as group(s) of people who share characteristics in common *and* experience adverse health and well-being outcomes. COO funded two cultural communities: the transgender/gender diverse (T/GD) community and Urban Native–led nonprofits in King County.

The Transgender Economic Empowerment Coalition (TEEC) is a coalition of organizations led by T/GD people and LGBTQ people of color, with the goal of empowering the T/GD community. When TEEC applied for COO funding, they were not confident that they would be funded. King County government and philanthropy funded LGBTQ communities but lacked a strong track record in funding T/GD organizations. In their proposal (2018), TEEC wrote the following: "We know working in coalition as organizations led by LGBTQ folks and specifically centering the leadership of transgender-led and LGBTQ people of color–led organizations, we are best suited to find solutions that address economic inequities that impact access to community connections, housing resources, affordable LGBTQ affirming healthcare" (TEEC, https://www.teecwa.org/). According to the executive director of the Ingersoll Gender Center, the lead agency for TEEC's COO funding, this was at the time one of the largest national awards ever for a regionally focused transgender-led organization. COO staff and PHSKC's RFP review committee, which included community partners, were impressed with how TEEC clearly articulated the T/GD community's needs and their commitment to ensuring that the T/GD community be heard and counted.

TEEC had a bold vision of this work being led by T/GD for T/GD people in King County. TEEC also understood the intersectionality of race, gender, sexual orientation, and gender identity. Thus, the activities chosen by TEEC sought to impact racism, transphobia, and homophobia. Unfortunately, like the many local health departments, PHSKC had limited quantitative data on the inequities that we knew were impacting the transgender community. However, in their application, TEEC was able to demonstrate the inequities faced by their community drawing from state and national sources. The data showed, for example, that 28 percent of transgender people live in poverty, and that number grows to 38 percent and 43 percent for Black and Latinx T/GD groups, respectively (James et al., 2016).

TEEC was focusing its efforts on advocating for policies and programs that support T/GD people returning from jail or prison to address the very high housing instability this population faces. Indeed, even among the general population of recently released persons, rates of unstable housing well above 70 percent are not uncommon (deVouno-Powell et al., 2018; Remster, 2019). TEEC was most recently working on building a youth advisory group to ensure that TEEC's policies and programs address the challenges youth are facing. To inform their implementation activities and help fill the data gap in T/GD communities, TEEC used COO funds and evaluation technical assistance provided by PHSKC to COO grantees, to develop and administer an assessment on economic status, education, employment history, experience with discrimination, and other areas. Completed by over 300 individuals, the survey provided a wealth of findings on the economic challenges and lived experiences of the T/GD community in King County and was analyzed with the help of a trans graduate student from the University of Washington. Key among the findings of the assessment survey (n = 351), were that 50 percent of respondents were employed full time, 13 percent were employed part time, and over 8 percent were unemployed, as compared to an unemployment rate of 3 percent in Seattle (TEEC, https://www.teecwa.org/). These findings were shared with TEEC members and other T/GD-serving partners to increase visibility of the issues impacting the T/GD community. TEEC also conducted an employer survey with over a hundred respondents to gauge employers' competency levels around gender-inclusion policies. Based on the findings, TEEC also developed an employment model policy, and employers began assessing their own policies and working with TEEC to ensure that T/GD employees felt safe and welcomed in their place of employment. Many of TEEC's organization partners are part of a King County working group trying to help the County figure out how to better serve LGBTQ persons—including providing avenues to get better data on trans experiences in King County.

Despite these and other successes over the past two years, TEEC also had to overcome some challenges. The lead organization that received and administered the funds had to be temporarily transferred from the Ingersoll Gender Center, a transgender-led organization that had served as the lead applicant on the proposal, to the Greater Seattle Business Association (GSBA), Washington State's LGBTQ and allied chamber of commerce. Although Ingersoll Gender Center was the lead applicant on the proposal, it, and most of the other trans-led organizations comprising TEEC, lacked the infrastructure to manage large government funding. The GSBA, a member of TEEC, took on the role of fiscal agent for the partnership. It was important to TEEC, however, that this work be led by a T/GD organization. The PHSKC/ COO was also committed to supporting trans-led partnership and worked with Ingersoll to develop the internal controls and systems needed to effectively manage large grants. Consequently, Ingersoll was able to return to the role of fiscal agent in the implementation phase of their work during 2018–2021. This commitment to TA and capacity building assistance to organizations is a common practice across COO.

Case Study 2: Seattle Urban Native Nonprofits (SUNN)

King County occupies Native lands and is home to a vibrant urban Indian community. However, this community has experienced persistent disparities rooted in historical oppression and institutional racism, including the expulsion, exclusion, and violence directed at the Duwamish and other tribal communities in the region. The impacts of the historic and ongoing legacy of colonization include unequitable access to funding and resources; gaps in culturally responsive services, investments, and programming; inadequate physical space dedicated to urban Indian communities; inadequate recognition and representation in decisionmaking; and continued violence. American Indian / Alaska Native (AI/AN) rates of heart disease, diabetes, low birth rate, and alcohol use (binge drinking) are higher than those for the general population (King County United Way, 2014).

With COO support, the Seattle Urban Native Nonprofits (SUNN), a fourteen-member leadership roundtable of nonprofit organizations serving the Native community, tackled the challenges facing Indigenous people in King County. The SUNN collaborative represented a unified public voice that advances equity for all its members and for the Native community throughout King County, envisioning an urban Native community "united in spirit and practice, trusting and compassionate in our relationships, and fully embracing the ancient wisdom and healing that will sustain us for generations" (Best Starts for Kids, 2019, p. 27).

With funding from COO to ensure that all members of the SUNN collaborative (i.e., organizations, groups, and individuals) are compensated for their time, wisdom, and commitment, SUNN was able to follow a deliberative process to (1) create a cohesive and unified policy agenda and platform; (2) create and sustain a visible presence; (3) strengthen and enhance the inherent skills of the SUNN collaborative; (4) develop a dedicated, motivated, and empowered base of community advocates; and (5) foster long-term sustainability and a collective vision. COO supported SUNN's vision through funding, trainings, and PHSKC staff support, which allowed SUNN the time and resources to build its organizational capacities, communications, and emerging policy platform. SUNN helped to convene community members from across King County and created new opportunities for Native professionals to collaborate and engage. Over a hundred people regularly attended SUNN's monthly events (which moved to virtual due to COVID-19), strengthening networks and relationships. These events were a time for members of the Native community to celebrate their history and traditions, support each other's work, and share their assets and challenges with decisionmakers and potential funders.

SUNN created a space for smaller organizations to join with larger organizations, amplifying the former's role in decisionmaking and their ability to advocate on behalf of the communities with which they worked. One such organization is the Native American Women's Dialog on Infant Mortality (NAWDIM) collective. NAWDIM was organized in 2000 by Native women and allies in Seattle/King County out of concern about AI/AN infant mortality rates in King County. NAWDIM members come from Native-led organizations, such as Seattle Indian Health Board and United Indians of All Tribes Foundation, as well as allies such as Open Arms Perinatal Services and PHSKC. NAWDIM is dedicated to Indigenous infant and cultural survival and engages community members and policymakers through critical dialogue, advocacy, education, and cultural activities, such as infant cradleboard classes. Cradleboards are a traditional practice in which an infant is secured to a frame with blankets or straps for sleeping or transport.

Another SUNN collaborative partner, Red Eagle Soaring Native Youth Theatre (RES), seeks to "empower AI/AN youth to express themselves with confidence and clarity through traditional and contemporary performing arts" (Red Eagle Soaring, n.d.). Seattle Indigenous Youth Arts & Performance (SIYAP) is a summer theatre workshop offered by RES in which youth explore and express themselves through traditional and contemporary performing arts and take creative action on issues affecting their lives. SIYAP's recent production, "Crack in the Wheel" (https://www.youtube.com/watch?v=DUXU_AbLHUY), integrated the healing power of Native arts and cultural lifeways that promote social, physical, and intellectual engagement.

SUNN collaborative partners also advanced policies to address the needs of urban AI/ANs. For example, the Seattle Indian Health Board educated policymakers about the need for behavioral health services that are accessible and appropriate to the Native community. These services included traditional and culturally specific peer support groups and addiction resources. Chief Seattle Club worked with All Home, a local organization working on Seattle's homeless crisis, to address the undercounting of Native populations experiencing homelessness during the annual Point-in-Time (PIT) Count. The primary purpose of the annual PIT Count— locally known as Count Us In—is to collect data on the needs of people experiencing homelessness and to spark action. A successful and accurate PIT Count that includes members of our AI/AN community is an essential component to informing our system response to homelessness.

From "Business as Usual" to High-Level Partnership: Changes in PHSKC's Processes

TEEC and SUNN's commitment to community-driven solutions has required that the local health department shift from doing business as usual to being the true partner that they demand. The first step was to name and acknowledge inequitable policies and practices that contributed to community distrust. For example, many of the trans/LGBTQ and Native organizations that comprised these two organizations had little experience or success in applying for or receiving health department funding. One way to rectify this was for PHSKC to hire capacity building consultants who provided technical assistance to grantees in writing their proposals. The RFP review process included community partners who reflected the communities PHSKC sought to reach, and all reviewers participated in an anti-bias training that was tailored for King County prior to reviewing applications.

To build the capacity of organizations, applicants who were not awarded grants were given the opportunity to meet with PHSKC staff to receive feedback on their proposal. Awarded partnerships were also able to access 25 percent of their first-year budget to assist with any start-up costs. This was vital for smaller organizations that tend to lack the financial reserves necessary for spending their own money up front and then waiting for reimbursement. In addition, PHSKC shifted from a cost reimbursement model to setting up a payment schedule where grantees receive the same payment amount monthly. The consistent monthly payments allowed organizations to better manage their cash flow.

The health department made a commitment to hire staff who reflected the communities we seek to serve. All strategy leads and the COO director are women of color, 80 percent of COO are BIPOC (Black, Indigenous, people of color) and 90 percent are residents of King County. PHSKC staff further viewed grantees as the experts of their communities and moved away from a more transactional approach to contract monitoring. Grantees thus met regularly with health department staff; these meetings provided grantees an opportunity to share their concerns about the initiative and to receive technical assistance. Staff conducted site visits to better understand partners' capacity for completing the contracted work and to identify ways to support the partners in meeting their goals. Site visits provided space for shared learning. Finally, when the COVID-19 pandemic hit, disproportionately impacting communities of color, followed by protests prompted by the murder of George Floyd and the killings of other unarmed Black people in the United States, the local health department was impelled to officially declare racism a public health crisis (Hayes, 2020). PHSKC recognized this as another opportunity to review our processes. In response to the pandemic, staff worked with community partners to adjust their timelines by moving grant deliverables to later in the contract period. Grantees were allowed to modify their scopes of work to respond to the immediate COVID-19 needs of their communities. Knowing that timelines would be impacted by social distancing and the need to work virtually,

COO offered grantees an opportunity to extend their contracts, allowing them more time to complete deliverables. Grantees were provided additional funding to help mitigate the challenges of working remotely, support staff and community needs, and maintain or expand on their work.

What's Next? A Community-Designed and COO-Funded Learning Community

While the COO partnerships have logged a considerable number of successes, including making some gains in the outcomes listed in box 9.1 (notably workforce development and increased civic engagement), there remain unresolved and deep challenges, including the following:

— How can the COO initiative counteract the strong forces of residential displacement and the suburbanization of poverty?
— Are investment levels enough to measurably respond to the challenges faced by low-income neighborhoods that are home to people of color?
— How can the business sector be brought more fully into this work on terms defined by the community?
— What is the best way to evaluate COO's institutional support for social change?

COO recognizes that this is an important and trying moment. In King County and across the country, people are fighting for greater justice, opportunity, and well-being on multiple fronts. COO's goal was, and remains, to provide resources that seed and strengthen ideas, make transformation real, dismantle embedded racial injustices, and provide platforms for connecting, learning, and networking. In fact, many public health departments, including Alameda County Public Health Department, New York City's Department of Health and Mental Hygiene, Multnomah County Health Department, and Public Health Madison & Dane County, have embedded racial equity and anti-bias work within their institutions. Toward this end, Alameda developed a Public Health 101 series that includes a module on undoing racism, a leadership fellows' program, and a strategic planning process that explicitly focused on addressing structural racism (Bingham et al., 2017).

In 2019, COO launched its Learning Community activities to build organizational capacities and fund community-driven and led innovations. Activities included Learning Circle cohorts focused on collaborative capacity building to support organizations' efforts in specific topic areas (e.g., economic and real estate development), skills-building trainings open to all community organizations on various topics (e.g., conflict resolution), an Equitable Development Summit, and Learning Community's Commercial Affordability Pilot, which sought to increase community ownership and support business owners at risk of displacement. In August 2020, PHSKC released two RFAs through COO's Learning Community arm, with two more RFAs to follow. The intention for the "Learning from Community

Stories—the Impact of COVID-19" RFA is to provide an opportunity to illustrate positive community resilience in response to the pandemic in BIPOC communities, and dismantle racism and oppression that lead to inequities (Griffith et al., 2007; Kendi, 2019). The funds provide an opportunity for groups to tell the stories of the intersections of the pandemic in low-income / communities of color / immigrant-refugee communities by collecting and analyzing data related to the health, social, and economic impacts of COVID-19. The Community of Practice RFA will support a contractor or organization to codesign with PHSKC staff a Community of Practice peer learning group for the lead agencies of COO partnerships. The group is intended to be a space to engage in peer learning and facilitated conversations to practice effective techniques and skills to build partnerships with deeper relationship, trust, and conflict resolution skills. As we all continue to adjust to relying more on virtual platforms for engagement, outreach and learning, and working within the preventive measures needed to be safe amid the COVID-19 pandemic, COO leadership will continue to look to its partners to help guide this work.

Conclusion and Lessons Learned

As one of our project partners noted early on, "'Go slow to go fast." The work of building a solid community–agency team with clear, shared outcomes is a key factor in COO's success. When health departments and funders reject relationships built on power imbalances and shift power to communities, they create the space for community leadership to cocreate goals and strategies with lasting impact. As illustrated in our TEEC and SUNN case studies, our communities and community organizations are best suited to identifying community-felt concerns and effective actions. Support from local health departments in the form of financial and staff resources and technical assistance can help propel this effort. Healthy community work based on sharing power and resources with community leaders has required our large health department to reflect, create, and make concrete and long-term changes to internal processes. The result is partnerships with a broader reach and the potential for more sustained change.

Questions for Further Discussion

1. What are some of the ways in which intentionally "going slow" might take place in a partnership? Thinking back on your own experience or that of an organization you are familiar with, can you think of an instance that illustrated how going slow enabled going fast?
2. The chapter states that COO funding–supported community organizations could navigate local political situations because the community had better access to elected officials than county staff. What are some of the ethical considerations here for the county? For the community organizations?

REFERENCES

Best Starts for Kids. (2019). *2018 Best Starts for Kids Annual Report*. https://kingcounty.gov/~ /media/depts/community-human-services/best-starts-kids/documents/2018%20 Best%20Starts%20for%20Kids%20Annual%20Report%20-%20Full.ashx.

Best Starts for Kids Blog. (2017a, October 12). Meet our technical assistance providers! https:// beststartsblog.com/2017/10/12/technical-assistance.

Best Starts for Kids Blog. (2017b, October 20). Watch the COO Systems & Policy Change Grants Webinar. https://beststartsblog.com/2017/10/20/coo-systems-policy-change-grants -webinar/.

Bingham, J., Gowler, R., Schaff, K., Gaonkar, R., Nelson, J., & Noor, S. (2017). Advancing racial equity: Strategic interventions using the leverage and power of local public health departments. *Nat Civic Rev, 106*(3), 48–54.

Butterfoss, F. D., & Kegler, M. C. (2012). A coalition model for community action. In M. Minkler (Ed.), *Community Organizing and Community Building for Health and Welfare* (3rd ed., pp. 309–328). Rutgers University Press.

Communities of Opportunity. (2015, November 30). People governance meeting materials. https://www.coopartnerships.org/meeting-materials/2018/7/17/2015-meeting-materials.

deVouno-Powell, S., Minkler, M., Bissell, E., Walker, T., Vaughn, L., & Moore, E. (2018). Criminal justice reform through participatory action research. In N. Wallerstein, B. Duran, J. G. Oetzel, & M. Minkler (Eds.), *Community-Based Participatory Research for Health: Advancing Social and Health Equity* (3rd ed., pp. 305–320). Jossey-Bass.

Freudenberg, N., Franzosa, E., Chisholm, J., & Libman, K. (2015). New approaches for moving upstream: How state and local health departments can transform practice to reduce health inequalities. *Health Educ Behav, 42*(1_suppl), 46S–56S.

Greene-Moton, E., & Minkler, M. (2020). Cultural competence or cultural humility? Moving beyond the debate. *Health Promot Pract, 21*(1), 142–145.

Griffith, D. M., Mason, M., Yonas, M., Eng, E., Jeffries, V., Plihcik, S., & Parks, B. (2007). Dismantling institutional racism: Theory and action. *Am J Community Psychol, 39*(3–4), 381–392.

Hayes, P. (2020, June 11). Racism is a public health crisis: The transformation starts here. It starts with us. *Public Health Insider*. https://publichealthinsider.com/2020/06/11/racism-is -a-public-health-crisis/.

Iton, A., & Ross, R. K. (2017). Understanding how health happens: Your zip code is more important than your genetic code. In R. Callahan & D. Bhattacharya (Eds.), *Public Health Leadership* (pp. 83–99). Routledge.

James, S., Herman, J., Rankin, S., Keisling, M., Mottet, L., & Anafi, M. A. (2016). *The Report of the 2015 US Transgender Survey*. National Center for Transgender Equality. https://trans equality.org/sites/default/files/docs/usts/USTS-Full-Report-Dec17.pdf.

Kendi, I. X. (2019). *How to Be an Antiracist*. One World.

King County. (2015, February 10). Press Release. The Seattle Foundation and King County to invest $1.5 million to expand successful community efforts that confront increasing inequity. https://kingcounty.gov/elected/executive/constantine/news/release/2015/Febru ary/10-opportunity-grants.aspx.

King County United Way. (2014). Assessment of assets and opportunities of the King County urban Indian population. https://philanthropynw.org/sites/default/files/files/events/A%20 Vision%20for%20the%20Urban%20Indian%20Community%20Report.pdf.

Kretzmann, J. P., & McKnight, J. L. (1993). *Building Communities from the Inside Out: A Path toward Finding and Mobilizing a Community's Assets*. Institute for Policy Research.

Minkler, M., Rebanal, R. D., Pearce, R., & Acosta, M. (2019). Growing equity and health equity in perilous times: Lessons from community organizers. *Health Educ Behav, 46*(1_supp), 9S–18S.

National Academies of Sciences, Engineering, and Medicine (NASEM). (2017). *Communities in Action: Pathways to Health Equity.* National Academies Press.

Red Eagle Soaring. (n.d.). Red Eagle Soaring Native Youth Theatre. https://www.redeaglesoaring .org/.

Remster, B. (2019). A life course analysis of homeless shelter use among the formerly incarcerated. *Justice Q, 36*(3), 437–465.

Somali Health Board. (2018). *2017 Annual Report.* https://somalihealthboard.org/wp-content /uploads/2019/01/annual-report-SHB-2017.pdf.

Tervalon, M., & Murray-Garcia, J. (1998). Cultural humility versus cultural competence: A critical distinction in defining physician training outcomes in multicultural education. *J Health Care Poor Underserved, 9*(2), 117–125.

Wolff, T., Minkler, M., Wolfe, S. M., Berkowitz, B., Bowen, L., Butterfoss, F. D., Christens, B. D., Francisco, V. T., Himmelman, S. T., & Lee, K.S. (2017). Collaborating for equity and justice: Moving beyond collective impact. *Nonprofit Q, 9,* 42–53.

PART FOUR

Community Assessment and Issue Selection

Fields such as public health, social work, and city and regional planning typically focus considerable attention on needs assessment and use a variety of methods to determine the problems and needs experienced by the groups or communities involved. Increasingly, however, the importance of shifting our gaze from a narrowly conceived needs assessment to a broader community assessment has been realized. Reflecting this change in emphasis, the first two chapters in this part of the book provide approaches to community assessment that go well beyond needs assessment as it is typically conceived and indeed reject the narrow needs assessment approach as rooted in a "deficit thinking" mentality that can harm, rather than enhance, efforts at community organizing and community building for health.

Trevor Hancock and Meredith Minkler begin in chapter 10 by posing a series of questions that get to the heart of the whys and hows of community assessment for health. Drawing in part on the former's extensive experience as a key architect of the healthy cities movement worldwide, they suggest that the very focus of such efforts should move from community health assessment to *healthy community assessment* if we are to pay adequate attention to the numerous factors affecting the health and well-being of communities. Arguing that community assessments are needed, not only for the information they provide for and about change but also for empowerment, the authors make the case for assessment that is truly of, by, and for the community. Expanding on John McKnight's oft-expressed belief that "institutions learn from studies, communities learn from stories," they further point to the need for collecting both stories and more traditional study data as part of a comprehensive assessment process.

Hancock and Minkler use Sylvia Marti-Costa and Irma Serrano-Garcia's (1983) classic categorization of assessment techniques according to the degree of contact with community members they entail (no contact, minimal contact, etc.) as a framework within which to explore a wide range of assessment techniques and approaches. The chapter makes a strong case for the use of multiple methods, with an accent placed on those methods, such as the development and use of community or neighborhood indicators (appendix 4) that can help individuals and communities become more empowered, in part through their active involvement in and ownership of the assessment process.

A critical part of the shift from a needs assessment to a community assessment focus involves appreciating that communities are not simply collections of needs or problems but vital entities possessing many strengths and assets. Chapter 11 presents and updates a classic contribution to the community assessment literature, namely, John Kretzmann and John McKnight's (1993) approach to "mapping community capacity." Pointing out that the needs-focused approach to low-income communities has led to deficiency-oriented policies and programs, they propose instead a capacity-oriented model (McKnight & Russell, 2018).

Their community mapping technique looks first to "primary building blocks"– those assets such as people and their talents and associations–located in the neighborhood and largely under its control. But they also have us consider nonprofit organizations, local businesses, and the like that are located in the neighborhood and that, although largely controlled by outsiders, nevertheless may constitute important "secondary building blocks."

Finally, and to further expand our thinking, Lionel J. Beaulieu, professor of rural and regional development at Purdue University, joins McKnight and Kretzmann in this new edition, adding both his perspectives on the utility of asset mapping in rural places and an additional set of assets, Flora and Flora's (2008) seven "community capitals." These include some already familiar concepts, such as social capital (Moore & Kawachi, 2017), and the built environment, but add others, such as natural capital, in reference to "the landscape, air, water, soil, and biodiversity of a community," which in turn are linked to weather and a healthy ecosystem (Beaulieu, 2014). Although this chapter addresses itself to geographic communities, the approach it demonstrates can clearly be adapted for use in a workplace or common interest community as well.

Closely connected to community assessment is working with communities in ways that enable the communities, rather than outsiders, to determine the goals and issues around which they wish to mobilize. In chapter 12, the final chapter in this part, veteran organizers and activists Lee Staples and Rinku Sen draw our attention to the pivotal area of issue selection with communities. Echoing a theme that runs throughout much of the book, Staples and Sen argue that issues should indeed come from the members and potential members of a community. At the same time, they see outside organizers as having a useful role to play in helping community groups become familiar with the criteria of "good issues" so that they can select issues for action that measure up against these important yardsticks for success. As the authors suggest, a good issue is one about which the community feels deeply. But it is also an issue that is winnable, provides opportunities for leadership development and broad-based member participation, and is consistent with the long-range goals and strategies of the organization (Sen, 2003; Staples, 2016; appendix 10).

Using diverse examples from social work and health-related organizing efforts in the United States, the authors describe and illustrate the process of "cutting" the issue and how this and related processes fit within the conduct of a broader strategic analysis (appendixes 10, 11). Four core concerns are discussed: appealing to diverse constituencies, testing alternative possible solutions and coming up with strong goals and objectives, selecting the right targets, and finding the "handles" (e.g., laws, regulatory processes, or broken campaign promises) that can be used to open an opportunity for change. The need for careful strategic analysis is also emphasized here, and illustrated elsewhere (chapter 19; appendix 11), as a critical part of the organizer's tool kit.

REFERENCES

Beaulieu, L. J. (2014, October). Promoting community vitality and sustainability: The Community Capitals Framework. Purdue University Center for Regional Development. https://docplayer .net/48294421-Community-vitality-sustainability-the-community-capitals-framework .html.

Flora, C. B., & Flora, J. L. (2008). *Rural Communities: Legacy and Change* (3rd ed.). Westview Press.

Kretzmann, J. P., & McKnight, J. L. (1993). *Building Communities from the Inside Out: A Path toward Finding and Mobilizing a Community's Assets*. ACTA Publications.

Marti-Costa, M., & Serrano-Garcia, I. (1983). Needs assessment and community development: An ideological perspective. *Prev Hum Serv, 2*(4), 75–88.

McKnight, J. L., & Russell, C. (2018). The four essential elements of an asset-based community development process. What is distinctive about asset-based community process? ABCD Institute, DePaul University.

Moore, S., & Kawachi, I. (2017). Twenty years of social capital and health research: A glossary. *J Epidemiol Community Health, 71*(5), 513–517.

Sen, R. (2003). *Stir It Up: Lessons in Community Organizing and Advocacy.* Jossey-Bass.

Staples, L. (2016). *Roots to Power: A Manual for Grassroots Organizing* (3rd ed.). Praeger.

10

Community Health Assessment or Healthy Community Assessment

Whose Community? Whose Health? Whose Assessment?

TREVOR HANCOCK

MEREDITH MINKLER

Many questions should be asked concerning the performance of a community health assessment. In this chapter, we discuss a number of these questions and provide examples of assessment processes that we believe illustrate promising approaches. As our title implies, we believe that to be truly empowering and health promoting, assessment should be of the community, by the community, and for the community.

Why Assess?

In a seminal article written almost forty years ago, Marti-Costa and Serrano-Garcia (1983) argued that, far from being neutral or objective, needs assessment is, in reality, an ideological process that can serve political purposes ranging from system maintenance and control to the promotion of social change and consciousness-raising. At one end of the ideological continuum are needs assessments designed to support and justify the status quo. Although they may include some efforts at "fine tuning" the way the system functions, they do not question or wish to change the ideological commitments on which that system is based (Marti-Costa & Serrano-Garcia, 1983). The health educator trying to increase attendance at agency-sponsored community health fairs, for example, might well conduct an assessment to determine whether the event's hours and location were problematic for local residents. But if the agency had already committed to health fairs as its modus operandi for community health outreach, the health educator would not be expected—or wanted—to determine residents' perceptions of whether the fairs really addressed their primary health needs.

In contrast, an assessment open to higher-level change would actively involve community residents not only in helping the agency or organization critically rethink its mission and activities, but in becoming more skilled and empowered themselves in the process. As Marti-Costa and Serrano-Garcia (1983) have suggested, such an assessment would have the following purposes:

- Measure, describe, and understand community lifestyles
- Assess community resources to lessen external dependency
- Return needs assessment data to facilitate residents' decisionmaking
- Provide skill training, leadership, and organizational skills
- Facilitate collective activities and group mobilization
- Enable consciousness-raising

Clearly, the values and assumptions underlying this process heavily influence the choice of assessment techniques, the interventions proposed, the utilization of data obtained, and the perceptions of who owns the data in the first place.

Rationale behind Community Health Assessment

For professionals concerned with community organizing and community building for health and welfare, there are two reasons for the imperative placed on effective and comprehensive community health assessments: information is needed both for change and for empowerment.

Information for Change

The first kind of information has three purposes: to stimulate change or action, to monitor change or action, and to assess the impact of change (Hancock et al., 1999). Information that will stimulate change must carry "social and political punch." Such information includes hard data and stories that point out differences, particularly inequalities in health and the social and environmental determinants of health among different groups and sectors in the community. Given the short-term basis of much social and political action, such data also must be sensitive to short-term change, focusing on inequalities where there is a reasonable chance of seeing some change in a comparatively brief time period. Although it is critical to document differences in mortality rates for lung cancer or heart disease, for example, this needs to be balanced by information on people's perceived state of health, their social and physical living conditions, and their behaviors, all of which may be more likely to reflect changes in the short term following some policy or community action.

The change rationale for community assessment also involves the need for information about the processes of change or of action. As a result, such assessment must put a heavy accent on stories and observations that can help unearth, for example, potential precursors to change. These might include widespread community knowledge of a new project, the establishment of participatory mechanisms (e.g., intersectoral committees), evidence of the development of new skills (e.g., in leadership and media advocacy), and indicators of political commitment to the project at the local level. Such intermediate-level activities may in turn lead to other actions (e.g., health-promoting policies) that will ultimately lead to better health.

Information that will assess the impact of change on health can function as a baseline of the individual and community dimensions of health. Here health is defined broadly to include physical, mental, and social well-being in both subjective and objective terms. Regular repetitions of the baseline measures via surveys and other instruments must be conducted to assess change.

Information for Empowerment

An entirely different, but equally important reason for wanting information about health is that knowledge is power and is thus a vital component of empowerment. As discussed in chapter 3, the process of empowerment is central to the World Health Organization's (WHO) (1986) definition of health promotion. Individuals and communities can become truly empowered only if they have the knowledge required to assess their situation and to take action—backed by sufficient power— to make change happen. The most obvious way of defining and obtaining information is to ask the community itself for its definition of a good or healthy community. In so doing, the health promotion professional may learn of important, yet often neglected, components about which information should be collected. But by asking the community how to define health, assess progress, and measure change, the health professional is also helping to further the process of empowerment.

A useful illustration of this approach may be found in the Building Healthy Communities initiative of The California Endowment (TCE), one of the largest philanthropic organizations in the United States, that for over ten years has committed 80 percent of its funding to enabling fourteen low-income neighborhoods and their community organizers and partners to radically reimagine and rebuild their communities. The initiative began from TCE's premise (Iton & Ross, 2017) that a person's zip code should not be their most important "health number" (more important than their blood pressure, cholesterol level, etc.) and asked and listened to the experts—local residents—to find out "what their neighborhoods look and feel like when they're healthy and when they're not" (www.TCE.org). The findings of the healthy community assessments they supported in community after community mirrored much of what public health professionals, city planners, and academic researchers already knew. These included, for example, the facts that kids won't do well academically if they go to school hungry, and that "neighbors won't get to know and trust each other unless they have common places to exercise, talk and meet up" (www.TCE.org; Iton & Ross, 2017). When community members were *at the center* of such assessments, however, and of reimagining their collective visions for their own healthy community—and when sufficient resources were provided to help—many important and sustainable changes took place on the community level as well as through the policy level (Iton & Ross, 2017; Minkler et al., 2010, 2012; Pastor et al., 2018; chapter 2).

Knowing how well one's community functions, how much it cares about the well-being and quality of life of its citizens, and how choices that affect health are made—and by whom—enables people to more fully and actively participate in the life of the community (Arnstein, 2019; Diers, 2004).

Whose Community, Whose Health?

We have referred thus far to "the community." But as earlier chapters have suggested, the real question is, "Whose community are we referring to?" Professionals working with geographic communities often focus on a particular neighborhood, and this is indeed the level with which people tend to identify. Yet, since one of the intents of the healthy city or community process is to stimulate local government involvement in and commitment to improving the health of the community, the boundaries for assessment may also be municipal. The first challenge, then, is to assess the healthy community process and situation at both the municipal and the community or neighborhood levels.

A second challenge is to conceptualize health in a broad enough manner that we can look well beyond such traditional indicators as morbidity and mortality to embrace the WHO's (1948) view of health as "a state of complete physical, mental and social well-being, and not merely the absence of disease and infirmity." As discussed below, community members often have creative and meaningful ways of conceptualizing health for themselves. The challenge for the health professional is to pay more attention to how the members of the community define health and to incorporate their definitions for assessing the health of the community.

Needs or Capacities?

Professor and community builder John McKnight (Kretzmann & McKnight, 1993; chapter 11) describes the importance of the "associational life," or the informal and formal community-based organizations and networks that form the underpinnings of the community. This is similar to what Robert Putnam (2000) calls "civicness" or social solidarity (Moore & Kawachi, 2017). McKnight and his colleagues have been particularly concerned with having professionals change their focus from individual and community deficits that require services to assets and capacities, including such "community capitals" as natural capital and the built environment (Flora & Flora, 2008) that enable community building (chapter 11).

The implications of such a 180-degree shift in how we view people and communities are profound. For they suggest that we should re-evaluate the entire way in which we conceive of the role of professionals in the community—as enablers and facilitators rather than as providers of services—and the purpose of those services. From the perspective of assessment of the community's health, McKnight's approach has two important implications. First, it underscores the importance of assessing capacity and not merely "needs," and second, it reminds us that *the process of that assessment* should itself contribute to the capacity of people and communities and to community health.

McKnight and his colleagues' approach (chapter 11) provides a useful corrective in ensuring that we don't in the process fail to engage communities themselves in identifying their assets, as well as the challenges they face. As Seattle-based community builder Jim Diers (2004) notes, "Communities have a knack for converting a problem into an asset, whether it is a graffiti-covered wall, a vacant lot, an abandoned building, a dead tree, garden waste, . . . or incessant rain" (p. 171). Community garden plots, of which an estimated 29,000 exist in parks in the 100 largest U.S. cities alone (The Trust for the Public Land, 2020), provide one such potent example. Community development, capacity building with respect to gardening and nutrition, economic development, intergenerational and intercultural action, improved nutrition, and the creation of green space are among the many benefits associated with these gardens (Ong et al., 2019; Ozer, 2007).

In emphasizing the importance of a focus on community assets and strengths, we do not mean to diminish the importance of also recognizing and addressing the very real needs faced by communities, particularly during times of large-scale health and social crises and diminishing resources. Early in the COVID-19 pandemic, for example, the Richmond, California–based Safe Return Project of, by, and for currently and formerly incarcerated persons and their families and communities, conducted a respectful online needs assessment of their members, asking questions such as the following: What are you most concerned about during this time? How has this situation impacted the quality of life in your community? What does support look like for you and your family during this time (e.g., food, rent, utilities, childcare, medications)? Members were then asked if any of their needs were urgent, and if so, how much money they would need to address them. The online survey asked about others in their care (e.g., children, people with disabilities, a child returned from college, foster youth, an elder or newborn, and currently or formerly incarcerated loved ones). Finally, participants were asked, *"How do you think we can get more support for our community?"* That last question implicitly underscored the Safe Return Project's appreciation of the lived experience and often deep community understanding of its members (deVuono-Powell et al., 2018), and invited their involvement in helping their community through an unprecedented time, and one particularly hard for currently and formerly incarcerated persons (www.safereturnprj.org).

Community Health Assessment or Healthy Community Assessment?

To understand the difference between a community health assessment and a healthy community assessment, it is necessary to begin with a clear understanding of the meaning of the term *healthy community*. The most commonly accepted definition was developed by Hancock and Duhl (1986, p. 24) for the WHO and continues to be used in the Healthy Cities movement globally and locally, as well as by numerous government and nongovernmental organizations (NGOs), coalitions, and funders: "A healthy [community] is one that is continually creating and improving those physical and social environments and expanding those community resources which enable people to mutually support each other in performing all the functions of life and in developing to their maximum potential."

As this definition suggests, a healthy community is a process, not a status. Although low mortality and morbidity are important, a healthy community is not necessarily one that has the highest health status in a conventional sense, but one that is striving with every fiber of its being to be more healthy. Ideally, this would be reflected in a commitment at all levels from the political to the personal, across all sectors, and involving all stakeholders around the common focus of improving the health, well-being, and quality of life of the community and its members. The closer a community is to this ideal, the closer it is to being a healthy community.

Almost forty years ago, and based on a wide range of literature, Hancock and Duhl (1986) suggested the following eleven key elements of a healthy community, which have stood the test of time:

1. A clean, safe, high-quality environment (including housing quality)
2. An ecosystem that is stable now and sustainable in the long term
3. A strong, mutually supportive, and nonexploitative community
4. A high degree of public participation in and control over the decisions affecting one's life, health, and well-being
5. The meeting of basic needs (food, water, shelter, income, safety, work) for all the city's people
6. Access to a wide variety of experiences and resources, with the possibility of multiple contacts, interaction, and communication
7. A diverse, vital, and innovative city economy
8. Encouragement of connectedness with the past, with the cultural and biological heritage, and with other groups and individuals
9. A city form that is compatible with and enhances the preceding parameters and behaviors
10. An optimum level of appropriate public health and sick care services accessible to all
11. High health status (both high positive health status and low disease status)

Importantly, *only one of these 11 refers directly to health status*, which is the usual focus of a community health assessment.

A good place to begin a healthy community assessment is to consider the classical epidemiological elements of place, time, and person. Here, however, *place* refers to the geography and environment of the community, *time* refers to its history and development, and *person* refers to the demographic profile of the community. Much can be learned about a community's health by understanding these three elements. The community's geography will reveal factors likely to affect health, such as climate, natural resources (especially water and food sources), natural hazards, air and water quality, and wind direction, all of which usually define where low-income populations will live (downwind, downstream, and downhill—or uphill if the hills are dangerous!). The community's history provides important information on the major economic, political, and social forces that have shaped the community's evolution and that explain many of the present circumstances that influence the health of the community. Finally, the community's present demography—such factors as age and gender distribution, and racial/ethnic and socioeconomic characteristics—provides further information that enables us to anticipate some of the health-related issues facing the community.

Specific issues can be examined regarding each of the eleven components of a healthy community and others that are considered important by the community.

- Do people in the community have access to such basic prerequisites for health as food, shelter, education, clean water and air, clean and safe environments, and sustainable resources?
- What is the degree of equity (or inequity) in the community?
- How strong is civic or associational life?
- How do urban design and architecture affect health in this community?
- What is being done to improve health?
- How rich is the cultural life of the community, its artistic, creative, and innovative elements?
- What is the environmental quality of the community, what is its impact on regional and local ecosystems, and what is being done to minimize that impact?
- Does everyone have access to basic primary care?

In the years since these questions were first developed, many new tools and approaches have been developed to aid in the assessment process (chapters 16, 21; appendixes 2, 3, 4). For example, and building on the second question regarding the degree of equity or inequity in the community, PolicyLink's Racial Equity Index (Langstron, 2020; www.policylink.org) enables public health professionals, community leaders, and policymakers to quickly access a summary score that provides "a snapshot of how well [their city] is performing on racial equity compared to its peers" (see table 10.1).

The index's two components are an *inclusion score* (e.g., the extent of racial gaps in outcomes on nine equity indicators) and a *prosperity score* (i.e., how their population as a whole is doing on those same indicators) (Langstron, 2020). Although the Racial Equity Index can also be applied to states and the nation as a whole, its utility for healthy city assessments in the country's 100 largest cities is particularly useful for our work.

A related and increasingly popular approach involves working with communities or other partners to develop community health indicators (CHIs) that characterize a neighborhood or community as a whole, rather than simply the individuals

TABLE 10.1

Indicators Included in the Racial Equity Index

Economic Vitality	Readiness	Connectedness
Median wages	Educational attainment	Air pollution exposure
Median hourly for full-time wage and salary workers ages 25–65	Share of population ages 25–64 with a BA or higher	Index of exposure to air toxics for cancer and noncancer risk
Unemployment	Disconnected youth	Commute time
Share of labor force ages 25–64 that is unemployed	Share of youth ages 16–24 who are not working and are not in school	Average travel time to work in minutes for workers ages 16 and older who work outside the home
Poverty (economic insecurity)	School poverty	Rent burden
Share of people with family incomes below 200% of the federal poverty level	Share of students in high-poverty schools (>75% of students eligible for free or reduced-price lunch)	Share of renter-occupied households spending more than 30% of income on housing costs

Sources: Langstron (2020); PolicyLink (2020).

or subgroups it comprises (https://ctb.ku.edu/en/table-of-contents, chap. 38; appendix 4). CHIs can also suggest how the community's health status, broadly defined, is changing over time. Good CHIs should reflect both *health determinants* (e.g., environmental quality and social cohesion) and *process dimensions* (e.g., education and civil rights). The CHIs developed by the nonprofit Human Impact Partners (discussed later in this chapter and presented in appendix 4) well meet these criteria.

Yet less-traditional indicators may also be usefully included in a healthy community assessment, as when the Sustainable Seattle indicators included wild salmon runs through local streams along with traditional measures, such as gallons or water consumed (Davey, 2017; Kisson, 1996). And in a classic example, a community in Hawaii identified the presence of Manapua trucks—small fast-food trucks that visit local communities—as an indicator of declining community health. They based this belief on four facts: (1) the fast food trucks replaced home cooking and family dining, (2) the nutritional quality of their food was poor,

(3) they made it easier for children to buy cigarettes, and (4) they harmed local businesses by undercutting them and taking money out of the community (Mendoza, 2016; personal communication from Marilyn Martinson, August 17, 2020). Examples like the latter are illustrative of how communities can offer thoughtful indicators of local health status that outside professionals would likely never consider.

A healthy community assessment would also need to look at the *processes* underway in the community that are believed to be related to health and the extent to which health is taken into account or is a focus for action. On the level of the city or formally defined municipality, for example, the following could be considered:

- Does the municipal council take health into account in its policy deliberations, explicitly developing healthy public policy?
- Is there a mechanism for health impact assessment?
- Do the local planning department and other government bodies understand the impacts of planning and design on health?
- Is the economic sector (e.g., the chamber of commerce, business improvement associations) part of the process?
- Do businesses understand the importance of health for their activities?
- Do they understand the importance of equitable access to the basic determinants of health for the entire population?
- Are neighborhood and resident groups involved? In what way?
- Are the environmental groups and organizations involved? The school boards? Faith-based organizations? The police? Local politicians at all levels of government?

The above perspectives on healthy community assessment laid important groundwork for the concept of "Health in All Policies" (HiAP), defined by Rudolph and colleagues (2013, p. 1) as "a collaborative approach to improving the health of all people by incorporating health considerations into decision-making across sectors and policy areas." The term *HiAP* was coined by global public health leader Ilona Kickbusch in 2007, building on the WHO's goal of engaging all government sectors in incorporating health considerations in their decisionmaking (Kickbusch & Buckett, 2010). Almost simultaneously, health officers across the large and diverse San Francisco Bay Area, were working across sectors and geographic divides to address regional Social Determinants of Health (SDOH) using a HiAP approach. Both the Public Health Institute / American Public Health Association (Rudolph et al., 2013) and the WHO (2015) published detailed manuals for others wishing to use this approach.

Finally, and in addition to reaching across sectors and regions, a healthy community assessment would take the time to determine not only formal leadership at the local level but also those informal leaders who can be identified through such methods as reputational and decisional analysis. The former technique involves having knowledgeable community members formally or informally "nominate" residents who play a powerful role in community affairs. The latter technique has informants describe recent community decisions and the roles played by various key participants in actually bringing about those decisions. The following questions are useful in identifying informal leaders:

- Who do people in this neighborhood go to for help or advice?
- Who do children go to?
- When the community has had a problem in the past, who has been involved in working to solve it?
- Who gets things done in the community?
- If I could talk to only three people in this community, who would they be? (Ellis & Walton, 2012; Eng & Blanchard, 1991; Sharpe et al., 2000; appendix 3).

By studying the processes of community action and change on multiple levels and uncovering multiple players in these processes, the healthy community assessment greatly broadens its potential for subsequently involving these diverse stakeholders in building a healthier community.

We have argued so far that several categories of information for and about health are needed for assessment at the local level. These include people's perceptions of the strengths and resources of their communities; their stories about the formal and informal processes of developing healthy cities and healthy communities; inequities in health and the SDoH; health status data, at the neighborhood or small-area level; and both subjective and objective assessments of physical, mental, and social well-being (Hancock et al., 1999; Plough & Chandra, 2015). Clearly, a *healthy community assessment* is much more than a *community health assessment*.

How Do We Assess?

Knowing what to assess is only part of the approach to healthy community assessment; we also need to determine how the process can contribute to the health of the community. This process question is vital, requiring that we consider carefully both the type of information that is collected and the degree of involvement with the community during the data collection process.

The Type of Information Collected

As John McKnight is fond of pointing out, "Institutions learn from studies; communities learn from stories." Studies are usually data rich and, with the important exception of community-based participatory approaches to research noted later in the chapter, tend to be carried out by academics and professionals working "on" rather than "with" communities (Minkler, 2014). The data are analyzed to yield information, but the knowledge that is acquired is seldom returned to the community, and as a result there is little increase in wisdom. Stories, in contrast, represent the accumulated and almost folkloric wisdom of a community, and because knowledge is power, the empowering potential of stories as a source of information about health becomes apparent.

Without discounting the importance of hard data in robust community assessments, the value of combining such data with the lay knowledge of community members has been well demonstrated (Cyril et al., 2015; Minkler, 2014; Wallerstein et al., 2018). People can learn much about the health of their communities by listening to and telling stories, whether around the kitchen table, at community meetings, through the internet or local media, or through events that celebrate successes or acknowledge loss. As discussed in chapter 17, community participation in the arts and literature can also be particularly potent means of gaining such insights (Sonke et al., 2019).

Stories can form the basis of studies, with qualitative ethnographic research often providing a more formal means of listening to and learning from stories. The classic early work of Penelope Cannan in Molokai is illustrative. When villagers were asked what they valued about their communities, they identified "the slow pace of life." When then asked how to measure the pace of life, community members suggested counting the number of alarm clocks in each village: if the number of alarm clocks went up, the villagers were clearly losing their slow pace of life. As this story illustrates, people know what is important to them, and have the ability to identify innovative and meaningful measures that make sense in their own community. In fact, it is doubtful if an army of academic and professional researchers would have ever come up with the "alarm clock indicator" on their own! Ethnographic studies and other means of gathering and really listening to people's stories can provide critical information for an assessment of community health and well-being.

Of course, quantitative approaches and studies also have an important role to play in assessing communities and community health, including documenting health inequities in infant mortality and other dimensions in and between communities. Quantitative methods often have the advantages of perceived scientific rigor, large denominators, and forms of data analysis that make the findings readily accessible to policymakers and others who "need the numbers" to make a case for new legislation or other proposed actions. For quantitative studies to live up to their potential as part of an empowering community assessment, however, they must measure health outcomes that are amenable to analysis at the small-area level and in a rapid timeframe. PolicyLink's earlier mentioned Racial Equity Index (Langstron, 2020) and the University of Kansas's Community Tool Box (http://ctb .ku.edu, chap. 38) with the plethora of quantitative and qualitative assessment resources it provides, enable communities to look in real time at multiple dimensions of their communities, and use the findings as the basis for further discussion and community and policy action for change.

Many of the resources described in this and other chapters attend to the empowerment goal of healthy community assessment, either through the transfer of information and knowledge to members of the community or, ideally, by actively engaging them in the research process itself. This participatory action research (PAR) or community-based participatory research (CBPR) process starts with a topic of concern to the community, "equitably" involves all partners throughout the research process, involves co-learning and local capacity building, balances research and action, and commits to sustainability over the long haul (Israel et al., 2013; Minkler, 2014; chapter 15). In one such project in a small Latinx community in San Diego County, California, which had become a "dumping ground" for local toxic polluters, the community's Environmental Health Coalition partnered with academic researchers and other allies to help uncover the "numbers and stories" to help make the case for policy-level change. In addition to powerful in-house Geographic Information Systems (GIS) data showing the disproportionate burden of pollution borne by residents, the Coalition hired neighborhood women as *promotoras de salud* (health promoters) and trained them in survey research methods, land-use planning, community organizing, and policy advocacy. Six of the *promotoras* designed and conducted a door-to-door survey, which uncovered high rates of childhood asthma, as well as overwhelming neighborhood interest in relocating polluting industries outside the town (Environmental Health Coalition, 2005; https://www.environmentalhealth.org). These multimethod findings, together with disease burden data from academic partners at the University of Southern California and the *promotoras'* own stories, which they presented in testimony before the city council, played a substantial role in getting several policy victories. Among these were the passage of an ordinance to phase out polluting industries and a specific plan requiring that health impacts and community input be included in all future city decisionmaking (Minkler et al., 2010, 2012). Equally important, however, was that one of the *promotoras* went on to become a member of the city council and later the vice-mayor of her small city, further enhancing community members' real and perceived sense of empowerment and ability to control their own destiny (Minkler et al., 2012; https://www.environmentalhealth.org).

In sum, a balance of studies and stories provides the information needed to assess communities and community health. How this information is collected, the purposes for which it is sought, and whether the findings are then returned to the community all play a critical role in determining the empowering potential of the assessment process.

The Degree of Involvement with the Community

The many diverse methods for conducting a healthy community assessment can usefully be grouped into categories defined by the extent to which they involve contact between the outside professional and members of the community. Since contact with and high-level involvement of community residents in the assessment process are vital parts of community organizing and community building for health, special attention should be given to methods that foster such involvement as part of the assessment process. At the same time, as noted earlier, the utility of studies that produce hard data, including some that may involve no-contact or minimal contact methods, should be appreciated.

No-Contact Methods

Demographic and social indicators, such as rates of substance abuse, unemployment, and morbidity and mortality, are often the first types of data looked at by health professionals charged with conducting a community needs assessment. Using methods like small-area analyses, or dynamic modeling, studies using such data often have the advantages of a large numerical base or a representative sample and an aura of "scientific objectivity." No-contact methods, such as multivariate analysis, can further document such factors as the impacts of race and class on mortality rates in neighboring communities and as such can provide information that may be vital in demonstrating health inequities in a format that legislators and advocacy groups can use in fighting for health resources.

However, utilization of such methods is based on the assumption that "the community needs and problems that appear in official statistics are representative of community problems"—an assumption not always warranted (Marti-Costa & Serrano-Garcia, 1983, p. 81). Statistics on mental health treatment, for example, may indicate a dramatic change in the types of mental illnesses in a given community when what in fact has changed are the service categories for which insurers provide funding. Thus mental health professionals may simply be creatively labeling what they see in order to continue treating persons they believe to be in need.

No-contact methods often include documents review, with pertinent "documents" including community newspapers or newsletters, written progress reports from health and social service departments, and community bulletin boards (both virtual and online), whose contents may give a flavor for the kinds of issues and resources represented in a given community. When used without community involvement, however, such methods, although providing some useful information, lack the potential to facilitate local empowerment or mobilization.

Moreover, the term *no-contact methods* is increasingly becoming something of a misnomer. With smartphones and other devices now more powerful than the huge corporate and university computers of the 1970s, opportunities have vastly expanded for community members to be involved in the collection and use of data that were formerly within the exclusive purview of researchers and professionals. Resources like the aforementioned Community Tool Box (http://ctb.ku.edu), which includes more than 9,000 pages of how-to information to assist communities and professionals alike, are among a wealth of new internet-based systems that greatly enhance the ability of local communities to effectively study, mobilize around, and address shared interests and concerns (chapter 16). By helping community members become conversant with such tools and their applications in the assessment process, professionals can greatly expand the empowering potential of many so-called no-contact methods.

Minimal Contact Observational Methods

A variety of observational methods may be useful for the health professional wishing to gain an initial impressionistic sense of the community with which he or she will be working. One such technique involves a neighborhood "windshield tour" or walk-through. Using this approach, the health educator or other social change professional or community member walks or drives slowly through a neighborhood, ideally on different days of the week and at different times of the day, while being "on the lookout" for a whole variety of potentially useful indicators of community health and well-being. Observing the condition of houses and automobiles, the nature and degree of activity level, and social interaction between residents and the like can provide valuable impressionistic information, as can sitting in a neighborhood coffee shop, or observing at a community forum or PTA meeting (Eng & Blanchard, 1991; appendix 3).

As in the case of no-contact methods, minimal contact approaches are increasingly being used in ways that promote community involvement and hold the potential for facilitating empowerment. Health department–sponsored efforts like the Healthy Neighborhood Project in Contra Costa County, California (Ellis & Walton, 2012), for example, trained neighborhood residents to use walk-throughs, asset mapping, and other techniques, viewing their community through fresh eyes as they gathered impressionistic data, which then were shared and compared with those of other members of the assessment team. Once again, if a goal in community assessment is to further empowerment, creating opportunities for increased community contact and involvement is critical.

Interactive Contact Methods

This category of methods includes techniques such as key informant interviews, door-to-door surveys, and a variety of small-group methods for eliciting data and stories about a local community. Among the latter, arguably the most popular is the focus group, which brings together, under the direction of a trained moderator, a small group of community members who, in a confidential and nonthreatening discussion, address a series of questions concerning their feelings, in this case about their community (Krueger & Casey, 2014). Employed by health agencies, philanthropic foundations, community-based organizations, and local policymakers, focus groups provide stories and perceptions that can greatly enrich the overall community assessment. Increasingly, they also engage community partners as co-facilitators and co-interpreters of findings, providing additional benefits to the process from both a data collection and an empowerment perspective. Many other interactive contact methods lend themselves to use with either small or larger groups and are discussed in chapters 5, 17, and 24, and in appendixes 2, 3, 10, and 11.

A common theme throughout this chapter has involved the importance of asking—and having community members ask themselves—the kinds of questions that provoke meaningful discussion about community, health, and healthy communities. Whether in the context of focus groups or key informant interviews, or as part of large town hall meetings or community dialogues, such questions might include the following:

- What do you like best about living in this community?
- What would you like to see changed?
- Is this a good place to raise children? (Why or why not?)
- Do people in the neighborhood socialize with one another often? Do you socialize with others here?
- If youth get into a fight in this community, are adult residents likely to intervene?
- How would you characterize the relationship between members of different racial or ethnic groups in the neighborhood?
- Who gets things done? (Ellis & Walton, 2012; Eng & Blanchard, 1991; Sharp et al., 2000; appendix 2)

Questions like these often generate a wealth of initial data and stories about a community and may also help in the identification of a core group of informal leaders who may then be brought together, engaged in a similar dialogue, and encouraged to be key participants in a community organizing or community building project (appendix 2). The results of such data collection may be presented in narrative form, charts and graphs, or a combination that summarizes key findings. As suggested earlier, however, the richest and most accurate findings may emerge when local residents themselves conduct the interviews and then help in analyzing or interpreting the results (Cashman et al., 2008; Minkler et al., 2012; chapter 15).

Although contact methods by definition involve community residents, their potential for truly facilitating empowerment depends on the how these methods are employed. Focus groups and key informant interviews, for example, can be disempowering if they only seek information about community needs and problems and ignore or discount the participants' knowledge of their community's resources and assets. In contrast, a contribution to community capacity building may be made when questions are asked that encourage residents to reflect on and contribute to a broader understanding of community strengths. Questions like, What makes this a good or healthy community in which to live? can help residents think positively about the strengths of their communities. *Community asset mapping techniques*, as described in chapter 11, similarly represent a powerful means for community members to work together in identifying the strengths and potential "building blocks" of their neighborhoods, and not merely their problems and deficiencies. By revealing an appreciation of the community by the outsider, and engaging informants in a process of thinking critically about the strengths and competencies of their community, such techniques and questions can make a real difference in the information obtained and in the community's willingness to be actively involved in the assessment process.

Multimethod Assessment

Clearly, no one method or approach to community assessment can capture the richness and complexity of communities and community health. A strong case should therefore be made for the use of multiple methods, or what researchers refer to as "triangulation." Mobilizing for Action through Planning and Partnerships, or MAPP (http://www.naccho.org/tools.chm) is one such approach and was developed by the National Association of County and City Health Officials (NACCHO) working collaboratively with the Centers for Disease Control and Prevention (CDC). Using this strategic planning tool, public health leaders help communities prioritize public health issues as well as resources for addressing them. Case vignettes, as well as a variety of user-friendly assessment techniques and resources, are available at the website for those wishing to apply this multimethod approach (https://toolbox.naccho.org/pages/index.html). Similarly, organizations like the National Neighborhood Indicators Partnership (https://www.neighborhoodindicators.org/) and Human Impact Partners (www.HIP.org) often serve as critical intermediaries, enabling the collection of local-level data that may then be harnessed and used to inform broader community building and the development of healthy public policy. The aforementioned community health indicators developed by Human Impact Partners (appendix 4) provide a particularly good case in point. Although developed by professionals, the indicators address each of eleven issue areas, from livelihood and housing to violence, social exclusion, environmental quality, and environmental stewardship, with each key area linked to several health determinants and outcomes, as well as measurable indicators, in a simple, easy-to-use format (appendix 4). They reflect both health determinants (e.g., environmental quality and social cohesion) and process dimensions (e.g., education). Finally, they meet key qualities of Hancock et al. (1999) for making such indicators relevant to both policymakers and the general public:

- Face validity—They make sense to people.
- Theoretical and empirical validity—They measure an important health determinant or dimension.
- Social value—They measure things people care about.
- Valency—They are powerful and carry social and political punch. (Hancock et al., 1999)

By helping community members become conversant with such tools and their applications in the assessment process, health and other professionals can greatly expand the empowering potential of the healthy community assessment process.

Regardless of the scale on which a community assessment is conducted, it is likely to be most effective if it combines multiple methods, respects both stories and studies, and places its heaviest emphasis on eliciting high-level community participation throughout the assessment process.

Summary

This chapter has attempted to build on the classic ideological framework provided by Marti-Costa and Serrano-Garcia (1983), as well as more recent insights developed through the Healthy Cities Movement, Health in All Policies, and numerous other examples to propose an empowering approach to community assessment for health. Both stories and studies are vital if we are to stimulate, monitor, and assess the impact of change and at the same time facilitate the empowerment that comes with knowledge, specifically with the transfer of knowledge to communities. Likewise, no single assessment tool or technique is sufficient in and of itself to sensitively and accurately capture community or community health. That is better accomplished by multiple methods, especially those whose use can help individuals and communities become more empowered while making explicit the realities of the community, its resources, and its health.

Questions for Further Discussion

1. The authors argue that "information for change" in a healthy community assessment must carry "social and political punch" if it is to stimulate action. Thinking of examples from media stories you have read, or from this or prior chapters of the book, what might be an example of either a community story or hard data that would capture a health or social inequity in a powerful enough way to get the attention of policymakers and stimulate them to want to act? What might be one way to help ensure that the information reaches them in a way that has a good chance of getting them to act? Try also writing a headline and the first two to three lines of a press release as an example of how you might share a story or hard data in a compelling and powerful way.

2. The chapter makes a strong case for engaging community members in helping to conduct a healthy community assessment (HCA), in part because their lived experience may lead to new indicators far different than those we as outside professionals might come up with. You want to involve some community members in your agency's HCA, but your supervisor is unconvinced. What arguments might you make as to the added value of their being included in the process? And how would you go about finding community members to invite?

REFERENCES

Arnstein, S. R. (2019). A ladder of citizen participation. *J Am Plann Assoc, 85*(1), 24–34.

Cashman, S., Adeky, B., Allen, A. J. III, Corburn, J., Israel, B. A., Montaño, J., Rafelito, A., Rhodes, S. D., Swanston, S., Wallerstein, N., & Eng, E. (2008). The power and the promise: Working with communities to analyze data, interpret findings, and get to outcomes. *Am J Public Health, 98,* 1407–1417.

Cyril, S., Smith, B. J., Possamai-Inesedy, A., & Renzaho, A. M. (2015). Exploring the role of community engagement in improving the health of disadvantaged populations: A systematic review. *Glob Health Action, 8*(1), 29842.

Davey, E. (2017). Recapturing the learning opportunities of university sustainability indicators. *J Environ Stud Sci, 7*(4), 540–549.

deVuono-Powell, S., Minkler, M., Bissell, E., Walker, T., Vaughn, L., & Moore, E. (2018). Criminal justice reform through participatory action research. In N. Wallerstein, B. Duran, J. G. Oetzel, & M. Minkler (Eds.), *Community-Based Participatory Research for Health: Advancing Social and Health Equity* (3rd ed., pp. 305–319). Jossey-Bass.

Diers, J. (2004). *Neighborhood Power: Building Community the Seattle Way.* University of Washington Press.

Ellis, G., & Walton, S. (2012). Building partnerships between health departments and communities: Case studies in capacity building and cultural humility. In M. Minkler (Ed.), *Community Organizing and Community Building for Health and Welfare* (3rd ed., pp. 130–147). Rutgers University Press.

Eng, E., & Blanchard, L. (1991). Action-oriented community diagnosis: A health education tool. *Int Q Community Health Educ, 26*(2), 141–158.

Environmental Health Coalition. (2005). Reclaiming Old Town National City: A Community Survey. Environmental Health Coalition. https://www.environmentalhealth.org/images/EHC_Toxinformer/ToxInformer_PDFs/ToxieSummer05_ENG_WEB.pdf.

Flora, C. B., & Flora, J. L. (2008). *Rural Communities: Legacy and Change* (3rd ed.). Westview Press.

Hancock, T., & Duhl, L. (1986). *Healthy Cities: Promoting Health in the Urban Context.* WHO Europe.

Hancock, T., Labonte, R., & Edwards, R. (1999). Indicators that count! Measuring population health at the community level. *Can J Public Health, 90* (Suppl. 1), 22–26.

Israel, B., Eng, E., Schulz, A. J., & Parker, E. A. (2013). *Methods in Community-Based Participatory Research for Health* (2nd ed.). Jossey-Bass.

Iton, A., & Ross, R. K. (2017). Understanding how health happens: Your zip code is more important than your genetic code. In R. Callahan & D. Bhattachara (Eds.), *Public Health Leadership* (pp. 83–99). Routledge.

Kickbusch, I., & Buckett, K. (2010). *Implementing Health in All Policies.* Government of South Australia.

Kisson, A. (1996). Developing indicators of sustainable community: Lessons from sustainable Seattle. *Environ Impact Assess Rev, 16*, 337–350.

Kretzmann, J. P., & McKnight, J. L. (1993). *Building Communities from Inside Out: A Path toward Finding and Mobilizing a Community's Assets.* Center for Urban Affairs and Policy Research.

Krueger, R. A., & Casey, M. A. (2014). *Focus Groups: A Practical Guide for Applied Research* (5th ed.). Sage.

Langstron, A. (2020). Introducing the National Equity Index. Oakland, CA. https://nationalequityatlas.org/research/introducingindex.

Marti-Costa, S., & Serrano-Garcia, I. (1983, Summer). Needs assessment and community development: An ideological perspective. *Prev Hum Serv, 2*(4), 75–88.

Mendoza, J. (2016). Community resilience and food equity: The case for the Honolulu Hawker Centre. https://scholarspace.manoa.hawaii.edu/handle/10125/45579.

Minkler, M. (2014). Enhancing data quality, relevance, and use through community-based participatory research. In N. Cytron, K. Petit, & G. T. Kingsley (Eds.), *What Counts? Harnessing Data for America's Communities* (pp. 245–259). Federal Reserve Bank of San Francisco and the Urban Institute.

Minkler, M., Garcia, A. P., Rubin, V., & Wallerstein, N. (2012). *Community-Based Participatory Research: A Strategy for Building Healthy Communities and Promoting Health through Policy*

Change. A report to the California Endowment. PolicyLink, University of California Berkeley. https://www.policylink.org/sites/default/files/CBPR.pdf.

Minkler, M., Garcia, A. P., Williams, J., LoPresti, T., & Lilly, J. (2010). Sí se puede: Using participatory research to promote environmental justice in a Latino community in San Diego, CA. *J Urban Health, 87*(5), 796–812.

Moore, S., & Kawachi, I. (2017). Twenty years of social capital in health research: A glossary. *J Epidemiol Community Health, 71*, 513–517.

Ong, M., Baker, A., Aguilar, A., & Stanley, M. (2019). The meanings attributed to community gardening: A qualitative study. *Health Place, 59*(1), 102190.

Ozer, E. (2007). The effects of school gardens on students and schools: Conceptualization and considerations for maximizing healthy development. *Health Educ Behav, 34*(6), 846–863.

Pastor, M., Terriquez, V., & Lin, M. (2018). How community organizing promotes health equity, and how health equity affects organizing. *Health Affairs, 37*(3), 358–363.

Plough, A., & Chandra, A. (2015). *From Vision to Action: Measures to Mobilize a Culture of Health.* Robert Wood Johnson Foundation.

PolicyLink. (2020). National Equity Axis. https://www.policylink.org/our-work/economy/national-equity-atlas.

Putnam, R. (2000). *Bowling Alone: The Collapse and Revival of American Community.* Simon and Schuster.

Rudolph, L., Caplan, J., Ben-Moshe, K., & Dillon, L. (2013). *Health in All Policies: A Guide for State and Local Governments.* American Public Health Association and Public Health Institute.

Sharpe, P. A., Greany, M. L., Lee, P. R., & Royce, S. W. (2000). Assets-oriented community assessment. *Public Health Rep, 113*(2–3), 205–211.

Sonke, J., Golden, T., Francois, S., Hand, J., Chandra, A., Clemmons, L., Fakunle, D., Jackson, M. R., Magsamen, S., Rubin, V., Sams, K., & Springs, S. (2019). *Creating Healthy Communities through Cross-Sector Collaboration* [White paper]. University of Florida Center for Arts in Medicine / ArtPlace America.

The Trust for the Public Land. (2020). Here's the dirt on park trends: Community gardens are growing. https://www.tpl.org/blog/here%E2%80%99s-dirt-park-trends-community-gardens-are-growing.

Wallerstein, N., Duran, B., Oetzel, J. G., & Minkler, M. (Eds.). (2018). *Community-Based Participatory Research for Health: Advancing Social and Health Equity* (3rd ed.). Jossey-Bass.

World Health Organization. (1948). *Constitution of the World Health Organization.* Adopted by the International Health Conference in New York in 1946 and entered into force on April 7, 1948.

World Health Organization. (1986). *Ottawa Charter for Health Promotion.* WHO Europe.

World Health Organization. (2015). *Health in All Policies Training Manual.* WHO Press.

11

Mapping Community Capacity

JOHN L. McKNIGHT

JOHN P. KRETZMANN

LIONEL J. BEAULIEU

Countless older cities in the United States have suffered for decades from massive economic shifts that have seen hundreds of thousands of often well-paying industrial jobs either disappear completely or move away, often to countries with cheaper labor and more lax workplace and environmental standards. Further, while many downtown areas in the cities left behind have experienced a "renaissance," the high-tech and other jobs created there are different from those that once sustained neighborhoods. Either these new jobs are highly professionalized, requiring advanced education and credentials, or they are routine, low-paying service and "gig economy" jobs offering little in the way of benefits and a pathway to upward mobility. In effect, these economic shifts, particularly the loss of decent employment possibilities from low-income neighborhoods, have removed the bottom rung from the fabled American "ladder of opportunity." With the coronavirus pandemic that disproportionately affected low-wage, frontline service workers and their families, and those without jobs to begin with, this picture has become even bleaker. For many people in older city neighborhoods, as well as the small places that dot rural America, innovative approaches for rebuilding their lives and communities, and new openings toward opportunity, are a necessity.

Focusing attention on urban neighborhoods makes sense since 83 percent of Americans now live in the nation's urban areas (Plecher, 2020). But the capacity building tools and orientations discussed in this chapter are equally applicable to our nation's rural settings, home to more than 46 million people (Johnson & Lichter, 2019). Rural towns and communities face equally compelling challenges, among them the aging of their populations, the out-migration of talented youth, the closure or departure of key industries, and the relative absence of quality health care and broadband services. Even prior to the COVID-19 pandemic, many urban and rural areas across the United States were bearing a heavy toll as population losses and economic stagnation produced hot spots of despair, including accelerated rates of substance abuse and suicides. Indeed, in 2019, the lifetime risk of deaths from drug overdose in West Virginia was fully one in thirty (Sehgal, 2020).

Given these realities, it is no surprise that most Americans viewed low-income urban neighborhoods and rural towns as a problem, even before the pandemic brought their plight into sharper focus. Both low-income urban and rural areas are typically noted for their deficiencies and needs—a view accepted by most elected officials who codify and program this perspective through deficiency-oriented policies and programs. Then human service systems translate the programs into local activities that teach people the nature of their problems and the value of services as the answer to their needs. As a result, many low-income urban neighborhoods and rural places have become environments of service where residents develop the mind-set that their well-being depends on being a client. They see themselves as people with needs to be met by outsiders. And gradually, they become primary consumers of services, lacking the training, skills, and other resources needed to be producers or creators of their own future or that of their community. Consumers of services focus vast amounts of creativity and intelligence on the survival-motivated challenge of outwitting the "system" or on finding ways—in the informal or even illegal economy—to bypass the system entirely.

There is nothing "natural" about this process. In fact, it is the predictable course of events when deficiency and needs-oriented programs dominate the lives of communities in which low-income people reside. To counter this trend, we discuss and illustrate the concept of "capacity building"—the process of identifying individual, organizational, and community capabilities that serve as the first step on the path toward community regeneration (chapter 3). We then introduce the concept of *community capitals*, a framework that is complementary to the asset-based community development (ABCD) approach (Kretzmann & McKnight, 1993) that has guided our work over many years. The community capitals framework expands our understanding of the distinct arenas in which important assets can be discovered—whether in urban, suburban, or rural settings.

The Capacity-Focused Alternative

The alternative to the more needs or deficit-based approach to community is to develop policies and activities based on the capacities, skills, and assets of low-income people and their neighborhoods or communities. There are two reasons for this capacity-oriented emphasis. First, a wealth of evidence indicates that significant community development rarely takes place unless community residents are committed to investing themselves and their resources in the effort (McKnight & Russell, 2018; Sonke et al., 2019; Wallerstein, 2006). This is why, while we cannot develop communities from the top down or from the outside in, we *can* provide valuable outside assistance to communities that are actively developing and mobilizing their own assets (chapters 3, 10).

The second reason for emphasizing the development of the internal assets of local urban neighborhoods and rural areas is that the likelihood of attracting a major firm to locate in a low-income community is at best remote. There are exceptions (e.g., Warsaw, Indiana, a city of 15,000 residents that has emerged as the orthopedic medical devices capital of the world). But far more often, the economic vitality of urban neighborhoods or rural towns is dependent on the ability of local people, organizations, and institutions to identify and build on their existing economic assets while simultaneously creating a climate where the entrepreneurial spirit of the local residents can be unleashed. Finally, and particularly during economic downturns, the ample and sustained flow of federal or state funds to tackle the major challenges affecting urban and rural America is unlikely. As the federal response to the COVID-19 pandemic underscored, federal funds may be particularly hard to access in communities of color, with The Center for Responsible Lending estimating that fully 95 percent of Black-owned businesses were unlikely to benefit from loans from the Payroll Protection Program (https://www.responsiblelending .org/sites/default/files/nodes/files/research-publication/crl-cares-act2-smallbusiness -apr2020.pdf?mod=article_inline). Yet, while it is critical that we work to end such discriminatory practices, it is also important to work within the community to promote its development.

Unfortunately, the dominance of the deficiency-oriented social service model has led many people in low-income neighborhoods to think in terms of local problems rather than assets—with these perceived deficits often identified, quantified, and mapped through "needs assessments" (chapter 10). The result is a map of low educational attainment, substance abuse, unemployment, and more. But in places where there are effective community development efforts, there is also a map of the community's assets, capacities, and abilities in recognition of the fact that even the poorest city neighborhood or low-income rural town have in place individuals and organizations that possess the resources upon which to rebuild. The key to local regeneration is not only to tap the resources that are already controlled but also to harness them for community development purposes.

The process of identifying capacities and assets, both individual and organizational, is the first step on the path toward community regeneration. Mapping these assets is still frequently done by local residents, with or without an outside professional, walking or driving slowly through their neighborhood or rural place, in pairs or small groups, and both listing and indicating on a tablet or old-fashioned paper map where they see these different assets, or liabilities that may be turned into assets (appendix 3). More recently, however, virtual and often free tools like Google's My Maps (maps.google.com) are being effectively used in this work. As Corburn and colleagues note in appendix 2, using such tools, "organizers and community residents can mark assets and liabilities in their community, share this information easily on the web with others and allow a number of users to edit or 'ground truth' this information over time" (Sadd et al., 2014).

Regardless of the method or methods used in its creation, however, once this new "map" has replaced the one focused on needs and deficiencies, the regenerating community can begin to assemble its assets and capacities into new combinations, new structures of opportunity, new sources of income and control, and new possibilities for production.

Mapping the Building Blocks for Regeneration

Of course, not all community assets are equally available for community building purposes. The most easily accessible assets, or building blocks, are those located in the neighborhood and small rural places controlled by those who live there. Next are those assets located in the neighborhood or rural community but controlled elsewhere. Finally, least accessible are those potential building blocks located outside these communities and controlled by those external to it. Our focus is on the first of these assets—those primary and secondary resources that are embedded in the community and can be activated to address the priorities of urban neighborhood and rural places.

Primary Building Blocks—Assets and Capacities Located inside the Neighborhood or Rural Places, Largely under Their Control

The two general categories of capacities most readily available for the regeneration of neighborhoods and rural localities are the assets and capacities of *individuals* and those of *organizations or associations* that are part of the fabric of these areas. The first step in capturing any of these resources is to assess them, which typically involves developing a capacity inventory.

Individual Capacities

Our greatest assets are our people, so the starting point for any serious development effort is identifying the variety and richness of skills, talents, knowledge, and experiences of people in low-income neighborhoods and communities to provide a base on which to build new approaches and enterprises.

An inventory of capacities can involve a simple survey designed to identify the multitude of abilities within each individual. Residents have used the "capacity inventory" to identify the talents available to start new enterprises, through which people become producers rather than "problems."

Personal Income

It is generally assumed that low-income neighborhoods and rural places are poor markets, and in many predominantly Black communities, histories of redlining and other discriminatory practices have indeed contributed to this reality. In 2019, for example, the median Black household wealth in the United States averaged less than 15 percent of that of White households (Bhutta et al., 2020), and small and medium-sized banks were still far less likely to make home and business loans to Blacks than they were to Whites (Blackwell & McAffee, 2020). A new and powerful national reckoning with racial injustice in the wake of the 2020 Black Lives Matter protests against police brutality quickly extended to include historic and continuing race-based economic injustices, which led to widespread calls for redress (Blackwell & McAffee, 2020). Similarly, discriminatory practices affecting the livelihoods of immigrant Latinx, Native Americans, and other, often low-income, communities of color also have received renewed attention.

Yet, even given these realities and the urgent need for addressing them, people in poor communities may have more income per capita than is assumed, but—often for perfectly rational reasons—use it in ways that do not support local economic development. For example, a 2012 survey of 640 residents of San Francisco's low-income Tenderloin neighborhood revealed that close to half were going outside the neighborhood to buy groceries and other staples that were not available (or prohibitively expensive) in the neighborhood's small corner stores (Minkler et al., 2019). Extrapolated to the community as a whole, this amounted to a loss of roughly $2 million per year from the local revenue base. In response, community members, aided by the health department and university partners, helped catalyze and implement a city program that incentivized local merchants to access and sell fresh produce and other healthy foods, while decreasing space allotted for tobacco and other unhealthy products. The positive impacts for residents, merchants, and community capacity have been well documented (Minkler et al., 2019; chapter 19). As this example suggests, effective local development efforts can inventory the income, savings, and expenditure patterns of their neighborhoods and use this information to both understand the neighborhood economy and develop new approaches to capturing local wealth for local development.

The Gifts of Labeled People

When the article on which this chapter was based was first written in the late 1980s, we highlighted the rich potential waiting to be identified and contributed by even the most marginalized individuals. We noted that service systems had labeled these people "retarded," "mentally ill," "disabled," "elderly," and so on, adding that such individuals were likely to become dependents of service systems, excluded from community life, and considered burdens rather than assets to community life. Clearly, much has changed over the ensuing decades, with some of these labels (e.g., "retarded') dropped for their pejorative connotations and others (e.g., "disabled") now proudly claimed by many of those affected, for whom terms like this one represent an important source of collective identity and pride. Indeed, just as many elders banded together to form the Gray Panthers and other organizations that celebrate their identity and work to affect needed policy changes, disability rights became a rallying cry among the disabled whose leaders and organizations played a key role in the passage of the historic Americans with Disabilities Act three decades ago (Warden, 2020). Concurrently with these larger and often policy-focused efforts, were a growing number of unique community efforts to incorporate "labeled" people into local organizations, enterprises, and community associations (Cooney, 2016; Research on Disabilities, 2019). Their gifts and abilities were, and continue to be, identified and introduced to groups that value these contributions (e.g. "second chance" employers who hire and train formerly incarcerated people for employment in their businesses, and grocery stores who contract for baked goods from programs whose workers are people with developmental disabilities).

Individual Local Businesses

The shops, stores, and businesses that survive in low-income neighborhoods—especially those owned and operated by local residents—are often more than economic ventures. They are usually centers for community life as well. Black-owned barbershops and beauty salons were among the earliest examples of such establishments and have served as ongoing sources of community identity and pride (Bristol, 2009; chapter 14). Any comprehensive approach to community regeneration should inventory such enterprises and incorporate their energies and resources into community development processes. The experience and insight of these individual entrepreneurs might also be shared with local not-for-profit groups and both educators and students.

Home-Based Enterprises

It is fairly simple to inventory the businesses in low-income neighborhoods and rural places. However, and particularly during economic downturns like that accompanying the pandemic, there has been an uptick in informal and home-based enterprise. These range from residents using their own cars to deliver food and other necessities as part of the gig economy, to others who work at home and, for example, make and sell baked goods. Making an effort to understand the nature of these individual entrepreneurs and their enterprises is particularly important in rural areas, where the lion's share of businesses are either proprietorships (one-person operations) or enterprises that employ fewer than ten people. After gathering information about such operations, development groups can identify the factors that helped initiate them and the additional capital or technical assistance that could increase their profits as well as the number of people they support.

Associational and Organizational Capacities

Beyond individual capacities are a wide range of local resident-controlled associations and organizations, of which the following are examples.

Local Clubs and Associations

In addition to businesses and enterprises, low-income communities have a variety of clubs and associations that do vital work in assuring productive neighborhoods and communities. These groups might include service clubs, fraternal organizations, women's organizations, artistic groups, and athletic clubs. They are the infrastructure of working neighborhoods or rural places. Those involved in the community building process can inventory the variety of these groups in their areas, the unique community activities they support, and their potential to become part of the local asset development process or affiliate in other ways (e.g., by creating a congress of neighborhood associations).

Associations of Businesses

In many older neighborhoods or rural communities, local businesspeople are either not organized or not aware of the potential for effective joint partnerships in economic development. Connecting local businesses with each other and expanding their vision of their self-interest in community development are major efforts of effective community building activities.

Financial Institutions

Relatively few older neighborhoods or rural areas have a community-oriented financial institution, such as a bank, savings institution, or credit union. But where they do exist, they are invaluable assets. A case in point is the Hope Credit Union based in Jackson, Mississippi, and dedicated to building economic opportunities in Black communities across the Deep South. In 2018, it received an award from the *Wall Street Journal*'s Financial Inclusion Challenge, in recognition of its efforts to improve the financial health and security of low- and moderate-income people in the United States.

Cultural Organizations

People in low-income neighborhoods and rural areas are increasingly giving public expression to their rich cultural inheritance. Celebrating the history of the neighborhood, and the peoples who have gathered there, can play a key role in forming a community identity and countering negative images that originate outside the community (Sonke et al., 2019). Neighborhood history fairs; block parties and other events featuring the foods, music, dancing, and games of diverse peoples; cross-cultural discussions and classes; oral history projects and theatrical productions based on such histories—all can build strong relationships among residents and for regaining definitional control of the community.

Communications Organizations

Strong neighborhoods and communities rely heavily on their capacity to exchange information and engage in discussions. Neighborhood or town newspapers, particularly those that are controlled by local residents, are invaluable public forums. So, too, are less comprehensive media, such as newsletters, fliers, and even physical or virtual bulletin boards. In addition, local access cable TV, local radio, and social media, now becoming commonplace, have shown promise as vehicles relevant to community building.

Faith-Based Organizations

Local parishes, congregations, mosques, and temples have increasingly involved themselves in the community building agenda, sometimes through community organizations or community development groups (Kotz, 2019; Schutz & Miller, 2015; chapter 5), sometimes simply building on the strengths of their own members and networks. Further, the ability of local faith-based institutions to access related external organizations for support and resources constitutes an important asset (for more on the work of two such faith-based community organizations, the Gamaliel Foundation [http://www.gamaliel.org/] and ISAIAH [http://www.isaiah.org/], see chapter 5).

Secondary Building Blocks

In asset-based community development, second only in importance to the primary building blocks in and controlled by the local community, are those assets—from local clinics to libraries to housing and energy resources—located in but typically controlled by entities outside the community, yet which can sometimes be developed and brought under a local community's control. Although a detailed exploration of these secondary building blocks is beyond the scope of this chapter, we identify the key categories and provide two illustrative examples. We then describe a Community Capitals Framework that captures some of these same assets but also encourages us to think more broadly about the wide range of capitals on which our communities—and community development work—can build. The following are secondary building blocks in communities:

- Private and nonprofit organizations—higher education institutions, hospitals, clinics, HMOs, social service agencies
- Public institutions and services—public schools, libraries, parks, police, fire departments
- Physical resources—vacant land, commercial and industrial structures, housing, energy and waste resources

In the category of public institutions and services that exist in and have an impact on low-income communities, consider local schools in rural or small urban areas. A local school may serve as a community epicenter, and, particularly if it is well rated educationally or is a large employer, it may also serve as a magnet for attracting families to the community. Such schools are also often hubs for social, educational and recreational activities, or the glue that strongly bonds teachers, families, business owners, and community organizers (Brown & Schafft, 2011).

Turning now to the category of physical resources, consider the example of vacant land, structures, and housing as potential secondary assets that at first may be seen as liabilities. Many older urban neighborhoods are thought to be "blighted," with vacant lots, empty sites of old industry, and unused industrial and commercial buildings. However, in some U.S. cities, local groups have found creative and productive methods to regenerate the usefulness of both the land and the buildings. The community gardens movement (chapter 10) is one such success story that frequently begins with publicly owned lots. Similarly, abandoned but structurally sound buildings may be candidates for locally controlled rehabilitation efforts. In some rural areas, vacant main street buildings or long-abandoned industrial facilities have been converted to business incubators, makerspace, or small business enterprises. Under the banner of the Community Heart & Soul initiative, for example, the Orton Foundation and its partners productively engaged local residents in regeneration efforts in dozens of small towns and cities across fourteen states (Karas, 2019).

The Community Capitals Framework: A Value-Added Process for Uncovering Local Assets

Taking stock of the assets of local people, organizations, and associations and then activating them in order to pursue positive improvements in an urban or rural community can be an empowering step for local residents. Not only does it serve to restore hope, it changes the mind-set of people who see what is possible when they look inward, building on existing local assets.

While the seminal work by Kretzmann and McKnight (1993) has been instrumental in shifting community work to asset-based community development, new ways of conceptualizing the mix of assets rooted in urban neighborhoods or rural communities have gained traction. One garnering significant interest is the Community Capitals Framework (CCF), a model developed in 1992 and fine-tuned over the ensuing years by Flora and colleagues (Flora & Flora; 2008; Flora et al., 2004) and others (Beaulieu, 2014).

The CCF states that the lifeblood of any neighborhood or community can be linked to the presence and strength of seven community capitals: natural, cultural, human, social, political, financial, and built. These resources, when mobilized, can advance the long-term well-being of neighborhoods and communities (Jacobs, 2011). The following is a brief description of each of the community capitals:

Natural Capital

Natural capital consists of "the landscape, air, water, soil, and biodiversity of both plants and animals" (Beaulieu, 2014), which in turn are linked to weather, geographic location, natural resources, and natural beauty (Emery et al., 2006). A healthy and functioning environment provides valuable ecosystem resources, such as food, timber, wildlife habitat, flood control, and recreational opportunities, all of which are essential for human life.

Cultural Capital

Culture is classically described as a "tool kit of symbols, stories, rituals, even the world-view that shapes individuals" (Swidler, 1986). Cultural capital includes the values and symbols reflected in clothing, music, industry, art, language, and customs. It encompasses events, materials (paintings, books), festivals, museums, and other activities and institutions found in communities (Beaulieu, 2014).

Human Capital

This critical capital reflects the investments people make in their education, on-the-job training, or health—activities that translate into improved knowledge, skills, and health status for individuals. Human capital also includes efforts by individuals to enhance their interpersonal and leadership skills in hopes of strengthening their ability to become active contributing members to the civic life of their communities (Beaulieu, 2014).

Social Capital

The "glue" that holds a community together, the presence of which can spur economic growth that brings benefits to an entire neighborhood or community, has been called its social capital (Moore & Kawachi, 2017; Putnam, 2000). *Bonding* social capital represents the strong interactions and ties that people have with family, friends, neighbors, and close work associates, whereas *bridging* social capital reflects the linkages that individuals have with people and groups within the community with whom they have only limited interactions or with individuals and organizations outside the locality. These latter types of relationships are what Granovetter (1973) and Gee et al. (2017) labeled as "weak ties" that can be accessed in times of need. Finally, *linking* social capital consists of the vertical connections that tie community members to organizations and resources located outside the community (Moore & Kawachi, 2017; Putnam, 2000). These vertical linkages offer avenues for local people, organizations, and communities to gain access to valuable resources and ideas from outside the community that can be used to support and guide local initiatives. As Woolcock (2001) and van Deth et al. (2016) noted, the presence of various combinations of bonding, bridging, and linking social capital can have positive impacts on the range of social and economic outcomes that are possible in neighborhoods and communities.

Political Capital

The concept of political capital has three dimensions, beginning with individuals in positions of power and influence in the community and with "the ability to affect the distribution of both public and private resources" (Flora & Flora, 2008, p. 145). The second dimension is the ability to gain access to individuals and organizations—the so-called power brokers or movers and shakers—with the resources to influence important decisions (Flora et al., 2004). Finally, the third aspect of political capital refers to efforts that are made to develop new leadership in the community or to expand the engagement of residents in discussions of important community matters with various strategies, such as deliberation forums.

Financial Capital

A community's financial capital comprises the resources needed to fund the construction and implementation of a variety of programs, projects, and activities that advance the community's economic, social, and infrastructure development. These include community development banks, credit unions, loan funds, venture capital funds, and microenterprise loan funds. Such entities serve as potential sources of a wide range of products and services, including housing, community facilities, small business loans, and other community services that can serve to revitalize economically distressed neighborhoods and communities. The availability of financial capital can contribute to wealth creation and to community economic development activities, especially in low- to moderate-income households or places.

Built Capital

Built capital (also referred to as the built environment) is the infrastructure that supports human society—our roads, bridges, airports, water treatment facilities, buildings (industries, schools, offices, stores), communication technologies, and public places. The built environment also includes design factors and land uses (i.e., how our neighborhoods, communities, and cities are laid out). Increasingly, philanthropic foundations like The California Endowment (TCE.org) and the Robert Wood Johnson Foundation (RWJF.org) are making significant investments in improving the built environments in which people live, work, and play, in recognition of the profound influence of these environments on human health and well-being (Iton & Ross, 2017; Plough & Ford, 2015; Satariano & Maus, 2017).

Table 11.1 provides a synthesis of the seven community capitals, including a sampling of the types of local assets that can be linked to each. While it is unlikely that urban neighborhoods or rural places will have the full slate of capitals available to deploy, striving to pursue a more balanced investment in the seven community capitals can ultimately result in the emergence of strong, resilient neighborhoods and communities. It is worth noting that the community capacity building assets highlighted in the earlier section of this chapter—those associated with people, organizations, and associations—remain relevant under the umbrella of the CCF. The key difference is that the CCF offers a more extensive typology under which a broader array of local assets can be discovered and marshaled by people and groups wishing to pursue neighborhood- and rural community-driven priorities. Further, and once a community's assets have been inventoried and "mapped," whether considered in terms of traditional individual, associational, and organizational assets or also including the broader CCF, community leaders and their partners need to ask several questions key to the rebuilding task:

1. Which organizations can act most effectively as asset development organizations in our neighborhood?

TABLE 11.1

The Seven Types of Community Capitals

Type	Definition	Examples
Natural	Quality and quantity of environmental and natural resources existing in a community	Farmland, parks, mountains, lakes, rivers, forests, wildlife, other natural resource amenities
Cultural	Values, norms, beliefs, and traditions inherited from family, school and community; includes material goods that are produced at a specific time and have historical or cultural significance	Cultural events/festivals, musical heritage, libraries, books, museums, pictures; multi-lingual populations, historical associations
Human	Attributes of individuals that enhance their ability to earn a living, strengthen community, contribute to self-improvement, families, and organizations; includes access to education, and knowledge development, training and skill building activities and efforts to strengthen local leadership	Educational credentials, informal on-the-job training, work force training programs, youth and adult leadership programs, lifelong learning activities
Social	Connections existing among people and organizations that help make things happen in the community; includes close ties that promote community cohesion (bonding) and weaker ties with local and outside people and organizations that promote broad-based action on key matters (bridging)	Activities that build trust among people and groups of different races and ethnic backgrounds, citizen involvement in community discussions, events, and celebrations, civic and service groups that connect diverse people and organizations
Political	Ability to influence and enforce rules, regulations, and standards; access to individuals and groups that participate in civic discourse on difficult public issues and have the power to influence decisions	Elected and appointed government officials and staffers, political organization leaders, citizens that participate in issue forums and their voting rates in local, state and national elections

(continued)

Table 11.1. (continued)

Type	Definition	Examples
Financial	Variety of financial resources available to invest in local projects or economic development initiatives; efforts to build wealth to support community development activities	Community foundations, grants, microloan programs, revolving loan funds, community development financial institutions, banks
Built	Represents community infrastructure, physical structures and services needed to support business, education, and health care sectors	Broadband, utilities, bridges, roads, educational institutions, buildings, facilities, health care clinics

Sources: Emery et al. (2006); Flage and Hauser-Lindstrom (2007); Flora and Flora (2008); Flora et al. (2004); Jacobs (2011).

2. What kinds of community-wide research, planning, and decisionmaking processes can most democratically and effectively advance this rebuilding process?
3. Having inventoried and enlisted the participation of major assets inside the community, how might we build useful bridges to resources outside the community?
4. How might the weak ties developed as part of the linking and bridging elements of social capital serve as conduits for accessing these internal and extra-local assets?

Asset Development Organizations

To begin with, who might lead the community building process? Where might the necessary asset development organizations be found? Two kinds of existing community associations are particularly well suited to the task of knitting together a neighborhood's various assets and capacities. The first, already central to the lives of many older urban neighborhoods, is the multi-issue community organization, built along the "organization of organizations" model of the late Saul Alinsky (Alinsky, 1971; Schutz & Miller, 2015). Community organizers already understand the importance of associational life to the well-being of the neighborhood and to empowerment of the local residents. Many now incorporate a capacity-oriented approach to community building in their ongoing activities (chapter 5).

The second potential asset development organization is the community development corporation. Groups that are dedicated to community economic development have often worked hard to assemble the business assets available to the neighborhood. Many have championed strategies emphasizing local purchasing and hiring and have encouraged homegrown enterprise development. All these approaches can only be strengthened as the local development corporation broadens and deepens its knowledge of community capacity.

Together or separately, these two types of community-based organizations are well suited to the challenge of asset development. But in many low-income urban and rural communities, neither the multi-issue organizing group nor the development corporation may exist. In these settings, neighborhood leaders face the challenge of creating a new asset development organization. This new organization may be built on the strengths and interests of existing citizen's associations and will challenge those associations to affiliate for these broader purposes.

The Community-Planning Process

Having identified or created the asset development organization, community leaders face the challenge of instituting a broad-based process of community planning and decisionmaking. Capacity-oriented community planning may take many different forms, but all of them will have at least these characteristics in common:

1. The neighborhood planning process will aim to involve as many representatives of internally located and controlled assets as possible in the discussion and decisions. In fact, the map of neighborhood assets and community capitals provides an initial list of potential participants in the planning effort.
2. The neighborhood planning process will incorporate some version of a community capacity inventory in its initial stages.
3. The neighborhood planning process will develop community building strategies that take full advantage of the interests and strengths of the participants and will aim toward building the power to define and control the future of the low-income urban neighborhood or rural community.

Building Bridges to Outside Resources

Finally, once the asset development organization has been identified and has begun to mobilize neighborhood stakeholders in a broad-based process of planning, participants will need to assemble the many additional resources needed to advance the community building process. This will involve constructing bridges to persons and organizations outside the neighborhood, including some of those described earlier.

It is clear that no low-income neighborhood can "go it alone." Indeed, every neighborhood or rural place is connected to the outside society and economy to some degree. It is a mark of many low-income urban neighborhoods, in particular, that they are uniquely dependent on outside and human service systems. What they need, however, is to develop their assets and become interdependent with people, groups, and economic activity outside their neighborhood or small town.

Organizations leading developing communities often create unique bridges to the outside including, but well beyond, government agencies. They bridge to banks, corporations, faith-based organizations, other neighborhood advocacy groups, and so on (McKnight & Russell, 2018). These bridged relationships in the nongovernmental sector are vital assets in opening new opportunities for the local residents and enterprises in both urban and rural communities.

The task of the asset development organization, then, involves both drawing the map and using it. It involves leading the community interests into capacity-oriented planning and creating the organizational power to enable that process to become the map of the neighborhood's future.

Concluding Comments

Our chapter is intended to offer hope to low-wealth urban neighborhoods and rural communities that have struggled to create better places in which their residents can live, work, and recreate. The message of this chapter is clear: building vibrant communities, whether urban or rural, begins with a systematic effort to identify and activate the assets that are embedded within them—the talents, skills, resources, and capabilities of people, organizations, and associations that form the fabric of their urban neighborhoods and rural towns.

The first portion of the chapter outlined the urgency of shifting from a deficit-mentality "needs assessment" process to one built on local assets. Next, a step-by-step process for mapping the myriad of assets present in neighborhoods or communities was presented and illustrated. The Community Capitals Framework was then shared as an approach that complements and may add value to the asset-based community development approach by noting the seven arenas in which assets and resources can be discovered.

Finally, and whether using the original ABCD approach or broadening it to include the seven community capitals, the task facing local participants in the place-based planning process, and the community organizations supporting them, is both daunting and filled with promise. But meeting this challenge to rebuild our urban neighborhoods and rural communities from the inside out is critical to the hopes and aspirations of people everywhere.

Questions for Further Discussion

1. You are a staff member in a small health department serving a predominantly low-income community with multiple health and social problems. Your supervisor has asked you to conduct a "needs assessment" to better understand the health challenges of concern to residents. Although you understand that this may provide some useful information, you have read a chapter by John McKnight and colleagues, and are convinced that community asset mapping should also be conducted. What arguments would you make for mapping community assets as part of a broader assessment process? And how would you justify the extra time and costs this would entail?

2. In their research on the community capitals framework, Flora and colleagues note that communities' long-term resilience rests on the presence and strength of seven community capitals. Recognizing that not all communities and neighborhoods are likely to have the full slate of community capitals in place, especially those in economically distressed areas, which of the seven community capital assets would you give primary attention to in your community building efforts, and why?

REFERENCES

Alinsky, S. D. (1971). *Rules for Radicals: A Pragmatic Primer for Realistic Radicals*. Random House.

Beaulieu, L. J. (2014, October). Promoting community vitality and sustainability: The Community Capitals Framework. Purdue Center for Regional Development and Purdue Extension. https://docplayer.net/48294421-Community-vitality-sustainability-the-community-capitals-framework.html.

Bhutta, N., Chang, A. C., Dettling, L. J, & Hsu, J.W., with assistance from J. Hewitt. (2020, September 28). Disparities in wealth by race and ethnicity in the 2019 Survey of Consumer Finances. Fed Notes. https://www.federalreserve.gov/econres/notes/feds-notes/disparities-in-wealth-by-race-and-ethnicity-in-the-2019-survey-of-consumer-finances-20200928.htm.

Blackwell, A. G., & McAffee, M. (2020, June 26). Banks should face history and pay reparations. *New York Times*. https://www.nytimes.com/2020/06/26/opinion/sunday/banks-reparations-racism-inequality.html.

Bristol, D. W. (2009). *Knights of the Razor: Black Barbers in Slavery and Freedom*. Johns Hopkins University Press.

Brown, D. L., & Schafft, K. A. (2011). *Rural People and Communities in the 21st Century: Resilience and Transformation*. Polity Press.

Cooney, K. (2016). Work integration social enterprises in the United States: Operating at the nexus of public policy, markets, and community. *Nonprofit Policy Forum, 7*(4), 435–460.

Emery, M., Fey, S., & Flora, C. B. (2006). *Using Community Capitals to Build Assets for Positive Community Change*. Community Development Society. https://www.comm-dev.org/images/pdf/Issue13-2006.pdf.

Flora, C. B., & Flora, J. L. (2008). *Rural Communities: Legacy and Change* (3rd ed.). Westview Press.

Flora, C. B., Flora, J. L., & Fey, S. (2004). *Rural Communities: Legacy and Change* (2nd ed.). Westview Press.

Gee, L. K., Jones, J. J., Fariss, C. J., Burke, M., & Fowler, J. H. (2017). The paradox of weak ties in 55 countries. *J Econ Behav Organ, 133*, 362–372.

Granovetter, M. (1973). The strength of weak ties. *Am J Sociol, 78*, 1360–1383.

Iton, A., & Ross, R. K. (2017). Understanding how health happens: Your zip code is more important than your genetic code. In R. Callahan & D. Bhattacharya (Eds.), *Public Health Leadership* (pp. 83–99). Routledge.

Jacobs, C. (2011). Measuring success in communities: Understanding the community capitals framework. Extension Extra. South Dakota State Cooperative Extension Service: Issue 16005 (Revised April).

Johnson, K., & Lichter, D. (2019, February 6). Rural depopulation in a rapidly urbanizing America. Carsey Research National Issue Brief 139 (pp. 1–6). University of New Hampshire Carsey School of Public Policy. https://carsey.unh.edu/publication/rural-depopulation.

Karas, D. (2019, January 6). One man's mission to revitalize small-town America. *Christian Science Monitor*. https://www.csmonitor.com/World/Making-a-difference/2019/0106/One-man-s-mission-to-revitalize-small-town-America.

Kotz, P. (2019, March 6). The Kindness Revolt: A not-so-secret plot to make a better Minnesota. CityPages. http://www.citypages.com/news/the-kindness-revolt-a-not-so-secret-plot-to-make-a-better-minnesota/506724471.

Kretzmann, J. P., & McKnight, J. L. (1993). *Building Communities from the Inside Out: A Path toward Finding and Mobilizing a Community's Assets.* ACTA Publications.

McKnight, J. L., & Russell, C. (2018). The four essential elements of an asset-based community development process. What is distinctive about asset-based community process? ABCD Institute, DePaul University. https://www.nurturedevelopment.org/wp-content/uploads/2018/09/4_Essential_Elements_of_ABCD_Process.pdf.

Minkler, M., Estrada, J., Dyer, S., Hennessey-Lavery, S., Wakimoto, P., & Falbe, J. (2019). Healthy retail as a strategy for improving food security and the built environment in San Francisco. *Am J Public Health, 109*(S2), S137–S140.

Moore, S., & Kawachi I. J. (2017). Twenty years of social capital and health research: A glossary. *J Epidemiol Community Health, 71,* 513–517.

Plecher, H. (2020, July 15). *Urbanization in the United States 1970 to 2019.* World Bank. https://www.statista.com/statistics/269967/urbanization-in-the-united-states/.

Plough, A., & Ford, C. (2015). *From Vision to Action: A Framework and Measures to Mobilize a Culture of Health.* Robert Wood Johnson Foundation.

Putnam, R. (2000). *Bowling Alone: The Collapse and Revival of American Community.* Simon and Schuster.

Research on Disabilities. (2019, August 2). July 2019 Jobs Report: Positive pattern continues for jobseekers with disabilities. National Trends in Disability Employment. Comparison of People with and without Disabilities. Kessler Foundation and University of New Hampshire's Institute on Disability (UNH-IOD). https://researchondisability-pre.sr.unh.edu/season4-episode8.

Sadd, J., Morello-Frosch, R., Pastor, M., Matsuoka, M., Prichard, M., & Carter, V. (2014). The truth, the whole truth, and nothing but the ground-truth: Methods to advance environmental justice and researcher–community partnerships. *Health Educ Behav, 41*(3), 281–290.

Satariano, W. A., & Maus, M. (2017). *Aging, Place, and Health: A Global Perspective.* Jones & Bartlett Learning.

Schutz, A., & Miller, M. (2015). *People Power: The Community Organizing Tradition of Saul Alinsky.* Vanderbilt University Press.

Sehgal, A. R. (2020). Lifetime risk of death from firearm injuries, drug overdoses, and motor vehicle accidents in the United States. *Am J Med, 133*(10), 1162–1167.

Sonke, J., Golden, T., Francois, S., Hand, J., Chandra, A., Clemmons, L., Fakunle, D., Jackson, M. R., Magsamen, S., Rubin, V., Sams, K., & Springs, S. (2019). *Creating Healthy Communities through Cross-Sector Collaboration* [White paper]. University of Florida Center for Arts in Medicine / ArtPlace America.

Swidler, A. (1986). Culture in action: Symbols and strategies. *Am Sociol Rev, 51,* 273–286.

van Deth, J. W., Edwards, B., Moldavanova, A., & Woolcock, M. (2016). Associations and social capital. In D. H. Smith, R. A. Stebbins, & G. Jurgen (Eds.), *The Palgrave Handbook of Volunteering, Civic Participation, and Nonprofit Associations* (vol. 1–2, pp. 178–197). Palgrave Macmillan.

Wallerstein, N. (2006, February). *What Is the Evidence on Effectiveness of Empowerment to Improve Health?* Health Evidence Network Report. WHO Regional Office for Europe. https://www.euro.who.int/__data/assets/pdf_file/0010/74656/E88086.pdf.

Warden, D. (2020). The Americans with Disabilities Act at thirty. *Calif L Rev Online, 11,* 308.

Woolcock, M. (2001). The place of social capital in understanding social and economic outcomes. *Can J Policy Res, 2*(1), 11–17.

12

Selecting the Issue

LEE STAPLES
RINKU SEN

Community organizer Mike Miller is fond of saying that there is an important difference between problems and issues: *problems* are things outsiders say are wrong with a community, while *issues* are things community members feel strongly enough about to want to do something about. For other organizers, problems refer to large-scale systems that are too large and vague to help community groups focus on real changes worth fighting for. They remind us that identifying specific issues within large-scale problems helps us define clear conflicts to which our group can propose a resolution.

Regardless of the exact definition we use, however, one of the most difficult and hotly contested organizing tasks is helping members decide which issues to take up and how—a process known as *issue selection* or *issue development*. Issues are the most public expression of an organization's values and worldview. Like all the other parts of organizing, issue selection is a craft, both science and art. As such, it has rules and logic, a language and systems. These can always be improved and adapted for a particular organization, but the need to develop issues is beyond dispute. Each organization and coalition must decide what values and precepts will guide its issue choices, how to frame those issues, and how to educate and engage its members in issue selection and framing.

We devote most of this chapter to the importance of, and strategies for, selecting and "cutting" or framing an issue for a successful campaign. But we begin with a related and often neglected topic: What happens when your group doesn't have the luxury of selecting an issue because the issue chooses them? We then discuss several areas critical in either situation, namely, strategic analysis in identifying targets and handles and moving into action.

Choosing the Issue, or Having It Choose You

Although in theory community groups should embark on new campaigns only after considerable discussion and analysis, sometimes they have little choice but to respond to a particular issue: that's when the issue chooses *them*, rather than vice versa. For instance, a neighborhood group would be expected to react quickly to the discovery of toxic waste dumping in the local river, or the suspension of weekly trash pickup. Similarly, an immigrant-rights group could hardly overlook a legislative proposal to eliminate state health coverage for low-income, legally registered noncitizens. The silver lining of such situations is that many people will be highly interested and ready to take action. In such instances, the community group really cannot afford to walk away if it wants to do the right thing while retaining its credibility. It is a time to fight the good fight—win, lose, or draw (Staples, 2016).

Years ago, as a student organizer, Rinku trained other students around the country as part of the Grassroots Organizing Weekends under the auspices of the United States Student Association and the famed Midwest Academy, a training institute founded in 1973 for community organizers and organizations committed to "advancing the struggle for social, economic, and racial justice" (https:// midwestacademy.com). In co-leading the Academy's session called "Choosing Issues," Rinku asked participants to review a set of criteria for good issues, apply them to campaign options, and rank the options to determine the best issue.

Students of color, women, and LGBT students, arguably the most explicitly marginalized constituencies on their campuses, frequently resisted our characterization of "good" issues. They asserted, quite correctly, that they rarely had the luxury of choosing issues. Rather, issues were thrust upon them by oppressive institutional policies and practices that forced them into survival mode. Furthermore, they said, choosing issues creates a hierarchy among oppressions: groups have to make implicit, if not explicit, judgments about which issues are important enough to work on and which are not, who deserves liberation and who does not.

These students had good reason to resist this framework. However wellmeaning, the criteria being used and the notion of prioritizing issues had been leveraged against these groups by less marginal groups to justify avoiding their controversial issues (chapter 8).

Today, we would suggest that those students create their own criteria for prioritizing issues. While it is true that some attacks must be answered immediately and forcefully, having clear criteria can help your group respond effectively, as well as move beyond defensive postures to victories that improve their sense of control and other quality-of-life markers. Without clear criteria to guide them, organizations tend to jump from issue to issue and thus have difficulty applying the successes and capacity built during one campaign to the next. As Marion Steeg, former staff director of Working Partnerships, likes to say, "Some issues you choose, some issues choose you." Even when issues choose you, however, you still have to decide whether or not to act like the "chosen people." When our opponents pick a fight that agitates everyone and has major implications, we risk becoming irrelevant if we *don't* respond. However, strong organizations cannot be driven entirely by the crises created by their opposition. A completely reactive stance produces stagnant organizations that can never get ahead of their opposition, and that are always running to shift a debate, the parameters of which have already been set.

Issues and Issue Campaigns

Issues have at least three elements: a constituency with a grievance, a set of demands that address that grievance, and an institutional target at whom the grievance is directed. If a group cannot identify these elements with specificity, then it is probably still dealing at the level of problems rather than carving out issues.

There are also four principles to crafting a good issue. First, we must have *clear criteria* that guide our issue choices. Second, and because they define the conflict and provide negotiating points, our *demands must be ambitious and specific*. Third, these *demands should be directed toward the individual decisionmakers* with the power to make change, and who constitute our targets (Sen, 2003; Staples, 2016; appendixes 8, 9, 11). All of these add up to the fourth principle: we must *pay attention to the frame* we put an issue in as well as the issue itself (Dorfman, 2009; Wallack et al., 1999; chapter 24).

Although these considerations are relevant to any group, whether formal or informal, when we are working as part of a coalition or other grassroots community organization (GCO), additional criteria also come into play. In this larger context, the issues selected will have long-lasting implications for organizational leadership, the ideas we advance in the larger society, and the kinds of institutional changes we are able to gain.

The importance of the interrelationship between organizational development and issue campaigns can't be overemphasized. Viewed from this broader perspective, issue campaigns are both ends and means. GCOs form as vehicles to address issues of concern. A GCO's ability to deal successfully with any issue is a function of its level of organizational development. Organizations grow through experience and practice; issue campaigns are the very lifeblood of that process. Through them, new people are attracted, existing members remain active, and leadership abilities come to flower (Staples, 2016).

Choosing Issues: Some Core Considerations

Of the many matters to consider in issue development, three stand out: *depth*, *breadth*, and *organizational mileage*. *Depth* refers to how intensely community members feel about an issue, while *breadth* relates to how widespread that concern is.

The strongest issues will be felt deeply by a broad cross section of the community (Bobo et al., 2010; Sen 2003; Staples, 2016). For instance, a proposal to close a popular community health clinic in a low-income urban neighborhood might be strongly opposed by virtually everyone living in the area. This issue would have *both depth and breadth*, thereby helping to ensure that large numbers of the affected constituency would participate in collective action to resist the closure. In the same neighborhood, people living on a street where street lights have been out for over a month as winter approaches would likely be deeply concerned and willing to take action. But residents living ten blocks away may not even be aware of the existence of this problem, greatly limiting the base from which to draw participants. Still another potential issue, such as beautification of parks in the area, might have wide support, yet likely would not be on many residents' top 10 list of concerns. Finally, if the appeal of an issue is neither broad nor deep (e.g., in this hypothetical low-income neighborhood, a proposal to limit offshore oil drilling), it should not even be up for consideration.

Along with the depth and breadth of community and member concern with a potential issue, a third core consideration in issue selection is that of *organizational mileage*. Coined half a century ago (Haggstrom, 1971) and a staple of organizing in the Alinsky (1971) tradition (Schutz & Miller, 2015), organizational mileage is an important means of assessing the degree of organizational development attained by a grassroots group. The best issue campaigns will develop *organizational mileage* while simultaneously appealing to the self-interests of community members. Therefore, when choosing an issue, a community organization must be concerned about *not only whether it can be won but also how the campaign will develop the group.*

Groups usually need large numbers of actively engaged people, both to achieve a victory on the issue and to increase organizational mileage. To assess the latter, consider ten dimensions: membership, leadership, staffing, structure, goal attainment, target systems influenced, strategy and tactics employed, finances, allies, and communications (Staples, 2016).

Before deciding to embark on a new issue campaign, it is helpful to address the following questions. Although not an exhaustive list, the questions illustrate the thought process that goes into a strategic analysis that maximizes an issue's potential for organizational mileage (Staples, 2016; appendixes 8, 9, 11).

- Is the issue consistent with the organization's long- and middle-range goals?
- Will the issue be unifying or divisive? Who will be unified or divided exactly?
- What is the community organization's capacity to undertake this issue campaign at the present time?
- Will the campaign help the GCO grow?
- Will the campaign provide a good educational experience for leaders and members, developing their critical consciousness, independence, and skills?
- Will the GCO receive credit for a victory on the issue, improve its credibility, and increase its overall visibility?

- How will the campaign affect organizational resources?
- Will the campaign develop new allies or enemies?
- Will the campaign emphasize collective action, producing new strategies, tactics, or issues?
- Will the campaign be crafting ambitious and specific demands?
- Will the campaign produce a significant victory?

Although the complete answers to questions like these may not be available until *after* the organization engages in a systematic postcampaign evaluation process, much can be determined and predicted ahead of time.

The Midwest Academy Criteria for Choosing Issues

The Midwest Academy (http://www.midwestacademy.com/), often described as the "gold standard" for issue selection in community organizing, developed a related set of propositions that can help groups consider diverse dimensions of issue selection. Indeed, of the many tools and strategies taught through the Academy's week-long courses (in which over 25,000 organizers have participated to date), among the best known are its criteria for choosing among different issues (box 12.1). Several of these criteria speak directly or indirectly to facets of organizational mileage, while others overlap with other core considerations (e.g., depth and breadth of support) captured in the questions outlined above (Staples, 2016).

Few issues perfectly meet all criteria, so we have to negotiate to find the most promising ones. A group might prioritize criteria differently depending on the phase of the organization's life. For example, "winnability" might be more important to a newer organization that is trying to establish a track record; therefore, it might choose smaller, less controversial issues. Because all organizations cannot be all things to all people at all times, most of us have to find compromises among choosing ideal criteria to guide our issue work, the need to react to our opposition, the limits of our organizational resources, and the imperatives of our organizational mission (Staples, 2016).

Elsewhere, Staples (2016) discusses in more detail each of several themes captured in and across the questions and criteria listed above. These include the following:

- Consistency—Is the issue consistent with the long-range goals of the organization?
- Capacity—What is the organization's capacity to undertake this issue at the present time?
- Education—Will the campaign provide a good educational experience for leaders and members?
- Tactics—Will the campaign emphasize collective action, producing new strategies, tactics, or issues? (p. 126).

BOX 12.1

Midwest Academy Criteria for Choosing Issues

1. The issue meets the principles of direct action organizing—that is, it leads to a real difference in people's everyday lives, it gives people a sense of their own power, and it changes the relations of power.

2. The issue is worthwhile, widely and deeply felt, nondivisive, and consistent with the organization's values and vision. Many people in your constituency must find it important enough to take some action on it.

3. The issue suggests clear demands. The changes you propose address the negative conditions you've identified.

4. The issue is winnable. You have determined the likelihood of getting your solutions adopted by a particular agency or institution; precedents in other places, the affordability of your plan, the strength of your legal arguments, a clear strategy, or some other advantage raises your chances of winning.

5. The issue is easy to understand. The common rule is that you should be able to explain it in one paragraph on a flyer.

6. The issue has a clear target. In organizing, the target is always an individual who can agree to meet your demands.

7. The issue has a clear time frame that works for you. Issue campaigns, like good novels or movies, should have a beginning, middle, and end, and you should know roughly how long each of those phases will last.

8. The issue gives you opportunities to build leadership. An issue campaign should have many roles for people to play because the issue itself lends itself to many different creative tactics. For example, an issue that can be won only through a lawsuit is not the kind that builds leadership, as the key decision-making and negotiation roles tend to be limited to lawyers and judges.

9. The issue sets up your organization to tackle additional and related issues. The issue should help build a track record, a base of people, and knowledge that the organization can easily transfer to other arenas.

Source: Bobo et al. (1991), p. 28.

Finally, considerable attention must be directed to the *nature of the demands*: Will the campaign develop ambitious and specific demands that define the conflict? Demands provide your organization's major negotiating points and help determine the ebb and flow of a campaign. Strong campaigns have multiple demands, letting the group carve out incremental victories that motivate your membership to stay together, put cracks in the system that can be widened with additional campaigns, attract allies to collaborate on more ambitious efforts, and raise your level of knowledge about a specific institution and arena.

Substantive demands often have a policy character. For example, and while still insufficient, major wins resulted from Black Lives Matter protests in several cities (e.g., ending school contracts with police, and redirecting millions of dollars from local police departments to health and welfare programs). Such wins were important, in part, in meeting such criteria as giving a sense of power, changing conditions, shifting power, helping address racial inequities, and using "race-based discrimination" as a handle (Sen, 2003; appendix 8).

However, *procedural demands* are also important, including securing meetings with targets, placing your organization's leaders on institutional planning committees, or forcing politicians to host public hearings on your issues (Staples, 2016).

Winning victories, empowering people, and bringing about change are what organizing is all about. Without good strategic thinking, however, none of this is possible.

Working from the Bottom Up in Issue Selection

Although the above tools are useful in helping groups assess potential new issues and strategies for success, there aren't any shortcuts in this process. For example, it may be tempting to discuss a possible issue among only the top leadership, but this common mistake overlooks one key factor. These leaders may be so committed to the organization that they are no longer typical of rank-and-file members and, as such, may be very poor judges of which issue campaigns will appeal most widely and deeply to the membership. Within the organization, issues should be tested and selected with as much bottom-up participation as possible. To do otherwise is to risk a campaign without a large base of committed people.

Finding and testing out organizing issues typically involve talking with community members and trying out various themes. Such exploration can take place through organizational meetings, actions, events, door knocking, house meetings, town halls, and, now more than ever, through online neighborhood surveys and social media (ideally followed up by community meetings to share and discuss findings).

For professionals in fields like health promotion and social work, focus groups or community forums are also popular methods for finding and testing issues and community-perceived needs (Krueger & Casey, 2014). Regardless of the particular means used, however, the role of the organizer, whether in the Alinsky (1971) or Freirean tradition, is one of active listening, asking questions, and facilitating the issue-selection process prior to the determination of targets and tactics, and action based on critical reflection (Freire, 1970, 1973; Schutz & Miller, 2015; Sen, 2003; Su, 2009; chapter 5).

Framing the Issue

Once an organization selects an issue, it still has to determine how to frame it in a compelling way. A good frame has two important characteristics. First, it is broad. It can move from issue to issue because it speaks to the shared values of our constituency and allies and, as much as possible, those of the larger public. Strong frames shape the membership's expectations about what kinds of issues fall within the organization's mission, reflecting ambitious definitions of justice. Second, because framing is largely a matter of working with language, a good frame will shape your media messages to greatest advantage (Dorfman & Bakal, 2018; Wallack et al., 1999; chapter 24). Frames can be expressed in various ways—through campaign slogans and names, the headlines of press releases, or simply the repetition of particular images, words, and phrases. Many politically conservative groups have a long track record of successfully framing their issues, in part, by investing resources in testing and evaluation to determine what frame provides the most fuel for their agenda. For example, attacks on welfare are framed as reducing "dependency," while affirmative action has been reframed as "special preferences." Among progressives, many of the most effective living wage campaigns stress the need for corporate accountability in exchange for tax subsidies, or subsidy accountability. Struggles to win higher wages and benefits for childcare workers have been attached to the goal of increasing quality by reducing turnover, well before COVID-19. Necessary higher baseline wages are framed as "self-sufficiency."

Our frames may also be heavily influenced by changing political, social, and cultural contexts (Dorfman, 2009; chapter 24). Indeed, one way we can measure progress is by noting the extent to which we can use more progressive frames over time. For example, the widespread use of "fighting systemic racism" as a frame got a huge boost in the public discourse in the aftermath of the police killing of George Floyd in 2020, the historic protests and continued attention to new police killings of unarmed people of color. Naming long-standing practices like racialized policing and redlining as systemic racism has made it possible to make successful demands, such as mandatory anti-racism training in many public and private sector organizations (Came & Griffin, 2018; Kendi, 2019; chapter 4; appendix 1).

Cutting and Framing in the Issue Campaign

To develop the basic outlines of an issue campaign, ask the classic question, "*Who* wants to get *what* from *whom* and *how* will this be accomplished?" Answers to this four-part question help us identify the action group that seeks change, what goals and objectives they are pursuing, the target system they intend to activate or influence, and how they will employ handles or leverage points to achieve their ends. The issue is *cut* and *framed* when these questions are answered.

Action Group

The people who participate in an issue campaign will feel it is in their own self-interest to do so. Obviously, issues appeal differently to different constituencies. For instance, climate change, and calls for things like more affordable solar power and electric vehicles to help combat it, have been of growing concern to many middle- and upper-class activists, as well as youth. But in a low-income neighborhood where issues of basic survival confront people daily (and where there is fear of lost jobs during the transition to a green economy), climate change, let alone electric cars and solar panels, may have little immediacy compared with inadequate housing, unemployment, and poor schools. If the issue is cut effectively, however, it may well attract both constituencies. For example, many low-income communities of color live near freeways and other polluting facilities and suffer high rates of asthma and related health problems. In these communities, talking instead about environmental justice and demands (such as more stringent regulation of carbon emissions to reduce asthma and improve air quality) may help residents feel self-interest in the broader issue. Specific issues must be "cut" to appeal to particular constituencies: rent control to resonate with tenants, low-interest home improvement loans to engage homeowners, or good quality public housing near public transportation for low-income and disabled residents.

The depth of an issue's appeal is partly a function of the emotional response it triggers. Frequently, *defensive* issues (e.g., "stop the cutbacks," "stop the oil pipeline") arouse more passion than efforts to win a positive reform or program. Fear is a powerful motivator. Like the proverbial straw that breaks the camel's back, such issues may be able to activate people who have never participated before. Often these are NIMBY ("not in my backyard") issues that provoke a strong emotional response from community members who perceive their interests as being threatened.

Of course, many campaigns to bring about proactive change also generate plenty of emotion, including outrage at lost opportunity, hope and excitement over moving forward, which are often more sustainable when outrage burns out. Issues such as a livable wage, preventing opioid overdoses, expanding affordable housing, gun control, women's reproductive rights, and protecting immigrants' rights have moved many thousands of people on both the left and the right into action in recent years. Furthermore, any GCO that seeks to empower people must move beyond defensive responses that simply "tame" the behavior of institutional decisionmakers, to proactive campaigns that transform power relationships (Schutz & Miller, 2015). But it is critical to frame these positive efforts in a manner that generates sufficient passion to motivate lots of people.

Goals and Objectives

Goals are broad statements about *what* people want done to solve a problem or to make a change, such as "end human rights violations in psychiatric hospitals." *Objectives* are *specific outcomes* that contribute to the achievement of goals and are time sensitive and measurable, such as "adoption of a new mental health department policy on the use of forced restraints and seclusion in state psychiatric hospitals by Memorial Day." The overall goals of an issue campaign should be clear, compelling, and enjoying strong community support.

Cutting and framing the issue necessitates determining *what specific objectives* will move the group toward its ultimate goal. *Objectives must be concrete and realistic.* Possible solutions to the problem at hand should be tested with a number of people as part of the issue-cutting and -framing process. *It is important to start by finding out which options community members really want.* As in issue selection, this should be a true bottom-up process, not merely a ratification of the goals and objectives of leaders, organizers, planners, politicians, or various interested parties. Testing different alternatives helps people develop ownership of both the issue and the strategy to resolve it. This investment is essential for the campaign to be truly broad based and participatory. Community members will invest time and energy only if they feel passionate about the issue's goals and objectives.

Once there is a general sense of the preferable solution(s), the group must determine how *realistic* the various possibilities are. This is an area where *action research* (Townsend, 2019) or *participatory research* (Minkler, 2014; Vincent & Fernandez, 2016; chapter 15) plays a key role. Good research is essential in order to predict the potential for accomplishing particular objectives. As much as possible, the GCO's leaders should be involved in the research process. They should share new information learned with the full action group. For example, as soon as it is discovered that the housing authority is sitting on an unspent sum of money provided by the Department of Housing and Urban Development to "solve the trash problems," public housing tenants who are unhappy with the dumpsters provided for trash collection should be informed. Formulating objectives is a dynamic process that continues to evolve as more information is gathered and various viable options are presented.

You will continue to shape and refine specifics as you weigh and analyze more factors. At the start, as you first cut and frame the issue, it is enough to draw the broad outline of demands. Again, remember that *what* the objectives will be is a function of *who* the action group is, *what* target system they intend to activate or influence, and *how* they can use *handles* to achieve their ends.

Target System

To pursue its objectives, the action group attempts to influence a *target system*, which may be internal (e.g., motivating community members to participate in a development project) or external (e.g., pressuring institutional decisionmakers to do what they otherwise would not do). There are many factors to consider when determining whom to target, beginning with identifying the person who has the power to make concrete, specific decisions on the action group's objectives and holding that person accountable. Identifying the right target, and understanding his or her self-interest, helps the action group assess the degree of leverage it can bring to bear (Falbe et al., 2018; appendixes 8, 9, 11). The group will be able to influence the target to the extent that it can affect positive or negative self-interests, such as votes, customers, public image, career advancement, or keeping a job.

Accurate targeting requires solid research. We must understand the decision-making process thoroughly, and then fix responsibility correctly on one or more key individuals who can meet our demands and who are vulnerable to pressure from the action group, such as the governor, a corporate CEO, the mayor, a commissioner, the city council, a hospital administrator, or a school committee.

Power mapping (Falbe et al., 2018; appendix II) is a useful tool at this stage for identifying relevant stakeholders who support or oppose the desired change, and their relative influence vis-à-vis the target. Be sure that you know the "chain of command" and can distinguish between formal and informal decisionmaking processes, remembering that those who wield the most power may not occupy the most visible positions. The action group may have to move first on those who are officially responsible to "smoke out" the powers that be. In other instances, the best strategy is to move directly on the hidden decisionmakers. In addition, the group may call for strict adherence to orthodox decisionmaking procedures, or it may push for creative changes in established practices.

There is nothing like a villain to energize a campaign. In one classic example, M-POWER (Massachusetts People / Patients Organized for Wellness, Empowerment and Rights) targeted the director of a large psychiatric hospital where patients were receiving poor care and where three deaths had occurred in one year. On Valentine's Day, the director was confronted by a large demonstration, during which M-POWER members passed out empty heart-shaped boxes that had contained chocolates, now holding cards asking him to "have a heart" and treat patients with dignity and proper care. Under continued pressure from this action group, the director soon resigned, and a new director took office and promised reform.

Sometimes a community organization has limited direct leverage vis-à-vis a particular target. In such instances, indirect secondary targets may be used. For example, a health care coalition might target a teaching hospital to pressure it to institute preventive programs for infant mortality, childhood obesity, adolescent smoking, and diabetes in the low-income neighborhood where it is located. If the hospital CEO was unresponsive to the action group, the group might then target individual members of the facility's board. The members might be more vulnerable to negative publicity than the CEO, and they might even support the coalition's goals and objectives. Or they might remain neutral on the matter, especially if the publicity would be bad for their business and individual reputations. The CEO might not respond to the direct action of the community coalition but would most likely pay attention to pressure from influential board members. It is of the utmost importance that indirect secondary targets should be chosen using two criteria: ability to influence the primary target and vulnerability to pressure from the action group. In these efforts, too, power mapping can be a valuable tool (Falbe et al., 2018; appendix II).

Handles

Just as you need a handle to open a door, you need a handle to grab hold of an organizing issue. *Handles* are points of leverage that an action group can use to influence or activate a target system. Handles may be *situations* that make a target more vulnerable to pressure from community members (e.g., upcoming elections, hazardous waste spills, or other crises). They may be *precedents* that set the stage for similar demands, or *regulatory processes* that can be used to gain new information or to mobilize large numbers of people to attend public hearings and testify. Handles may also be *incidents*, such as an abuse of power when a police officer shoots an unarmed person of color.

Handles provide a means for *how* change efforts move from the realm of hope to real accomplishments; they enable proponents of change to *overcome resistance or inertia.* The leverage of handles gets target systems moving in the right direction, making decisions and taking action in ways that are consistent with the action group's goals and objectives for social change. Handles can be either positive incentives (carrots) or negative sanctions (sticks). All things being equal, carrots are preferable to sticks, since positive incentives make it more likely that the affected target system will really internalize changes with positive payoffs. Community development projects frequently use a wide variety of positive *internal* incentives to encourage people to get involved in a change effort. For instance, inducements such as food, music, awards, certificates of participation, tickets to an amusement park, or prizes might be handles to encourage youth to participate in a neighborhood cleanup. A community clinic might hold a health fair with similar attractions, as well as face painting for kids, a radio or social media personality, and local entertainment.

Positive incentives might also be used to help frame issues in "win-win" terms for *external* target systems. Judy Meredith's "hero opportunity" concept is relevant here (Meredith & Dunham, 2016). The idea is that individual decision-makers can look good and gain a measure of credit by agreeing to help an action group meet its objectives. Thus, an elected official—especially one facing a strong challenger in an upcoming election—might act to meet a community group's request to open a new youth center or to sponsor an inclusionary zoning ordinance. While this phenomenon is inconsistent with the discussion above regarding the importance of community groups receiving credit for their accomplishments, there are times when the trade-off for support and ultimate success is worth the sacrifice.

Unfortunately, all things *are not* equal, which is often why a GCO is formed in the first place. Under such circumstances, stronger forms of collective action are necessary; we use handles to pressure targets to act in a manner or to modify or stop certain activities. Handles can also provide a reason for *why* the action group's position is justifiable, such as a broken promise, an existing law that hasn't been enforced, or a contradiction. Thus, the concept entails both a *tool* that an action group can use to maximize its power on an issue as well as a *rationale* that underscores the legitimacy of the campaign when the issue is framed (chapter 24). For instance, a study or report releasing new information can place target systems on the defensive. The data could be produced by a third party, such as the Action

Center for Race & the Economy (https://acrecampaigns.org/), which helps translate data into accessible, user-friendly formats or by the organization's own research and communications team members (chapter 15).

Bureaucratic regulations often allow great latitude in interpretation. At times, a strict interpretation may serve organizational interests, while frequently a broad definition may be more advantageous for the action group. Louis Lowy, one of Lee's mentors and former colleagues, often pointed out that bureaucrats operate in three arenas: what they *must* do to fulfill the basic requirements of their positions, what they *must not* do to exceed their authority, and what they *may* do at their discretion. Handles can be found in all three areas.

For example, since housing inspectors *must* enforce the state sanitary code, a tenants' group can use this handle to hold their feet to the fire, making sure that absentee slumlords are held properly accountable. Discretionary judgments made by those in authority can have profound impacts on whether community members get access to health care, housing, education, safety, social services, benefits, employment, or training. The fact that these individuals *may* act in a way that is consistent with the objectives of an action group provides a handle of possibility. Similar to broken promises, *contradictions* present a clear case of a disconnection or gap between rhetoric and reality. When an action group frames its issues to publicize such gaps, it can usually operate from a stance of "moral superiority," enabling it to place the target in a defensive, if not indefensible, position. Generally, the media are quick to pick up on stories depicting contradictory behavior, strengthening the group's leverage in the process (chapter 24).

In contrast to incidents, *events* (as defined here) are usually scheduled and fairly predictable. Using them allows for more forethought and planning. Events provide handles and excellent opportunities for direct action because they occur at a fixed time and place where an organization can go to frame an issue and gain access to and confront a target. High-profile events already will be covered by the media, thereby providing a "news peg" that enables the action group to frame its message for a larger audience (chapter 24). Typical examples are a corporation's annual stockholder's meeting, a speech or visit by a public official, the dedication of a new building, a special public hearing, or a political fund-raising dinner. City Life/Vida Urbana dramatically illustrated this handle by using strong direct action organizing to physically block scheduled auctions of foreclosed buildings in Greater Boston neighborhoods.

Handles are the single most important variable in cutting and framing an issue. Handles are usually present in some form, although they may not be readily apparent. It is very often not a question of *whether* they exist, but rather *where* and *when* they can be found (Staples, 2016).

These four elements—action group, goals and objectives, target system, and handles—are interrelated, and we should not try to separate or sequence them. Work on all of them simultaneously. They define the basic outline of a potential issue, which you have now cut and framed.

Issue Selection and Strategic Analysis: A Final Note

This chapter has focused on the criteria that community organizations should consider when selecting new issues. It has also examined the elements that constitute the process of cutting the issue—a vital part of strategic development. Issue development is a task that encompasses all aspects of organizing practice—outreach, research, ideology, and strategy. Requiring that any new issue meets every one of our criteria greatly limits our choices. However, having a clear set of criteria and being flexible about which of these is most important at a particular stage in the organization's history can help us make more ambitious issue choices. When the community is involved in researching issues and designing the solutions, our organizations are also more likely to be able to sustain longer and more ambitious struggles.

While a full discussion of strategic analysis is beyond the scope of this chapter (see Homan, 2016; Staples, 2016; appendixes 8, 9, 11), a few key points follow. First, a SWOT analysis, to examine strengths, weaknesses, opportunities, and threats (Chermack & Kasshanna, 2007; Gürel & Tat, 2017; appendix 11), can help a group lay out the internal strengths and weaknesses of the action group and the opportunities and threats in the external environment, and provides an excellent tool for initial analysis. This approach enables proponents of a social change to make a rigorous assessment of the positive and negative factors that will directly affect chances for success. Second, a force field analysis (Dubey, 2017; Lewin, 1947; Minnesota State Health Department, 2020; appendix 11) is a valuable tool for assessing the level of agreement that exists between an action group and a target system, and the helping and hindering forces that will affect the change effort. Conducting a force field analysis helps inform the selection of appropriate strategies. These and other tools and guidelines for strategic analysis are discussed in detail in the KU Community Tool Box, chapter 14 and section 14 (https://ctb.ku.edu/en/table-of-contents /assessment/assessing-community-needs-and-resources/swot-analysis/main).

Warren's (1975) classic strategic guidelines suggest three major types of change strategies: *collaborative strategies* (where there is broad agreement), *campaign strategies* (when differences among parties exist), and *adversarial strategies* (when persuasive arguments are unlikely to be effective). While the mechanics of a strategic analysis are quite simple (appendix 11), the various factors should be viewed dynamically rather than statically, with action and change as the goals.

Other key factors of any strategic analysis are opposition, objective conditions, organizational capacity, and support. The analysis should answer several basic questions: Who is against you? What is beyond your control that affects chances for success (both positively and negatively)? What is your action group capable of doing? What is the possibility of assistance from allies or from joining a coalition? Whether it is done formally through a strategic analysis or more informally, analysis of these factors, in conjunction with the process of cutting the issue, should give a reasonably accurate picture of the level of organizational action and clout necessary to achieve success.

In sum, your organization must weigh multiple factors and consider many variables when choosing and cutting issues, in addition to developing effective strategies. But the group should be careful not to analyze and strategize to the point where no action can materialize. It is impossible to plan for or imagine every single possibility. There is a time to act!

Questions for Further Discussion

1. One of the many core criteria discussed in issue selection is whether the issue being considered will be unifying or divisive for your grassroots organization or coalition. Identify an issue that may be of relevance and importance for your group or organization. What do you think are the most compelling arguments for ensuring that the issue will promote unity in your group?

2. Can you think of an instance in which an issue that might be more controversial (e.g., popular with some members but disliked by others) might be important to take up even if it didn't fully meet the unity criterion? Or is it always a mistake to do so?

Acknowledgments

Portions of this chapter are adapted from the following: Staples, L. (2016). Analyze, strategize, and catalyze: Issues and strategies. In *Roots to Power: A Manual of Grassroots Organizing* (3rd ed., pp. 123–175). Praeger. Copyright © 2016 by Praeger Publishers. Reproduced with permission of the publisher; and Sen, R. (2003). Picking the good fight. In *Stir It Up: Lessons in Community Organizing and Advocacy* (pp. 48–78). Copyright © 2003 by Jossey-Bass and John Wiley & Sons. Reproduced with permission of the publisher.

REFERENCES

Alinsky, S. D. (1971). *Rules for Radicals: A Practical Primer for Realistic Radicals.* Random House.

Bobo, K., Kendall, J., & Max, S. (1991). *Organizing for Social Change: A Manual for Activists in the 1990s.* Seven Locks Press.

Bobo, K., Kendall, J., & Max, S. (2010). *Organizing for Social Change: Midwest Academy Manual for Activists* (4th ed.). Forum Press.

Came, H., & Griffin, D. (2018). Tackling racism as a "wicked" public health problem: Enabling allies in anti-racism praxis. *Soc Sci Med, 199,* 181–188.

Chermack, T. J., & Kasshanna, B. K. (2007). The use and misuse of SWOT analysis and implications for HRD professionals. *Hum Resour Dev Int, 10*(4), 383–399.

Dorfman, L. (2009). Using media advocacy to influence policy. In R. J. Bensley & J. Brookins-Fisher (Eds.), *Community Health Education Methods: A Practical Guide* (3rd ed., pp. 181–203). Jones & Bartlett Publishers.

Dorfman, L., & Bakal, M. (2018). Using media advocacy to influence policy. In R. J. Bensley & J. Brookins-Fisher (Eds.), *Community Health Education Methods: A Practical Guide* (4th ed., pp. 267–292). Jones & Bartlett Publishers.

Dubey, S. (2017). Force field analysis for community organizing. *Proceedings from ICMC 2017: The 4th International Communications Management Conference.* MICA.

Falbe, J., Minkler, M., Dean, R., & Cordeiro, A. J. (2018). Power mapping: A useful tool for understanding the policy environment and its application to a local soda tax initiative. In N. Wallerstein, B. Duran, J. G. Oetzel, & M. Minkler (Eds.), *Community-Based Participatory Research for Health: Advancing Social and Health Equity* (3rd ed., pp. 405–410). Jossey-Bass.

Freire, P. (1970). *Pedagogy of the Oppressed.* Translated by M. B. Ramos. Seabury Press.

Freire, P. (1973). *Education for Critical Consciousness.* Seabury Press.

Gürel, E., & Tat, M. (2017). SWOT analysis: A theoretical review. *J Int Soc Res, 10*(51), 993–1006.

Haggstrom, W. C. (1971). The theory of social work method. [Unpublished paper].

Homan, M. S. (2016). *Promoting Community Change: Making It Happen in the Real World* (6th ed.). Cengage Learning.

Kendi, I. X. (2019). *How to Be an Antiracist.* One World.

Krueger, R. A., & Casey, M. A. (2014). *Focus Groups: A Practical Guide for Applied Research* (5th ed.). Sage.

Lewin, K. (1947). Quasi-stationary social equilibria and the problem of social change. In T. M. Newcomb & E. L. Hartley (Eds.), *Readings in Social Psychology* (pp. 340–344). Holt, Rinehart and Winston.

Meredith, J. C., & Dunham, C. (2016). Real clout: Rules and tools for winning public policy campaigns. In L. Staples, *Roots to Power: A Manual for Grassroots Organizing* (3rd ed., pp. 361–380). Praeger.

Minkler, M. (2014). Enhancing data quality, relevance, and use through community-based participatory research. In N. Cytron, K. Petit, & G. T. Kinglsey (Senior Eds.), *What Counts? Harvesting Data for American's Communities* (pp. 245–259). Federal Reserve Bank of San Francisco and the Urban Institute.

Minnesota State Health Department. (2020). Force field analysis. https://www.health.state.mn.us/communities/practice/resources/phqitoolbox/forcefield.html.

Schutz, A., & Miller, M. (2015). *People Power: The Community Organizing Tradition of Saul Alinsky.* Vanderbilt University Press.

Sen, R. (2003). *Stir It Up: Lessons in Community Organizing and Advocacy.* Jossey-Bass.

Staples, L. (2016). *Roots to Power: A Manual for Grassroots Organization* (3rd ed.). Praeger.

Su, C. (2009). *Streetwise for Book Smarts: Grassroots Organizing and Education Reform in the Bronx.* Cornell University Press.

Townsend, A. (2019). Who does action research and what responsibilities do they have to others? *Educ Action Res, 27*(2), 149–151.

Vinent, I., & Fernandez, R. (2016). Popular education and participatory action research. In L. Staples, *Roots to Power: A Manual for Grassroots Organizing* (3rd ed., pp. 318–337). Praeger.

Wallack, L., Woodruff, K., Dorfman, L., & Diaz, I. (1999). *News for a Change: An Advocate's Guide to Working with the Media.* Sage.

Warren, R. (1975). Types of purposive social change at the community level. In R. M. Kramer and H. S. Specht (Eds.), *Readings in Community Organization Practice* (2nd ed., pp. 134–149). Prentice-Hall.

PART FIVE

Community Organizing and Community Building within and across Diverse Groups and Cultures

The last three decades have witnessed, as seldom before, a real appreciation (and for some, a genuine fear) of the effective community organizing and community building efforts taking place among and with women, Blacks and other people of color, LGBTQ people, immigrants, Indigenous people, the disabled, and others. Many on the political right feared and disparaged such organizing, particularly as it played out in the Black Lives Matter protests that shined a harsh and overdue spotlight on police brutality against Black people and caused an even longer overdue national reckoning with systemic racism. On the left, such organizing was often enthusiastically heralded, albeit sometimes problematic, as when "White allies" ended up outnumbering the very people whose visibility and rights they had shown up to support (Minkler et al., 2019; chapter 8).

Professionals in fields like public health, social work, urban and regional planning, and community psychology have increasingly been among those urging our own fields of practice to take a hard look at our traditional ways of operating and to make genuine change. As Iton and Shrimali (2016) urge those of us in public health, "Take action now: whether it is reflecting on your power in relation to the communities you serve, implementing dialogues in your organization on how to incorporate power-sharing with those you serve, or designing new programs to build collective power for change" (p. 1757), we cannot wait any longer.

For the most part, however, and with some notable exceptions (Bester & Jean, 2012; Sen et al., 2010; Su, 2009) the wealth of experience of often marginalized groups in building community and organizing for change has not been well represented in the literature. Furthermore, what literature does exist has suggested that traditional models of community organizing are often ill suited to work with marginalized groups, whose reality tends to differ markedly from that of the architects of many of these models.

This part begins with chapter 13, Lorraine M. Gutiérrez and Edith A. Lewis's thoughtful approach to organizing with women of color, which stresses the utility of feminist perspectives for developing a culture- and gender-relevant model of practice. The special accent placed on both the theory development and the lived experience of women of color in their model have led to its becoming a classic in the field; this updated presentation of their work underscores its continued relevance.

Using as a framework interrelated principles of education, participation, and capacity building, the authors draw on the literature, and on a wealth of personal experience in social work, to develop an approach that acknowledges and confronts the combined effects of racism, classism, and sexism. Building in part on the early work of Felix Rivera and John Erlich (1995), Gutiérrez and Lewis's model views varying roles for organizers, depending, in part, on their degree of oneness and identification with the community in question. Regardless of the role played, however, they argue that a number of precepts are critical to effective organizing with women of color, among them learning actively, recognizing and embracing the conflict inherent in cross-cultural work, involving women of color early on in leadership roles, and in other ways contributing to community capacity.

The roles of history and culture in community practice with people of color is then developed by Laura A. Linnan, Stephen B. Thomas, and Susan R. Passmore in chapter 14, which presents an in-depth look at the historical and present-day significance of barbershops and beauty salons as cultural sites of meaning, community education, and organizing that extend well beyond their surface roles. Indeed, when professor and social commentator Melissa Harris-Perry (2011) joked that she left Princeton for Tulane University so that she could get her hair done, she was speaking to much deeper than personal grooming. As Linnan and her coauthors describe, Black barbershops and beauty salons were among the first Black-owned businesses in the country, with the former also important safe meeting places during both the Underground Railroad and the civil rights movement (Bristol, 2009). Not surprisingly, they were also quick to join the community response to the pandemic, even with their own often severe loss of revenue and the fact that they were far less likely than White businesses to receive federal or bank loans to help them stay afloat (Phillips, 2020).

As described in this chapter, the comfort of entering a Black-owned and -run beauty salon or barbershop in the lives of Black women and men and the unique and intimate relationships between these practitioners and their customers made them a critical resource and venue for health education to help reduce health disparities. Most of chapter 14 explores the more than two decades of the BEAUTY project in central North Carolina and the HAIR project in Pittsburgh, Pennsylvania that have done just that, by both starting where the people are and developing educational messages in and with community members in places of strength, safety, rich cultural heritage, and social connections. In addition to making available a wide range of health-promoting programs and services, both programs have helped build the capacity of shop owners as effective community health advocates, but also as successful members of both the business community and the larger community. Although incorporating some different elements (e.g., the use of an active community advisory board in the BEAUTY project), both programs have demonstrated measurable changes along multiple axes (e.g., from increasing the number of conversations with clients about a range of health topics and participation in screenings to the involvement of dozens more beauty salons and barbershops in the projects).

The authors also discuss several recent systematic reviews and randomized controlled trials that have further built the evidence on the effectiveness of such approaches to addressing health disparities (Linnan et al., 2014). Finally, they share a wide range of lessons learned, from the utility of community advisory boards in trust building and recruitment, to the value of getting media attention for participating shops, to the importance of both working within shop owners' severe time constraints and helping them bring in needed resources as they continue to serve during the difficult times ahead.

In chapter 15, Charlotte Chang, Alicia L. Salvatore, Pam Tau Lee, Shaw San Liu, and Meredith Minkler illustrate the potent combination of popular education, community organizing, and participatory research in work with an immigrant population–low-wage restaurant workers in San Francisco's Chinatown–to build individual and community capacity while studying and addressing some of the major problems facing this community. The Chinatown project included multiple partners: the Chinese Progressive Association (CPA), the local health department, two major universities, and immigrant workers themselves. The chapter demonstrates the goodness-of-fit between community organizing and participatory or community-based participatory research (CBPR), as well as the grounding of such work in a popular education approach based on the lived experience of community members themselves and accenting individual and community empowerment and action based on critical reflection (Freire, 1994; Garzón-Galvis et al., 2019; Su 2009; chapter 5). Chang and her colleagues also illustrate the utility of an ecological and multimethod approach stressing worker training in organizing and research, data collection on multiple levels, and participatory evaluation as an approach to both collectively studying the project's processes and outcomes and helping improve its processes and dynamics along the way. But they also emphasize the partnership's commitment to action for social change, particularly on the issue of greatest concern to workers: documenting and ending the widespread practice of wage theft. Whether in their receipt of far below minimum wage, having their wages held up for months at a time, being denied breaks and paid overtime, and having the boss take some of their tips, the workers pointed out that wage theft was their greatest health problem. From collecting solid quantitative and qualitative data to getting the media and policymakers' attention, to the pivotal role the CPA and its partners played in helping craft, pass, implement, and enforce one of the nation's first municipal wage theft ordinances, the community-led partnership helped address this problem, while also creating a low-wage-worker bill of rights.

Chang and her colleagues talk candidly about the challenges this work entailed, from conflicting community–academic timelines and power differentials to the labor-intensive nature of the work. But they stress above all the power of this approach as a force for change, grounded in the experience of workers and their growing ability to articulate their concerns in the corridors of power, and strong and collaborative data collection for developing the evidence base needed to use community organizing to best advantage for change.

In an epilogue looking back over the ten years since the project's official end, the authors note that more than $10.6 in lost wages has been recovered by and for workers in and beyond Chinatown, and that numerous organizations and communities across the country have sought consultation in their own work on this and related health and safety issues facing workers. The authors also note that individual and community capacity building so central to the original study has continued to contribute to CPA and its work in multiple ways, from two of the original project partners serving on the origination's board of directors to worker partners forming a critical part of the organization's leadership. The longer-term outcomes of the project are presented as a testament to Israel et al.'s (2013) CBPR principle stressing the importance of being engaged over the long haul—a principle equally relevant in community organizing for social change.

REFERENCES

Bester, D., & Jean, V. (2012, September). Strengthening Black organizing across the United States. *Mobilizing Community Power*. Philanthropic Initiative for Racial Equity: Critical Issues Forum. https://racialequity.org/wp-content/uploads/2018/11/CIF4strengtheningBlack.pdf.

Bristol, D. W. (2009). *Knights of the Razor: Black Barbers in Slavery and Freedom*. Johns Hopkins University Press.

Freire, P. (1994). *Pedagogy of Hope*. Continuum.

Garzón-Galvis, C., Wong, M., Madrigal, D., Olmedo, L., Brown, M., & English, P. (2019). Advancing environmental health literacy through community-engaged research and popular education. In S. Finn & L. O'Fallon (Eds.), *Environmental Health Literacy* (pp. 97–134). Springer.

Harris-Perry, M. (2011). *Sister Citizen: Shame, Stereotypes, and the Black Woman in America*. Yale University Press.

Israel, B. A., Eng, E., Schulz, A. J., & Parker, E. A. (2013). Introduction to methods for CBPR for health. In B. A. Israel, E. Eng, A. J. Schultz, & E. A. Parker (Eds.), *Methods for Community-Based Participatory Research in Public Health* (pp. 3–38). Jossey-Bass.

Iton, A., & Shrimali, B. P. (2016). Power, politics, and health: A new public health practice targeting the root causes of health equity. *Matern Child Health J, 20*(8), 1753–1758.

Linnan, L., D'Angelo, H., & Harrington, C. (2014). Health promotion research in beauty salons and barbershops: A synthesis of the literature. *Am J Prev Med, 47*(1), 77–85.

Minkler, M., Rebanal, R. D., Pearce, R., & Acosta, M. (2019). Growing equity and health equity in perilous times: Lessons from community organizers. *Health Educ Behav, 46*(1_suppl), 9S–18S.

Phillips, J. (2020, May 8). Why the Black barbershop experience may be a causality of the coronavirus pandemic. *San Francisco Chronicle*. https://www.sfchronicle.com/opinion/article/Why-the-black-barbershop-experience-may-be-a-15256927.php.

Rivera, F., & Erlich, J. (1995). *Community Organizing in a Diverse Society* (2nd ed.). Allyn and Bacon.

Sen, R., Wessler, S., & Apollon, D. (2010). *Better Together: Research Findings on the Relationship between Racial Justice Organizations and LGBT Communities.* Report. Applied Research Center.

Su, C. (2009). *Streetwise for Book Smarts: Grassroots Organizing and Education Reform in the Bronx.* Cornell University Press.

13

Education, Participation, and Capacity Building in Community Organizing with Women of Color

LORRAINE M. GUTIÉRREZ
EDITH A. LEWIS

The field of community organizing has increasingly addressed the need for an approach to practice that respects and builds on the special challenges posed by our diverse society. Yet although much community organizing has taken place among women and communities of color, too little attention has been paid to the ways in which race, gender, ethnicity, along with social class affect the organizing effort. *Intersectionality*, or the ways in which aspects of identify, such as race, gender and class, combine in diverse ways to construct a social reality (Sanchez-Hucles & Davis, 2010), is a useful concept for our work as organizers with and by women of color. As described by Kimberlé Crenshaw, the law professor who coined this term, intersectional feminism is "a prism for seeing the way in which various forms of inequality often operate together and exacerbate each other" (UN Women, 2020).

Also critical is paying attention to those often overlooked federal and state policies and practices through which "the social exclusion of Black women has been instituted and perpetuated" (Carter & Lautier, 2018; chapter 4). Such oversights have often prevented organizers from working effectively with women or communities of color (Gutiérrez & Creekmore, 2008; McGoldrick & Hardy, 2008; Minkler et al., 2019). By failing to recognize and account for the many ways in which issues of oppression affect organizing work, organizers can perpetuate the objectification and exploitation of these groups. Organizers whose own racial or ethnic stereotypes distort their view of communities of color, for example, will be ineffective in building leadership or working in partnership (Abram et al., 2005; Few-Demo, 2016; Jones, 2010). In this way, community organizing efforts can perpetuate the very problems they were designed to solve.

This chapter begins by examining several contributions to our thinking about organizing with women of color, with special attention to the contributions of feminist perspectives on organizing. An empowerment framework stressing education, participation, and capacity building is then developed and used to explore different dimensions of effective community organizing with women of color.

Examples of organizing both within and across racial/ethnic groups are provided to illustrate many of the points made and offer lessons for social change professionals in their roles as organizers.

Multicultural Perspectives on Community Organizing

Much of the literature that does exist on multicultural organizing emphasizes the ways in which organizers can develop cultural competence and cultural humility for working in partnership with communities (Chávez, 2018; Greene-Moton & Minkler, 2020). This literature stressed the ways in which organizers can use their own self-awareness to build bridges for work within communities. Organizers are encouraged to examine their own biases and take the role of the learner in approaching a community and discovering its strengths and concerns (Chávez, 2018; Guadalupe & Lum, 2005; Gutiérrez et al., 2005; appendix 1).

Several scholars, most notably Felix Rivera and John Erlich (1998), made early and critical contributions to organizing with communities of color by positing that the appropriate roles for organizers are best determined by their relationship to the community (Midgley, 2007; Spencer et al., 2000; Yoshihama & Carr, 2003). If an organizer is a member of the community, they argue, the most intimate or primary contact is appropriate. Primary contact would involve immediate and personal grassroots work with the community. In contrast, an organizer who is of a similar ethnic or racial background but not of the community should instead be involved on the secondary level. This level would involve participation as a liaison between the community and the larger society (Grittner, 2019). The tertiary level of contact would be most appropriate for those organizers who are not members of the group. They can provide valuable contributions to the community through consultation, the sharing of technical knowledge, and the hands-on work in the background that is also critical to effective organizing. For example, outside professionals interested in participating in community work with a local Black neighborhood could first establish relationships with key individuals in the community (chapter 10). The professional as organizer's responsibilities would be those *defined by the community*, no matter how insignificant these might seem on the surface. Efforts to learn the strengths of the community as they are exemplified in daily learning activities within the community would be a primary activity for the organizer (chapter 11). In this way, the organizer's willingness to use the ethno-conscious perspective of "noninterference" would be recognized in time by residents, and more opportunities for work with that community might be revealed (Lewis, 2009).

Over twenty-five years ago, Bradshaw and colleagues (1994) proposed that a "hybrid model" of organizing which integrates aspects of the Saul Alinsky (1971) approach to social action organizing with relevant perspectives from feminist organizing be used with communities of color. Flexibility, leadership identification and training, the appropriate use of both collaborative and confrontational tactics, and the role of the organizer as a learner and facilitator are among the characteristics of this hybrid model. Of importance in this model are skills for developing cultural competence and cultural humility that enable the outside organizer to better understand, respect, and learn from the community (Greene-Moton & Minkler, 2020; Hyde, 2008). These skills involve (1) cultivating awareness of one's own understanding of the community, (2) finding ways to learn more about the local community through informal leaders, (3) working as partners to develop local leadership, and (4) focusing on ways to build cohesiveness within and between racial/ethnic communities. As is by now clear, the most critical role of the organizer indeed is that of a culturally humble learner who reflects on their own assumptions and biases, recognizes the gifts and lived experiences of the group, approaches the community to better understand and honor the group's concerns, and helps facilitate change (Chávez et al., 2010; Greene-Moton & Minkler, 2020; Lewis & Gutiérrez, 2003).

Contributions from Feminism

Much of the conceptual and practice-based literature on organizing with women has been written from a Western feminist perspective (Few-Demo, 2016; Hyde, 2008; Lewis, 2009). Feminist approaches can contribute to organizing with women of color through their emphasis on integrating personal and political issues through dialogue. Feminist organizing assumes that sexism is a significant force in the experiences of all women and one that lies at the root of many of the problems they face (Demos et al., 2019). Therefore, a major focus for organizing with women of color is to identify ways in which sexism, racism, and other forms of oppression are affecting their lives (Carter & Lautier, 2018; Reed et al., 2011). Common methods for feminist organizing include the development of consciousness-raising groups, engagement in reflexive practice, creation of alternative services, and social action that incorporates street theater and other holistic methods (Hyde, 2008; Jones, 2010; Lewis & Gutiérrez, 2003).

An important focus of feminist approaches is reflected in their concern with developing ways to work across differences. All women are thought to be a part of a "community" of women, as well as members of their own specific communities. Therefore, organizers need to work to bridge differences between women based on such factors as race, class, physical ability, sexual orientation, and gender identity on the principle that diversity is strength (Wilson et al., 2010). The goal for feminist organizing has been most effectively met when carried out from a multicultural perspective and with attention to the role of intersectionality (Lewis et al., 2014; Sanchez-Hucles & Davis, 2010; Stall & Stoecker, 2012).

Organizing with Women of Color

Organizing by women within racial/ethnic communities in the United States has a rich and diverse history. For example, the organization of Black Women's Clubs in the United States a century ago by leaders such as Ida B. Wells Barnett was instrumental in developing nursing homes, day care centers, and orphanages within African American communities. These clubs also organized for social change, particularly on antilynching and antirape campaigns and in the foundation of organizations such as the National Urban League (Collins, 2000; Sen, 2020; Stall & Stoecker, 2012; Taylor, 2005).

Women of color have always worked to improve conditions within their communities and in society in general and have been more likely than White middle-class women to see community activism as a natural outgrowth of their gender role (Bracho et al., 2016; Carter & Lautier, 2018; Lewis, 2009; Minkler et al., 2019). During the mid- to late twentieth century, for example, women played important roles in the movement for equality and civil rights within racial/ethnic communities (Lewis, 2009; Lewis & Gutiérrez, 2003). Neighborhood violence, economic issues, and environmental concerns, including climate change, are but a few of the areas on which women of color in urban and some rural communities (e.g., Native American women whose lands are threatened by oil pipelines) have organized, and often served as movement leaders (Byrne et al., 2002; Segal & Martinez, 2007; Taylor, 2005).

Effective community organizing efforts build on these traditions. By looking at such historical and contemporary efforts, we can identify ways to draw on their strengths and learn from and adapt the strategies that already exist. As noted earlier, the role of the organizer can and should vary according to their relationship to the community or the issue being addressed (Rivera & Erlich, 1998). To determine the appropriate role, we must involve the community in defining the issues it wishes to address and the strategies it feels will be most effective and culturally appropriate in attempting to achieve collectively set goals. For example, a Native American woman may be able to use her role as a member of the community and a designated leader to work on the primary level with her community to bring about change (McCammon et al., 2018). A Latinx or Japanese American organizer could provide important technical assistance or research skills but would not work on this primary level and would take a very different role in relation to the community. Although we emphasize the necessity of participation by community members in primary roles, the important roles that can be played by nonmembers of the community on the secondary and tertiary levels should not be underestimated (Chun, 2016; Hyde, 2004; Yoshihama & Carr, 2003).

Education, Participation, and Capacity Building

What does this analysis suggest about community organizing with women of color? Utilizing an empowerment framework that stresses the core concepts of education, participation, and capacity building, we can develop sensitive and effective methods for community practice (Gutiérrez & Lewis, 1999). Many of the methods described here are equally relevant to organizers and community members, and the processes of education, participation, and capacity building should take place with the organizer as well as with community members (Bracho et al., 2016; chapter 9). These reciprocal process methods can be summarized as follows:

Education

1. Learn about, understand, and participate in the women's racial/ethnic community.
2. Recognize and build on ways in which women of color have worked effectively within their own communities; build on existing structures.
3. Serve as a facilitator, and view the situation through the lens or vision of women of color.

Participation

4. Use the process of praxis, or action based on critical reflection (Freire, 1970) to understand the historical, political, and social context of the organizing effort.
5. Begin with the formation of small groups.
6. Recognize and embrace the conflict that characterizes cross-cultural work.

Capacity Building

7. Involve women of color in leadership roles.
8. Understand and support the need that women of color may have for their own separate programs and organizations.

Education

Educational efforts toward community organizing and change need to be grounded in the ways in which women of color share similarities and differences with European American women and men of color. Community organizers have often recognized the impact of powerlessness on women of color from the perspective of institutional racism. Frequently overlooked in this process, however, is the role of gender inequity in influencing the life chances of women of color. The field has often ignored the history of community participation by women of color (Bracho et al., 2016; Minkler et al., 2019). When women of color are viewed solely as members of their racial or ethnic group and gender is not taken into account, community organizers may alienate women of color and reinforce ways in which sexism, both in the larger society and within ethnic minority communities, is a form of oppression (Abu-Lughod, 2002; Collins, 2000; Harris-Perry, 2011).

As suggested in earlier chapters, an important first step in effective community organizing involves defining the community (chapters 7, 10, 11). The fact that women of color can be members of multiple communities and hold multiple identities based on race, gender, geography, and other factors presents both a challenge and an opportunity for organizers. From an organizing perspective, however, the central issue for organizing will often define the community. For example, if the issue is toxic waste dumping in a community, then the neighborhood or city may be an appropriate level for work. If the issue is reproductive rights, then gender may be the focus. Awareness of these memberships in multiple communities can be helpful when an organizer is building coalitions or alliances between different groups.

An organizer who is from a different racial, ethnic, or class background than the women she works with must recognize how her life experience has colored her perceptions and how her status has affected her power relative to the political structure. Her beliefs and perceptions should not dominate the organizing effort. She must work toward serving as a co-facilitator and view the situation through the "lens" or "vision" of women of color. In part, this requires allowing this vision to alter the way the organizer views their own work and sharing that new information with others hoping to organize and work within communities of color (Gutiérrez et al., 2013; Lewis, 2009; Zetzer, 2018).

When organizing with low-income women in a housing project, one of the authors initially attempted to separate individual from community concerns. She believed at first that group members would work on individual problem resolution for eight weeks and then, having established a pattern of interaction within the group, would be able to work cooperatively on analysis and resolution of community concerns. It became clear within the first two meetings that the group could not separate and sequentially work with individual and community concerns. As one participant put it, "My individual problems are the community's problems." The flexibility to alter the design based on the realities of the community allowed the group to continue working toward resolution of its identified goals, not those of the facilitator/researcher. This example illustrates the importance of understanding the community's lens on reality and the process of praxis, or action based on critical reflection, to unravel and address the salient historical, social, and political forces at work. In the preceding example, had the outside organizer insisted on separating the individual from the community problem, she would have alienated and probably lost committed community activists for whom this separation was an artificial and inappropriate one. By respecting the community's vision of the intimate interdependence of these levels, however, she was able to facilitate a process through which participants proceeded to make change on both the individual and community levels (Lewis, 2009).

Organizers should also use the process of praxis to understand and address the historical, political, and social contexts of the organizing effort. This means that the organizing process as well as the outcome will inform both the organized community and the "community" of the organizer. As organizers and community groups analyze the process and outcome of organizing efforts, the outcome of a tactic often emerges as less important than what the community and organizer learn about the nature of the problem being addressed. In this way, community issues are often redefined.

The involvement of women of color in the movement against gender-based violence clearly illustrates this principle. When many feminist shelters observed that they were unsuccessful in reaching women of color, they defined the problem as that of inadequate outreach. When this outreach was unsuccessful, women of color in some localities provided feedback to many shelter programs that their approach was alienating and foreign to communities of color. They often identified the lack of women of color in administrative or permanent staff positions as one way in which the program indicated a lack of commitment to their community. Programs that have been most successful with women of color have been those that addressed their own racism, classism, and ethnocentrism in the development of alternative programs (Wilson et al., 2010; Zetzer, 2018).

Participation

Participating in the women's racial/ethnic community is an important step for educating the organizer and building bridges for future work. This participation can result in an analysis of societal institutions, including the one represented by the organizer, and how they might ultimately benefit or hurt the community. Churches, community centers, schools, and social clubs can be avenues for reaching women of color and effecting change within the community. Knowledge can also be gained about specific communities of color through reading and participation in community events. When an organizer is not an ongoing member of the community of women with whom she will be working, developing an understanding of the community's cultural context is vital (Abram et al., 2005; Few-Demo, 2016; Suarez & Lewis, 2020).

In an effort to become involved in the community, one organizer participated in activities sponsored by the local community center. She worked for several months in enrichment programming for the children of the community before proceeding to work with the women. During this time, she became aware of community members' patterns of interaction, their relationships with agencies in the city, and other potential issues in the community. Community members and group participants had the opportunity to meet and talk with the community worker and to watch her interact with their children. Many of the initial participants in subsequent organizing efforts later mentioned that their decision to participate in the work was directly related to their approval of the facilitator's work with their children and the nature of her presence in the community.

Effective organizing often begins with the formation of small groups. The small group provides the ideal environment for exploring the social and political aspects of "personal" problems and for developing strategies for work toward social change (Abu-Lughod, 2002; Bracho et al., 2016; Gutiérrez et al., 2005). It can also be a forum for identifying common goals among diverse groups of women.

The small group, or house meeting strategy, has historically been the primary way in which women of color have been organizing movements to improve conditions in ghettos and barrios and global communities (Dolphyne et al., 2001). This strategy involves organizing small groups of individuals to work on specific problems and later coordinating these small groups so that they can work in coalition with others on joint issues. Many grassroots movements for women of color around the world emerged from initially informal discussion groups. The building of these alliances to develop community efforts can be particularly challenging when they involve more than one ethnic group. This is particularly true because the United States remains a highly segregated society, due in part to systemic racism baked into systems like housing, banking, and education that result in many people experiencing little meaningful interaction with those outside their own race, class, or ethnic group (Harris-Perry, 2011; Solomon et al., 2019). Effective organizing across diverse groups requires breaking down societal boundaries to build alliances (Gutiérrez et al., 2013; Hyde, 2004; Jones, 2010). Furthermore, it necessitates recognizing and embracing the conflict that characterizes cross-cultural work. Conflicts will inevitably arise both within those organizations that have been successful in reaching a diverse group and between the organization and a larger community that may be threatened by the absence of expected boundaries. In some respects, the emergence of conflict is an indication that meaningful cross-cultural work is taking place. However, the sources and resolution of conflict will affect the outcomes of the organizing effort. The extent to which the organizer anticipates conflict related to group interaction, the effects of internalized oppression, wider political strategies to hinder or destroy the community change effort, and similar factors will often determine whether organizing efforts are successful (Jones, 2010).

Conflict includes the discomfort many organizers feel when they find themselves the sole person from a different ethnic or class background in a group of women of color or when they attempt to participate for the first time in a community event that has previously been attended solely by persons from the community. It is important for organizers to recognize that they will be "tested" by community members to determine whether they, as others who came before, are present only to "take." Giving on the community's terms, as illustrated in the earlier example of the author's work with children, is one example of the testing process experienced by someone attempting to enter the community.

It is our experience that White organizers are often less comfortable than women of color with the conflict engendered by the development of a multicultural organization. Conflicts are a part of our everyday lives. They reflect choices about fact, value, and strategy alternatives that we face intra- or interpersonally (Lewis, 2009; Morelli & Spencer, 2000). Too often, women have been socialized into conflict-avoidance behaviors. These behaviors only temporarily delay conflicts, which will resurface when issues are not addressed directly. Addressing a conflict has often been misconstrued as synonymous with confrontation, another conflict-resolution strategy. They are, however, quite different. Confrontation often means the minimization of or an attack on a party with which there is conflict. This minimization, either at the personal or political levels, can easily be perceived as a threat, which inevitably leads to an escalation of the conflict rather than a dialogue about its nature (Few-Demo, 2016).

Addressing conflict directly means employing interpersonal skills, such as engagement, active listening, and consensus building. It means viewing the situation through various lenses in the presence of all who are involved in the conflict and then managing to reach some consensus about how to proceed. The process of reaching this consensus often involves being open about our differing conflict styles and managing to hear the content, rather than just the effect, of the messages being presented (Chávez et al., 2010). To do so also requires taking a strengths-based approach—in this case, acknowledging the capacity or strengths in the conflict style of the group—on the part of those who have been privy to only one way of handling conflicts. In this way, conflict-avoidance techniques may be valued for their ability to offset the attack, whereas confrontation approaches may be valued for their ability to focus immediate attention on the conflict (Stevens, 2002; Suarez & Lewis, 2020).

Conflict management that results in genuine dialogue and analysis of the basis of difference will have a direct effect on the outcome of an organizing effort. For example, only after White Americans involved women of color in their organizations did many White American women encounter a different view of gender roles and how they translate into different strategies and goals. Once women of color were included in such organizations, work around sexual assault had to recognize and deal with the fears of many White women concerning men of color. In one organization, it was only after the group began a campaign confronting "the myth of the black rapist" that women of color within the organization and in the larger community came to believe that the organization represented their needs.

Dealing with such conflict is difficult but valuable. If we are to work toward a more equitable society, this vision must be integral to the work of our organizations (Wolff et al., 2017). We must know ourselves and be open to knowing others. Dealing with community backlash and conflict also requires taking risks to speak out in support of our vision. The inability to resolve these conflicts has resulted in the death of some organizations and has minimized our ability to work in coalition.

Capacity Building

Contemporary organizing by women of color has often taken a grassroots approach based on existing networks of family, friends, or informal and formal ethnic community institutions. In this way, individual, family, and community interests are viewed as compatible and integrated with one another. Many African American women, Latinx, and other women of color describe themselves as motivated to engage in activism *because* of their commitment to their communities and ethnic group (Bracho et al., 2016; Collins, 2000; Dolphyne et al., 2001). Women have also often been active in the mutual aid societies within ethnic communities, such as the Hui among the Chinese, the Ko among the Japanese, and the tribal councils among Native Americans. Each of these organizations has served as a vehicle for assisting individual ethnic group members, families, and entire communities through the establishment of business loans, funerals, and community programs.

Organizers must recognize and build on these networks and the myriad ways in which women of color have worked effectively within their own communities. Outside organizers, regardless of their own race or ethnicity, need to work with community leaders and learn from them the most effective ways of working in particular communities. Working with existing leaders may involve organizers in types of activities that are different than those in which they may usually engage. For example, to provide survival services, existing community leaders may be active in church-related activities or with municipal agencies (Gutiérrez et al., 2005). Organizers can learn from these women the ways that they have found to survive and leverage political power.

Organizers also need to recognize how women of color have been involved in advocating for women's rights since the beginning of the feminist movement. For example, many of the first shelters for battered women were founded by women of color responding to the needs in their communities (Demos et al., 2019; Lewis & Gutiérrez, 2003; Taylor, 2005). Recognition of the contributions of women of color to feminist causes can help to break down some of the barriers and difficulties that exist in this work.

As suggested earlier, however, community organizing with women of color may involve a broader perspective than the one initially envisioned by the organizer. This broader perspective would recognize the many ways in which race, gender, class, and ethnicity are intertwined. Consequently, it would underscore the impossibility of separating the needs of women from those of their families and communities (Demos et al., 2019). The role of women in the civil rights movements of the 1950s and 1960s and more recently in the founding of #Black Lives Matter and its large-scale mobilizations against police killings of Black and Brown people nationally and globally well illustrate the importance of gender to mobilization efforts. Too often, however, the role of women of color in such work has not received the visibility it deserves. The successful Montgomery, Alabama, bus boycott, for example, is usually credited to African American male ministers who were in public leadership positions. However, the impetus for the boycott was a group of African American women who impressed on the ministers that the cause was just and that they would launch the boycott themselves if the ministers did not take a public stance. The women raised the consciousness of the ministers and in this way contributed significantly to social action. However, they were willing to work behind the scenes, rather than spearheading the boycott themselves, because they thought it was imperative that Black men's leadership be supported. The delicate intersections of race, ethnicity, class, and gender must be in the forefront of the organizer's praxis perspective. But we can also take heart in the fact that women of color are now often in the leadership of community organizing and social movements. Indeed, all three cofounders of Black Lives Matter were Black women

(Szetela, 2020), and as noted above, women of color played prominent roles in the national protests following the police killings of George Floyd and other unarmed Black men, and also of Breonna Taylor, Sandra Bland, Aura Rosser, and other Black women. These facts represent an important step forward.

On the scale of community or neighborhood organizing, leadership of women of color in organizing today is also an important corrective to the earlier unidirectional "outreach approach," in which communities of color have long been targets of change rather than active participants and collaborators (Cossyleon, 2019). When the latter approach is used, women of color often resist organizing efforts and, in some cases, undermine them (Rotramel, 2020; Stevens, 2002). It is crucial, therefore, to involve women of color in leadership roles from the outset. Predominantly White American organizations wishing to collaborate with women of color need to incorporate women of color as leaders and active participants before engaging in this kind of work (Minkler et al., 2019). Such collaboration may require redefining the kind of work the organization does, as well as looking critically at its members' attitudes toward institutions such as the church and family. The history of attempts at collaboration suggests that cross-cultural work requires identifying how racism may exclude women of color from leadership roles (Gutiérrez et al., 2013; Minkler et al., 2019). Successful collaboration will require that White organizers change their interactions with women of color and be capable of sharing power and control of their programs. This type of organizational work embraces the tenets of feminist organizing that emphasize the importance of using an intersectional lens to better understand the historical contexts surrounding an issue of concern and recognizing that "diversity is strength."

Issues of perceived or actual social class differences must be taken into account, even when organizers are from the same ethnic or gender background as the community in which they are working. As noted earlier, the definition of community may be psychological as well as geographic. Those entering, or re-entering, communities need to be cognizant that their economic or educational backgrounds may be perceived as making them somehow different from other community members. They must anticipate suspicion or backlash as a possible consequence. As in other conflict situations, a process of dialogue and action can be used to work through this problem, such that the organizer can then participate in the community on the latter's own terms. Perhaps one of the highest compliments paid to one of the authors was in a community meeting in which she was introduced to others as "not an educated fool."

One method for building effective coalitions is the incorporation of informal "debriefing" groups for community workers. These groups would include all members of the community and would provide opportunities for input and clarification of the organizing process. Those in key leadership positions would model their ongoing praxis experiences by being open about the choices made in the organizing effort and the assumptions upon which these choices rested. Debriefing sessions would allow for community members who are not an integral part of the organizing effort to share additional strategies and to evaluate the impact of the design on the community to date. Some groups have used the house meeting strategy to provide debriefing opportunities, whereas others have relied on formal written materials, such as community newsletters, to keep community members informed. Consistent ongoing debriefing efforts need to be built into the organizing design and expanded as needed.

Within the realm of organizing, there is room for multiethnic organizations and cross-ethnic coalitions, but also for organizations developed by and for women of color. In the latter regard, organizers need to understand and support the need that women of color may have for their own separate programs and organizations. For women of color, a separate group or organization in which we can explore who we are in relation to the communities in which we live can often provide the basis for creating a vision for future work. A separate organization is one means for building on strengths and nurturing capacity within a community. In work with women of color in an educational setting, the formation of a women of color caucus had a positive impact on the ability of a women's studies program to hire more faculty of color and to develop courses that were more racially and ethnically inclusive. Although the formation was initially viewed by some as divisive, all participants in the program ultimately recognized that the caucus was a critical element in the empowerment of women of color and their capacity to work for positive change for all.

Summary

This chapter has used a framework of education, participation, and capacity building to explore empowering strategies and approaches for community organizing with women of color. Based in part on the pioneering work of Rivera and Erlich (1998), we have argued that different roles are appropriate for organizers, depending on their relationship to the community (e.g., whether they are a member, a nonmember with a similar racial or ethnic background, or a person of a different racial or ethnic group).

Regardless of the role played, however, several principles are critical in effective organizing with women of color. These include being an active learner and facilitator who can view a given situation through the "lenses" of women of color, recognizing and embracing the conflict that characterizes cross-cultural work, involving women of color in leadership roles, and in other ways contributing to the building of community capacity. Both feminist perspectives and cultural perspectives on organizing in communities of color offer valuable lessons for organizers who cross race, ethnic, gender, class, and other lines in their organizing efforts. Finally, and particularly in these fraught times of overlapping crises which place in sharp focus the structural inequalities shaping our lives, an intersectional feminist approach can help women of color and other organizers use this opportunity, in their own work and in work across differences, to help create more resilient—and more equitable—communities and societies (UN Women, 2020).

Questions for Further Discussion

1. What effective strategies can community organizers use when contemplating projects that will include women of color?
2. Identify two examples of ways in which capacity building utilizing the lenses of women of color may alter the behaviors of facilitators from different ethnic groups.

REFERENCES

Abram, F. Y., Slosar, J. A., & Walls, R. (2005). Reverse mission: A model for international social work education and transformative intra-national practice. *Int Soc Work, 48*(2), 161–176.

Abu-Lughod, L. (2002). Do Muslim women really need saving? Anthropological reflections on cultural relativism and its others. *Am Anthropol, 104*(3), 783–790.

Alinsky, S. D. (1971). *Rules for Radicals: A Pragmatic Primer for Realistic Radicals.* Random House.

Bracho, A., Lee, G., Giraldo, G. P., De Prado, R. M., & Latino Health Access. (2016). *Recruiting the Heart, Training the Brain: The Work of Latino Health Access.* Hesperian Health Guides.

Bradshaw, C. P., Soifer, S., & Gutiérrez, L. (1994). Toward a hybrid model for effective organizing in communities of color. *J Community Pract, 1*(1), 25–42.

Byrne, J., Martinez, C., & Glover, L. (2002). A brief on environmental justice. In J. Byrne, C. Martinez, & L. Glover (Eds.), *Environmental Justice: Discourses in International Political Economy* (pp. 3–17). Transaction Publishers.

Carter, C., & Lautier, C. (2018, November 20). Taking our seat at the table: Black women overcoming social exclusion in politics. Demos. https://www.demos.org/research/taking-our-seat-table-black-women-overcoming-social-exclusion-politics.

Chávez, V. (2018). Cultural humility: Reflections and relevance for CBPR. In N. Wallerstein, B. Duran, J. G. Oetzel, & M. Minkler (Eds.), *Community-Based Participatory Research for Health: Advancing Social and Health Equity* (3rd ed., pp. 357–362). Jossey-Bass.

Chávez, V., Minkler, M., Wallerstein, N., & Spencer, M. S. (2010). Community organizing for health and social justice. In L. Cohen, V. Chávez, & S. Chehimi (Eds.), *Prevention Is Primary: Strategies for Community Well-Being* (2nd ed., pp. 87–112). Jossey-Bass.

Chun, J. J. (2016). Building political agency and movement leadership: The grassroots organizing model of Asian immigrant women advocates. *Citizen Stud, 20*(3–4), 379–395.

Collins, P. (2000). *Black Feminist Thought: Knowledge, Consciousness, and the Politics of Empowerment* (2nd ed.). Routledge.

Cossyleon, J. E. (2019). "Power in numbers": Marginalized mothers contesting individualization through grassroots community organizing. In V. Demos, M. T. Segal, & K. Kelly (Eds.), *Gender and Practice: Insights from the Field* (pp. 115–127). Emerald Publishing.

Demos, V., Segal, M. T., & Kelly, K. (Eds.). (2019). *Gender and Practice: Insights from the Field.* Emerald Publishing.

Few-Demo, A. L. (2016). But some of us are brave: All the women are White, all the Blacks are men—Black Women's Studies. *J Fam Theory Rev, 8*(2), 247–253.

Freire, P. (1970). *Pedagogy of the Oppressed.* Translated by M. B. Ramos. Seabury Press.

Greene-Moton, E., & Minkler, M. (2020). Cultural competence or cultural humility? Moving beyond the debate. *Health Promot Pract, 21*(1), 142–145.

Grittner, A. L. (2019). The Victoria Mxenge: Gendered formalizing housing and community design strategies out of Cape Town, South Africa. *J Housing Built Environ, 34*(2), 599–618.

Guadalupe, K. L., & Lum, D. (2005). *Multidimensional Contextual Practice: Diversity and Transcendence.* Brooks/Cole.

Gutiérrez, L., & Creekmore, M. (2008). Cultural institutions and the arts. In T. Mizrahi & L. Davis (Eds.), *Encyclopedia of Social Work* (20th ed., vol. 1, pp. 492–497). Oxford University Press.

Gutiérrez, L., Dessel, A., Lewis, E., & Spencer, M. (2013). Principles, skills, and practice strategies for promoting multicultural communication and collaboration. In M. Weil, M. Reisch, & M. Ohmer (Eds.), *Handbook of Community Practice* (2nd ed., pp. 445–460). Sage.

Gutiérrez, L., & Lewis, E. (1999). *Empowering Women of Color.* Columbia University Press.

Gutiérrez, L., Lewis, E., Nagda, B. A, Wernick, L., Nagda, B. A., & Shore, N. (2005). Multicultural community practice strategies and intergroup empowerment. In M. Weil, M. Reisch, D. N. Gamble, L. Gutiérrez, E. A. Mulroy, & R. A. Cnaan (Eds.), *Handbook of Community Practice* (pp. 341–359). Sage.

Harris-Perry, M. (2011). *Sister Citizen: Shame, Stereotypes, and the Black Woman in America.* Yale University Press.

Hyde, C. A. (2004). Gendered perceptions of community needs and concerns: An exploratory analysis. *J Hum Behav Soc Environ, 8*(4), 45–65.

Hyde, C. A. (2008). Feminist social work practice. In T. Mizrahi & L. Davis (Eds.), *Encyclopedia of Social Work* (20th ed., vol. 2, pp. 216–221). Oxford University Press.

Jones, R. G. (2010). Putting privilege into practice through "Intersectional Reflexivity": Ruminations, interventions and possibilities. *Reflections: Narratives of Professional Helping, 10*(1), 122–125.

Lewis, E. A. (2009). Group- versus individual-based intersectionality and praxis in feminist and womynist research foundations. In S. A. Lloyd, A. L Few, & K. R. Allen (Eds.), *Handbook of Feminist Family Studies* (pp. 304–315). Sage.

Lewis, E. A., & Gutiérrez, L. (2003). Intersections of gender and race in group work. In M. B. Cohen & A. Mullender (Eds.), *Gender and Groupwork* (pp. 132–143). Routledge.

Lewis, E. A., Sakamoto, I., & Gutiérrez, L., (2014). Women of color. In A. Gitterman (Ed.), *Handbook of Social Work Practice with Vulnerable and Resilient Populations* (3rd ed., pp. 561–579). Columbia University Press.

McCammon, H. J., McGrath, A., Hess, D. J., & Moon, M. (2018). Women, leadership, and the US environmental movement. In H. J. McCammon & L. A. Banaszak (Eds.), *100 Years of the Nineteenth Amendment: An Appraisal of Women's Political Activism* (pp. 312–339). Oxford University Press.

McGoldrick, M., & Hardy, K. (2008). *Re-visioning Family Therapy: Race, Culture and Gender in Clinical Practice.* Guilford Press.

Midgley, J. (2007). Global inequality, power, and the unipolar world. *Int Soc Work, 50*(5), 613–626.

Minkler, M., Rebanal, R. D., Pearce, R., & Acosta, M. (2019). Growing equity and health equity in perilous times: Lessons from community organizers. *Health Educ Behav, 46*(1_suppl), 9S–18S.

Morelli, P. T., & Spencer, M. S. (2000). Use and support of multicultural and antiracist education: Research-informed interdisciplinary social work practice. *Social Work, 45*(2), 166–175.

Reed, B. G., Newman, P. A., Suarez, Z. E., & Lewis, E. A. (2011). Interpersonal practice beyond diversity and towards social justice: The importance of critical consciousness. In B. Seabury, B. H. Seabury, & C. D. Garvin (Eds.), *Foundations of Interpersonal Practice in Social Work: Promoting Competence in Generalist Practice* (3rd ed., pp. 60–98). Sage.

Rivera, F., & Erlich, J. (1998). *Community Organizing in a Diverse Society* (3rd ed.). Allyn & Bacon.

Rotramel, A. (2020). *Pushing Back: Women of Color–Led Grassroots Activism in New York City.* University of Georgia Press.

Sanchez-Hucles, J. V., & Davis, D. D. (2010). Women and women of color in leadership: Complexity, identity, and intersectionality. *Amer Psychol, 65*, 171–181. https://doi.org/10.1037/a0017459.

Segal, M. T., & Martinez, T. A. (2007). *Intersections of Gender, Race, and Class.* Roxbury.

Sen, R. (2020, July 1). Why today's social revolutions include kale, medical care, and help with the rent. Zócalo Public Square. https://www.zocalopublicsquare.org/2020/07/01/mutual-aid-societies-self-determination-pandemic-community-organizing/ideas/essay/.

Solomon, D., Maxwell, C., & Castro, A. (2019). Systemic inequality: Displacement, exclusion, and segregation; How America's housing system undermines wealth building in communities of color. Center for American Progress.

Spencer, M., Lewis, E., & Gutiérrez, L. (2000). Multicultural perspectives on direct practice in social work. In P. Allen-Meares & C. D. Garvin (Eds.), *Handbook of Social Work Direct Practice* (pp. 131–150). Sage.

Stall, S., & Stoecker, R. (2012). Community organizing or organizing community? Gender and the crafts of empowerment. In J. DeFilippis & S. Saegert (Eds.), *The Community Development Reader* (2nd ed., pp. 201–208). Routledge.

Stevens, J. W. (2002). *Smart and Sassy: The Strengths of Inner-City Black Girls.* Oxford University Press.

Suarez, Z. E., & Lewis, E. A. (2020). Spiritually and culturally diverse families: The intersection of cultural, religion and spirituality. In E. P. Congress & M. J. Gonzales (Eds.), *Multicultural Perspectives in Working with Families* (4th ed., pp. 295–314). Springer.

Szetela, A. (2020). Black Lives Matter at five: Limits and possibilities. *Ethn Racial Stud, 43*(8), 1358–1383.

Taylor, D. (2005). American environmentalism: The role of race, class and gender in shaping activism 1820–1995. In L. King & D. McCarthy (Eds.), *Environmental Sociology: From Analysis to Action* (pp. 87–106). Roman and Littlefield.

UN Women. (2020, July 1). Intersectional feminism: What it means and why it matters right now. Originally published at Medium.com/@UN_Women. https://www.unwomen.org/en/news/stories/2020/6/explainer-intersectional-feminism-what-it-means-and-why-it-matters.

Wilson, R. J., Abram, F. Y., & Anderson, J. L. (2010). Exploring a feminist-based empowerment model of community building. *Qual Soc Work, 9*(4), 519–535.

Wolff, T., Minkler, M., Wolfe, S. M., Berkowitz, B., Bowen, L., Butterfoss, F. D., Christens, B. D., Francisco, V. T., Himmelman, A. T., .& Lee, K. S. (2017). Collaborating for equity and justice: Moving beyond collective impact. *Nonprofit Q, 9*, 42–53.

Yoshihama, M., & Carr, E. S. (2003). Community participation reconsidered feminist participatory action research with Hmong women. *J Community Pract, 10*(3), 85–103.

Zetzer, H. A. (2018). Whiteout: Growing out of the problem of white privilege. In S. K. Anderson & V. A. Middleton (Eds.), *Explorations in Diversity: Examining the Complexities of Discrimination, Privilege, and Oppression* (3rd ed., pp. 9–24). Oxford University Press.

14

Mobilizing Black Barbershops and Beauty Salons to Eliminate Health Disparities

Lessons Learned on the Road to Health Equity during a Global Pandemic

LAURA A. LINNAN
STEPHEN B. THOMAS
SUSAN R. PASSMORE

Among the goals of Healthy People 2030 are to promote, strengthen, and evaluate the nation's efforts to improve the health and well-being of all people, including a focus on achieving efforts to "eliminate health disparities, achieve health equity, and attain health literacy to improve the health and well-being of all" (U.S. Department of Health and Human Services, 2020). Yet despite decades of gains in the overall health status for the general population, racial and ethnic health disparities persist across a broad spectrum of health outcomes and behavioral risk factors. There is growing consensus that accelerating efforts to eliminate racial and ethnic health disparities will require innovative community-based interventions and substantial trust building with respected community partners among racial and ethnic minorities, who suffer disproportionately from the leading causes of death.

The COVID-19 pandemic has shed a disturbing light on these disparities in both incidence and mortality among specific racial and ethnic minorities. For example, cases of COVID-19 are 2.6 times higher for Blacks, 2.6 times higher for Latinos, and 2.8 times higher among American Indians compared with Whites. And, while the COVID-19 mortality rates for all of these groups are higher than those for Whites, Blacks are experiencing the highest rate, at 2.1 times the death rate of Whites (Centers for Disease Control and Prevention, 2019).

According to Hooper and colleagues (2020), there are at least two major explanations for this alarming reality. First, racial/ethnic minority populations have a disproportionate burden of underlying comorbidities, such as diabetes, cardiovascular disease, asthma, HIV, morbid obesity, liver disease, and kidney disease, but not for chronic lower respiratory disease or chronic obstructive pulmonary disease (COPD). Second, racial/ethnic minorities typically live in more crowded, urban conditions and are more likely to be employed in public-facing, lower-wage occupations (e.g., services and transportation) that make physical distancing more difficult and increase exposure to the virus. In fact, Yancey (2020) acknowledges that "social distancing is a privilege" and the ability to isolate in a safe home, work remotely with full digital access, and sustain monthly income are components of this privilege that many racial and ethnic minorities do not enjoy.

Unequal access to health care and underlying unequal treatment due to systemic racism will exacerbate these differences. Black, Latino, and Native American patients disproportionately report experiences with discrimination in health care settings across the nation.

Moreover, many studies have demonstrated bias among health care professionals to include perceptions of Black, Latino, and Native American patients as less valued and cooperative, which have also been shown to be conveyed in their interactions with patients. Such mistreatment experienced through time and generations has resulted in an understandable deep distrust for health professionals, which continues to play out in delays in care seeking and hesitancy to engage in health prevention screenings. In the context of COVID-19, such distrust threatens to shape testing and vaccine uptake as well as the engagement in COVID vaccine trials.

To make progress toward eliminating racial and ethnic health disparities from COVID-19 and other leading causes of death, communities must be engaged in exploring the context of existing health disparities, formulating solutions, and ultimately making the decisions that affect their health. Strategies for community building and community organizing lie at the heart of addressing racial health disparities. Building community capacity by engaging with community members at each step of the process is essential for creating a shared vision, ensuring successful implementation, and promoting long-term sustainability of effective interventions (Giachello et al., 2003; Wallerstein & Duran, 2010). The involvement of community members as equals in decisionmaking processes can help build relationships based on trust, which promote the type of changes that are the foundation of a serious effort to affect health disparities (Wallerstein & Duran, 2010).

A promising approach is to begin with shared, trusted spaces that exist in the community, not in clinical or academic settings. Every ethnic group has "safe zones" or "sacred spaces" that represent community empowerment centers where they gather, share cultural traditions, connect with their historical narrative, and engage in writing new chapters of that story. The Black church is one example that has been well documented (Campbell et al., 2007); however, not all members of the Black community attend church regularly. We urgently need to find new partners, new places, and more effective interventions to close the health disparity gap. This chapter focuses on partnerships with Black barbershops and beauty salons as increasingly important places for promoting health and reducing health disparities. Barbershops and beauty salons have a legacy of community building and community organizing and are places where community members and researchers can come together to address health disparities while building community capacity. It is not surprising then that barbershops and salons have joined in the community response to COVID-19 despite the difficulties they have faced in loss of revenue as small businesses less likely than others to receive emergency loans. In the pages that follow, we review the important social, political, and economic history of U.S.-based Black beauty salons and barbershops, as well as the evidence for community-engaged research done in partnership with salons and shops designed to address health disparities. We share examples of two research teams that have used community-organizing strategies to engage with Black beauty salons and barbershops, as well as key lessons learned from this work. Finally, we highlight how beauty salons and barbershops, despite the many challenges of the COVID-19 pandemic for small businesses, are uniquely positioned to play key roles in addressing the alarming disparities in deaths related to COVID-19 among Blacks, with prevention and control interventions.

Beauty Salons and Barbershops: Contemporary and Historical Perspective

I think that barbershops from the beginning of time have always been a place of self-healing, self-awareness and just love. So I feel like we needed to be open.

–Troy D. Johnson, cited in Cabrera (2020)

Beauty salons and barbershops are found in almost every city, town, and rural community in the United States. More than 80,000 establishments (77,000 beauty salons, 4,500 barbershops) had a reported combined annual revenue of about $20 billion in May 2020; 722,600 barbers, hairstylists and cosmetologists were employed in these businesses, and 66,500 were barbers, with the remaining 656,100 as hairstylists, hairdressers, or cosmetologists (Bureau of Labor Statistics, 2020). Unfortunately, the COVID-19 pandemic has had a serious impact on all businesses, and especially small businesses like barbershops and beauty salons. According to Safegraph (Paton, 2020), a data firm that determines which businesses people visit by tracking aggregated and anonymized cellphone data, foot traffic to hair and beauty salons and barbershops dropped 60 percent nationwide by mid-April 2020. Moreover, a survey of 2,500 salons revealed that although 14.5 percent of owners said they had enough savings to survive three months without revenue, one-third said they could only survive one month, and nearly half said they have no emergency funds at all. The economic viability of these important places of community connection and fellowship is clearly at risk.

However, with a rich history and prominent role in the lives of Blacks, beauty salons and barbershops have served (and will continue to serve) as places for community building and community organizing beginning in the 1800s and continuing through today (Bristol, 2009). Originally a place where Black barbers provided shaves, haircuts, and wigs to elite men, such as Thomas Jefferson and Benjamin Franklin, barbershops evolved and adapted to the racial climate and policies of the United States. Barbershops provided an essential vehicle of economic mobility for Black men who lacked other means. Financial stability, especially compounded through generations, provided the independence necessary to support resistance to unjust social norms (Mills, 2005).

Although their history does not date as far back as that of barbershops, hair-dressing services as well as owning a beauty salon provided one of a limited number of avenues for Black women to become entrepreneurs at a time when the majority of Black were marginalized with limited access to economic opportunities (Byrd & Tharps, 2001). In fact, Annie Turnbo Malone and Madam C. J. Walker, both pioneers in the hair-care and beauty industry, are documented as being the wealthiest Black women during the early 1900s, with the latter becoming the first Black millionaire (Bundles, 1990; Byrd & Tharps, 2001). Historically, improving the overall health and well-being of Blacks has been an integral part of the community organizing and community building functions of Black-owned barbershops and beauty salons (Bristol, 2009; Bundles, 1990). As early as the 1830s, some Black barbershops became centers for abolitionists, soliciting customers to sign antislavery petitions and carrying abolitionist publications (Bristol, 2009). Barbershops also served as part of the Underground Railroad (Bristol, 2009). During the civil rights movement, the Black beauty salon was utilized as a meeting place for activities because, unlike the church and other prominent Black institutions, it was a less "visible" institution within the community. Serving as a natural setting for information sharing is one of the critical attributes of the Black barbershop and beauty salon that historically made them optimal sites for socializing, organizing, and building community (Mills, 2005) as well as addressing health disparities (Linnan et al., 2014; Luque et al., 2010a).

Another critical attribute of the Black barbershop and beauty salon is the uniquely intimate relationship between the barbers and stylists and their customers (Bristol, 2009; Hart et al., 2008). Often, customers establish long-term, friendly, trusted relationships with their preferred barber or stylist (Bristol, 2009). The high number of repeat contacts between customers and their barber or stylist form the type of "weak ties" that are thought to fill important gaps in social support that are accessible to everyone, extending beyond close family bonds that might be geographically displaced (Adelman et al., 1987; Granovetter, 1973). From conversations about politics, sports and the economy, to health and personal relationships, barbers and stylists have routinely served as sounding boards for their customers (Bristol, 2009) and as trusted confidants.

We have established that barbershops and beauty salons provide a safe haven for addressing social justice issues (Bristol, 2009; Mills, 2005) and that barbers and stylists serve as natural helpers in the community for their customers (Hess et al., 2007; Johnson et al., 2010; Luque et al., 2010a). Yet it is equally important to emphasize that barbershop and salon owners tend to be deeply concerned about the health and well-being of their communities (Britto, 2018; NPREd, 2020). Engaging with owners as "gatekeepers" to their stylists or barbers and their customers is critically important for implementing successful health-related interventions that address disparities in the Black community (Linnan et al., 2001; Luque et al., 2010a).

For more than twenty years we have led teams in Pennsylvania and Maryland (Thomas), and in North Carolina (Linnan), working in collaboration with barbershop and salon owners, stylists and barbers and their customers on a wide array of health-related programs and services designed to eliminate health disparities. This work has further placed a heavy emphasis on building the capacity of these owners to be successful members of the business community as well as the larger community. However, we are mindful of the caution of Musa who emphasizes that these same informal networks in the Black community are also potential means for the spread of rumors, concerns, and conspiracy theories (Musa et al., 2009). These, in turn, may reduce health care service utilization or create rumors that work against prevention strategies. However, Solomon and colleagues conducted an observational study in Black and White beauty salons and determined that less than 2 percent of observed health-related conversations were false (Solomon et al., 2004). Our efforts have not only monitored the quality and accuracy of the information provided, we have addressed myths and misconceptions about health risks and the causes of health problems, and worked to build trust and authentic relationships with barbershop and salon owners, stylists and barbers, and their customers.

Given all of the evidence that points to the importance of these small businesses in all communities, but particularly in the Black community, now more than ever, we need to find ways to preserve beauty salons and barbershops and mobilize them in the fight against COVID-19 and in other health-related priorities.

Overview of Beauty Salon and Barbershop Interventions

There have been two separate reviews of the literature on beauty salon and barbershop interventions (Linnan et al., 2014; Luque et al., 2010a). In brief, we have learned that barbershop and salon interventions have addressed a variety of health problems, including cancer, hypertension, diabetes, kidney disease, stroke, and cardiovascular disease, and health behaviors, such as diet, physical activity, and smoking. We have also learned that shops can provide ideal settings to explore topics such as occupational exposure to toxins and willingness to participate in clinical research. Passmore and colleagues (2019, 2021) showed that barbershops were culturally appropriate venues for promoting health but could not make strong conclusions on effectiveness. However, Linnan and colleagues (2014) concluded that 73.3 percent of intervention studies involving barbershops and salons demonstrated statistically significant health outcomes and enrolled primarily underrepresented minorities. Moreover, they demonstrated that the level and type of stylist or barber engagement varied but higher levels of involvement were associated with better health outcomes. Predominant themes in this early literature on partnerships to address health issues through beauty salons and barbershops included that (1) barbers and stylists felt it important to them personally that they help their clients by sharing health information with them; (2) many already talk to their clients about health; (3) customers are interested in receiving health information from their stylists or barbers; and (4) male customers showed a willingness to obtain not only education but also medical services, such as prostate cancer screening tests, blood pressure and blood glucose measurements, physical measurements, and fitness assessments in the barbershop (Linnan et al., 2014; Luque et al., 2010b).

In the years since those early reviews were published, several rigorously evaluated randomized controlled trials have been completed to further build the evidence of effectiveness for beauty salon and barbershop interventions. For example, Victor et al. (2010) have conducted several cluster randomized trials in Black barbershops designed to address hypertension. Overall, 63.6 percent of participants in the intervention group achieved a healthy blood pressure level (below 130/80 mmHg), as compared with 11.7 percent of participants in the control group ($p < .001$), and the intervention increased appropriate use of antihypertensive medications among participants. A more recent group randomized trial in barbershops by Wilson and colleagues (2019) tested a strengths-based, peer-led small group session designed to reduce condomless sexual behavior as a means of preventing HIV among heterosexual men (intervention) versus a prostate cancer screening with similar coaching (control). Intervention participants (64.4 percent) were significantly more likely than control participants (54.1 percent) to report no condomless sex (adjusted odds ratio [OR] = 1.61; 95% confidence interval [CI] = 1.05, 2.47).

Although there is a growing literature on the effectiveness of interventions in beauty salons and barbershops, some challenges remain. With a few exceptions, many interventions are taken to the salons or shops and are "community-placed" rather than community-based. That is, even when community partnerships are formed, the issues addressed by interventions have been largely selected by researchers rather than in partnership with owners, barbers and stylists, and customers. In this chapter, we focus on two different approaches to working with beauty salons and barbershops (physical activity, colorectal and prostate cancer screening, smoking cessation) and the ways in which these settings and their owners, stylists, and barbers were mobilized to address health disparities while building community capacity. In North Carolina, we consider a twenty-two-year partnership with the NC BEAUTY and Barbershop Advisory Board and resulting in more than two decades of rigorously evaluated research specifically addressing disparities in a variety of health outcomes (e.g., smoking, physical activity, healthy eating, cancer and cardiovascular disease screening tests, and falls prevention) in both beauty salons and barbershops. In Maryland, we explore the history and achievements of the Health Advocates In-Reach and Research (HAIR) initiative, which began in Pittsburgh, Pennsylvania, over two decades ago and now includes ten barbershops and salons. Over this time, HAIR has been home to a wide range of research studies and ongoing partnerships with local health care providers, and because the HAIR network of shops and salons was already established, it has become home to recent work dispelling myths about COVID-19 and promoting testing and vaccine uptake.

The North Carolina BEAUTY and Health Project: Preventing Cancer and Promoting Health in Beauty Salons

The North Carolina Bringing Education and Understanding to You (BEAUTY) and Health Project (hereafter the BEAUTY Project) is a twenty-two-year-old, ongoing partnership between researchers at the University of North Carolina at Chapel Hill (UNC) and beauty salon owners, licensed stylists, and their customers. In 2000, Dr. Linnan led an interdisciplinary team of researchers from the UNC Gillings School of Global Public Health and convened an advisory board that consisted of a group of salon owners, stylists, directors of local beauty schools, and product distributors to ask them the following question: "What do you think of the idea of promoting health in beauty salons?" A community-based participatory research (CPBR) approach (Wallerstein & Duran, 2010) was used to help answer this question, including a series of steps to gather data that was reviewed with the board, and then to work collaboratively with salon owners and their customers to build a series of participatory research projects. Over the last decade, this initial effort has blossomed to include work with over a hundred beauty salons and more than 2,500 of their customers. Although not a focus of this chapter, we also expanded efforts in to work with more than 80 Black barbershops and over 1,500 of their customers in North Carolina and have consulted with other programs, both domestically and internationally. From this original partnership, we have expanded projects to salons serving new populations (Latinx), using new methods (online continuing education courses for licensed stylists), and addressing new health issues (occupational exposures and falls prevention), as well as the sustainability of these efforts.

Brief History of the BEAUTY Project: Building Trust to Build Capacity

Consistent with the community organizing principle of starting where the people are and to understand whether the idea of promoting health in the salons was even viable, board members emphasized that the cooperation of licensed stylists would be essential. Together, we developed a survey of all fifty-eight licensed stylists in one North Carolina county (see Linnan et al., 2001 for detailed findings). Briefly, findings revealed that (1) stylists routinely talked with their customers during visits, including talking about health; (2) stylists were interested in attending training about how to deliver health messages in the salon; and (3) stylists were most comfortable and willing to talk with their customers about exercise, healthy eating, and healthy weight. Since these behaviors are related to preventable risk factors for many chronic diseases and were the most comfortable for stylists to talk about, they were selected as the first issues to be addressed. The survey results were also used to develop the initial stylist training workshop, which was the preferred method for receiving training as reported by cosmetologists.

While stylists were clearly supportive of the idea of promoting health, the advisory board and research team embarked on a second formative study to observe "how things worked" in the salon so as to create the most culturally and contextually appropriate intervention. Using a standardized protocol, an observational study in ten salons (five Black and five White salons) was conducted to assess which health topics were talked about most, which were not discussed, who initiated the conversations, how much time was spent in the salon, and what health myths and misconceptions were raised (Solomon et al., 2004). Observational findings confirmed that (1) health topics were discussed in approximately one in five conversations; (2) diet, exercise, and stress were among the most commonly discussed health topics; and (3) there were few differences in the topics discussed in Black versus White salons, but Black women spent more time in the salons, on average, than did White customers (Solomon et al., 2004). We processed the results with board members and worked together to create an intervention that was appropriate for the salon and effective for initiating conversation between the stylist and customer about health. Once again, the advisory board's review of initial findings provided important insights and guidance. For example, when we shared our data, advisory board members pointed out that health talk was initiated equally by customers and stylists, so we decided that our intervention focus must be twofold and include (1) mirror stickers with the slogan, "Ask me about the BEAUTY Project," prompting customers to begin a discussion with their stylist, and (2) training for the stylists on how to start the conversation during a typical visit.

Separate focus group discussions were also conducted with salon customers to understand their thoughts about health, beauty, and the possibility of promoting health in the salons (Kim et al., 2007). These results revealed that women were very interested in receiving health information in the salons and that at different ages women had different thoughts about beauty and health. Using this formative research, we developed an intervention that included a training workshop for stylists with role-plays addressing women of different ages, as well as interactive educational displays and print materials for customers linking beauty and health with stories from women of all ages. The stylist training workshop dispelled common myths and misconceptions about health and how to prevent leading causes of death and discussed the "good news" about prevention with specific messages about physical activity and healthy eating. Key messages introduced at the stylist training workshop demonstrated how stylists might weave messages into a typical visit with a customer. Stylists then tried out the messages via role-play during a typical customer appointment. The interactive educational displays encouraged customers to ask stylists questions about key health messages.

Next, the BEAUTY Board and research team recruited two salons to participate in a pilot test of the intervention we developed (Linnan et al., 2005). Results of this eight-week pilot study revealed that stylists were enthusiastic partners in the training workshops and reported a willingness to deliver the targeted health information in conversations with their customers. In addition, customers reported an increase in self-efficacy and actual behavior changes in diet and physical activity, with these changes significantly more likely among customers who had more contact with their stylists. Changes were evident both at immediate postintervention and as part of a twelve-month follow-up. These results provided encouraging support for a larger effectiveness trial funded in forty Black beauty salons by the American Cancer Society as well as several intervention studies based in beauty salons and barbershops and funded by the Centers for Disease Control and Prevention and the National Institutes of Health over the past two decades. Topics included promoting physical activity in Black barbershops (Linnan et al., 2010), falls prevention in beauty salons (Arandia et al., 2017), and planning for sustainability of these interventions (Linnan, 2014).

Maryland Health Advocates In-Reach and Research (HAIR): Mobilizing Black Barbershops to Promote COVID-19 Mitigation Behaviors and Vaccines

HAIR began with a community-focused revision of the national public awareness campaign "Take a Loved One to the Doctor Day." Dr. Stephen Thomas and his colleagues at the Center for Minority Health in the University of Pittsburgh's Graduate School of Public Health (Pittsburgh Research Center), partnered with a network of Black barbershops and salons in Pittsburgh, Pennsylvania, to launch the more community focused "Take A Health Professional to the People Day." This innovative twist on the U.S. Department of Health and Human Services campaign evolved over time from three barbershops and 10 health professionals in 2001 to ten barbershops and salons and over 200 health professionals screening approximately 700 people in one day at the height of the program in 2008. The campaign ultimately became a year-round community-engaged research program, Health Advocates In-Reach and Research (HAIR). In time, HAIR grew as a venue for public health education, clinical screenings, and assessments.

From the beginning, HAIR included a focus on a broad, holistic definition of health and wellness as well as having a strong emphasis on trust building. Key to the HAIR approach was respect for barbers' needs to run a business as well as their knowledge of both the community and the health problems plaguing it. Over time, the HAIR shops in Pittsburgh became sites for wellness in the community. HAIR supported training for barbers as lay health advocates so that they became certified in cardiopulmonary resuscitation and partnered with clinicians to provide services. Blood pressure screenings, depression screenings, echocardiograms, and even prostate exams were conducted throughout the HAIR barbershop network. In 2011, the team moved to the University of Maryland, College Park, to establish the Maryland Center for Health Equity in the School of Public Health and built a new network. MD HAIR includes ten shops and salons where screenings (carbon dioxide, blood pressure, and hemoglobin A1c) take place regularly through a collaboration with a local health care system. Maryland barbers and stylists have also been trained as lay health advocates in an intervention to promote colorectal cancer screening. In partnership with Cigna Healthcare, thirty-six barbers and stylists from all ten shops attended educational sessions on health disparities, health equity, research ethics, colorectal cancer knowledge and screening, and local health care resources. This knowledge equipped barbers and stylists with the ability to pass on knowledge to clients and provide them with a referral to Cigna or other no-cost, locally available screening services.

HAIR also supported other activities in the shops. For example, in Pittsburgh, a local playwright created a one-act play, *A Healthy Day in the Neighborhood*, which was presented to barbers and stylists, among other audiences. Once HAIR was established in Maryland, the focus on the arts continued through collaborations with the University of Maryland, Clarice Smith Performing Arts Center, to produce art installations and poetry readings. The HAIR network has also supported participation in clinical trials to counter the ongoing lack of diversity in biomedical research, which places unnecessary limitations on our knowledge of human variation and disease, the generalizability of research findings, and our ability to address health disparities (Knepper & McLeod, 2018; Oh et al., 2015). Clinical trials supported by HAIR have investigated topics including environmental health, mental health, and asthma in both Pittsburgh and Maryland. The HAIR shops have also provided a venue to gather community views of participation in genomics research (Passmore et al., 2019).

Finally, in recognition of the resources and knowledge in the shops, HAIR has played a productive role in the education of health professionals. In Pittsburgh, HAIR shops served as venues to train pharmacy students in communication skills, train dentistry students in community-implemented oral examinations, and serve as a clinical rotation for nursing students. In 2007, the Mayo Clinic's Center for Translational Science Activities (CTSA) established a formal course with the Pittsburgh Research Center, which included a one-week rotation course known as "Urban Immersion." Physician scientists from the CTSA were integrated with teams of clinicians who worked in the barbershops. The aim was to build their "cultural confidence" and conduct simulations of advanced screening techniques. For example, a Mayo physician demonstrated the use of a laptop echocardiogram on thirteen participants in one of the participating barbershops (Huskins et al., 2008), benefiting customers with diagnosed or suspected heart problems while further demonstrating the viability of the barbershop as an important venue for using sophisticated diagnostic methods designed to improve health care access.

Colors of the COVID-19 Pandemic: Impact on Barbershops and Beauty Salons

After decades of incremental progress documenting the value of barbershops and salons as venues for advancing health promotion and disease prevention, focused largely on risk factors for preventable chronic diseases, we are now confronting a global pandemic where these underlying medical conditions make COVID-19 a leading cause of death in the United States. In so many ways the pandemic's community spread has warped time itself. For example, in eight months (March–October 2020) COVID-19 had reversed a decade of global gains against poverty. In the United States, it had (1) produced the worst monthly unemployment figures since the Great Depression; (2) caused over 200,000 deaths; and (3) exposed how politics during a presidential election year can marginalize science and undermine trust in our public health institutions. This social carnage was abetted by inadequate government planning before and responses during, the pandemic. Where there had been a shortage of goodwill toward government, there was also insufficient voluntary cooperation with public health protocols (e.g., social distancing, wearing masks, etc.). On October 2, 2020, Donald J. Trump, the 45th president of the United States of America, was medevaced on Marine One from the White House to Walter Reed National Military Medical Center for emergency treatment related to complications from COVID-19 infection. This situation riveted the nation and global community as we all witnessed the indiscriminate tenacity of COVID-19.

In 1967, at the height of the civil rights movement, Dr. Martin Luther King Jr. posed the question, "Where do we go from here: chaos or community?" (King, 1967). The COVID-19 global pandemic has brought us to this poignant fork in the road once again. Who could have imagined how humble Black barbershops and salons could generate lifesaving insight we so desperately need today and into the future. In Black communities, we need to engage people who are already trusted sources. Black barbers and stylists have tremendous credibility, and they are seen as trustworthy pillars of the community. The credibility and trust they have is something we in public health now need in our efforts to eliminate racial and ethnic health disparities, the underlying conditions making COVID-19 so deadly. At a time of a global pandemic it is not just the mitigation message that matters, it is also the messenger that matters, and this is the context where we can reimagine the societal role of barbershops and salons. What better place to role model how to practice COVID-19 mitigation behaviors, what better trusted venue to receive a COVID-19 test and a seasonal flu shot—all while receiving personal care in the barbershop and salon? There is a growing body of scientific evidence that it is (1) feasible to deliver lifesaving medical screenings and public health services in barbershops and salons and (2) these activities are acceptable to and welcomed by the Black community. Given these facts, we have a scientific and ethical obligation to scale barbershop and salon health campaigns across the nation (Linnan et al., 2014; Thomas et al., 2011).

We believe the lessons learned from decades of research on Black barbershops and salons (see box 14.1) will help lead us toward what Dr. King called the "Beloved Community," a society based on justice, equal opportunity, and love of one's fellow human beings (https://thekingcenter.org/king-philosophy/). In the post-pandemic

BOX 14.1

Charting a Path Forward: Lessons Learned from Barbershop and Beauty Salon Partnerships

Building trust is essential, and it takes time and effort. There is a history of mistrust with the medical community and in some cases with researchers who represent academic institutions.

An advisory board that comprises beauty salon and barbershop owners, stylists and barbers, and customers can be extremely helpful for the process of building trust. Consistent with community-based participatory research approaches, the board can help plan, prioritize, implement, and evaluate health-related activities that occur in beauty salons and barbershops.

Advisory board members can help with recruitment of salons and barbershops and will improve participation in all sponsored programs and activities. In the BEAUTY Project, members created a video that enhanced participation among beauty salon owners, stylists and their customers over time (Linnan, 2014).

Salon and barbershop owners, stylists, and barbers tend to be community minded, eager to work collaboratively on efforts that will improve their customers' health. They are willing and able to be key spokespersons for prioritized projects and are well connected with other owners, stylists, and barbers.

Owners, stylists, and barbers tend to be busy, entrepreneurial people. Do not assume they have a lot of time to participate in trainings or delivering a complicated intervention. Instead, find ways to integrate brief messages into typical customer interactions or with materials they can share with customers in their chair. Recognize that their goal is to see as many customers as possible in a day—the health intervention will need to "fit" within, before, or after a typical visit.

Salons and barbershops are unlike other settings (e.g., worksites, schools, or churches) where individuals come on a certain day or time for a specific amount of time. Most women schedule a salon appointment, but others walk in for required services. The time spent depends on the hair care services provided. Nearly 20 percent of women in the initial BEAUTY study visited the salons weekly, and up to 80 percent returned at least once every eight weeks. Thus, determine how often customers visit, and make sure materials are updated regularly to keep things new and interesting for customers.

Consider ways to recognize salons and barbershops for project participation using local media or newspapers. Local publicity is helpful to small businesses and can help their financial bottom line by strengthening bonds with existing customers and attracting new customers.

To build capacity in these small businesses, and continue to build trust that strengthens partnership with owners of barbershops and salons, offer economic development opportunities in return for participating in health-related

(continued)

BOX 14.1 (continued)

research. For example, in North Carolina, we teamed up with the Minority Economic Development Center to offer free workshops for owners on tax preparation for small businesses, how to get credit, how to best do marketing using social media, and more. Strengthening economic viability of businesses helps ensure long-term viability of this work.

HAIR has been community driven, which has been a large part of our success. We have not imposed a clinical or academic definition of health on HAIR. In this way, we have been driven to explore new ideas and ways of expression through the arts, which have been powerful vehicles for communication. It is important to enter the community with an authentic appreciation for what the community can teach us as public health professionals.

Attention must be paid to differences in culture and perspective between the world of the shops and the typical world of clinicians. For some HAIR shops located in high-crime neighborhoods, the clear apprehension felt by some health care professionals entering the community was observed by the barbers, often creating tension. In time, a mandatory successful orientation for health professionals was instituted, but it placed another demand on staff time and budget.

Networks like HAIR require a sustainable investment, which puts them at odds with funding sources typically available from federal grants and foundations, which are project focused and time limited. This work requires innovation, collaboration, and resource leveraging. For example, the need to implement community-based health promotion projects for a local health care system provides opportunities for screenings in the HAIR network. Finding ways to support the work in the times between grant awards is also essential for establishing authentic and sustainable trust and partnership.

Beloved Community of the future the Black barbershop and salon will be a place to receive quality health care—imagine that. What do we have to lose?

Summary

This chapter presented the history of interventions based in beauty salons and barbershops and offered examples of two such interventions guided by community organizing principles and community-based participatory research approaches. In addition, we offered lessons learned from these efforts. Beauty salons and barbershops have a unique historical, political, economic, and social reality and a growing evidence base of effectiveness for promoting health and preventing disease. As a result, they often serve as the lifeblood for the Black community and may serve a uniquely important role during the COVID-19 pandemic. We believe that these important settings are integral places where prevention and control efforts should be mobilized. This is true in all U.S. communities and around the world. COVID-19 has brought into stark reality the need for addressing the underlying causes of health disparities—by reaching and engaging members in dialogue based on trust. Recognizing and building on the role of beauty salons and barbershops as places of strength, safety, rich cultural heritage, and social connections, there is growing evidence in support of working collaboratively with owners, stylists and barbers, and their customers to address disparities in health by instituting or supporting testing, contact tracing, and vaccine distribution, when available. In this way, the path forward for partnerships with beauty salon and barbershop owners remains strong and essential.

Questions for Further Discussion

1. The authors note that every ethnic group has safe zones or safe spaces that serve as community empowerment centers, with barbershops and beauty salons key among those places in Black communities. Thinking about your own ethnic group or community of identity, or those of others you may be familiar with (e.g., LGBTQ youth), what might be an example of a safe space? What makes it safe?

2. This evidence suggests that interventions based in beauty salons and barbershops have been successful in enrolling participants in a wide array of health promotion and disease prevention activities, and have proven effective in achieving desired outcomes. What can be done to get more communities to engage with beauty salon and barbershop owners? What can be done to sustain effective interventions over time?

REFERENCES

Adelman, M. B., Parks, M. R., & Albrecht, T. L. (1987). Beyond close relationships: Support in weak ties. In T. L. Albrecht & M. B. Adelman (Eds.), *Communicating Social Support* (pp. 126–147). Sage.

Arandia, G., Jones, J., Shubert, T., Bangdiwala, K., & Linnan, L. (2017). Feasibility of assessing falls risk and promoting falls prevention in beauty salons. *J Prim Prev, 38*(6), 567–581.

Bristol, D. W. (2009). *Knights of the Razor: Black Barbers in Slavery and Freedom.* Johns Hopkins University Press.

Britto, B. (2018, July 26). Baltimore's homeless veterans get their own free barber shop. *Baltimore Sun.* https://www.baltimoresun.com/features/baltimore-insider/bs-fe-barber-shop-mcvet-20180619-story.html.

Bundles, A. P. (1990). *Madam C. J. Walker.* Chelsea House.

Bureau of Labor Statistics, U.S. Department of Labor. (2020). Occupational outlook handbook, barbers, cosmetologists, hairstylists on the internet. https://www.bls.gov/ooh/personal-care-and-service/barbers-hairstylists-and-cosmetologists.htm.

Byrd, A. D., & Tharps, L. L. (2001). *Hair Story: Untangling the Roots of Black Hair in America.* St. Martin's Press.

Cabrera, C. E. (2020, June 25). 3 long (haired) months: Barbershop before-and-afters. *New York Times.* https://www.nytimes.com/2020/06/25/nyregion/nyc-barber-shops-coronavirus.html.

Campbell, M. K., Hudson, M. A., Resnicow, K., Blakeney, N., Paxton, A., & Baskin, M. (2007). Church-based health promotion interventions: Evidence and lessons learned. *Public Health, 28*(1), 213.

Centers for Disease Control and Prevention. (2019). Hospitalization and death by race/ethnicity. https://www.cdc.gov/coronavirus/2019-ncov/covid-data/investigations-discovery /hospitalization-death-by-race-ethnicity.html.

Giachello, A. L., Arrom, J. O., Davis, M., Sayad, J. V., Ramirez, D., Nandi, C., & Chicago Southeast Diabetes Community Action Coalition. (2003). Reducing diabetes health disparities through community-based participatory action research: The Chicago southeast diabetes community action coalition. *Public Health Rep, 118*(4), 309–323.

Granovetter, M. S. (1973). The strength of weak ties. *Am J Sociol, 78*(6), 1360–1380.

Hart, A., Underwood, S. M., Smith, W. R., Bowen, D. J., Rivers, B. M., Jones, R. A., & Allen, J. C. (2008). Recruiting African-American barbershops for prostate cancer education. *J Natl Med Assoc, 100*(9), 1012–1020.

Hess, P. L., Reingold, J. S., Jones, J., Fellman, M. A., Knowles, P., Ravenell, J. E., & Victor, R. G. (2007). Barbershops as hypertension detection, referral, and follow-up centers for black men. *Hyperten, 49*(5), 1040–1046.

Hooper, M. W., Naples, A. M., & Perez-Stable, J. (2020). COVID-19 and racial ethnic disparities. *JAMA, 323*(24), 2466–2467.

Huskins, C., Thomas, B., Ford, F., Browne, C., Greene, E. L., Robins, G., & Gabriel, E. (2008). Using innovative community engagement strategies to enhance the education and training of scholars in minority health and health disparities research. Institute of Medicine.

Johnson, L. T., Ralston, P. A., & Jones, E. (2010). Beauty salon health intervention increases fruit and vegetable consumption in African-American women. *J Am Diet Assoc, 110*(6), 941–945.

Kim, K., Linnan, L., Kulik, N., Carlisle, V., Enga, Z., & Bentley, M. (2007). Linking beauty and health among African American women: Using focus group results to build culturally and contextually appropriate interventions. *J Soc Behav Health Sci, 1*(1), 41–59.

King, M. L. (1967). *Where Do We Go from Here: Chaos or Community?* Beacon Press.

Knepper, T. C., & McLeod, H. L. (2018). When will clinical trials finally reflect diversity? *Nature, 557*(7704), 157–159.

Linnan, L. (2014). Planning for sustainability: Lessons learned from the North Carolina BEAUTY and Health Project. *Revista Familia Ciclos deVida e Saude no Contexto Sociale (REEF-ACS)* (online), *2*(2), 214–220. http://seer.uftm.edu.br/revistaeletronica/index.php/refacs /article/viewFile/1172/pdf.

Linnan, L., D'Angelo, H., & Harrington, C. (2014). Health promotion research in beauty salons and barbershops: A synthesis of the literature. *Am J Prev Medicine, 47*(1), 77–85.

Linnan, L., Ferguson, Y., Wasilewski, Y., Lee, A. M., Yang, J., Solomon, F., & Katz, M. (2005). Using community-based participatory research methods to reach women with health messages: Results from the North Carolina BEAUTY and health pilot project. *Health Promot Pract, 6*(2), 164–173.

Linnan, L. A., Kim, A. E., Wasilewski, Y., Lee, A. M., Yang, J., & Solomon, F. (2001). Working with licensed cosmetologists to promote health: Results from the North Carolina BEAUTY and health pilot study. *Prev Med, 33*(6), 606–612.

Linnan, L. A., Reiter, P. L., Duffy, C., Hales, D., Ward, D. S., & Viera, A. J. (2010). Assessing and promoting physical activity in Black barbershops: Results of the FITStop pilot study. *Am J Men's Health, 5*(1), 38–46.

Luque, J. S., Rivers, B., Gwede, C., Kambon, M., Green, B. L., & Meade, C. (2010b). Barbershop communications on prostate cancer screening using barber health advisers. *Am J Men's Health, 5*(2), 129–139.

Luque, J. S., Rivers, B. M., Kambon, M., Brookins, R., Green, B. L., & Meade, C. D. (2010a). Barbers against prostate cancer: A feasibility study for training barbers to deliver prostate cancer education in an urban Black community. *J Cancer Educ, 25*(1), 96–100.

Mills, Q. T. (2005). "I've got something to say": The public square, public discourse, and the barbershop. *Radic Hist Rev, 93*, 192–199.

Musa, D., Schulz, R., Harris, R., Silverman, M., & Thomas, S. B. (2009). Trust in the health care system and the use of preventive health services by older black and white adults. *Am J Public Health, 99*(7), 1293–1299.

NPREd. (2020, March 29). Turning kids into readers, one barbershop at a time. https://www.npr.org/sections/ed/2018/03/29/595180210/turning-kids-into-readers-one-barbershop-at-a-time.

Oh, S. S., Galanter J., Thakur N., Pino-Yanes, M., Barcelo, N. E., White, M. J., deBruin, D. M., Greenblatt, R. M., Biggins-Domingo, K., Wu, A. H. B., Borrell, L. N., Gunter, C., Powe, N. R., & Burchard, E. G. (2015). Diversity in clinical and biomedical research: A promise yet to be fulfilled. *PLOS Med, 12*(12), e1001918.

Passmore, S. R. (2021). Use of a qualitative story deck to create scenarios and uncover factors associated with African American participation in genomics research. *Field Methods, 33*(2), 159–174.

Passmore, S. R., Jamison, A. M., Hancock, G. R., Abdelwadoud, M., Mullins, C. D., Rogers, T. B., & Thomas, S. B. (2019). "I'm a little more trusting": Components of trustworthiness in the decision to participate in genomics research for African Americans. *Public Health Genomics, 22*(5–6), 215–226.

Paton, E. (2020, June 12). Hair salons reopen, and Americans rush back. *New York Times.* https://www.nytimes.com/2020/06/12/fashion/haircut-salon-reopening.html.

Solomon, F. M., Linnan, L. A., Wasilewski, Y., Lee, A. M., Katz, M. L., & Yang, J. (2004). Observational study in ten beauty salons: Results informing development of the North Carolina BEAUTY and health project. *Health Educ Behav, 31*(6), 790–807.

Thomas, S. B., Quinn, S. C., Butler J., Fryer C. S., & Garza M. A. (2011). Toward a fourth generation of disparities research to achieve health equity. *Ann Rev Public Health, 32*, 399–416.

U.S. Department of Health and Human Services. (2020). Healthy People 2030 Framework. https://www.healthypeople.gov/2020/About-Healthy-People/Development-Healthy-People-2030/Framework.

Victor, R. G., Ravenell, J. E., Freeman, A., Leonard, D., Bhat, D. G., Shafiq, M., Knowles, P., Storm, J. S., Adhikari, E., Bibbins-Domingo, K., Coxson, P. G., Pletcher, M. J., Hannan, P., & Haley, R. W. (2010). Effectiveness of a barber-based intervention for improving hypertension control in black men: The BARBER-1 study; A cluster randomized trial. *Arch Intern Med, 171*(4), 342–350.

Wallerstein, N. B., & Duran, B. (2010). Community-based participatory research contributions to intervention research: The intersection of science and practice to improve health equity. *Am J Public Health, 100* (Suppl. 1), S40–S46.

Wilson T., Gousse, Y., Joseph, M. J., Browne, R. C., Camililien, B., McFarlane, D., Mitchell, S., Brow, H., Urraca, N, Romeo, D., Johnson, S., Salifu, M., Stewart, M, Vavagiakis, P., & Fraswer, M. (2019). HIV prevention for Black heterosexual men: The Barbershop Talk with Brothers Cluster randomized trial. *Am J Public Health, 109*(8), 1131–1137.

Yancey, C. W. (2020). COVID-19 and African Americans. *J Natl Med Assoc, 323*(19), 1891–1892.

15

Popular Education, Participatory Research, and Community Organizing with Immigrant Restaurant Workers in San Francisco's Chinatown

A Case Study

CHARLOTTE CHANG
ALICIA L. SALVATORE
PAM TAU LEE
SHAW SAN LIU
MEREDITH MINKLER

Popular education, participatory research, and community organizing have been used across diverse settings, cultures, and populations. Each has had a major influence on the development of social movements and social change processes worldwide (Brown et al., 2011; Della Porta & Diani, 2015). As illustrated in this chapter, these approaches, used together, can create synergy and increased momentum for both community capacity building and multilevel empowerment and social change.

We briefly review the shared roots and influences of popular education, community organizing, and participatory research, which is also known as community-based participatory research (CBPR). We then present a case study from San Francisco's Chinatown that illustrates how popular education was applied by a CBPR partnership investigating the working conditions and health of immigrant restaurant workers and collaboratively advocating for equitable and sustainable change. This approach helped weave together broader goals common to both community organizing and participatory research, such as leadership development, empowerment, social justice through action, and improvements in worker health and well-being (Chang, Minkler et al., 2013; Minkler et al., 2018). We describe the project's short- and intermediate-term outcomes and lessons learned from the partnership about how popular education, participatory research, and community organizing can be mutually reinforcing in the struggle for social justice and health equity for marginalized populations.

Finally, looking back over the decade since this project officially ended, we highlight the longer-term outcomes to which it contributed, both locally and beyond, with a particular focus on building community capacity and addressing wage theft, the workers' greatest health concern and a major public health problem.

Popular Education

As discussed in chapter 5, popular education focuses on the experience of the learners themselves. As classically described by Arnold and colleagues (1995), it "serves the interests of the popular classes (exploited sectors of society), [and] involves them in critically analyzing their social situation and in organizing to act collectively to change the oppressive conditions of their lives" (p. 5). Inherent in popular education are the emphases on the perspective of the learner, as well as larger educational and social change goals (Beder, 1996; Garzón-Galvis et al., 2019; Wallerstein & Duran, 2018; chapter 5). Beder (1996) identifies three key components of popular education approaches: *praxis, collective and participatory orientation*, and *action*. Briefly, praxis is action based on critical reflection (Freire, 1973) and involves an iterative process that permeates decisionmaking in popular education (Beder, 1996; Streck, 2016). The collective and participatory orientation of popular education underscores its focus on group process, including ownership of the process and the information uncovered by the members themselves. It further recognizes the need for generation of group solutions and for a sustainable infrastructure for collective social action, including community capacity building and the development and nurturing of new leaders (Beder, 1996; Garzón-Galvis et al., 2019; Su, 2009; Wallerstein & Duran, 2018). Finally, the action component of popular education is reflected in the fact that this approach "is always rooted in struggles for democratic social change" and the belief that "ordinary people can make that change" (Garzón-Galvis et al., 2019; Richard, 2004, p. 48; chapter 5).

Participatory Research

When communities find that they require data to support their organizing needs and efforts to improve their health and welfare, participatory research can provide an important alternative to traditional outside expert–driven research paradigms. Over twenty five years ago, participatory research was concisely defined as "systematic investigation with the collaboration of those affected by the issue being studied for purposes of education and taking action or effecting social change" by George et al. (1996, p. 7). Popular education and similar approaches question traditional conceptualizations of the nature and production of knowledge and emphasize the need for knowledge generation to be democratic and emancipatory in its processes and outcomes (Fine et al., 2021; Streck, 2016; Wallerstein & Duran, 2018). Among the central principles of participatory research are that it should involve co-learning, be mutually beneficial, involve an empowering process that contributes to community capacity, and balance research and action (Israel et al., 2013).

While community organizing and participatory research have many similar goals, their users may also have differing aims. For example, unlike traditional community organizing, participatory research frequently involves academic or other professionally trained partners whose research occurs along a spectrum. At one end are researchers who focus heavily on knowledge generation and pragmatic improvements to organizational functioning. At the other end may be key players who focus primarily on the social change action that is central to community organizing and involves a high degree of community participation (Balazs & Morello-Frosch, 2013). Although "balancing research and action" is a core participatory research principle (Israel et al., 2013), tensions between the knowledge generation and community action commonly arise. Despite such challenges, real opportunities exist for merging participatory research and community organizing efforts, particularly as more critical perspectives on the former are gaining greater adherence. Fine and her colleagues (2021) recently noted that such research (which they term *critical participatory action research*) must be grounded in the saying "nothing on us without us," which has long been a mantra of the Maori people of New Zealand, Black and Colored South Africans, the disabled, and AIDS activists in the United States (345). As Fine and her colleagues note, that simple but powerful phrase "translates into the belief that research questions and designs must be crafted by research collectives that include and center the perspectives of those most marginalized and with the least sociopolitical power, [and] research teams must always ask, 'to whom are we accountable?'" (p. 345). Finally, the action imperative inherent in truly community-centered and community-driven participatory research also stresses that the research process is not over until research-based and equity-focused community and/or policy outcomes have been achieved—typically well after the funding for such research has ended (Minkler, 2014).

Popular education can be a powerful means for integrating the paradigms of participatory research and community organizing and for more effectively promoting their shared commitments to community capacity building, empowerment, and action to address community-identified goals.

Case Study: Engaging Immigrant Chinese Restaurant Workers in Popular Education, Participatory Research, and Organizing to Change Working Conditions

An example of the successful integration of participatory research, community organizing, and popular education may be found in a CBPR study of immigrant restaurant workers' working conditions and health, conducted in San Francisco's Chinatown, and the subsequent organizing campaign in which all of us authors participated. Combining critical analysis and consciousness-raising with action helped improve the quality and salience of the research and the effectiveness of concomitant organizing efforts (Chang, Minkler et al., 2013; Minkler et al., 2018). This process also strengthened community capacity through the enhancement of restaurant worker leadership and the increased visibility of the Chinese Progressive Association (CPA), a community-based organization located in the heart of Chinatown and the project lead, as a potent resource for change in the community and beyond.

The Community and Partnership

San Francisco's Chinatown is the cultural hub of the city's Chinese immigrant community and a vibrant, dynamic neighborhood home to over 13,000 residents and numerous local businesses (Tom, 2019). In increasingly service-oriented urban economies, and notwithstanding the significant loss of restaurant jobs during the COVID-19 pandemic, restaurants have historically been an important source of work, employing approximately one-third of residents in Chinatowns across the county. Health and safety problems abound in restaurants and include traditional occupational health concerns, such as cuts, burns, falls, and on-the-job stress (U.S. Bureau of Labor Statistics, 2018). But health problems also encompass serious economic and other social vulnerabilities when employers do not pay the legal minimum wage and in other ways engage in wage theft (e.g., by delaying or evading payment of wages earned, sometimes for periods as long as several months, not paying overtime, etc.) (Minkler et al., 2014; Restaurant Opportunities Center United, 2018).

The CPA had been organizing and addressing such issues for over thirty-five years. In 2007 it formed a partnership with the University of California, Berkeley (UCB) School of Public Health and its Labor Occupational Health Program (LOHP); the San Francisco Department of Public Health (SFDPH); and the University of California, San Francisco (UCSF), Division of Occupational and Environmental Medicine. Initiated by the CPA and building on previous collaborations between various partners on separate efforts, the new partnership formed to carry out a participatory research study of working conditions and health among Chinatown restaurant workers. The project was funded by a Centers for Disease Control and Prevention (CDC) grant to UCB, the primary university partner, with the majority of funding subcontracted to the CPA and UCSF. A second grant from The California Endowment, the state's largest health philanthropic foundation, went directly to the CPA. The partnership subsequently expanded to include a group of six current and former Chinese restaurant workers who provided on-the-ground community expertise for the research and the focal point of the CPA's efforts to develop leaders for its campaign to address the working conditions of Chinese immigrant workers.

The study was ecological in nature and included focus groups with restaurant workers, a detailed survey of working conditions and health among 433 Chinatown restaurant workers, and SFDPH partner observations of working conditions in 106 of the 108 neighborhood restaurants (Gaydos et al., 2011; Minkler et al., 2014; Salvatore & Krause, 2010). A comprehensive and ongoing evaluation of the partnership was also a critical part of the research process (Chang, Minkler et al., 2013; Chang, Salvatore et al., 2013).

Integrating Participatory Research and Community Organizing

As Kathleen M. Roe and Brick Lancaster (2005) have pointed out, "Research and practice are best understood as a partnership, learning from and informing each other" (p. 129). Integrating participatory research and community organizing requires open communication, mutual consideration, and careful planning on the part of all collaborators. In the Chinatown project, many hours of informal and formal partnership meetings were dedicated to discussing and reflecting on the varying needs, strengths, and visions for community change of different partners, the goals of the partnership, and adaptations needed. Adoption by the CPA was needed to recruit worker partners, who could then be leaders for the citywide organizing campaign. This made it possible to use time and resources more efficiently and form more cohesive connections between the research and organizing components of the worker partners' training.

Critical to the integration of the participatory research and organizing aspects of the project was the project director herself, a university partner at LOHP, long-time community organizer in Chinatown, and founding board member of the CPA. A veteran of previous participatory research collaborations between labor organizations and academic researchers and an experienced popular educator, the project director served several critical roles. As an "insider" in both the university and community, she understood the differing needs and complementary goals of the research and organizing and acted as a bridge between the different partners. She worked closely with CPA organizers to coordinate and conduct partnership meetings, worker trainings, research and organizing activities, and actions involved (Chang, Salvatore et al., 2013). Although the CPA had decades of experience organizing in the community, it had never before conducted research with academic and health department professionals. The mentorship provided by the project director was doubly important, as it enabled CPA organizers, in turn, to facilitate the worker partners' participation in the study.

Popular Education Approach

Popular education permeated all stages of the Chinatown project. Two organizers at the CPA and the project director developed an evolving, progressively more intensive curriculum for worker partners that drew heavily from popular education practices to address the dual needs of the research and the organizing.

INTERACTIVE, PARTICIPATORY, AND LEARNER-CENTERED TRAININGS. To introduce and prepare worker partners who had no prior experience conducting research, CPA organizers and the project director developed trainings designed to teach them about participatory research and facilitate greater familiarity and comfort with the CPA and the other project partners.

All trainings were conducted at the CPA office in Chinatown. Training activities focused on workplace health and safety, workers' rights, recruitment of participants, survey design, interviewing, confidentiality, and informed consent and on taking part in CPA organizing activities. Interactive activities, such as risk mapping (Brown, 2008; Mujica, 1992), neighborhood mapping (appendix 2), workshops on policymaking and power mapping (chapter 22; appendix 11), and mock food inspections in a simulated kitchen were used in training sessions. The exercises enhanced worker partners' participation, assisted them in drawing connections between their own lives and study and organizing goals, and elicited their knowledge and expertise.

One exercise, which was designed to trigger workers' reflections about their experiences and generate new knowledge, began by displaying pictures of Chinese restaurant workers in various work-related situations and providing the prompt, "What kind of questions would these workers have about their working conditions?" One worker partner shared a story of a coworker who suffered a head injury after slipping on the floor. The coworkers who walked the injured worker to the hospital were yelled at by the boss for leaving work, and the injured worker was fired upon her return to work. When asked for assistance with medical bills for the work-related injury, the boss told the injured worker that the incident was her own fault, and the expenses were her sole responsibility. This story and others led not only to additional questions being added to the worker survey regarding such abuses but also to training on how to handle emergency situations at work.

CRITICAL REFLECTION. Critical reflection was a central component of the worker trainings throughout all stages of the research and organizing. Worker partners were engaged in facilitated reflections about the larger political and economic contexts of the specific issues they were discussing. After learning about CBPR involving other communities of immigrant women workers, the worker partners took part in a critical analysis of the status of immigrant workers in the restaurant industry and in the country in general. In discussing the root causes of workplace hazards and their health impacts, worker partners concluded that it is important to use the law to protect people.

Research ethics training, which is required for all federally funded research involving human subjects, was also used to raise workers' consciousness about the human rights and social justice abuses that made such a formal review process important. When atrocities committed by Nazi forces in World War II in the name of science were discussed, worker partners reflected on their own historical trauma when "Japan did the same to China" during World War II. The discussion went on to explore how participatory research can help protect the safety of study participants in part through the active engagement of workers as study partners and not simply research subjects.

Worker partners also engaged in critical reflection during six monthly data interpretation workshops following the worker survey and restaurant observations.

Workshops were conducted in different languages, including Cantonese, by the project director and CPA organizers, with additional support from university and health department partners, who wore simultaneous transition equipment. Worker partners provided many insights into the data that were originally apparent to other partners. For example, they explained that the relatively high proportion of workers who reported receiving sick leave benefits (58 percent) most likely reflected the misconception that making up an unpaid sick day with an extra day of work without pay was in fact sick leave (Minkler et al., 2014) They suggested that the apparent underreporting of workplace abuses, such as being yelled at (reported by 42 percent) could be because workers were constantly being yelled at by their supervisors (Chinese Progressive Association, 2010) and would only have responded in the affirmative if the "yelling had made them cry." Similarly, when asked for a definition of "good health," a worker partner explained that "health doesn't impact your [ability to] go to work. Unless you're in the hospital and you can't move."

ACTION. Along with interactive, learner-centered activities and critical reflection, action was a central popular education component in the worker partners' leadership development training. As one CPA organizer remarked, "Experiencing the struggle and directly confronting power" was an indispensable step, particularly among low-income, immigrant workers, some of whom may also be undocumented.

Activities requiring worker partners to take action in the community were introduced incrementally. Early on, they passed out fliers on topics such as wage and hour violations, a task that some found challenging because of its public nature, later moving on to a wider range of activities and issues (e.g., supporting workers from a poultry market in Chinatown that owed thousands of dollars in back wages to its employees). The worker partners joined the campaign picket lines and attended planning sessions. With time, they took on increasingly visible roles, sharing their personal experiences at public hearings on city budget cuts and participating in demonstrations for immigrant rights.

Throughout their involvement, the project director and CPA organizers continued providing opportunities for reflection to reinforce critical analysis and further consciousness-raising and learning. In these discussions, worker partners reflected on the inspiring example of the poultry workers organizing for their rights, and considered the incentives for employers to withhold wages within the larger economic and political context. Such reflections, together with their experiences with action, were the foundation for subsequent recommendations for change and organizing demands made by CPA organizers and worker partners.

PARTICIPATORY RESEARCH: TRANSLATING RESEARCH TO ACTION. Consistent with both participatory research principles and community organizing goals, the partnership recognized the importance of translating research into action. Results from the survey of 433 restaurants corroborated the expressed concerns of the workers: that wage theft and pay-related violations were widespread and the problems of greatest concern to workers. Fifty percent of workers surveyed did not receive minimum wage, 17 percent were not paid on time, and 76 percent of those who worked over forty hours per week were not paid overtime wages (Chinese Progressive Association, 2010; Minkler et al., 2014; Salvatore & Krause, 2010). Approximately a third of workers indicated that their bosses took some portion of the tips. High proportions of respondents reported accidents and injuries; 48 percent had been burned on the job in the previous year, 40 percent had suffered cuts, and 17 percent had slipped or fallen (Chinese Progressive Association, 2010; Minkler et al., 2014).

The study's observations of working conditions in 106 of the 108 restaurants supported worker-reported data. Checklist findings indicated multiple preventable hazards, including an absence of anti-slip mats (52 percent), wet and greasy floors (62 percent), lack of posting of required labor laws (65 percent), and lack of fully stocked first aid kits (82 percent) (Chinese Progressive Association 2010; Gaydos et al., 2011; Minkler et al., 2014; Salvatore & Krause, 2010).

The dissemination and action phase of the project involved organizing initiatives taken on by the CPA and allies, with the worker partners playing important roles, as well as activities undertaken by the health department and university partners to translate findings into action. A key step in translating the research into action was the CPA's drafting and launch of a comprehensive report called *Check, Please!* This report summarized findings of the participatory research and worker focus groups (Chinese Progressive Association, 2010). The CPA also drew upon additional studies to illustrate how working conditions in Chinatown reflected broader trends in the city and across the country for low-wage workers (Bernhardt et al., 2009; Mujeres Unidas y Activas, 2007; Restaurant Opportunities Center of New York, 2005). Recommendations for improving the conditions of low-wage workers citywide included adopting the low-wage worker bill of rights that was developed by the San Francisco Progressive Workers Alliance (PWA), a coalition founded by the CPA and other local worker centers and organizations.

Worker partners played a prominent leadership role in the large public press conference held to launch the CPA's report (Chinese Progressive Association, 2010). Research findings and recommended actions were presented to over 200 members of the community, four of the eleven city supervisors, and approximately twenty members of the press. Several worker partners spoke at the event, were interviewed by local and ethnic media reporters, and quoted in media outlets. A front-page article describing the workers was published in the *San Francisco Chronicle* the next day (Coté, 2011).

Following the launch event, the CPA, worker partners, the PWA, and the board of supervisors worked together to prepare the San Francisco Wage Theft Prevention Ordinance. The CPA and the PWA introduced this novel legislation with a kickoff press event on the steps of city hall and a public hearing in which worker partners and other members of the original study team participated. Provisions of the ordinance aimed to improve the processing and handling of workers' labor violation claims and holding employers accountable (e.g., by enhancing the city's ability to investigate and address problems, eliminating delays in citations, imposing penalties for failure to post the legal minimum wage, and requiring public notification when violations are found). The ordinance also called for better education for workers on their rights, information on investigations of their employers, and increased protection from employer retaliation. In introducing the legislation, Supervisor Eric Mar remarked, "I am proud to be introducing local legislation that is drawn from action-based research and bottom-up grassroots organizing that will help strengthen labor law enforcement in San Francisco and give workers a meaningful voice in stopping wage theft in our City" (Eric Mar, personal communication, May 12, 2011) The board of supervisors unanimously passed the ordinance, which the late Mayor Ed Lee then signed into law. The CPA and the PWA later successfully organized for the creation of a citywide task force to improve the interorganizational coordination of agencies responsible for enforcing labor laws and workers' rights and consider ways to reward "high-road" employers, who want to do the right thing but must compete against those who ignore even basic labor standards. Finally, the CPA and community partners stressed a citywide approach that would bring together the voices of all low-wage worker communities.

Along with policy action, the CPA and worker partners scaled up educational activities. Efforts included "worker teas," held monthly at the CPA, in which worker partners played a central role in planning, defining issues and topics to be discussed, facilitating education sessions, and conducting outreach with community members.

Other members of the participatory research partnership also led efforts to translate study findings into sustainable improvements for restaurant workers. In part as a result of the significant lack of labor law postings documented in this research, for example, the health department began requiring proof of workers' compensation insurance coverage for all new and change-of-business health permits, and worked to improve citywide compliance with such policies. These efforts included sending formal letters to regulatory bodies, such as the city's Office of Labor Standards Enforcement (OLSE), to inform them of the study's findings and hold meetings about improving enforcement of these laws. The OLSE and the SFDPH went on to explore mechanisms to improve violator identification and enforcement (Gaydos et al. 2011).

PERSONAL TRANSFORMATION AND ORGANIZATIONAL GROWTH. Although community organizing and participatory research guided by popular education are heavily focused on engaging participants in taking action and changing identified drivers of inequity, there is an equally strong emphasis on personal and collective transformation. Through the Chinatown project, worker partners reported overcoming fears of engaging with new people, learning to speak in public, a greater sense of courage and confidence, and a deepened analysis of and perspective on social issues (Chang, Salvatore et al., 2013). In Freire's (1973) words, the changes worker partners noted in themselves were part of developing a critical consciousness and a belief in their ability to transform their world.

Evidence of the worker partners' transformation emerged at the project midpoint, when they began to feel comfortable discussing their own leadership potential, a dramatic change from the beginning of the project, when they shied away from use of the word *leader*. As the project continued, further shifts were observed, with worker partners moving from simply "wanting to help other workers" to owning issues and solutions themselves through the public sharing of their own stories and experiences working in restaurants and living in the community (Chang, Salvatore et al., 2013).

Worker partners directly attributed their changes to the experiences they had with the CPA and the project (Chang, Salvatore et al., 2013). One commented, "[My leadership skills] increased a lot. . . . It's like yesterday at the hearing, I went and spoke. In the beginning, I was really scared. If I had never been to CPA before, I would have been more afraid. Yesterday I wasn't afraid at all." Another worker leader reported that the trainings, activities, and experiences with CPA and the project had changed her thinking, noting, "[Previously,] I didn't dare to fight for anything. When I was working, [the boss] said, 'Work,' and I would work. Later, when my old boss asked me to go back, I would tell him I wanted minimum wage, I did not want to be owed wages."

Several worker partners also mentioned that friends and family began to view them as people who help new immigrants and restaurant workers. They served as resources to friends and acquaintances who were owed back wages or needed help with housing or employment. Some even inspired their family members to begin participating in community activities as well.

Several worker partners became an integral part of the CPA's Worker Organizing Committee, the leadership core of the organization. They took on increasingly higher-profile roles and were largely responsible for activities that fostered community and built the CPA's membership base among the city's Chinese immigrants. Worker partners frequently spoke at public events, such as demonstrations on wage theft and immigration; facilitated CPA events; and represented the organization at educational exchanges with other workers and community groups in San Francisco and beyond. Several were part of the CPA's 2011 U.S.-Mexico Border Exchange Trip, where they learned from and built community with area workers, organizations, and activists working on immigration, housing, and environmental justice issues.

Throughout this transformational process, worker partners reflected on a very positive environment, which they described as being just like family. The mutual support provided by this community was noted by the worker partners because, as one worker put it "sometimes they are bolder than I am and I can learn some skills from them" (Chang, Salvatore et al., 2013).

At the organizational level, CPA staff cited capacity built through their involvement in the project. For example, the two research grants allowed them to obtain resources to develop community leaders more proactively and prospectively than in prior, more reactive efforts dictated by the tight time pressures of earlier campaigns. The outreach and recruitment efforts of the worker partners, as well as the research findings and subsequent CPA report and launch, raised the CPA's profile and brought greater visibility to workers' rights in Chinatown, and in San Francisco's larger Chinese immigrant community.

Finally, the data generated in the study also helped the CPA to be more effective in obtaining grants and raising additional resources to support their mission to "educate, organize, and empower" the low-income and working-class immigrant Chinese community in San Francisco and to build collective power with other oppressed communities to demand better living and working conditions and justice for all people (Chinese Progressive Association 2010).

Lessons Learned

The integration of popular education, participatory research, and community organizing can be a potent means of studying and addressing collective health and social problems. These approaches can complement and strengthen each other by improving the relevance and quality of research, helping in more effectively working toward shared goals of empowerment and capacity building, and creating a stronger foundation for promoting action for change.

Benefits to Participatory Research

Popular education and community organizing orientations provide many benefits for the research process (Streck, 2016). Involving members of the community most affected by the health issue being studied can increase the relevance of the research, and improve instruments, participant recruitment, data collection, and interpretation of findings (Balazs & Morello-Frosch, 2013; Israel et al. 2013; Minkler, 2014). In the Chinatown study, worker partners expanded the focus of the investigation to include a careful look at wage theft as a major health issue and helped develop research instruments that were culturally and linguistically appropriate. Worker partners' lay knowledge and experiences were also key to identifying and addressing such ethical concerns as fear of employer retaliation and the imperative of improving the relevance and cultural sensitivity of both survey items and the restaurant-level occupational checklist (Gaydos et al., 2011; Minkler et al., 2010, 2014). Additionally, the high-level community participation helped to ensure that the research findings were both communicated back to the community and used as the basis of action to address issues of concern.

Empowerment and Community Capacity

Empowerment and capacity building at both individual and organizational levels are central goals of both action-oriented participatory research and community organizing (Israel et al., 2013; Minkler, 2014; Wallerstein & Duran, 2018). The use of a popular education approach combining critical reflection and action enhanced the development of a core group of worker leaders in the Chinese immigrant worker community, furthered the expansion of the CPA's com- munity and worker networks, and resulted in a higher profile for the organization and its causes. This process also greatly facilitated translation of the research findings into action, as with the launch and dissemination of the community report on the research, the creation of legislation to prevent wage theft, and the development of coalitions and alliances with other worker and community groups facing similar issues across city, country, and international borders.

On an individual level, in participatory research and in community organizing informed by popular education, community partners should themselves see changes in their capacity and power. The dramatic changes often described by worker partners in the Chinatown project were a critical outcome of this project. As mentioned earlier, several thus described how they went from eschewing the title of *leader* to testifying before the board of supervisors, participating in rallies, telling their own stories to the media, and actively working for change for and with other low-wage workers. (Chang, Minkler et al., 2013; Minkler et al., 2018).

Yet the co-learning critical to participatory research and popular education further suggests the importance of ensuring that outside researcher partners are also growing through their collaboration in the work. Both university and health department partners in the Chinatown project commented on how much their work with the CPA and the worker partners had increased their own understanding of problems, such as wage theft, and the immense benefits that community partners, with their expert knowledge of their community, brought to the research and its action outcomes. As Bernard (2002) reminds us, "For Freirians in occupational health concerned with generating an assertive, critically thinking, united workforce . . . we need to unleash the full power of popular education and not limit ourselves to promoting the form without the critical—including self-critical—content" (p. 7).

At the organizational level, enhanced capacity and strength should be a key outcome of such work. In the Chinatown project, the integral role that the worker partners hired and trained through the study went on to play as a Worker Committee leadership core for the CPA, and the organization's enhanced visibility and increased resource base, provide important examples of such growth and change.

Conclusion

The case study from San Francisco's Chinatown discussed in this chapter illustrates how integrating participatory research and community organizing efforts can support the distinct yet complementary ends of each while also furthering shared goals of community empowerment, capacity building, and social change. Popular education, a key philosophical tradition shaping the development of both participatory research and Freirian approaches to organizing in and of itself, can help to weave together the common threads of these two related but distinct paradigms. Popular education can enable participatory research partnerships to better study and address community-identified problems through community organizing and related social action (Beder, 1996; Garzón-Galvis et al., 2019). At the same time, it can provide community organizers with the philosophical grounding, skills, and resources needed to promote true, member-led action based on critical reflection, while using data gathered collaboratively that reflect lay and professional ways of knowing.

The Chinatown case study demonstrates the fluid boundaries that exist between popular education, community organizing, and participatory research as well as the potential of such fluidity for achieving change on multiple levels (Minkler, 2014; Richard, 2004). From these efforts come additional ripple effects as the individuals who participate in the process come to internalize the struggles and take ownership over the conceptualization of community issues and their solutions and begin to influence their families, friends, colleagues, and community. Discussions of the "good life" and "good jobs" initiated in worker trainings laid the foundation for recommendations for policy change and for building the base of support and leadership in the community, which, in turn, led to stronger linkages and alliances with diverse workers and communities across the city and beyond. The multilevel changes described included individual workers feeling a new sense of power and empowerment, the CPA's being increasingly recognized as a strong worker voice within and well beyond Chinatown, new anti–wage theft legislation, and the health department's use of the data collected to help pressure for real changes in restaurant working conditions. Through its work on each of these levels, the project helped lay the foundation for improving the health and lives of Chinese immigrant workers in the community and low-wage workers across the city. The project incorporated the critical expert knowledge of immigrant workers and facilitated their ability to work in genuine partnership with academic researchers in gaining new knowledge for change. This all occurred through a process that was itself empowering, helping to pave the way for more transformative change in the years ahead and demonstrating that knowledge is indeed power in community organizing (Alinsky, 1971; Garzón-Galvis et al., 2019; Sen, 2003; chapters 5, 22). Reflecting on her experience, one worker partner summed this up well: "When I first got involved in this survey project, I thought it was impossible to change anything in Chinatown. But now that we have done so much work in the community and helped other workers recover wages, I see that change is possible. We can improve things. We must!" (Chinese Progressive Association 2010, p. 25).

Epilogue: Ten Years Later

In the more than a decade since the Chinatown Health and Safety Study drew to an official close in 2010, numerous additional developments have taken place that can be linked, in part, to the original project. The central concern of the CPA and its worker partners then—as now—is wage theft in all its forms. By mid-2020, the CPA had helped low-wage restaurant workers recover over $10.6 million in owed wages in Chinatown and the broader San Francisco Bay Area, including most recently, $2.6 million recovered for the 133 workers in a single restaurant (Echeverria, 2020). The CPA is recognized as a national leader in anti–wage theft organizing and enforcement strategy

Although only a few of the original worker partners remain active with the CPA today, given other work commitments, health problems, and caregiving responsibilities, many continue to express support for the organization and its work. A former surveyor with the study, for example, went on to become an at first reluctant, and then a deeply committed and enthusiastic, leader of one of the largest wage theft victories, helping win back $4 million for workers in a single dim sum restaurant. She was also actively involved in the fight for a $15 minimum wage, and social justice campaigns on issues including the right to unionize and climate justice (https://cpasf.org/media-resources/san-francisco-chronicle-wage-theft-a-scourge-for-low-income-workers).

The partnership's study and the report on its findings were key to building the CPA's current worker organizing program, in part by establishing an initial worker leadership base through the intense training and leadership development it provided for a small but critical group of workers. As the CPA's executive director remarked, "[The research] armed us with documentation of the community's reality that was an untold story—the statistics we needed to get policymakers' attention. That information became the key part of our campaign to end wage theft." The CPA staff's introduction to a major funder (The California Endowment) through an academic partner also helped in "seeding fundraising for our work and programs" well beyond the study.

The CPA staff also commented on the value of continued relationships with some of the academic and health department partners. A doctoral student later became a full time researcher and trainer at LOHP and an active member of the CPA's board of directors in 2014, while another LOHP partner with long roots in Chinatown served, until recently, as chair of the CPA's board. An SFDPH staff member from the original study remained a "steadfast supporter," following up on enforcement regarding health and other violations in the restaurants, while she and other academic and health department partners continue to show up for events like the CPA's annual Lunar New Year celebration and fundraiser, and provide financial donations and consultation, as desired, to the organization.

Finally, CPA staff and academic and health department partners have contributed to expanding the work in other parts of the state and country by sharing the methods, outcomes, and lessons learned, with interested community-based organizations, universities, and health departments. CPA staff reported doing "a ton of sharing about the research and the report, plus the ways we used it in the [wage theft ordinance] campaign, and the connection to local labor enforcement work."

Their presentations at conferences as well as gatherings of worker organizations led to further follow-up and requests for technical assistance and consultation. Academic, community, and health department partners shared the project's processes and outcomes through close to a dozen peer-reviewed academic and professional journal articles and book chapters. With few exceptions (e.g., a technical report on statistical findings), community partners served as coauthors on these publications and were frequently invited to co-present talks at professional organizations and university forums and classes.

As a result of the wide dissemination of study methods and findings, including media coverage of new wage theft victories (Echeverria, 2020), the academic and health department partners and their community counterparts were asked for help in adapting aspects of the study to new research in other regions. The principal investigator helped colleagues in Southern California, New York, and Massachusetts to develop a wage theft measurement tool as part of a national study of work organization risk assessment (Choi et al., 2019). Based on the CPA-led study and its findings, wage theft was one of seven core justice-related items (along with discrimination, harassment, bullying, etc.) on which data is now being collected nationally using this tool. Most of the wage theft questions were taken directly from the CPA survey instrument to enable comparison of findings.

With the advent of the COVID-19 pandemic, the CPA, like many other social justice–focused community organizations (Sen, 2020; chapter 6), quickly pivoted to provide mutual aid to the most vulnerable members of the community, including distribution of cash assistance and supplies through its COVID-19 Pandemic Emergency Stabilization Fund, while ensuring that the people most affected by the crisis remained at the center of the decisionmaking process. At the same time, the CPA continued to fight on the policy level for paid sick leave and universal health care, issues that were cast into even sharper relief by the socioeconomic and racial/ethnic inequities in COVID-19 cases, hospitalizations and fatalities.

At this writing, the CPA is also playing a leading role in fighting the increasing xenophobic attacks against Chinatown's low-income workers and seniors, as well as hate crimes against Asian American and Pacific islanders (AAPI) in the city and beyond, that are often a response to the fear and retaliatory anger over the so-called China virus stoked by former president Donald Trump and his supporters. As part of its work with the Coalition for Community Safety and Justice of which it is a part, the CPA further helped to get a $700,000 allocation in the 2021 city budget for restorative justice, victims services and related needs.

Against the backdrop of the pandemic and the many fraught developments during and in its aftermath, the story of the CPA, its participatory research partnership, and the ripple effects of the work provide a consistent ray of hope. The CPA has become even more widely known and respected for its leadership on numerous critical issues both in Chinatown and beyond on worker and tenant rights, but also in the fight against AAPI hate crimes. The participatory research partnership it co-created and led well illustrates Fine et al.'s (2021) call for a more critical approach to such research, that truly centers and is accountable to the community. Finally, as Barbara Israel and her colleagues (2013) remind us, a core principle of CBPR is the commitment of partners for the long haul. This epilogue attempts to illustrate the value of heeding that call in our work for equity and justice with, for, and led by, marginalized communities and their organizations.

Questions for Further Discussion

1. The authors note that while a core principle of participatory research calls for balancing research and action, tensions often emerge in practice, particularly when community partners are anxious to share preliminary findings and academic partners want to wait for further analysis and publication of results. Assume you are part of a partnership where this tension has arisen. What steps might you suggest the partnership take to try to reach a compromise? And what could they do to prevent such problems in the future?
2. The SF Chinatown Restaurant Worker Health and Safety Study offered informative examples of ways in which the lived experience of worker partners improved research instruments, the interpretation of findings, and their effective dissemination and use to affect change. Think back on an example from this case study that resonated with you and why it did. Did the chapter make you think differently about your own comfort level in collaborating with community residents on an issue of strong local concern? If so, in what ways?

Acknowledgments

Funding for this work was provided by the CDC's National Institute of Occupational Safety and Health, The California Endowment, and the Occupational Health Internship Program. We are also deeply grateful to our project partners, Alex T. Tom, Alvaro Morales, Fei Yi Chen, Niklas Krause, Megan Gaydos, Robin Baker, and Rajiv Bhatia; CPA worker leaders, Hu Li Nong, Gan Lin, Li Li Shuang, Rong Wen Lan, Michelle Xiong, Zhu Bing Shu, and Li Zhen He; and the seventeen community surveyors who were critical to the project's success. Sincere thanks are also extended to the many Chinatown restaurant workers who took part in this study and its subsequent action component. Finally, we are very grateful to the Progressive Workers Alliance, Young Workers United, Mujeres Unitas y Activas, the Data Center, and other organizational allies, as well as the San Francisco Department of Public Health, the board of supervisors, and the late mayor for their help in translating this work into action.

REFERENCES

Alinsky, S. D. (1971). *Rules for Radicals: A Pragmatic Primer for Realistic Radicals.* Random House.
Arnold, R., Barndt, D., & Burke, B. (1995). *A New Weave: Popular Education in Canada and Central America.* CUSO Development Education and Ontario Institute for Studies in Education, Adult Education Department.

Balazs, C. L., & Morello-Frosch, R. (2013). The three R's: How community-based research strengthens the relevance, rigor and reach of science. *Environ Justice, 6*(1), 9–16.

Beder, H. (1996). Popular education: An appropriate educational strategy for community-based organizations. *New Dir Adult Cont Educ, 70*, 73–83.

Bernard, E. (2002). Popular education: Training rebels with a cause. In L. Delp, M. Outman-Kramer, S. J. Schurman, & K. Wong (Eds.), *Teaching for Change: Popular Education and the Labor Movement* (pp. 6–8). UCLA Center for Labor Research and Education.

Bernhardt, A., Milkman, R., Theodore, N., Heckathorn, D., Auer, M., Defilippis, J., Gonzalez, A. L., Narro, V., Perelshteyn, J., Polson, D., & Spiller, M. (2009). *Broken Laws, Unprotected Workers: Violations of Employment and Labor Laws in America's Cities*. National Employment Law Project.

Brown, M. P. (2008). Risk mapping as a tool for community-based participatory research and organizing. In M. Minkler & N. Wallerstein (Eds.), *Community-Based Participatory Research for Health: From Process to Outcomes* (pp. 453–457). Jossey-Bass.

Brown, P., Morello-Frosch, R., & Zavestoski, S. (2011). *Contested Illnesses: Citizens, Science, and Health Social Movements*. University of California Press.

Chang, C., Minkler, M., Salvatore, A. L., Lee, P. T., Gaydos, M., & San Liu, S. (2013). Studying and addressing urban immigrant restaurant worker health and safety in San Francisco's Chinatown district: A CBPR case study. *J Urban Health, 90*(6), 1026–1040.

Chang, C., Salvatore, A. L., Lee, P. T., San Liu, S., Tom, A. T., Morales, A., Baker, R., & Minkler, M. (2013). Adapting to context in community-based participatory research: "Participatory starting points" in a Chinese immigrant worker community. *Am J Community Psychol, 51*(3–4), 480–491.

Chinese Progressive Association (CPA). (2010). *Check, Please! Health and Working Conditions in San Francisco Chinatown*. San Francisco Chinese Progressive Association.

Choi, B., Landsbergis, P., Seo, Y., Dobson, M., & Schnall, P. (2019, November 2–6). Creating a new instrument for work organization risk assessment in the United States: The Healthy Work Survey (HWS) project. In *APHA's 2019 Annual Meeting and Expo*. American Public Health Association. https://apha.confex.com/apha/2019/meetingapp.cgi/Paper/445883.

Coté, J. (2011, July 18). Wage theft a scourge for low income workers. *San Francisco Chronicle*. https://www.sfgate.com/news/article/Wage-theft-a-scourge-for-low-income-workers-2354262.php.

Della Porta, D., & Diani, M. (2015). *Oxford Handbook of Social Movements*. Oxford University Press.

Echeverria, D. (2020, August 14). Workers win $2.6 million wage theft settlement with Bay Area restaurant. *San Francisco Chronicle*. https://www.sfchronicle.com/food/article/Workers-win-2-6-million-wage-theft-settlement-15482120.php#:~:text=More%20than%20130%20restaurant%20workers,between%20workers%20and%20the%20restaurant.

Fine, M., Torre, M. E., Oswald, A. G., & Avory, S. (2021). Critical participatory action research: Methods and praxis for intersectional knowledge production. *J Couns Psychol, 68*(3), 344–356.

Freire, P. (1973). *Education for Critical Consciousness*. Seabury Press.

Garzón-Galvis, C., Wong, M., Madrigal, D., Olmedo, L., Brown, M., & English, P. (2019). Advancing environmental health literacy through community-engaged research and popular education. In S. Finn & L. O'Fallon (Eds.), *Environmental Health Literacy* (pp. 97–134). Springer.

Gaydos, M., Bhatia, R., Morales, A., Lee, P. T., Liu, S. S., Chang, C., Salvatore, A. L., Krause, N., & Minkler, M. (2011). Promoting health and safety in San Francisco's Chinatown restaurants: Findings and lessons learned from a pilot observational checklist. *Public Health Rep, 126*(3_suppl), 62–69.

George, M. A., Green, L. W., & Daniel, M. (1996). Evolution and implications of P.A.R. for public health. *Health Promot Educ, 3*(4),6–10.

Israel, B. A., Eng, E., Schulz, A. J., & Parker, E. A. (2013). Introduction to methods for CBPR for health. In B. A. Israel, E. Eng, A. J. Schultz, & E. A. Parker (Eds.), *Methods for Community-Based Participatory Research in Public Health* (pp. 3–38). Jossey-Bass.

Minkler, M. (2014). Enhancing data quality, relevance, and use through community-based participatory research. In N. Cytron, K. Petit, G. T. Kingsley, D. Erickson, & E. S. Seiman (Eds.), *What Counts? Harvesting Data for American's Communities* (pp. 245–259). Federal Reserve Bank of San Francisco and the Urban Institute.

Minkler, M., Lee, P. T., Tom, A., Chang, C., Morales, A., Liu, S. S., Salvatore, A., Baker, R., Chen, F., Bhatia, R., & Krause, N., (2010). Using community-based participatory research to design and initiate a study on immigrant worker health and safety in San Francisco's Chinatown restaurants. *Am J Ind Med, 53*(4), 361–371.

Minkler, M., Salvatore, A., & Chang, C. Y. (2018). Participatory approaches for study design and analysis. In R. Brownson, G. Colditz, & E. Proctor (Eds.), *Dissemination and Implementation Research in Health: Translating Science to Practice* (2nd ed., pp. 175–190). Oxford University Press.

Minkler, M., Salvatore, A. L., Chang, C., Gaydos, M., San Liu, S., Lee, P. T., Bhatia, R., & Krause, N. (2014). Wage theft as a neglected public health problem: An overview and case study from San Francisco's Chinatown District. *Am J Public Health, 104*(6), 1010–1020.

Mujeres Unidas y Activas. (2007). Day Labor Program Women's Collective of La Raza Centro Legal and the DataCenter. In *Behind Closed Doors: Working Conditions of California Household Workers* (pp. 1–8). Mujeres Unidas y Activas.

Mujica, J. (1992). Coloring the hazards: Risk maps research and education to fight health hazards. *Am J Ind Med, 2*(5), 767–770.

Restaurant Opportunities Center of New York. (2005). *Behind the Kitchen Door: Pervasive Inequality in New York City's Thriving Restaurant Industry.* New York City Restaurant Industry Coalition.

Restaurant Opportunities Center United. (2018). Better wages, better tips restaurants flourish with one fair wage. https://chapters.rocunited.org/wp-content/uploads/2018/02/OneFair Wage_W.pdf.

Richard, A. M. (2004). *Learning to Change: A Case Study of Popular Education among Immigrant Women* [Doctoral dissertation, University of California, Berkeley]. Dissertation Abstracts International (UMI No. 3165538).

Roe, K. M., & Lancaster, B. (2005). Mind the gap! Insights from the first five years of the circle of research and practice. *Health Promot Pract, 6*(2), 129–133.

Salvatore, A. L., & Krause, N. (2010). Health and working conditions of restaurant workers in San Francisco's Chinatown: Report of survey findings. Unpublished report. University of California, Berkeley, and University of California, San Francisco.

Sen, R. (2003). *Stir It Up: Lessons in Community Organizing and Advocacy.* Jossey-Bass.

Sen, R. (2020, July 1). Why today's social revolutions include kale, medical care, and help with rent. Zócalo Public Square. https://www.zocalopublicsquare.org/2020/07/01/mutual-aid -societies-self-determination-pandemic-community-organizing/ideas/essay/.

Streck, D. R. (2016). Participatory research methodologies and popular education: Reflections on quality criteria. *Interface-Comunicação, Saúde, Educação, 20,* 537–547. https://www .scielosp.org/article/icse/2016.v20n58/537-547/en/.

Su, C. (2009). *Streetwise for Book Smarts: Grassroots Organizing and Education Reform in the Bronx.* Cornell University Press.

Tom, A. (2019). Chinese Progressive Association, San Francisco, CA. *J Asian Am Stud, 22*(I), 79–84.

U.S. Bureau of Labor Statistics. (2018). Nonfatal occupational injuries and illnesses data by industry and case type. https://www.bls.gov/iif/soii-chart-data-2018.htm.

Wallerstein, N., & Duran, B. (2018). Theoretical, historical, and practice roots of CBPR. In N. B. Wallerstein, B. Duran, J. G. Oetzel, & M. Minkler (Eds.), *Community-Based Participatory Research for Health: Advancing Social and Health Equity* (3rd ed., pp. 17–30). Jossey-Bass.

PART SIX

Using the Arts and the Internet as Tools for Community Organizing and Community Building

The past few decades have seen the application of many innovative new tools and approaches that have enriched community building and organizing, and some of these, such as user-friendly approaches to developing and using neighborhood health and social indicators (chapters 10, 20; appendix 4) and digital technologies for community mapping (appendix 2) are discussed elsewhere in this book. This part focuses on two, very different approaches that nonetheless have in common enormous and proven potential for enhancing community building and organizing and reaching new and expanded populations with our work. These seemingly polar opposite approaches are harnessing the power of the internet to create online strategies for community building and organizing, and using the age-old power of the arts to engage new partners and reach new audiences with our campaigns and initiatives for promoting health and social equity through community organizing and community building.

In chapter 16, public health trainers and practitioners Nickie Bazell and Evan vanDommelen-Gonzalez consider the powerful roles of the internet and social media in community building, organizing, and advocacy. As they note, with over half of the world's population now online, and the average user spending six hours a day on the internet (International Telecommunications Union, 2020), often via social media, *not* to create and use a careful online strategy as part of an organization or coalition's overall strategy may well doom it to irrelevance. Unlike most treatments of this topic, however, Bazell and vanDommelen-Gonzalez purposely do not include in this chapter a long list of currently popular web links and other resources since, as they correctly suggest, the very rapidity of change in the virtual universe suggests that many of these sites and resources will likely be extinct in short order. Instead, they focus on the bigger issues and questions and remind us that such tools are effective only when embedded in a broader and carefully designed strategy that includes "real world" engagement as well as cyberactivism. Among the broader-picture questions that they challenge us to think about are the following: What are our objectives? Do we want to disseminate information? Raise funds? Get the attention of journalists? What do we know about our audience and environment? What is our message and how will it resonate with our target audience(s)? For example, which messages are most likely to be shared online? What action steps might we see? And of critical importance in community organizing, how can we get our viewers to engage beyond the hashtag? Finally, how do we evaluate our online efforts? As Bazell and vanDommelen-Gonzalez point out, although there are many useful tools, such as Google Analytics, for helping us in this latter task, having a carefully thought out evaluation strategy is as important for our online work as it is when we are working in communities in real time.

The authors share powerful examples of dramatic changes brought about through online organizing, particularly in times of crisis. They highlight, for example, the #NeverAgain campaign in 2018, organized by students at Marjory Stoneman Douglas High School in Parkland, Florida, within days of the shooting that left seventeen of their classmates dead and seventeen more injured. The combination of political action on the ground and their online activism made possible coordination with a national March for Our Lives and massive school walk-outs across the country. And in Florida, it played a major role in the swift passage of legislation raising the age to buy firearms from 18 to 21 and requiring a three-day waiting period for most weapons (Rahman-Jones, 2018).

As the authors go on to note, however, just as online organizing has extraordinary potential, it also carries risks, particularly if no carefully developed strategy for its use is in place. Some of these, including the digital divide, were brought into sharper relief during the COVID-19 pandemic, when the proportion of low-income youth, tribal members, and rural residents with no or unstable internet access created still greater inequities during a time of distance learning and working from home (Vogels et al., 2020). Other risks were highlighted after events like the brutal police killing of George

Floyd, when images of a White officer with his knee on the neck of an unarmed Black man pleading, "I can't breathe!" were constantly replayed, and many Black people, in particular, relived this deeply personal trauma with each viewing.

Such challenges and many others demand our attention and action, but so, too, do the internet and social media's power for good. The chapter's closing case study of the youth job training and placement program, Enterprise for Youth, is shared to illustrate the latter, including how the reach and effectiveness of an already impressive community-based program can increase exponentially with a solid online strategy. Finally, as Bazell and vanDommelen- Gonzalez remind us, to be effective in any of our online work for change, attention to the basic principles of community building and organizing (Chávez et al., 2010) will be no less important than they are in our work with communities on the ground.

If the internet represents one of our most recent tools for community building and organizing, using the arts as a vehicle for such work remains among the oldest. Yet texts on community organizing tend largely to overlook the potential and the impressive track record of the arts in this work. In chapter 17, Caricia Catalani and her colleagues examine the arts as a vehicle for organizing and social change, their importance in social movements nationally and globally, and the theoretical bases for using the arts to stimulate community organizing and community building. When used by and with communities, the arts are seen as promoting organizing for health and welfare through a wide variety of often interrelated means, including getting people involved, facilitating assessment and health education, helping heal the wounds of historical trauma, and offering culturally sensitive approaches to addressing health inequities. Vivid case studies include the historic NAMES Project AIDS Memorial Quilt—the single largest art installation in the world—and the Clothesline Project, which, for over thirty years has been provocatively promoting awareness of violence against women and children around the world through art that "airs society's dirty laundry" (Hippe, 2000).

The cases include, as well, such contemporary examples as famed cellist Yo-Yo Ma's #Songs of Comfort, through which musicians around the world perform and upload their own musical offerings to bring a sense of community and reduce the social isolation many experienced during the COVID-19 pandemic. The chapter then turns to three case studies that capture diverse approaches to community building and organizing through the arts. These include a videovoice project (Catalani et al., 2012) two years after Hurricane Katrina devastated the ninth ward in New Orleans, and its use in enabling a team of survivors to capture and share the stories of the storm and its aftermath through graphic images and narratives. Their video, *In Harmony*, helped promote dialogue among diverse audiences locally and beyond, built individual and community capacity, and was used to press policymakers for needed change.

Chapter 17 then moves to San Francisco's Tenderloin Neighborhood, and the efforts of a women-and-queer-centered multiethnic dance company (ABD Productions), dedicated to inspiring social change through the arts. Beginning over a decade ago, the Skywatchers Project was created in tandem with a "Values-Based Methodology and Guidance for Practice" (appendix 5), which stressed such truths as "time moves at the speed of trust" (Brown, 2017) and the relational, conversational, durational, and structural dimensions of community practice. We learn how, as the group expanded, Skywatchers became a mixed-ability, intergenerational arts ensemble of Tenderloin residents and professional artists that continues today (Epstein et al., 2021). The forms of art created by this group include movement-based and visual arts, music, and the spoken word. Participants share a full range of life experiences, stories, talents, and struggles, and both the processes and outcomes of the work are explored, including its pivot to virtual and phone contact during the pandemic, when a new series of works were created shedding light on this moment in time in the city's most heavily impacted area.

The chapter concludes by arguing that in the face of the often substantial challenges to organizing that communities and their professional partners confront today, the particular strengths of the arts as effective organizing tools should not be overlooked.

REFERENCES

Brown, A. M. (2017). *Emergent Strategy*. AK Press.
Catalani, C. E., Veneziale, A., Campbell, L., Herbst, S., Butler, B., Springgate, B., & Minkler, M. (2012). Videovoice: Community assessment in post-Katrina New Orleans. *Health Promot Pract, 13*(1), 18–28.
Chávez, V., Minkler, M., Wallerstein, N., & Spencer, M. (2010). Community organizing for health and social justice. In V. Chávez, L. Cohen, & S. Chehimi (Eds.), *Prevention Is Primary: Strategies for Community Well-Being* (2nd ed., pp. 87–112). Jossey-Bass.

Epstein, N. E., Bluethenthal, A., Visser, D., Pinsky, C., & Minkler, M. (2021). Leveraging arts for justice, equity and public health: The Skywatchers program and its implications for community-
based health promotion practice and research. *Health Promot Pract 22*(1_suppl), 91S–100S.

Hippe, P. C. (2000). Clothing their resistance in hegemonic dress: The Clothesline Project's
response to violence against women. *Cloth Text Res J, 18*(3), 163–177.

International Telecommunication Union (ITU). (2020). Statistics. https://www.itu.int/en/ITU-D/Sta
tistics/Pages/stat/default.aspx.

Rahman-Jones, I. (2018, March 19). Florida shooting: How teenagers started a political campaign in
30 days. *BBC News*. https://www.bbc.co.uk/news/newsbeat-43392821.

Vogels, E. A., Perrin, A., Rainie, L., & Anderson M. (2020, April 30). 53% of Americans say the internet has been essential during the COVID-19 outbreak. Pew Research Center. https://www
.pewresearch.org/internet/2020/04/30/53-of-americans-say-the-internet-has-been
-essential-during-the-covid-19-outbreak/.

16

Creating an Online Strategy to Enhance Effective Community Building and Organizing

Harnessing the Power of the Internet

NICKIE BAZELL

EVAN VANDOMMELEN-GONZALEZ

Just as the internet is transforming how we communicate, work, shop, and learn about the world, it is reshaping how groups and individuals promote social change. The most successful advocacy work will leverage online tools to organize and build support, participate in important debates, and reach a wider audience. The internet and social media bring unmatched potential for organizers, but also carry important risks for those who do not think carefully about harnessing these tools properly.

Nearly 54 percent of the global population, or 4.1 billion people, use the internet (International Telecommunications Union, 2020), with the average internet user spending 6 hours online per day. The Western world now lives in what van Dijck and colleagues (2018) argue is a "platform society," dependent on the infrastructure of online platforms (e.g., Google, Facebook, Apple, Amazon, and Microsoft) that are permeating our communities and transforming the economy. Much of the time we spend online is accessing social media, on average 2 hours and 23 minutes a day (GlobalWebIndex, 2019). *Social media are online platforms that promote dynamic, real-time communication among many actors* (Barker et al., 2013; Lovejoy & Saxton, 2012). These platforms and tools allow us to forge and nurture relationships, create and share information and ideas, and promote social expression and change with unprecedented ease and reach (Kanter & Fine, 2010; Kaplan & Haenlein, 2010).

Social media are effectively being used to engage millions of people in a variety of issues to create social change as well as support the strategic management of nonprofits. Studies have demonstrated that social media are useful for creating dialogue, building community, and disseminating advocacy messages (Bortree & Seltzer, 2009; Briones et al., 2011; Greenberg & MacAulay, 2009; Guo & Saxton, 2014; Lovejoy & Saxton, 2012). As well, "social media have the potential of enabling nonprofits to participate in the collective evolution of communication by providing them with a faster, more cost-effective way to provide information, generate collective action, and promote sharing of resources" (Sun & Ascenio, 2019, p. 393). With so much information available through numerous venues, donors and supporters today are better equipped to access a wider variety of causes and organizations than at any time in the past (Guo & Saxton, 2018). As Jamie Smith describes, "Social media have the potential to not only put a face on nonprofit organizations but also to expand their capacity, reach and effectiveness" (Smith, 2018, p. 297). In fact, Barns and Andonian (2011) found that nonprofits more actively engage in social media than for-profit brands.

Given the central role that online organizing has played in political and social campaigns and movements, it is important to understand how these tools can be harnessed. In Barack Obama's 2008 presidential campaign, the strategic use of social media tapped into formerly politically inactive populations by engaging key stakeholders in each community, and was the single biggest factor in his winning the race (Rainie & Smith, 2008). Thousands of Obama's online supporters had never been politically active. They joined his campaign's online social network because of friends, traditional media messages, and talking to activists. Now these practices are standard in all political campaigns. During the Arab Spring, social media were central to bringing tens of thousands of people into the streets during the youth-led revolt that led to the ousting of Egyptian president Hosni Mubarak in 2011. The Occupy Wall Street movement in 2011 also showed how social media can be used to organize groups and individuals behind income inequality. In 2018, the #NeverAgain campaign was organized by student survivors within a few days of the school shooting at Marjory Stoneman Douglas High School in Parkland, Florida, in which seventeen students were killed and seventeen others injured. The direct political action on the ground and online spurred coordination with the March for Our Lives in a demonstration in Washington, DC, inspired schools nationwide to stage walkouts, and less than one month after the shooting, the Florida Senate voted to approve and the governor of Florida signed into law legislation that raised the age to buy a firearm from 18 to 21 and required a three-day waiting period for most weapons (Rahman-Jones, 2018). These examples illustrate that while internet tools must be central to an organizing strategy, they require organizers to be thoughtful and intentional about how such tools are leveraged within the context of larger goals.

With the demonstrated success of online organizing, the question facing community organizers and nonprofits today is not whether they *should* use social media for community building and advocacy, but *when* and *how* they should. Community organizers and nonprofits occupy space on a broad spectrum, and there is no one-size-fits-all approach to online organizing. Therefore the approach will largely result from the mission and vision of the organization or group. Unfortunately, many groups today have succumbed to the lure of easy-to-create social media accounts without taking the time to think about "how to establish a consistent, sustainable, and easily recognizable presence that integrates and enhances both online and real-world activities" (Turner, 2002, p. 55). As nonprofit organizations increasingly turn to social media to engage their communities, it is critical that they develop effective strategies that make better usage of their limited organizational resources and capacities (Guo & Saxton, 2018). This is especially important because a static online presence is almost as dangerous as no web presence at all (Smith, 2018). In this chapter we discuss the potential for using the internet for community organizing and outline the steps for creating an online strategy. We illustrate this through examples of social movements and a nonprofit case study. We also highlight precautions with using social media, emphasizing that social media serve as an outlet that should be used by organizers who are directed by time-tested community-organizing principles.

Online Advocacy and Activism

The countless communities and social networks we maintain via the internet have been increasingly used for online advocacy and activism. However, Smith and colleagues (2019) describe how doubts have been raised about the effectiveness of advocacy campaigns carried out in online forums or organized through social media, referring to them as slacktivism. The term "slacktivism" refers to the "low-cost, low-risk participation in a protest effort" whereby individuals "confine their outrage to the computer screen" (Bastos et al., 2015, p. 322), and "limit their support to online participation." While Smith and colleagues (2019) argue that research is not definitive in terms of social media's influence on the level of participation in a protest movement, they confer that social media magnify social pressure to get involved, leading to onsite participation via factors of empowerment, competence, social stake, and quality of engagement experience. That said, social media use may be less influential in a less volatile climate, and it could be the "red hot climate" (Smith et al., 2019, p. 194) that influenced the outcomes, such as during the Arab Spring uprising and Black Lives Matter movement during the COVID-19 pandemic discussed later in the chapter.

Online advocacy requires both careful organizing and the ability to relinquish power to constituents. Becky Bond and Zach Exley argue that advocacy organizations should have a centralized plan but distribute the work, combining digital campaigning with offline actions (Bond & Exley, 2016; Dennis & Hall, 2020). Vegh (2003) defines three types of Internet mobilization: calling for offline action (e.g., attending a rally), calling for an offline action that may be more effective online (e.g., e-mailing a policymaker), and calling for online action that is only possible online (e.g., campaigns through Facebook messaging and other social media apps).

And let us not take for granted the power of an image or video in increasing the visibility of an issue and encouraging people to act. For instance, Alan Kurdi was the three-year-old boy who fled Syria with his family amid the European refugee crisis and washed up on the shore of the Turkish coast in 2015. His tiny body lying in the water was an image that provided a visual representation of the collective loss of forced migration and moved many around the globe to donate to humanitarian efforts (Henley, 2015). While these often unplanned images can galvanize support for a cause, some organizations are taking a more proactive approach through digital storytelling or by using storybanking, "the systematic and on-going large-scale collection, digital archiving, and cataloging of personal stories for future development and incorporation in advocacy initiatives" (Trevisan et al., 2019, p. 5). Storybanking is a strategic, crowd-sourced practice that allows organizations to determine when these stories are deployed (Trevisan et al., 2019).

The ease of mass action via the internet is seductive. But using the internet to push hundreds of thousands of people into the streets to create change still requires a comprehensive strategy. In fact, most groups are not trying to overthrow a government. Most groups are small, and the metrics of success should correspond to what they are trying to accomplish, be it raising money, drawing awareness to a local issue, or urging local leaders to change a specific policy. Having a comprehensive organizing strategy is essential regardless of scale. While the ouster of Egyptian president Hosni Mubarak was one of the great successes of the Arab Spring, the uprising showed that protesters were collectively against the incumbent regime, but not definitive on how to replace it (Freelon et al., 2016). As Engler and Engler describe in *This Is an Uprising* (2016), "Egypt shows that widespread revolts can do amazing things, but uprising alone is not enough" (p. 253). While the internet can be a highly effective tool to mobilize large groups of people, a nimble and longer-term strategy is required to make lasting change.

Understanding Social Media and Social Movements

Why are social media so useful for community organizing? Beth Kanter and Allison Fine (2010) propose "social media powers social networks for social change" (p. 9). Consistent with the messages of Saul Alinsky (1971) and Paulo Freire (1973), who showed us that activism is most successful when organizers listen to and engage existing communities, social media offer new venues for such engagement. In fact, "social media can provide both a voice and a community to marginalized groups who either cannot or chose not to operate through traditional means" (Smith, 2018). For example, the "It Gets Better" movement provided a platform for individuals and communities to share their LGBTQ stories (Ciszek, 2013). The #MeToo movement raised awareness of the prevalence of sexual violence, providing space to share stories of personal trauma, connect with others, and provide support (Bogen et al., 2019). These examples highlight how marginalized groups used social media to create safe spaces for dialogue, amplify voices, and connect people with essential resources. The most effective internet organizers are using traditional techniques to tap into existing social networks. They are just using a different medium.

The reach of online networks continues to grow and is becoming more diverse. In addition, networks have become uniquely "searchable," which allows us to better target key individuals and rapidly spread ideas and issues through online social networks. With a well-tailored message, organizers are more likely to find the most valuable resource of the internet: attention. "Public attention is a necessary step for achieving social outcomes, for it is through attention that advocacy organizations are able to convince, connect, counteract, recruit, and mobilize" (Guo & Saxton, 2018, p. 8). Community organizing principles, such as listening to and assessing the community (see chapters 10 and 11), developing a long-term action strategy (Alinsky, 1971), "starting where the people are" (Nyswander, 1956), building community capacity and social capital (Chávez et al., 2010), and using social network mapping to assess and promote community identity (Amsden & VanWynsberghe, 2005) still apply in online organizing. The offline tactics of traditional organizing are still the key components of your toolbox; social media are merely a way to enhance, reinforce, and amplify them. Fortunately, social media are more nimble than traditional offline organizing (Guo and Saxton, 2018), so when organized and integrated tactically, the two can be effective at supporting a cause. The rise of Black Lives Matter online and offline offers an example of this complexity as well as the power of creating an online platform for social movement.

The Black Lives Matter Movement

In 2013, Alicia Garza, Patrisse Cullors, and Opal Tometi cofounded Black Lives Matter (BLM) in response to the murder of Trayvon Martin, an unarmed, Black, seventeen-year-old young man in Florida. Garza, building on an established social media presence, introduced "Black Lives Matter" via a Facebook post titled "a love letter to Black people," and Cullors created the hashtag: #BlackLivesMatter (Cobb, 2016). While BLM founders characterize the movement as a departure from "the old guard" in bringing to the foreground the experience of trans Black people and police violence against Black women, the evolution of BLM is also embedded in and is an extension of a long history of organizing to address police violence (Solomon & Rankin, 2019). Freelon and colleagues (2016) highlight how BLM social media expansion and impact followed the Ferguson protests that unfolded in response to the 2014 police shooting of Michael Brown, an unarmed, Black, eighteen-year-old. BLM did not organize the protests per se, nor are Garza, Cullors, and Tometi identified as the key leaders of the movement in Ferguson, but rather the *messaging strategy* of BLM evolved to offer an online platform for a broader offline racial justice movement—one that moved from police brutality as individual incidents to one of systemic racism (Freelon et al., 2016, p. 63).

A unique and tragic convergence of events unfolded creating a moment for BLM, whose leaders and members were prepared to take advantage of social media by using video sharing, harnessing media coverage, and escalating the impact of immense offline protests. On May 25, 2020, witness videos were released across devices and through social media apps throughout the country, showing police officer Derek Chauvin kneeling on George Floyd's neck and killing him. This moment was preceded by several other killings of unarmed Black people, including Breonna

Taylor, fatally shot by police in her home on March 13, 2020. At the same time the COVID-19 pandemic had taken hold of the country. The synergistic effects of BLM protest action shared through social media coupled with BLM pressure offline exposed how the country was fighting not one but two pandemics, one viral and one social. By May 2020, 15 to 26 million people, including younger, wealthier, and first-time protesters, had participated in BLM protests in the United States, making this the "largest movement in the country's history"—most protesters reported that they had *watched a video* of police violence toward protestors or the Black community in the last year (Bucchanana et al., 2020).

BLM's online strategy also includes a member-led network of more than forty BLM chapters across the United States and Canada, with a growing global network and a well-maintained, dynamic website that augments their social media presence. The BLM website showcases an animated slide deck of posts on various apps with different functions that include images, calls to action (including when and where to take the streets), and videos as well as quick links to articles, ways "to follow" the movement, and how to sign up for "special launches, network actions, programs and partnerships," donate to the cause, and access resources, including social media graphics for social media profiles, petitions, and resources for COVID-19, and downloadable reports and toolkits.

Online and social media tools can be used, to varying effect, to accomplish common organizing activities, such as community assessment, community and coalition building, political activism, fundraising, and sustainability. However, you must first create an online strategy that will dictate which tools to use, as well as how and why to use them.

Creating an Online Strategy for Nonprofit Community Organizing

Developing an online strategy is essential to creating an effective online presence that helps further the mission of an organization. Just as nonprofits are guided by strategic plans, online efforts should be guided by a broader strategy. Before launching any online initiative, it is important to know what you want to accomplish and then match the appropriate tools to achieve those goals by creating a strategy (Kanter & Fine, 2010). It should be noted that some online campaigns that go viral are organic campaigns that were not the product of a planned strategy, but rather generated through urgency. In addition, social media can facilitate relationships that have traditionally been face-to-face. But moving from going viral to achieving a long-term impact will require a strategy.

Nonprofits that implement a social media plan can improve their organizational capacity, both at the internal level of increased staff collaboration and at the organizational level raising more funds during their signature fundraising events (Sun et al., 2015). However, barriers to using social media are also linked to components of organizational capacity, including resources, expertise, leadership, and constituency (Sun & Asencio, 2019). Often, organizations or community groups hire a consultant or find a tech-savvy person to design their website or create their Facebook page, expecting dramatic results from a few hours of work. But successfully organizing through internet engagement requires building a dedicated internal team, from the executive director to line staff, that understands the strategy and purpose of the work. The case study of Enterprise for Youth at the end of the chapter will provide an example of how a nonprofit employed an online strategy to support its program goals.

We now walk through the steps to devising your strategy: identifying objectives, assessing your audience and environment, identifying your message in a fluid platform, and evaluating your online activities.

Identifying Objectives

The first step is identifying what you want to accomplish with an internet presence and how it will support a longer-term mission. Do you want to disseminate information about a specific topic? Do you want to draw traffic to your website so followers access your new publications and resources, or to promote an event or protest? Solicit donations? Or lure journalists for media coverage?

Like successful community organizing, internet organizing is not a stand-alone event; activities should build on each other to move toward a larger goal (chapters 12, 24). Raising awareness of an issue should be an overarching goal, but clearly defined objectives will be necessary to get you there. Using George Doran's (1981) SMART (specific, measurable, attainable, relevant, timely) criteria can guide you in developing objectives, but you will need to gather some more contextual information first. For BLM, while the online presence is robust and contributes to awareness, it is the specific actions and objectives of aligned organizations, such as the Black Organizing Project in Oakland, which won the George Floyd Resolution in June 2020 to remove police from the Oakland Unified School District (2020), and chapters of the BLM Global Network that impact social change at the local level.

Assessing Your Audience and Your Environment

Once you choose your objectives, define your audience by identifying the groups that will help you to reach these objectives. Your ultimate targets may be key decision-makers, policymakers, and "influencers" who can help you achieve your larger goal. But there are likely several intermediate layers of target audiences. For example, you may not have direct access to the policymakers you hope to influence. But mobilizing your online supporters may well generate the attention you need to reach policymakers. The people you hope to attract to your event are your immediate communities of focus. As shown in the following list, all your targets should be identified in detail:

- How old are they?
- What do they use the internet for?
- What social media tools are they currently using, and how often do they use them?
- Who are the key decisionmakers you want to influence, and whom do they listen to?

In order to answer many of these questions, you will need to assess your target audience by doing the online equivalent of listening to their conversations. As discussed in chapter 10, core principles of community assessment apply here: you must first listen to the general perceptions and beliefs of your target audience.

Listening to conversations online requires a fair amount of time. For starters, search for keywords on the internet related to your topic of interest, and divert them to a central reading place as they pop up, using feed readers—services that troll the web for keywords and topics you define and aggregate them in one place for you to read. Use these services to answer questions such as the following:

- What is being said about the topic you care about?
- What are other groups doing to make change?
- What are the most up-to-date health or other relevant statistics?
- What seems to be working?
- What are your partners and opponents doing?

To assess your target audience, go to the sites they are using and read what they are reading. Your youth audience may be reading and posting on one or more social media platforms many times a day, whereas your political officeholder targets may be using different platforms to inform their vote on a measure. And if your targets are congregating in certain online locales, what are they talking about in relation to your goals/issues/partners/competitors? What messages are they sharing or reposting?

Primary research can be conducted via surveys, focus groups, or interviews by asking your current supporters how often they engage through social media tools and if they would be willing to engage with your social media tools around specific issues. Sample templates of online surveys can be found online and adapted and sent out through various online survey sites. While you are likely to gather some useful information from primary research, direct observations will tell you the most about what your audience is actually doing. If your targets are congregating in certain online spaces, what are they talking about in relation to your goals, issues, partners, and competitors? What are your opponents saying about you, and what are they specifically saying that causes the most reaction or following? Empathy mapping from the field of design thinking is another way to listen and is a process to synthesize how to align your messaging with the needs of your audience or community of focus based on what users say, think, do, and feel.

Although listening takes time, the payoff can be enormous. Some of the most successful social media awareness campaigns in recent years have started as grassroots movements that nonprofits have successfully co-opted for organizational success (Smith, 2018). One striking example is the Amyotrophic Lateral Sclerosis Association's (ALS Association) use of the Ice Bucket Challenge. This challenge was inspired by three young men living with the disease who created videos of a bucket of ice being dumped over their own or someone else's head. What started with a meme to focus attention on this organization resulted in 17 million people uploading their videos to Facebook, which were watched by over 440 million people, 10 billion times. Within a six-week period, the ALS Association received $115 million from people all over the world (ALS Association, 2016). Constant listening and assessing allowed this group to take early action that resulted in tangible results.

When describing your target audience, be as specific as possible. To avoid a common mistake, remember that "the 'general public' is never a target audience" (Spitfire Strategies, 2011). If you are talking to everyone, you have failed to target anyone.

Framing Your Message in a Fluid Platform

Before you implement your online strategy, you need strong, clear, direct messages that your audience will embrace. This should be part of your existing communications strategy (Dorfman, 2010). Postal mail, flyers or posters, and meeting with influencers in person are still critical parts of your communications strategy that can be supported by, but not replace, your online activities (for more details on framing messages, see chapter 24, on media advocacy). Just as you will focus on different audiences for different goals, you will create tailored messages specific to your audiences. Messages directed toward volunteers may aim to inspire participation in a campaign, whereas messages directed toward policymakers may focus on demanding responsibility and accountability. Similarly, the strategic use of hashtags, a word or phrase preceded by the pound sign (#) used in a social media message, can aid in classifying messages, improving searchability, and allowing the organizations to link messages to existing knowledge and action communities (Saxton et al., 2015). Hashtags can be timely and effective, especially in response to emergencies and crises, as well as quickly getting out a message related to a rally or protest.

In addition, the nature of social media can have an impact on the framing of messages. In an analysis of 66,159 tweets using #BlackLivesMatter in 2014, Ince and colleagues (2017) examine how BLM framing is distributed through a decentralized movement over time from before the murder of Michael Brown to the nonindictment of Darren Wilson. The authors highlight how using social media to advocate for your cause across a wide audience is important because how people and communities interact with social media can impact the evolution and outcomes of the movement. That is, users, which include the general public and not necessarily the leaders of the movement, can generate content and can group and associate ideas, sort and flag content, and make it feasible to search streams of specific topics. "When hashtags are extremely successful, such as #BlackLivesMatter, they can create a community of like-minded people who can sustain a conversation and even mobilize offline" (Ince et al., 2017, p. 1818).

As before, crafting this message requires listening to your audience, knowing where they converse, and seeing what is most likely to elicit a positive response. We know that stakeholders are more likely to be engaged in two-way dialogic communication when stakeholders are involved in discussions that matter to them (Maxwell & Carboni, 2016). That is, the most effective messaging in organizing is driven by values. Therefore, what kinds of messages resonate with your target audience? What messages are most likely to be shared online? What kinds of action steps are people most likely to take part in? What are people most interested in hearing about? What will get communities to engage in offline action or "beyond the hashtag"?

Evaluating Your Impact and Your Strategy

Once you have created your online strategy, it is essential to pick the right metrics to match your strategy so you know if your methods are working. The good news is that most online activity can be measured. You just have to know how to set up your indicators and other measurement tools to enable you to gather the information that you need. You want to know who your audience is, and which individuals are engaged, and how they engage with your online content. The deeper the relationships that you have built with your audience, the more your efforts will pay off.

There are many resources to help you measure your impact. For instance, you can use Google Analytics to measure your reader growth, counting the number of subscribers versus visitors. It will also report to you whether those who accessed your page did so directly from a URL or if they were directed there from certain other sites and which pages they spent the most time on. Other tools can be used to measure your reader engagement, that is, how much readers are interacting with you and your content and sharing the content with others across social media tools. Most social media tools will have built-in metrics. Social media dashboards can be used to update, monitor, manage, and maintain several communication outlets at once.

But there is a difference between measuring your social media activity and measuring the actual impact on your issue. For instance, online engagement around a specific event may drive participants to show up at an event. However, the number of people who sign petitions at the event does not necessarily correlate well with the online engagement that drove the participants to the event.

To gauge the effectiveness of your social media activity in promoting offline action, consider polling your donors, event attendees, and volunteers about how they heard about your organization or cause. Did they hear about you through a friend? And if so, did this friend tell them in person or via an online platform or forwarded email? There are numerous easy-to-use online survey tools that provide a free or low-cost method of tracking such information. In addition to metrics and data collection, policy change and cultural shifts as a result of combined social media and offline efforts provide tangible evidence of impact. The nonprofit, Enterprise for Youth, discussed in the case study that follows, has closely integrated their online strategy with their programming, so the impact assessment process for program uptake and completion is a reflection of and accounts for this integrated relationship.

The impacts of BLM protests and organizing have resulted in concrete social actions related to police reform, health care (e.g., White Coats for Black Lives), curricular reform in higher education, as well as cultural shifts in industry, such as professional sports. Across the country there are growing pledges to reform policing and policy initiatives to redirect funding to community services in cities such as Minneapolis, New York, Los Angeles, and San Francisco. Though promising and overdue, as The Marshall Project highlights, these actions will require careful planning with various stakeholders, with attention to the unintended outcomes of past efforts (Weichselbaum & Lewis, 2020). Forging a national agenda and composed of organizations and individuals committed to a shared vision, the Movement for Black Lives (M4BL) through their Electoral Justice Project, has organized to get the Breath Act, which proposes divestment of federal resources from criminal justice and investment in noncarceral approaches to community safety, to the congressional floor (Chisholm, 2020). The thread of social media presence, the linking of BLM as the emblem of the mass demand for change, and subsequent actions in the name of BLM create a flexible and powerful organizing strategy.

If you have answered most of the questions in the preceding sections and have a clear, specific picture of whom to talk to, why you are talking to them, and how to talk to them, then you are well on your way to a successful online strategy. For a more detailed step-by-step walk-through, you may want to find interactive worksheets for creating an online communications strategy.

Engaging Your Audience Using Social Media and Addressing Performative Allies

Just as community organizing theories inform your online strategy, engaging your audience through social media requires etiquette. Part of building your network involves recognizing and rewarding people for passing your message on to their networks. This can take the form of sharing their links on your sites, or mentioning their event or cause in a blog. Reciprocal online support is an investment in relationships that may someday be fruitful.

As in offline conversations, most social media posts are continuous streams. You must seek opportunities to share expertise on topics where your organization is focused. Such posts help you direct the conversation, attract new supports, and provide information and details for offline actions. Attention to how quickly a social media post can take hold and travel is vital to careful online organizing efforts. One example of social media posting that had conflicting and even opposing effects for the BLM movement was the #blackouttuesday that captioned Instagram posts of black screens or black tiles. While the initial goal of this social media action was to encourage major music brands and industries to pause and consider the contributions Black people have made in these spaces as well as to prompt White and non-Black people to take action in sharing resources and links to organizations supporting the movement, thousands of people posted only black tiles. Whereas action-based posts became buried in a stream of silence, #blackoutuesday required activists to clear up misconceptions (Attiah, 2020). This is also a case of "performative allyship," which falls into the category of slacktivism discussed earlier in this chapter, and involves creating a social media presence to align with a cause without taking the steps to actively engage in social change.

Remember that your online strategy should not be composed purely of social media tools. There is a role for every platform you use that will connect to your greater strategy. Websites, e-mail lists, and searchable online databases are components of your online strategy that are just as important as your social media tools. This is especially true as many individuals and organizations tether their social media accounts and websites to freely circulate content between them, further enabling amplification of information on each platform (Freelon et al., 2016).

While there are many free and low-cost tools available on the internet to help you get out your message or to help viewers to take an action, all tools are not created equal—they meet different needs and require different amounts of staff time and financial resources. Social media may be inexpensive, but their effective use requires time and dedication.

Case Study: Enterprise for Youth

In 1969 Gladys Thatcher, a counselor by training and critical of adult authoritarianism, sat with young people in her San Francisco living room, listening intently to their career aspirations and matching them with jobs listed on index cards. This was the beginning of Enterprise for Youth, which by 2020 had served over 25,000 under-resourced young people. Governor Newsom of California recognized Enterprise as the first nonprofit to focus on the importance of job experience for emerging adults. Currently, Enterprise serves 500 young people a year through job readiness training; paid internships in fields such as health care, art and design, and city government; the Youth Council leadership program; and access to a job bank that matches young people with employers. To amplify youth voice, forge connections with job and internship hosts, and build their brand, it became apparent that a robust online strategy would be necessary. Over the course of three years, the CEO worked to make this a priority.

With buy-in from the staff at all levels, Enterprise began mapping an online strategy. To support this significant shift, it was key to secure and allocate resources to create a communications director position to develop and maintain the online strategy. Enterprise felt it was essential for the communications director to be integrated within the organization's programming and so the position joined regular program meetings, including one-on-ones with the senior program director. Ensuring strong connections between programming and communications allowed for an integrated approach to generating content for online messaging aligned with program impact goals. For example, Youth Council members collaborated with communications to generate video stories on what it meant for them to be in the Council, which were then shared via social media. When youth take over social media in this way, Enterprise sees increased participation in their programming.

Overseeing Enterprise's communication strategy, the communications director curates social media content, maintains the organization's website, and leads efforts to develop and evaluate long- and short-term goals for their online strategy. A key part of an online strategy is to identify your audience in order to decide what social media apps to employ. For Enterprise, their key audiences include current and prospective youth participants, internship hosts and career mentors, as well as donors. Enterprise employs four social media apps with different purposes based on the audience they want to reach and the type of information they want to share. LinkedIn, Twitter, and Facebook are used to share or link to longer forms of communication, such as Enterprises's program blog with features about the impact outcomes of internships as well as articles about issues such as income inequality that demonstrate the urgency of Enterprise's mission. Through Facebook, they also aim to generate an interactive experience and create a sense of community. For Instagram, the purpose is to share motivating content and celebrate youth, events, or partners, further creating awareness around their brand and amplifying youth voice through inspiring quotes from youth reflection essays that showcase the impact of their programming. A final aspect of their online strategy is to leverage social media to connect young people to opportunities and build networks. One way this is done is through Medium, an online publishing tool. Youth participants learn to become published thought leaders, have content to enhance their LinkedIn profiles, and make their voices heard.

Enterprise uses different tools to measure the impact of their online and program efforts. While it is possible to download user data, for now they direct their audiences, such as volunteers, youth, and donors, through their website and social media to forms they complete that then feed into Salesforce, a customer relationship management platform. They also use business plan software, Upmetrics, to assess program impact. When there were challenges due to COVID-19, the team focused on expanding their reach through social media and ways to deliver programming online. Trends in program participation during the pandemic indicated that Enterprise was well positioned to pivot and successfully engage remotely with youth participants. These successes did not come easily. The communications director maintained that for a small- to midsized nonprofit, one of the biggest challenges is time given the demands of careful social media management, though knowing a few tips can help. In addition to becoming familiar with basic design principles, it is essential to know where your audience engages in the social media landscape and focus on those channels, and to be clear about what makes your organization unique as part of your messaging. For Enterprise, a key message is that youth are powerful, and as the founder often states, "the promise of youth is our best and only incubator for our community's future and well-being of our imperiled planet."

Challenges with Online Organizing

The Digital Divide

As we have emphasized, social media and the internet are tools for organizing. The online strategy that guides your online activities should be informed by your comprehensive, and mostly offline, organizing plan that builds on the tenets of community organizing. Some of the communities we hope to reach may not be using the internet at all, or they may not have regular access to the internet. The "digital divide" is the gap between or uneven distribution of digital technology and internet access among communities and is created by factors such as generational gaps, literacy, geographic location, mental and physical disabilities, and traditional socioeconomic barriers that marginalized communities face (Herbert, 2005; Jansen, 2010). The requirement for remote learning and access to services, including health care, during COVID-19, put a spotlight on the digital divide. With the vast majority of K–12 schools closed and offering only remote instruction, a Pew Research report in 2020 found that 43 percent of lower-income families compared to 10 percent of upper-income families reported their children having to do homework on cell phones, 40 percent compared to 6 percent reported having to rely on public Wi-Fi due to internet instability, and 36 percent compared to 4 percent reported their children would not be able to complete homework due to no access to a computer at home (Vogels et al., 2020). Although school districts across the country set up systems to loan computers to students and families to support distance learning, this was not a long-term solution to address the divide. Jonathan Nez (2020), president of Navajo Nation, with COVID-19 disproportionately impacting Indigenous communities, addressed Congress in July 2020, stating that 60 percent of Navajo Nation residents do not have fixed internet or broadband access, with implications for telehealth, remote work and education, job opportunities, and skills training. An online organizing strategy requires how you will reach members of a community who may be offline, not by choice, but by the very inequities you may be trying to dismantle.

Trauma

On May 28, 2020, three days after George Floyd's death, Shenequa Golding wrote in Medium, "I just witnessed the lynching of a Black man, but don't worry Ted, I'll have those deliverables to you end of day" to characterize the experience of Black people maintaining professionalism "in the age of Black death." Dr. Janet Helms of the Institute for the Study of Race and Culture at Boston College described how the trauma from repeatedly watching the video of the killing of George Floyd contributes to the cumulative effects of racism and racial trauma (McLaughlin, 2020). While a video or image shared through social media can spark social action, we must also be mindful of how these videos or images fall on communities and how they might encapsulate a history of oppression, including state-sanctioned violence and other traumatic experiences, and what this means for how we incorporate healing, cultural humility, and steps to address fatigue in our comprehensive on- and offline community organizing and building strategy.

Digital Security

Activists must be aware of the surveillance and other risks posed by opponent groups and government authorities. It is becoming increasingly common to harass and wage online campaigns against activists, including publicly sharing the names, addresses, and photos of activists online in an attempt to create harassment campaigns, a practice known as doxing. Activists should understand their digital footprint and control what information is publicly available and do their best to scrub personal data from the internet.

Activists should take steps to protect the privacy of others participating in protests. Organizers such as the nonprofit Social Media Technologies have trained activists to use encrypted and anonymous platforms to communicate; livestream protests without law enforcement being able to track you; share photos that do not reveal personal features of others such as their faces or other physical features; secure a phone to deter tracking; and use privacy settings to reduce your social media footprint.

Groups must also be cautious about sharing false or misleading information. Unfortunately, social media rewards posts that stoke outrage and emotion. But that creates an incentive for individuals and groups to share potentially inflammatory material of dubious accuracy. Activists can undermine their long-term credibility if they fall victim to this trap. Misinformation experts have published guides to "think before you share" on social media, including checking the accuracy of content spreading online before engaging with it yourself.

Social Media Regulation

Organizers must be mindful of a shifting regulatory landscape related to digital technology. For instance, data-protection laws in the European Union and California set rules about how organizations can collect and share information about individuals. This could affect fundraising and other organizing efforts.

Additionally, activists should be cautious about relying too heavily on any one social media tool and remain open to experimentation on emerging platforms. As social media companies grow in power and influence, they will come under more political pressure for their business practices. This could result in people who activists are trying to reach using a service less. For example, a boycott of Facebook over a particular policy could limit an organization's ability to communicate effectively on the platform (Isaac & Hsu, 2020).

Conclusion

This chapter introduces a framework through which social movements and non-profit organizations can benefit from wielding the power of the internet by engaging the public and work partners. But while using the internet can be essential to furthering your cause, remember to stick to your community organizing principles. Your online efforts are not effective without your offline efforts, where in-person communications and engagement with your target audience are essential to moving toward your mission and meeting your objectives.

Just as your community organizing activities may change, so will the online tools that are available. New social media tools are introduced every day, and remaining static in your online strategy and implementation will only result in static support and results. Just as you need to remain agile in responding to opponents and the changing political landscape, it is essential to be flexible in consistently evaluating and adapting your online strategy to best meet the needs of your supporters and your mission. Since the last edition of this book was published in 2012, there have been countless examples of how online organizing has been an effective tool in influencing political and social change, connecting people to essential resources, and furthering the mission and reach of nonprofits around the globe. With ever-evolving opportunities for our online capacity to support community organizing and mobilizing, how will you harness these tools to fuel social change and sustainable impact in your communities?

Disclaimer: The internet is in constant evolution. By the time this book is in print, there will undoubtedly be new developments that affect how community organizing is supported by the internet, from new tools and new mechanisms to how new and existing tools are used. Therefore, this chapter intentionally avoids acting as a guide for which online organizing tools to use and how best to use them. Instead we highlight the importance of creating a flexible and evolving online strategy based on organizing principles and goals and available human, financial, and technological resources.

Questions for Further Discussion

1. As part of assessing the impact of your online organizing strategy, how will you monitor and communicate to stakeholders about potential unintended consequences of social media use related to privacy?
2. How can you ensure a sustainable and flexible online organizing strategy? Who is responsible for leading your efforts and what system is in place if, for instance, the communications director or team vacates their role(s)?

Acknowledgments

We are extremely grateful to Adam Satariano, AJ Titong, Bonnie Kwan, and Akiba Solomon for lending their expertise to this chapter and providing guidance on assessing online strategies for nonprofits and social movements. We want to express our utmost gratitude to Nínive Calegari, Rizal Adanza, and Carlo Solis of Enterprise for Youth, for sharing their online strategy and for their amazing work with young people in San Francisco.

REFERENCES

Alinsky, S. D. (1971). *Rules for Radicals: A Practical Primer for Realistic Radicals.* Random House.

The ALS Association. (2016). *2015 Annual Report: The Ice Bucket Miracle.* http://www.alsa.org/assets/pdfs/040516-annual-report-online.pdf.

Amsden, J., & VanWynsberghe, R. (2005). Community mapping as a research tool with youth. *Action Res, 3*(4), 357–381.

Attiah, K. (2020, June 3). #BlackOutTuesday was a case study in how performative solidarity goes awry. *Washington Post.* https://www.washingtonpost.com/opinions/blackouttuesday-was-a-case-study-in-how-performative-solidarity-goes-awry/2020/06/03/0b9c42b8-a5e4-11ea-b473-04905b1af82b_story.html.

Barker, M., Barker, D. I., Bormann, N. F., & Neher, K. E. (2013). *Social Media Marketing: A Strategic Approach.* South-Western Cengage Learning.

Barns, N. G., & Andonian, J. (2011). The 2011 Fortune 500 and social media adoption: Have America's largest companies reached a social media plateau? Center for Marketing Research, University of Massachusetts, Dartmouth. https://fayebsg.com/wp-content/uploads/2011/11/The-2011-Fortune-500-and-Social-Media-Adoption-Have-Americas-Largest-Companies-Reached-a-Social-Media-Plateau.pdf.

Bastos, M. T., Mercea, D., & Charpentier, A. (2015). Tents, tweets, and events: The interplay between ongoing protests and social media. *J Commun, 65,* 320–350.

Bogen, K. W., Bleiweiss, K. K., Leach, N. R., & Orchowski, L. M. (2019, May 22). #MeToo: Disclosure and response to sexual victimization on Twitter. *J Interpers Violence.* https://doi.org/10.1177/0886260519851211.

Bond, B., & Exley, Z. (2016). *Rules for Revolutionaries: How Big Organizing Can Change Everything.* Chelsea Green Publishing.

Bortree, D., & Seltzer, T. (2009). Dialogic strategies and outcomes: An analysis of environmental advocacy groups' Facebook profiles. *Public Relat Rev, 35,* 317–319.

Briones, R. L., Kuch, B., Fisher, L., & Jin, Y. (2011). Keeping up with the digital age: How the American Red Cross uses social media to build relationships. *Public Relat Rev, 37,* 37–43.

Bucchanana, L., Bui, Q., & Patel, J. K. (2020, July 3). Black Lives Matter may be the largest movement in history. *New York Times.* https://www.nytimes.com/interactive/2020/07/03/us/george-floyd-protests-crowd-size.html.

Chávez, V., Minkler, M., Wallerstein, N., & Spencer, M. (2010). Community organizing for health and social justice. In V. Chávez, L. Cohen, & S. Chehimi (Eds.), *Prevention Is Primary: Strategies for Community Well-Being* (2nd ed., pp. 87–112). Jossey-Bass.

Chisholm, N. J. (2020, July 7). The movement for Black lives introduces the Breath Act. *Colorlines.* https://www.colorlines.com/articles/movement-black-lives-introduces-breathe-act.

Ciszek, E. (2013). Advocacy and amplification: Nonprofit outreach and empowerment through participatory media. *Public Relat J, 7*(2), 187–213.

Cobb, J. (2016, March 7). The matter of Black lives. *The New Yorker*. https://www.newyorker.com /magazine/2016/03/14/where-is-black-lives-matter-headed.

Dennis, J., & Hall, N. (2020). Innovation and adaptation in advocacy organizations throughout the digital eras. *J Inf Technol Politics, 17*(2), 79–86.

Doran, G. T. (1981). There's a S.M.A.R.T. way to write management's goals and objectives. *Manage Rev, 70*(11), 35–36.

Dorfman, L. (2010). Using media advocacy to influence policy. In V. Chávez, L. Cohen, & S. Chehimi (Eds.), *Prevention Is Primary: Strategies for Community Well-Being* (2nd ed., pp. 157–180). Jossey-Bass.

Engler, M., & Engler, P. (2016). *This Is an Uprising: How Nonviolent Revolt Is Shaping the Twenty-First Century*. Bold Type Books.

Freelon, D., McIlwain, C. D., & Clark, M. D. (2016). *Beyond the Hashtags*. Technical Report. Washington, DC: Center for Media and Social Impact, School of Communication, American University. https://cmsimpact.org/resource/beyond-hashtags-ferguson-blacklivesmatter -online-struggle-offline-justice/.

Freire, P. (1973). *Education for Critical Consciousness*. Seabury Press.

GlobalWebIndex. (2019). *Flagship Report 2019*. https://www.globalwebindex.com/hubfs/Downloads /2019%20Q1%20Social%20Flagship%20Report.pdf.

Golding, S. (2020, May 29). Maintaining professionalism in the age of Black death is . . . a lot. *Medium*. https://medium.com/@shenequagolding/maintaining-professionalism-in-the-age -of-black-death-is-a-lot-5eaec5e17585.

Greenberg, J., & MacAulay, M. (2009). NPO 2.0? Exploring the web presence of environmental nonprofit organizations in Canada. *Glob Media J Can Ed, 2*(1), 63–88.

Guo, C., & Saxton, G. (2014). Tweeting social change: How social media are changing nonprofit advocacy. *Nonprofit Volunt Sect Q, 43*(1), 57–79.

Guo, C., & Saxton, G. D. (2018). Speaking and being heard: How nonprofit advocacy organizations gain attention on social media. *Nonprofit Volunt Sect Q, 47*(1), 5–26.

Henley, J. (2015, September 3). Britons rally to help people fleeing war and terror in Middle East. *The Guardian*. https://www.theguardian.com/uk-news/2015/sep/03/britons-rally-to -help-people-fleeing-war-and-terror-in-middle-east.

Herbert, S. (2005). Harnessing the power of the internet for advocacy and organizing. In M. Minkler (Ed.), *Community Organizing and Community Building for Health and Welfare* (3rd ed., pp. 331–345). Rutgers University Press.

Ince, J., Rojas, F., & Davis, C. A. (2017). The social media response to Black Lives Matter: How Twitter users interact with Black Lives Matter through hashtag use. *Ethn Racial Stud, 40*, 1814–1830.

International Telecommunication Union (ITU). (2020). Statistics. https://www.itu.int/en/ITU -D/Statistics/Pages/stat/default.aspx.

Isaac, M., & Hsu, T. (2020, July 7). Facebook fails to appease organizers of ad boycott. *New York Times*. https://www.nytimes.com/2020/07/07/technology/facebook-ad-boycott-civil-rights .html.

Jansen, J. (2010). *Use of the Internet in Higher-Income Households*. Pew Internet and American Life Project.

Kanter, B., & Fine, A. (2010). *The Networked Nonprofit: Connecting with Social Media to Drive Change*. Jossey-Bass.

Kaplan, A. M., & Haenlein, M. (2010). Users of the world, unite! The challenges and opportunities of social media. *Bus Horiz, 53*(1), 59–68.

Lovejoy, K., & Saxton, G. D. (2012). Information, community, and action: How nonprofit organizations use social media. *J Comput Mediat Commun, 17*(3), 337–353.

Maxwell, S. P., & Carboni, J. (2016). Social media management: Exploring Facebook engagement among high-asset foundations. *Nonprofit Manag Leadersh, 27*(2), 251–260.

McLaughlin, E. C. (2020, August). How George Floyd's death ignites a racial reckoning that shows no signs of slowing down. CNN. https://edition.cnn.com/2020/08/09/us/george -floyd-protests-different-why/index.html.

Nez, J. (2020, July 8). Addressing the urgent needs of our tribal communities. Testimony of Jonathan Nez. 116th Congress, U.S. House of Representatives. https://docs.house.gov /meetings/IF/IF00/20200708/110874/HHRG-116-IF00-Wstate-NezJ-20200708.pdf.

Nyswander, D. (1956). Education for health: Some principles and their application. *California Health, 14*, 65–70.

Oakland Unified School District. (2020, June 24). Resolution No. 1920-0260: George Floyd Resolution to Eliminate the Oakland Schools Police Department. https://ousd.legistar.com /LegislationDetail.aspx?ID=4564122&GUID=C591BB69-6054-4DCC-8548-69AA1623E643 &Options=&Search=.

Rahman-Jones, I. (2018, March 19). Florida shooting: How teenagers started a political campaign in 30 days. BBC News. https://www.bbc.co.uk/news/newsbeat-43392821.

Rainie, L., & Smith, A. (2008*). The Internet and the 2008 Election.* Pew Internet and American Life Project.

Saxton, G. D., Niyirora, J. N., Guo, C., & Waters, R. D. (2015). #AdvocatingForChange: The strategic use of hashtags in social media advocacy. *Adv Soc Work, 16*(1), 154–169.

Smith, B. G., Krishna, A., & Al-Sinan, R. (2019). Beyond Slacktivism: Examining the entanglement between social media engagement, empowerment, and participation in activism. *Int J Strateg Commun, 13*(3), 182–196.

Smith, J. N. (2018). The social network? Nonprofit constituent engagement through social media. *J Nonprofit Public Sect Mark, 30*(3), 294–316.

Solomon, A., & Rankin, K. (2019). *How We Fight White Supremacy: A Field Guide to Black Resistance.* Bold Type Books.

Spitfire Strategies. (2011). Smart Chart 3.0: An interactive tool to help nonprofits make smart communications choices. http://smartchart.org.

Sun, R., & Asencio, H. D. (2019). Using social media to increase nonprofit organizational capacity. *Int J Public Admin, 42*(5), 392–404.

Sun, R., Asencio, H., & Reid, J. (2015). Enhancing organizational capacity through the use of social media. In H. Ascencio & R. Sun (Eds.), *Cases on Strategic Social Media Utilization in the Nonprofit Sector* (pp. 262–300). IGI Global.

Trevisan, F., Vromen, A., Bello, B., & Vaughan, M. (2019). Mobilizing personal narratives: The rise of digital "story banking" in U.S. grassroots advocacy. *J Inf Technol Politics, 2*, 146–160.

Turner, R. (2002). Public policy, technology, and the nonprofit sector: Notes from the field. In S. Hick & J. McNutt (Eds.), *Activism, Advocacy, and the Internet* (pp. 43–57). Lyceum.

van Dijck, J., Poell, T., & de Waal, M. (2018). *The Platform Society: Public Values in a Connective World.* Oxford University Press.

Vegh, S. (2003). Classifying forms of online activism: The case of cyberprotests against the World Bank. In M. McCaughey & M. Ayers (Eds.), *Cyberactivism: Online Activism in Theory and Practice* (pp. 71–95). Routledge.

Vogels, E. A., Perrin, A., Rainie, L., & Anderson, M. (2020, April 30). 53% of Americans say the internet has been essential during the COVID-19 outbreak. Pew Research Center. https:// www.pewresearch.org/internet/2020/04/30/53-of-americans-say-the-internet-has-been -essential-during-the-covid-19-outbreak/.

Weichselbaum, S., & Lewis, N. (2020, June 9). Support for defunding the police department is growing. Here's why it's not a silver bullet. The Marshall Project. https://www.the marshallproject.org/2020/06/09/support-for-defunding-the-police-department-is -growing-here-s-why-it-s-not-a-silver-bullet.

17

Using the Arts in Community Organizing and Community Building

An Overview and Case Studies

CARICIA CATALANI
ANNE BLUETHENTHAL
DIERDRE VISSER
MARÍA ELENA TORRE
MEREDITH MINKLER

The arts, from literature to music, dance to painting, photography to textile work and sculpture, are powerful tools for community organizing and community building in health and related areas (Chin, 2017; McDonald et al., 1998; Romig, 2018; Sonke et al., 2019). They can draw attention to an issue, offer catharsis for a community after a crisis, unite communities to create art, communicate across cultural and language barriers, and in the process, promote health and well-being.

In this chapter, we illustrate how the arts have served as vehicles for change, highlight their legacy in social movements nationally and globally, and discuss and illustrate the theoretical basis of their use in community organizing and community building for health.

The Arts as a Vehicle for Community Organizing

The power of art for community building and organizing lies in its ability to communicate a message and elicit an emotional response, as well as in the process of creation itself. The arts and literature have always played a role in community organizing and social change. Poet and activist Audre Lorde (1984) expressed this view in her classic essay on the importance of poetry in people's lives, especially the lives of women: "For women . . . poetry is not a luxury. It is a vital necessity of our existence. It forms the quality of the light within which we predicate our hopes and dreams toward survival and change, first made into language, then into idea, then into more tangible action" (p. 37). Her view has been shared by many artists, educators, and advocates throughout history and across the globe. Black jazz singer

Billie Holiday insisted on singing a song about lynchings in the South to the shock (and often anger) of audiences. Chinese American architect, Maya Lin, designed the Vietnam War Memorial—a stark wall etched with approximately 58,000 names of the nation's war dead—to be a place for grieving and remembrance, as well as national healing after a war that had bitterly divided the country (www.thewall-usa .com). More recently, artists have shown their support for the Black Lives Matter (BLM) protests in murals and street art at the BLM Plaza in Washington, DC, and across the nation. Through boldly colored paintings and photographs, music, poems, and other art forms, they have memorialized the lives of George Floyd, Breonna Taylor, and other Black people lost to police violence and created new opportunities for communities to come together in the call for racial justice (Samayeen et al., 2020).

Legacy of the Arts in Social Movements in the United States and Beyond

The arts have played an important role in social movements in the United States and globally (Dunaway & Beer, 2010). Woody Guthrie's tributes to working people in songs like "This Land Is Your Land" in the 1940s and his harsh spotlight on injustice ("Deportees") won him a lasting place in U.S. culture (McDonald et al., 1998; Seely, 2020). And through his enduring performances renouncing racial hatred and oppression in the 1950s, Black actor and singer Paul Robeson helped set the stage for the civil rights movement. As McDonald and her colleagues note, "The forceful refrain of the gospel-turned-civil-rights song 'We Shall Overcome' became an anthem of the fight against segregation and for civil rights and later was embraced by the labor, peace, and women's movements" (p. 267). As Dunaway and Beer (2010), point out, however, it was not just individual singers and actors who made their voices for change heard, but folk music revivals that began in the late 1800s. They highlight in particular the work of Alan Lomax and Pete Seeger in the 1940s, who would together "help make folk respectable and fun," but more important, "to sing their way to action, to build labor unions, to remind people the world over that they were brothers and sisters" (p. 2).

In Nicaragua, the victory over dictator Anastasio Somoza in 1979 helped put into place new and popular forms of expression, from a grassroots literacy campaign to a new song movement and the flourishing of murals and poetry workshops (Randall, 1991). It is further telling that when the revolutionary Sandinista government was overthrown in 1990, one of the first orders of business of the capital city's conservative new mayor was to paint over some of Managua's most impressive pro-Sandinista murals (McDonald et al., 1998). More recently, both traditional art forms and new technology have facilitated artistic expression and citizen media in the Middle East, Africa, and Asia. In addition to videos and photographs recorded on protesters' mobile phones and shared through sites like YouTube, TikTok, and Facebook, for example, the proliferation of protest art in Hong Kong spoke volumes as well (https:// www.nytimes.com/2019/10/11/world/asia/hong-kong-protest-art). These same images are shared across public places, from subway stations to Facebook pages to TikTok, allowing an inside look at artistic renderings of repression that is usually largely closed off to the outside world (Herrman, 2020; Preston & Stelter, 2011).

Conceptual Bases for Using the Arts in Community Organizing for Health

To be effective, community organizing for health and social equity needs to begin with a people's reality. Central to that reality is culture, including people's collective past and hopes for the future. As Brazilian adult educator and passionate scholar/activist Paulo Freire put it, "How is it possible for us to work in a community without feeling the spirit of the culture that has been there for many years, without trying to understand the soul of the culture?" (Horton & Freire, 1990, p. 131).

The international women's movement has long demonstrated, through a wide array of literary and other art forms, the indispensable role of culture in the development of consciousness and identity (hooks, 1994; Lykes & Hershberg, 2012; McDonald et al., 1998; Ohmer, 2019). In particular, the concept of the development of *the voice* has been advanced as a key element in the process of transforming women's lives (Ohmer, 2019; Randall, 1991).

The critical role of voice is also integral to theories of individual and community empowerment, which form an important part of the theoretical base of both health promotion and community building and organizing. As described by Wallerstein (1992; chapter 3) empowerment is a social action process through which individuals and communities gain mastery over their lives *in the context of changing their social and political environments* to improve equity and quality of life.

The empowering potential of the arts and literature, in part, through use of the voice to articulate dreams and shared concerns as the basis of reflection, dialogue, and *praxis*, or action based on critical reflection (Freire, 1973), has been well documented (Romig, 2018; Sonke et al., 2019). Of note in its contributions to both theory and practice is the concept of photovoice, developed in the mid-1990s and subsequently used in many parts of the world to help people visually capture their concerns and dreams, engage in critical dialogue, and use their photographs and deeper reflections as a basis for action to promote change (Catalani & Minkler, 2010; Greene et al., 2018; Wang & Burris, 1997; Wang & Pies, 2004; box 17.1).

Whether in the virtual or physical world, the arts also promote health through the development and expansion of social support. With the exception of more collaborative arts, such as film, music, and theater, the arts are often solitary activities in the creation stage. However, the act of sharing the arts through community events, online social-networking and media-sharing sites, or person-to-person exchanges can be profoundly social and collective. By creating common reference points through culture, communities begin to break down isolation, share common experiences, and build collective vision. Early in the COVID-19 pandemic, famed cellist Yo-Yo Ma created what quickly grew into a global phenomenon when he posted to social media videos of himself performing songs like Antonín Dvořák's "Going Home," using the hashtag #SongsOfComfort, and then calling on other musicians around the world to do the same. Available on diverse social media platforms, #SongsOfComfort was a powerful source of hope, social support, and yes, comfort, reminding millions of people who were socially isolating in their homes that they were part of a much larger community.

The Arts in Urban Life

The arts play an important role in urban community building and organizing for health and well-being. In urban areas, the physical environment—with its sidewalks, buildings, subways, and parks—provides public opportunities for expression. Additionally, the population density of cities brings people into frequent contact, creating endless opportunities for shared experiences. Urban spaces give rise to diverse art forms from diverse voices, including murals, guerrilla theater, poetry slams, dance brigades, hip-hop music, storytelling, graffiti, and drama (Chávez et al., 2004; Taylor & Wei, 2020; Wang, 2010). These forms of diverse public expression can break down barriers and weave unity among the community's different threads.

The Arts in the Practice of Community Organizing for Health

Health education leader Dorothy Nyswander's (1956) admonition to "start where the people are" suggests that organizers, as part of their work, need to familiarize themselves with a people's cultural expressions. In the community, the arts can promote organizing for health in multiple ways, often simultaneously:

1. *To get people involved.* The use of art forms and activities involves people who might otherwise be disinterested or intimidated by more explicitly health-oriented or community-organizing activities. Simply put, the arts make getting involved fun. For example, rap and dance contests have been used to involve both LGBTQ and straight youth in building awareness of the prevention, early-stage diagnosis, and treatment of HIV/AIDS and sexually transmitted diseases (Mathews et al., 2020).

2. *To find out about a community.* The arts can be a valuable strategy as part of community assessments (chapter 10). In her role as director of Family, Maternal, and Child Health Programs at a large local department, Dr. Cheri Pies supplemented the state's mandated MCH "needs assessment" with a photovoice project (see box 17.1), through which sixty residents aged 13–50 were given disposable cameras and asked to take pictures reflecting *their* understandings of the key MCH strengths and challenges of their neighborhoods. Participants then shared one of two of their favorite pictures in smaller groups using critical questions to dig deeper into the images they captured, followed by group discussion (Wang & Pies, 2004).

BOX 17.1

The Photovoice Method

Of the many new community arts methodologies introduced in recent decades, few have been more widely used—or resonated more deeply—with health promotion practitioners engaged in community building, assessment, and organizing than photovoice. Developed by Caroline C. Wang and Mary Ann Burris, photovoice was described in their seminal paper (1997) as having three goals: "(1) to enable people to record and reflect their community's strengths and concerns, (2) to promote critical dialogue and knowledge about important issues through large and small group discussion of photographs, and (3) to reach policymakers" (p. 369). Rural women in Yunnan, China, joined by a broad coalition of policymakers, technical consultants, donors, and public health researchers and advocates, first used the photovoice method in the Chinese countryside, and its powerful impact was captured in a book that was widely shared the world over (Wang et al., 1995; figure 17.1).

The approach involves providing people with cameras (or having participants use their cell phones) and asking them to photograph their everyday reality or an issue of shared concern, typically including pictures of both assets and problems or challenges. They often use as an aid the mnemonic SHOWeD (Shaffer, 1984): *What do you See here? What's really Happening? How does this relate to Our lives? Why does this problem, concern, or strength Exist? What can we Do about it?* Participants then engage in critical reflective dialogue about the pictures and their context.

In the twenty-five years since its inception, photovoice has been widely used around the world to study and address a diversity of public health and social justice concerns, and it has proved particularly useful in helping oppressed or exploited groups share the nuances of their lived experience. The process itself may promote healing, while also shining a spotlight on—and ideally helping to change—some of the policies and underlying conditions that contribute to poor health and well-being in the first place. The exact number of photovoice projects is difficult to gauge, but a recent Google Scholar search identified roughly 16,500 reports published between 2004 and 2020 that had photovoice in the title. Several reviews of the photovoice literature (Catalani & Minkler, 2010; Derr & Simons, 2020; Suprapto et al., 2020; Teti et al., 2018) have found that photovoice projects frequently contribute to several outcomes associated with policy change, including enhanced community involvement in action and advocacy, enriched public health research, and individual empowerment, as well as sometimes being directly cited by policymakers as a catalyst spurring them to action.

In stark contrast to the issues that arise in a typical MCH needs assessment (e.g., low birth weight babies and teen pregnancy prevention) the two major themes generated through photovoice were the need for "safe recreation for children" and improvement in the broader community environment in their neighborhoods (Wang & Pies, 2004, p. 98). One resident's picture of a sign in front of the community's only park that read, "Danger—Enter at your own risk" was indeed so powerful that members of the city council quickly worked to have the park refurbished and made safe for reopening. As Drs. Wang and Pies note,

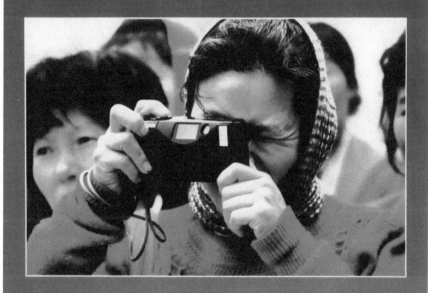

中 国 云 南 农 村
妇 女 自 我 写 真 集

Visual Voices
100 Photographs of Village China by the Women of Yunnan Province

FIGURE 17.1 Photograph of a Woman from Yunnan, China.

Source: The cover of the book *Visual Voices: 100 Photographs of Village China by the Women of Yunnan Province* (1995), with permission of C. C. Wang, photographer and lead author.

this project was a dramatic reminder of how much communities know and can show and tell "the experts" about what matters, when given the opportunity.

3. *To increase awareness and relay health education messages.* The arts are powerful messengers. Visual and oral representations are easy to grasp, regardless of literacy level, and health promotion messages can be developed and spread

throughout popular culture. In Spanish-speaking communities throughout the Americas during the HIV/AIDS epidemic, the song "Ponte el Sombrero" (put on your hat) was sung as a playful, nonthreatening way to encourage condom use (McDonald et al., 1998). Similarly, during the Ebola outbreak in West Africa in 2014, a popular rap group performed live and on a widely heard radio station to dispel rumors, encourage safety precautions, and bring hope (Marais et al., 2016). Bringing health messages through already established mediums of popular culture, such as movies and television (sometimes referred to as "edutainment" or "enter-education" (Wang & Singhal, 2016; Zeedyk & Wallace, 2003), have sometimes been successful in sparking conversations and action through their portrayals of community struggles with substance abuse or violence, or story lines about diabetes on a Spanish-language soap opera. The arts, when combined with media advocacy (chapter 24) or participatory media production, can further enable community members to express their concerns.

4. *To bring attention to an issue.* A cultural rendering of an issue will often catch people's attention, and may help change their perceptions. The Clothesline Project, begun in 1990 by women in Massachusetts to promote awareness of violence against women, provides a classic example. The project urges victims and survivors of violence against women to create a T-shirt that expresses their feelings: a white T-shirt in memory of a murdered woman, a blue one for survivors of childhood sexual abuse, a yellow one for a battered woman, and so on. When a series of these T-shirts are made and are displayed on a clothesline in a public place, they provide a graphic and moving statement about the realities so many women and children face, and they are also a powerful way of "airing society's dirty laundry" (Hippe, 2000). The project, which today includes some 50,000 to 60,000 shirts in forty-one states and five countries, took a simple, accessible medium and transformed it into a powerful voice against the pervasive problems of child sexual abuse, intimate partner violence, and other forms of violence against women (http://www.clotheslineproject .info/about.html).

5. *To promote community building.* Cultural forms of expression rooted in the community may not only give voice to shared concerns, they may also contribute to the community's collective life, whether through celebration, ritual, or mourning. Such community expressions, using methods such as digital storytelling (Greene et al., 2018), can be powerful tools in achieving organizing goals, particularly in communities of color, where oppression has often entailed the belittling or outright suppression of traditional cultural forms of expression (Duncombe & Lambert, 2017; Smith, 2008).

For the Healthy Native Communities Partnership, Inc. (HNCP), in Shiprock, New Mexico, digital storytelling honors and complements their community's centuries-old tradition of "using stories to make sense of the world [and] to inspire community change" (hncpartners.org). Since 2009, under the leadership of Shelley Frazier, Chris Percy, and Marita Jones, over 400 members of

diverse tribes have participated in HNCP's three-day digital storytelling trainings, building trust, engaging in meaningful conversations, and using digital
technology to amplify authentic community voices while inspiring "increased
community engagement around local priorities and issues" (hncpartners.org).
In 2017, HNCP provided training for the University of New Mexico's Center for
Participatory Research and three tribal research teams in digital storytelling
to highlight their New Mexico Family Listening Program's efforts to build community through cultural connections by engaging children and families and
sharing Family Listening Program stories with other community members and
tribal leaders (https://cpr.unm.edu/research-projects/flcp/digital-stories-.html).

6. *To promote healing from intergenerational and collective trauma.* Although the
restorative and healing powers of the arts for individuals have long been
acknowledged (Bang, 2016; Sonke et al., 2019; Stuckey, 2010), the role arts can
play in helping address collective and intergenerational trauma is gaining
attention (Sonke et al., 2019). Defined as "traumatic experiences that perme-
ate communities that share history, identity, or a sense of place" (Sonke et al.,
2019, p. 18; Yehuda & Lehrner, 2018), collective trauma, including the compounded and cumulative emotional wounds experienced as a result of slavery,
genocide, war, poverty, and forced relocation, is often carried from one generation to the next (https://sainta.org/5-observations-about-trauma/).

A powerful example of using the arts to address such trauma can be found
in "Colored to Black," a multimodal dramatic production drawing on eighty
years of Black oral histories from North Central Florida. Through showings in
schools and other physical and virtual spaces, Colored to Black juxtaposes dra-
matized vignettes from decades past with current issues that are having an
impact on the Black community, in a way that "exposes the origins, mechanisms, and health impacts of systemic racism on Black communities in America" (Sonke et al., 2019, p. 25).

Using a very different art form, the 9/11 Memorial design features twin
waterfall pools surrounded by bronze parapets that list the names of the 2,983
victims of the 9/11 attacks and the 1993 World Trade Center bombing. The pools
are set within a plaza where more than 400 swamp white oak trees grow. This
powerful memorial has become a beacon for millions who need to reflect on,
and cry over, loved ones and fellow Americans and others lost in the attacks,
while helping promote healing, understanding, and forgiveness (https://www
.911memorial.org/visit/memorial/about-memorial).

7. *To promote a culture of health.* In 2014, the Robert Wood Johnson Foundation,
together with the RAND Corporation and other partners, launched a bold new
initiative to create a national culture of health, through which everyone in our
diverse society "has a fair and just opportunity to live the healthiest life possible" (Plough & Gandhi, 2019, p. 490). Among its many approaches to this work
was providing support for efforts to integrate the arts and culture in public
health. As Sonke et al. (2019) note, "Because cultural norms are most effectively

shifted via cultural practices" (p. 16), investment in such work may be an important and underappreciated means of "making health a shared value, fostering cross-sector collaboration, and creating healthier and more equitable communities" (p. 15), all central components of the Culture of Health's Action Framework (Plough & Ford, 2015).

The Leaders from Louisville in Kentucky program won an RWJF Culture of Health Prize in 2016 for its creative use of the arts in working for healthier, more equitable communities. Residents of the Smoketown neighborhood, who live adjacent to the largest concentration of health care services in the state, have a life expectancy nine years lower than that of Louisville residents as a whole. To help shine a spotlight on that disparity, Andrew Cozzens's Smoketown Life Line Project documented the impact of trauma on many aspects of people's lives and health. Based, in part, on interviews with more than twenty local residents, his art form uses metal rods of different lengths—each representing the length of one community member's life. Crimps in the rods marked with different color bands represent adverse experiences (e.g., violence, addiction, incarceration, and trauma) to graphically show how lives have been needlessly shortened. Cozzens's project was created as part of Project HEAL (Health Equity Art Learning), a three-year effort that trained artists to help communities identify their health priorities and dig deeper to discuss complex underlying issues through sometimes difficult conversations. Project HEAL uses the arts to enable communities to work toward health equity, hand-in-hand with policymakers, health care institutions, nonprofits, and others (https://www.rwjf .org/en/blog/2017/03/four_ways_artistsca.html).

8. *To empower.* Perhaps the most important aspect of using the arts in community building and organizing for health and well-being lies in the ways that the creative process can help create the conditions in which individuals and communities can become empowered. Involvement in a creative process can be exhilarating. When one *becomes* the video maker, the poet, the dancer, or the muralist, and is transformed through that process, change can take place in both the messenger and the audience (Bublitz et al., 2019; Catalani et al., 2012).

    Perhaps the best-known example of this process is the Names Project's AIDS Memorial Quilt (https://www.aidsmemorial.org/interactive-aids-quilt) (Cherasia, 2020). Begun in San Francisco in 1987 by gay activist Cleve Jones and others to commemorate those who had died of AIDS, the Names Project attracted tens of thousands of others and grew from a memorial into a method for activism. To understand the role of this project in helping to create the conditions for empowerment, it is important to remember that particularly during the early 1980s, the mysterious and terrifying epidemic, almost always fatal and at first believed to be limited to gay and bisexual men, amplified homophobia and fear that led to many victims being denied traditional burials or being charged extra for them (Bass, 1987). The creation of each quilt piece, roughly the size of a coffin, and commemorating a loved one in a deeply personal rendering, was both personally healing and empowering as part of a much larger whole. The quilt October 1996 display in Washington, DC, constituted both the largest AIDS event and the largest community art event in history, with panels representing contributors from over forty nations. By 2020, the quilt included 48,000 panels representing 125,000 people and weighed 54 tons. The AIDS Quilt project reflects the feminist precept that the personal is political, while also representing a grassroots community arts and organizing effort on an almost unprecedented scale with people, often from marginalized groups, coming together to grieve while becoming more empowered through their involvement and that of thousands of others.

Using the Arts in Building Community and Promoting Change: Three Concluding Illustrations

As discussed earlier, a wide range of artistic approaches have been used in community organizing and community building for health, often in the process engaging groups and populations for whom more traditional health education approaches have held little appeal.

We conclude with three examples, each of which shows the power and the promise of a different approach to community building and organizing with the arts as a vehicle.

The first exemplifies the power of videovoice, an approach that builds on and complements the photovoice method illustrated earlier (see box 17.1), as well as participatory media and participatory video as developed and used by Chávez et al. (2004) and others (Benkler, 2006; Sitter, 2015). Videovoice is defined as "a research and advocacy approach through which people, who are usually the consumers of mainstream media, get behind video cameras to research issues of concern, communicate their knowledge, and advocate for change" (Catalani et al., 2012, p. 18).

Like photovoice, it is action oriented and facilitates the use of media as "an advocacy tool to reach policy makers, health planners, community leaders, and other people who can be mobilized to make change" (Wang & Pies, 2004, p. 96). Unlike photovoice, however, videovoice is able to capture movement, audio, and sequential narrative and, during the dissemination stage, to be shared in theaters, living rooms, classrooms, and websites, such as YouTube.com (Catalani et al., 2012).

The second example, the Skywatchers Program, illustrates how the co-creation of art in a new and challenging setting helped illuminate and was guided by a *values-based methodology for art and community practice*, the usefulness of which extends well beyond the arts. Because of the helpful lessons for health promotion and other practitioners as they engage with new communities, the Skywatchers methodology is presented in appendix 5, as a supplement to the story of the project and its methodology's unfolding and application presented later in this chapter.

The third and final example, the Morris Justice Project (MJP) in the Bronx, New York, is illustrative of how art often plays a powerful role in capturing some of the impetus for and the findings of participatory action research (PAR) on some of the most wrenching problems of our times. In the case of the MJP, these included police harassment of Black and Latinx people doing ordinary, and often perfectly legal, things in their own neighborhoods.

The New Orleans Videovoice Project:
Community Building, Assessment, and Capacity Building
in Post-Katrina New Orleans

Natural disasters caused or exacerbated by climate change, from catastrophic wild-fires in California to unprecedented floods on the Eastern Seaboard and beyond, are increasingly important causes of collective as well as individual trauma (Sonke et al., 2019). In one of the worst such events to date, when Hurricane Katrina hit New Orleans in August 2005, the historic flooding resulted in 1,500 deaths and the loss of 200,000 homes, 850 schools, 18,700 businesses, and some 220,000 jobs (LRA, 2006). These losses were disproportionately endured by low-income Black and other often marginalized communities (Drury et al., 2008) and resulted in the great-est forced migration in the history of the country (LaVeist, 2020).

Two years after the hurricane, the New Orleans videovoice project was imple-mented by a partnership of academic researchers, independent filmmakers, and community members from the hardest hit Central City neighborhood. The project began during the development of the city's master plan for rebuilding, a time when community partners sought to influence the local agenda, discourse, and action.

Community members of the partnership were trained in videography and helped gather assessment data through video interviews with residents, leaders, and policymakers, as well as footage covering both environmental and commu-nity events. Their participatory editing process and production resulted in several short films, and a final, longer one, titled *In Harmony*, highlighted the city's his-tory, current neighborhood conditions, and community members' hopes for the future (Catalani et al., 2009).

Partners premiered the film to over 200 city leaders and residents, followed by lively audience engagement. At the event, an elderly Black woman remarked that this was the first time in her life that she had been engaged in an open and frank discussion of race and racism in the presence of White people. Eighty percent of the audience members who submitted evaluations at the first showing (n=78) indi-cated that they were interested in joining with others to act on the issues raised by the film. The final films were shared online through YouTube (www.youtube .com/VideoVoiceCollective).

Participatory evaluation of the full project revealed a range of outcomes, from individual empowerment to community capacity building. All eleven partners reported that they were more engaged in community action and had more confi-dence in their ability to carry out community projects. In keeping with a project objective of transferring skills to the community, four local partners went on to gain employment that used their newfound video skills, and several continued to initiate new projects without the aid of outside filmmakers or researchers. A former teacher and member of the team thus created and became the director of a new organization called New Orleans Videovoices, funded by the W.K. Kellogg Foundation, through which she and other team members led four additional videovoice projects in both New Orleans and Mississippi. The New Orleans videovoice project, in sum, built local capacity to produce media and work collaboratively on social justice projects while enhancing understanding of local concerns through a rich and innovative community assessment and the engagement of policymakers and residents to work for change.

The Skywatchers Program and Its Values-Based Methodology for Collaborative Community Arts Practice

Skywatchers is a collaborative community arts ensemble of artists and residents of the Tenderloin, a neighborhood rich in art and culture, but economically the most impoverished in San Francisco (Haveman & Massaro, 2015; chapter 19). It is also the only remaining neighborhood in the center of any major city in the United States with a significant number of single-room-occupancy hotels (SROs) (Krentzman, 2017), which represent the bottom rung of the housing ladder. The program builds relationships of caring and reciprocity (appendix 5), co-creating art works and promoting arts-based advocacy with SRO and other low-income residents.

Skywatchers is a program of ABD Productions, a women- and queer-centered multiethnic dance company dedicated to inspiring social change through the arts. More than a decade ago, the ABD artistic director, Anne Bluethenthal, began visiting the Tenderloin National Forest, a small, community-created arts and green space in the heart of this densely populated neighborhood, and meeting with residents of nearby SRO hotels, slowly building connections through relationships of "trust across multiple axes of difference" (Epstein et al., 2021). As trust grew, some residents brought musical instruments, and increasing numbers of residents joined the musical jam and conversational circles from week to week. Younger master of fine arts students joined the project as well, honoring its relational and durational aspects through their regular presence and understanding that in community and in relationship building "time moves at the speed of trust" (Brown, 2017; appendix 5).

As the group expanded, Skywatchers became a mixed-ability, intergenerational arts ensemble of Tenderloin residents and professional artists that continues today. The forms of art created by this group include movement-based and visual arts, music, and the spoken word. Participants share a full range of life experiences, stories, talents, and struggles, as exemplified in the song "Dirty Water" about the filthy water coming from the artist and her neighbors' SRO hotel faucets and getting the attention of the city inspection committee when the song was performed on stage. Another resident artist, Proud Rita, wrote the poem "Not One of Us," making meaning of her own struggle to save her leg, transformed by a large tumor, by linking her personal experience (the potential loss of a limb and autonomy) to that of many low-income patients subject to medical expedience and amputation. The last stanza of her poem reads:

> I am here! Survivor among survivors
> Of the poverty industrial complex
> And I will roll my beautiful legs down this street
> And I will sing my songs of survival and love
> Because NOT ONE OF US IS DISPENSIBLE!
>
> —Proud Rita, 2016

Such works, and the emergent process through which they were created, underscore the relational, durational, and conversational dimensions of the Skywatchers methodology (appendix 5). The final, structural, dimension includes embodying and confronting difficult political issues in humanizing forms; developing strategic partnerships with neighborhood organizations; and working across sectors to make a tangible commitment to community leadership. In 2017, Skywatchers partnered with the Glide Foundation to launch the neighborhood's Leadership and Political Education Program, which graduated over forty community residents in three years who continue to engage in creative protest, community organizing, and advocacy (Epstein et al., 2021).

During the COVID pandemic, the Skywatchers team continued to collaborate through phone or Zoom calls, creating a collection of works titled *Life in the Containment Zone under Quarantine.* Many artistic projects emerged, from dialogues about social isolation and reparations and the need for new monuments, to the production of eye-catching posters about the most urgent and immediate issue of social distancing and public health. Further, and to feed the hearts and souls of people near and far toward the end of the pandemic, two outdoor mixed-media performances were held for small audiences in late May 2021. A third, which includes a discussion of the Skywatchers approach, was recorded and launched on YouTube (https://www.youtube.com/watch?v=9AaB8Cablmk).

As described in appendix 5, the Skywatchers values-based methodology continues to serve as a useful bridge to help disrupt problematic social narratives and highlight and address underlying conditions that adversely affect community health and well-being.

Using the Arts in Participatory Action Research to Address Police Harassment of Black and Latinx People in the South Bronx: The Morris Justice Project

The arts and activists are also vital contributors to the Morris Justice Project (MJP), a participatory action research (PAR) collective in New York City's South Bronx. Over several years, the project gathered, analyzed, and shared community-level data about police brutality and "broken windows policing." The latter term refers to policing practices that target "low-level "crimes" and create racialized patterns of

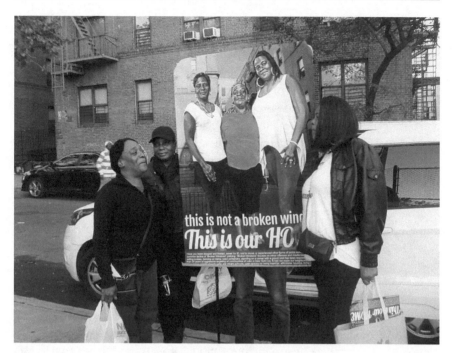

FIGURE 17.2 This is not a broken window. This is our home. Not a Broken Window Poster Series photo featuring (*left to right*) Morris Justice Project researchers Nadine Sheppard, Fawn Bracy, and Jaqueline Yates.

Photo credit: María Elena Torre. Poster: Evan Bissell with Morris Justice Project.

profiling, harassment, and violence in the lives of residents in low-income, Black and Latinx communities. Under these policies, residents of color are aggressively policed with stops, tickets, and arrests for everyday activities, such as running errands in the neighborhood or gathering with friends in front of their homes (deVuono-Powell et al., 2018).

The findings of MJP's "stats-n-action" collaborative data analysis (Stoudt & Torre, 2014) of a survey of over 1,000 local residents revealed that fully 75 percent of participants had been stopped by police, with a quarter of them stopped for the first time when they were age 13 or younger. These and other findings were shared, in part, through colorful posters wheat-pasted around the neighborhood and other art installations with powerful quotes from residents and statistics that helped tell the story of what this neighborhood endures at the hands of police. An evocative painting by artist and activist Evan Bissell became a centerpiece of one of MJP's powerful posters (figure 17.2). Using the painting as a starting point to catch the attention of passersby, MJP members added a collaboratively written paragraph, explaining the connection between the NYPD's new language of "broken windows policing" and the more familiar language of the ("officially" phased out) police policy of "stop and frisk." Written before current national calls to defund the police, the text points to the city's choice to heavily fund policing rather than the more critical needs of the neighborhood, such as affordable, stable housing, engaging schools, living-wage jobs, and accessible health care.

Both the art installations and other forms of data sharing frequently took place in what MJP's María Elena Torre termed "participatory contact zones" (Torre & Fine, 2010). These zones were places of communication and relationship building, debate, and more data collection. They brought out many residents, supporters, skeptics, and observers, both day and night. What held the group together as they wrestled through very real clashes of different experiences and beliefs that might have otherwise splintered them, was their deep commitment to the purpose of the work, and the collective desire *to be there*, gathering data that would speak aloud the dismissed story of the police abuse the neighborhood was enduring. Participation was not an afterthought, but part of the glue that allowed for the extraordinary work of engaging and navigating power as part of the methods used in the research.

The experience of the MJP research was so intense and intimate that members became a kind of family, whose relationships carried on after the research and sidewalk science and its artistic expression went on hiatus in 2016, and project meetings transitioned to educational presentations and research justice workshops for academics and community organizers. The importance of the project and its contributions have not diminished, however, with the very act of so many diverse people coming together—even with interruptions from time to time—seen by MJP members as also being implicit "reclamations of public space and an assertion of the need for public safety beyond policing" (deVuono-Powell et al., 2018, p. 306).

Conclusion

The arts have been a catalyst for change and growth in wide-ranging circumstances, providing a rich legacy for health organizers and promoters to draw on in their community-organizing and community-building efforts. Further, as Jill Sonke and her colleagues (2019) note, "Arts and culture can expose root issues, incorporate and amplify the voices and concerns of those who have been underrepresented and change our very interpretation and configuration of a given health reality" by bringing a new dimension into play (p. 9). In the process, they can improve communication while motivating and inspiring both artists and a growing array of audiences, as well as promoting cross-fertilization and collaboration between these diverse groups. Given the enormity of the challenges confronting professionals across disciplines working to promote health and social equity, combining the arts with community building and organizing can be an effective tool now and in the coming decades.

Questions for Further Discussion

1. The chapter provided many concrete examples of ways in which the arts can contribute to health and well-being, as well as to effective community

organizing and community. Thinking back on the examples provided, pick one that you found particularly appealing. What made it resonate with you? And beyond the particular way in which this example was seen as being useful (e.g., in getting people involved, finding out about a community, increasing awareness, and relaying health education messages, etc.), what other ways might the example you chose also contribute (e.g., might it also attract attention to an issue, promote healing, or help empower?). Explain why and how you believe the example you chose would be helpful in this other way or ways as well?

2. Community-based art *is* community practice. Providing opportunities for co-creation and partnership building among health professionals, artists, social activists, and neighborhood residents, community-based art provides creative avenues for identifying local concerns, restoring neighborhood vitality, and advocating for social justice. In what ways can you envision local health projects embracing arts and artists as creative forces for community organizing and neighborhood well-being?

Acknowledgments

The authors gratefully acknowledge Marian McDonald, Giovanni Antunez, and Megan Gottemoeller for their important early work in this area, and Jill Sonke and her partners for their 2019 white paper *Creating Healthy Communities through Cross-Sector Collaboration* and the inspiration it provided. Our deepest gratitude goes to the many artists whose work has moved and inspired us and countless others, and has also illustrated the powerful ways in which art can contribute to healthier lives and communities, in part through its roles in community organizing and community building for change.

REFERENCES

Bang, A. H. (2016). The restorative and transformative power of the arts in conflict resolution. *J Transform Educ, 14*(4), 355–376.

Bass, S. (1987, November 15). Funeral homes accused of bias on AIDS. *New York Times.* https://www.nytimes.com/1987/11/15/nyregion/funeral-homes-accused-of-bias-on-aids.html.

Benkler, Y. (2006). *The Wealth of Networks: How Social Production Transforms Markets and Freedom.* Yale University Press.

Brown, A. M. (2017). *Emergent Strategy.* AK Press.

Bublitz, M. G., Rank-Christman, T., Cian, L., Cortada, X., Madzharov, A., Patrick, V. M., Peracchio, L. A., Scott, M. L., Sundar, A., To, N., & Townsend, C. (2019). Collaborative art: A transformational force within communities. *J Consum Res, 4*(4), 313–331.

Catalani, C., & Minkler, M. (2010). Photovoice: A review of the literature in health and public health. *Health Educ Behav, 37*(3), 424–451.

Catalani, C. E., Veneziale, A., Campbell, L., Herbst, S., Butler, B., Springgate, B., & Minkler, M. (2012). Videovoice: Community assessment in post-Katrina New Orleans. *Health Promot Pract, 13*(1), 18–28.

Catalani, C., Veneziale, A., Campbell, L., Herbst, S., Springgate, B., & Minkler, M. (2009). In harmony: Reflections, thoughts, and hopes of Central City, New Orleans. Community Engaged Scholarship for Health. www.youtube.com/VideoVoiceCollective.

Chávez, V., Israel, B., Allen, A. J. III, DeCarlo, M. F., Lichtenstein, R., Schulz, A., Bayer, I. S., & McGranaghan, R. (2004). A bridge between communities: Video-making using principles of community-based participatory research. *Health Promot Pract, 5*(4), 395–403.

Cherasia, S. P. (2020, January 6). Affordances, remediation, and digital mourning: A comparative case study of two AIDS memorials. *Memory Studies.* https://doi.org/10.1177/1750698019 894686.

Chin, M. (2017). Feelings, safe space, and LGBTQ of color community arts organizing. *J Community Pract, 25*(3–4), 391–407.

Derr, V., & Simons, J. (2020). A review of photovoice applications in environment, sustainability, and conservation contexts: Is the method maintaining its emancipatory intents? *Environ Educ Res, 26*(3), 359–380.

deVuono-Powell, S., Minkler, M., Bissell, E., Walker, T., Vaughn, L., & Moore, E. (2018). Criminal justice reform through participatory action research. In N. Wallerstein, B. Duran, J. G. Oeztel, & M. Minkler (Eds.), *Community-Based Participatory Research for Health: Advancing Social and Health Equity* (3rd ed., pp. 305–320). Jossey-Bass.

Drury, S., Scheeringa, M. S., & Zeahan, C. H. (2008). The traumatic impact of Hurricane Katrina on children in New Orleans. *Child Adolesc Psychiatr Clin N Am, 17*(3), 685–702.

Dunaway, D. K., & Beer, M. (2010). *Singing Out: An Oral History of America's Folk Music Revivals.* Oxford University Press.

Duncombe, S., & Lambert, S. (2017). Lessons from Utopia. *Vis Inquiry, 6*(2), 253–272.

Epstein, N., Bluethenthal, A., Visser, D., Pinsky, C., & Minkler, M. (2021). Leveraging arts for justice, equity and public health: The Skywatchers Program and its implications for community-based health promotion practice and research. *Health Promot Pract, 22*(1_suppl), 91S–100S.

Freire, P. (1973). *Education for Critical Consciousness.* Seabury Press.

Greene, S., Burke, K. J., & McKenna, M. K. (2018). A review of research connecting digital storytelling, photovoice, and civic engagement. *Rev Educ Res, 88*(6), 844–878.

Haveman, J., & Massaro, R. (2015). *Poverty in the San Francisco Bay Area: Silicon Valley.* Research Brief. Institute for Regional Studies. https://jointventure.org/images/stories/pdf/poverty -brief-2015-03.pdf.

Herrman, J. (2020, June 28). TikTok is shaping politics. But how? *New York Times.* https://www .nytimes.com/2020/06/28/style/tiktok-teen-politics-gen-z.html.

Hippe, P. C. (2000). Clothing their resistance in hegemonic dress: The Clothesline Project's response to violence against women. *Cloth Tex Res J, 18*(3), 163–177.

hooks, b. (1994). *Outlaw Culture: Resisting Representations.* Routledge.

Horton, M., & Freire. P. (1990). *We Make the Road by Walking: Conversations on Education and Social Change.* Temple University Press.

Krentzman, J. (2017). *TNDC at 35. San Francisco, CA.* Tenderloin Neighborhood Development Corporation.

LaVeist, T. A. (2020). Katrina's lesson: Time to imagine an after COVID-19. *Am J Public Health, 110*(10), 1445.

Lorde, A. (1984). *Sister Outsider.* Crossing Press.

Louisiana Recovery Authority (LRA). (2006, February–May). Quarterly Report. Louisiana Recovery Authority, State of Louisiana. http://lra.louisiana.gov/assets/docs/.

Lykes, M. B., & Hershberg, R. M. (2012). Participatory action research and feminisms: Social inequalities and transformative praxis. In S. N. Hesse-Biber (Ed.), *Handbook of Feminist Research: Theory and Praxis* (pp. 331–367). Sage.

Marais, F., Minkler, M., Gibson, N., Mwau, B., Mehtar, S., Ogunsola, F., Banya, S. S., & Corburn, J. (2016). A community-engaged infection prevention and control approach to Ebola. *Health Promot Int, 31*(2), 440–449.

Mathews, A., Farley, S., Conserve, D. F., Knight, K., Le'Marus, A., Blumberg, M., Rennie, S., & Tucker, J. (2020). "Meet people where they are": A qualitative study of community barriers and facilitators to HIV testing and HIV self-testing among African Americans in urban and rural areas in North Carolina. *BMC Public Health, 20*, 1–10.

McDonald, M., Antunez, G., & Gottemoeller, M. (1998). Using the arts and literature in health education. *Int Q Community Health Educ, 18*(3), 269–282.

Nyswander, D. B. (1956). Education for health: Some principles and their application. *Health Educ Monogr, 14*, 65–70.

Ohmer, S. (2019). The making and silencing of "Axé-Ocracy" in Brazil: Black women writers' spiritual, political and literary movement in São Paulo. *J Int Women's Stud, 20*(8), 40–63.

Plough, A., & Ford, C. (2015). *From Vision to Action: A Framework and Measures to Mobilize a Culture of Health*. Robert Wood Johnson Foundation.

Plough, A. L., & Gandhi, P. (2019). Promoting social justice through public health practice. In B. S. Levy (Ed.), *Social Injustice and Public Health* (3rd ed, pp. 481–494). Oxford University Press.

Preston, J., & Stelter, B. (2011, February 18). Cellphones become the world's eyes and ears on protests. *New York Times*. http://www.nytimes.com/2011/02/19/world/middleeast/19video.html?partner=rss&emc=rss.

Randall, M. (1991). *Walking to the Edge: Essays of Resistance*. South End Press.

Romig, H. (2018). *Arts and Social Justice: The Role of Art Organizations in Building Community* [Unpublished master's thesis, Clark University].

Samayeen, N., Wong, A., & McCarthy, C. (2020, July). Space to breathe: George Floyd, BLM Plaza and the monumentalization of divided American urban landscapes. *J Educ Philos Theory*, 1–11.

Seely, P. (2020). Racism, fascism, and leftist movements in American popular music. In E. G. Dobbins, M. L. Piga, & L. Manca (Eds.), *Environment, Social Justice, and the Media in the Age of the Anthropocene* (pp. 289–320). Lexington Books.

Shaffer, R. (1984). *Beyond the Dispensary*. Nairobi: African Medical and Research Foundation.

Sitter, K. C. (2015). Participatory video analysis in disability research. *Disabil Soc, 30*(6), 910–923.

Smith, L. T. (2008). *Decolonizing Methodologies: Research and Indigenous People*. Zed Books.

Sonke, J., Golden, T., Francois, S., Hand, J., Chandra, A., Clemmons, L., Fakunle, D., Jackson, M. R., Magsamen, S., Rubin, V., Sams, K., & Springs, S. (2019). *Creating Healthy Communities through Cross-Sector Collaboration* [White paper]. University of Florida Center for Arts in Medicine / ArtPlace America, LLC.

Stoudt, B. G., & Torre, M. E. (2014). *The Morris Justice Project: Participatory Action Research*. Sage.

Stuckey, H. L. (2010). The connection between art, healing, and public health: A review of current literature. *Am J Public Health, 100*(2), 254–263.

Suprapto, N., Sunarti, T., Suliyanah, D. W., Hidayaatullaah, H. N., Adam, A. S., & Mubarok, H. (2020). A systematic review of photovoice as participatory action research strategies. *Int J Eval Res Educ, 9*(3), 675–683.

Taylor, C., & Wei, Q. (2020). Storytelling and arts to facilitate community capacity building for urban planning and social work. *Societies, 10*(3), 64.

Teti, M., Koegler, E., Conserve, D. F., Handler, L., & Bedford, M. (2018). A scoping review of photovoice research among people with HIV. *J Assoc Nurses AIDS Care, 29*(4), 504–527.

Torre, M. E., & Fine, M. (2010). Participatory action research in the contact zone. In J. Cammarota & M. Fine (Eds.), *Revolutionizing Education: Youth Participatory Action Research in Motion* (pp. 31–52). Routledge.

Wallerstein, N. (1992). Powerlessness, empowerment, and health: Implications for health promotion programs. *Am J Health Promot, 6*, 197–205.

Wang, C., & Burris, M. A. (1997). Photovoice: Concept, methodology, and use for participatory needs assessment. *Health Educ Behav, 24*(3), 369–387.

Wang, C., Wu, K. Y., Burris, M., Li, V., Zhan, W. T., & Xiang, Y. P. (1995). *Visual Voices: 100 Photographs of Village China by the Women of Yunnan Province.* Yunnan People's Publishing House.

Wang, C. C., & Pies, C. A. (2004). Family, maternal, and child health through photovoice. *Matern Child Health, 8*(2), 95–102.

Wang, E. L. (2010). The Beat of Boyle Street: Empowering Aboriginal youth through music making. *New Dir Youth Dev, 125,* 61–70.

Wang, H., & Singhal, A. (2016). East Los High: Transmedia edutainment to promote the sexual and reproductive health of young Latina/o Americans. *Am J Public Health, 106*(6), 1002–1010.

Yehuda, R., & Lehrner, A. (2018). Intergenerational transmission of trauma effects: Putative role of epigenetic mechanisms. *World Psychiatry, 17*(3), 243–257.

Zeedyk, M. S., & Wallace, L. (2003). Tackling children's road safety through edutainment: An evaluation of effectiveness. *Health Educ Res, 18*(4), 493–505.

PART SEVEN

Building, Maintaining, and Evaluating Effective Coalitions and Community Organizing Efforts

Skeptics have described partnerships as unnatural acts between nonconsenting adults. And indeed, many of us have seen partnerships (or more formal coalitions) fall apart when they have come together primarily because of the stipulation of a funding agency and do not represent any genuine shared concern with working collaboratively to help bring about change. Even when the commitment is there, however, the challenges to coalitions and other partnerships are many. As public health leader Lawrence W. Green (2000) pointed out over twenty years ago, for example, "Most organizations will resist giving up resources, credit, visibility and autonomy" and further, "Not everyone insists on being the coordinator, but nobody wishes to be the coordinatee" (pp. 64–65).

Although the challenges to coalitions and other partnerships are indeed numerous, when grounded in shared values and a strong theoretical base, coalitions and other partnerships can both function effectively and make real equity-focused impacts on the community, organizational, and policy levels (Wolfe et al., 2020; Wolff et al., 2016). Early efforts to provide such frameworks include Wallerstein et al.'s (2002) participatory evaluation model for coalitions with its accent on developing and using systems indicators. Kathleen Roe and her colleagues' (2005) early effort to build community though empowerment evaluation with one of the early mandated HIV Prevention Planning Councils provides another early and thoughtful example, and one highlighting some of the extraordinary challenges in this work, particularly during crises like the HIV/AIDS epidemic.

Since those early efforts, many new tools for participatory or empowerment evaluation have been developed, many of which have proved useful in the evaluation of community coalitions, and the reader is encouraged to see chapter 21 and appendix 10 for more details on such tools and their applications in this regard.

In chapter 18, we explore a model explicitly designed for use in evaluating community coalitions, and one that has stood the test of time, Frances D. Butterfoss and Michelle C. Kegler's (2009) widely used Community Coalition Action Theory (CCAT). Building on a classic definition by Feighery and Rogers (1990), the authors describe coalitions as "formal, long-term collaborations that are composed of diverse organizations, factions, or constituencies who agree to work together to achieve a common goal." They stress in particular the action orientation of community coalitions and the importance of a guiding theory that is not simply an academic exercise but rather is aimed at improving how coalitions work in practice.

After introducing some of the earlier thinking that contributed to CCAT, Butterfoss and Kegler discuss the benefits and costs of coalitions and lay out a set of constructs and "practice-proven propositions" for understanding coalition development, maintenance, and effective functioning. The various stages of coalitions, and the tasks associated with each, are described, with attention to such key issues as coalition context, leadership and staffing, and member engagement. Further, the theory's frequently circling back to the value of multilevel strategies that can help improve health and social outcomes on the community and other levels is an important factor differentiating CCAT from coalition models that are not community based, and that may have very different underlying values, goals, and guiding principles.

Many of the propositions and challenges laid out in chapter 18 are illustrated within a real-world context in chapter 19. Patricia Wakimoto and her colleagues present a case study of coalition building and community organizing to address the interrelated problems of food insecurity and tobacco saturation in San Francisco's culturally rich but economically poor Tenderloin neighborhood, a quarter of whose residents lived below the poverty line even before the pandemic. Without a single full-service grocery store, local residents are dependent on the neighborhood's dozens of small corner stores, which tend to stock primarily heavily processed foods, tobacco, alcohol, and sodas. Yet, as described in chapter 19, the neighborhood also has a long history of activism that served it well when local community based organizations (CBOs) and residents, catalyzed by local youths' research-based Google Map of half of the neighborhood's seventy corner stores, showed just how bleak the problem was and spurred them to action (Flood et al., 2015).

Using CCAT's three stages in coalition development—formation, maintenance, and institutionalization—Wakimoto and her colleagues illustrate how the Tenderloin Healthy Corner Store Coalition (the Coalition), was founded by a core group of diverse local CBOs and agencies, and co-led by two of them from its founding until well into the institutionalization phase. They also discuss the key role of concerned local residents, who, by virtue of their majority presence at monthly meetings and the Coalition's commitment to a majority rules decisionmaking process, ensured from the start the residents' real power and sense of ownership.

Indeed, it was the Coalition's commitment to community power and justice that led Wakimoto and her colleagues to include a second conceptual tool in their analysis: principles for Collaborating for Equity and Justice (CEJ) (Wolff et al., 2017). The six principles, stressing things like the use of approaches "in which residents have equal power in determining . . . the agenda and resource allocation," "work to build resident leadership and power," and "focus on policy, systems, and structural change," along with a seventh added in this book, emphasizing the importance of cultural humility and striving for cultural competence, proved a useful and often complementary addition to CCAT. Further, their incorporation was in keeping with Susan Wolfe and her partners' (2020) call for "using a principles-focused evaluation approach to evaluate coalitions and collaboratives working toward equity and social justice" (p. 45).

Of particular importance in Wakimoto et al.'s assessment of the Coalition was CCAT's emphasis on the heavy influence of context at every stage in a coalition's development. With attention to this and numerous other relevant propositions, the authors were able to better understand and discuss the formation, maintenance, and institutionalization stages of the Coalition. But they also explored areas where the Coalition deviated from CCAT, for example, in playing a key role, while still in its own organizational development, in helping craft, pass, and then implement and assess a municipal ordinance establishing a program, Healthy Retail SF (HRSF), incentivizing selected corner stores in food insecure neighborhoods that change their business model to healthy retail. Outcomes of this work on the community level include the successful conversion of nine stores to healthy retail, six of them in the Tenderloin, the first four of which showed a 35 percent increase in the sales of fresh produce (Minkler, Estrada et al., 2019). Also important, and in keeping with CCAT's emphasis on the importance of "community gatekeepers," was the pivotal role of "Food Justice Leaders," residents hired and trained in research, education, and advocacy, and whose store-level data collection was critical to both making the case for HRSF and monitoring its effectiveness. These and other Coalition accomplishments and obstacles faced are discussed in chapter 19, as is the utility of both CCAT and the CEJ principles for critically analyzing this unique community coalition.

In chapter 20, R. David Rebanal offers a helpful look at a topic typically overlooked in books and articles on community organizing, namely the importance of fundraising as a critical part of the work itself. As he notes, although most funders still tend to support primarily direct service, and many are hesitant to embrace controversial causes, growing numbers of foundations and other donors *are* supporting community organizing and related strategies that can help promote health equity and address the Social Determinants of Health (Iton & Ross, 2017; Minkler, Rebanal et al., 2019; Plough & Ford, 2015). Rebanal begins the chapter with a brief look at the historical roles and regulations that shaped philanthropic funding. He then discusses some of the more recent events—such as the movement for Black lives and for continued fights for the rights of immigrant and Indigenous people, and for climate justice and food security—that have helped to increase support for community organizing. He further highlights some of the major private philanthropies, including the Robert Wood Johnson Foundation, The California Endowment, the W.K. Kellogg Foundation, and the Seattle Foundation (chapter 9), which have deepened their support for community organizing that centers equity and racial healing as an important part of their work.

Rebanal devotes most of the chapter to providing a wealth of tips and strategies that can help community organizers and their agencies increase their success in fundraising from diverse sources, while also leveraging greater and wider financial support for this work.

Among the topics covered are how to find and reach out to prospective donors and build a diversified funding strategy that ideally includes some individual and corporate donors (provided no conflicts of interest are presented), as well as the philanthropic foundations on which most nonprofit community organizing groups tend to depend. Online resources for locating funding for work in particular areas (e.g., Grantmakers in Health and Funders for Justice) or with special population groups (e.g., Funders for LGBTQ Issues and Grantmakers for Girls of Color), as well as geographically focused funders, are among the resources highlighted. A detailed table with additional tips for fundraising is provided. New trends in philanthropy, including participatory "Giving Circles," through which groups of donors pool their funds and think strategically about what they want to support) are also discussed in this chapter.

Finally, Rebanal reminds us that despite the importance of being able to effectively raise funds to support our work, philanthropy and the private sector should not be seen as substituting for "large scale public financing and accompanying accountability necessary for more a more equitable society and the fundamental and systematic changes needed to achieve it." Indeed, for those of us engaged in community organizing for health equity and social justice, he correctly sees part of our work as helping to move a sometimes reluctant government further in this direction.

The last chapter in this part focuses on another topic seminal to our effective work in community organizing and community building, or in fields such as public health and social work, in which such approaches may be critical to our efforts to promote health and social equity. For whether we are building and working with coalitions or making the case to a prospective funder about the worthiness of our project, being able to demonstrate the efficacy of our agency, coalition, or program in meeting its objectives and making a measurable difference through its efforts is a critical part of our work. In chapter 21, Chris M. Coombe, Patricia Wakimoto, and Zachary Rowe describe how the process of evaluation—often one of the least favorite parts of a public health or other practitioner's work—can be used as a capacity building tool in organizing, as well as a source of knowledge for project improvement. Participatory or empowerment evaluation is described as a partnership approach to evaluation that engages those who have a stake in the project, program, or initiative in all aspects of evaluation design and implementation. Findings are applied as they emerge to solve problems and adjust course. Further, and unlike more conventional evaluation approaches, participatory evaluation, particularly in the "emancipatory tradition" (Cousins & Whitmore, 1998; Wiggins et al., 2018), argues that both the evaluation process and its results or products are shared, and can be used to create more equitable power relationships while promoting social action and change.

Coombe and her colleagues begin by discussing the limitations of conventional evaluation approaches and their grounding in the positivist paradigm of the natural sciences, which views knowledge "as an objective reality that can be discovered by 'impartial' observers, using quantitative experimental design as the gold standard." Although, as they note, this is a powerful research model that works well for things like assessing vaccine efficacy, its usefulness in evaluating community organizing, community building, and the like is more open to question. For example, when an outside expert conducts the evaluation, predetermined measures of success may miss the things community members care about most, and their understanding of what is really happening. Short-term indicators of success that community members of an organization or coalition may be best able to identify can also be missed. And without sharing of findings along the way, valuable opportunities for midcourse correction may be missed as well.

For these reasons and more, participatory evaluation is increasingly gaining appreciation. Coombe and her colleagues share an eight-stage model of participatory evaluation that draws on the work of Springett (2017), Wandersman (2015), and others. The process begins with identifying the purpose of the evaluation and committing to a participatory approach, and includes articulating goals and objectives and identifying change indicators; selecting methods for tracking progress; collecting and then collectively analyzing the data; communicating the results to relevant audiences; and finally, translating the findings into actions, systems, or policy changes.

As the authors make clear, the engagement of community partners at every stage of the process has a number of advantages. It can decrease distrust of the process, help in the development of new indicators and instruments, increase community capacity in areas such as systematic data collection and analysis, and provide both a deeper understanding of the role of context, and a greater likelihood of policymakers being able to hear from community members themselves about the work.

Although Coombe and her coauthors discuss some of the challenges posed by participatory evaluation, they conclude that it can be a powerful tool for community organizing and other efforts that have empowerment, capacity building, and social change as goals, while paying attention to the real voices of community members and demystifying the evaluation process.

REFERENCES

Butterfoss, F. D., & Kegler, M. C. (2009). Community coalition action theory. In R. DiClemente, L. Crosby, and M. C. Kegler (Eds.), *Emerging Theories in Health Promotion Practice and Research* (2nd ed., pp. 236–276). Jossey-Bass.

Cousins, J. B., & Whitmore, E. (1998). Framing participatory evaluation. *New Dir Eval, 80*, 5–23.

Feighery, E., & Rogers, T. (1990). *Building and Maintaining Effective Coalitions*. Stanford Health Promotion Resource Center.

Flood, J., Minkler, M., Hennessey Lavery, S., Estrada, J., & Falbe, J. (2015). The Collective Impact Model and its potential for health promotion: Overview and case study of a healthy retail initiative in San Francisco. *Health Educ Behav, 42*(5), 654–668.

Green, L. W. (2000). Caveats on coalitions: In praise of partnerships. *Health Promot Pract, 1*(1), 64–65.

Iton, A., & Ross, R. K. (2017). Understanding how health happens: Your zip code is more important than your genetic code. In R. Callahan & D. Bhattachara (Eds.), *Public Health Leadership* (pp. 83–99). Routledge.

Minkler, M., Estrada, J., Dyer, S., Hennessey Lavery, S., Wakimoto, P., & Falbe, J. (2019). Healthy retail as a strategy for improving food security and the built environment in San Francisco. *Am J Public Health, 109*(suppl_2), S137–S140.

Minkler, M., Rebanal, R. D., Pearce, R., & Acosta, M. (2019). Growing equity and health equity in perilous times: Lessons from community organizers. *Health Educ Behav, 46*(1_suppl), 9S–18S.

Plough, A., & Ford, C. (2015). *From Vision to Action: A Framework and Measures to Mobilize a Culture of Health*. Robert Wood Johnson Foundation.

Roe, K. M., Roe, K., Carpenter, C. G., & Sibley, C. B. (2005). Community building through empowering evaluation: A case study of community planning for HIV prevention. In M. Minkler (Ed.), *Community Organizing and Community Building for Health* (2nd ed., pp. 386–402). Rutgers University Press.

Springett, J. (2017). Impact in participatory health research: What can we learn from research on participatory evaluation? *Educ Action Res, 25*(4), 560–574.

Wallerstein, N., Polascek, M., & Maltrud, K. (2002). Participatory evaluation model for coalitions: The development of systems indicators. *Health Promot Pract, 3*(3), 361–373.

Wandersman, A. (2015). *Getting to Outcomes: An Empowerment Evaluation Approach for Capacity Building and Accountability*. Sage.

Wiggins, N., Parajon, L., Coombe, C. M., Duldulao, A., Wang, P., & Rodriguez Garcia, L. (2018). Participatory evaluation as a process of empowerment: Experiences with community health workers in the US and Latin America. In N. Wallerstein, B. Duran, J. Oetzel, & M. Minkler (Eds.), *Community-Based Participatory Research for Health* (3rd ed., pp. 251–264). Jossey-Bass.

Wolfe, S. M., Long, P. D., & Brown, K. K. (2020). Using a principles-focused evaluation approach to evaluate coalitions and collaboratives working toward equity and social justice. *New Dir Eval, 2020*(165), 45–65.

Wolff, T., Minkler, M., Wolfe, S. M., Berkowitz, B., Bowen, L., Butterfoss, F. D., Christens, B. D., Francisco, V. T., Himmelman, A. T., & Lee, K. S. (2017). Collaborating for equity and justice: Moving beyond collective impact. *Nonprofit Q, 9*, 42–53.

18

Community Coalition Action Theory

Designing and Evaluating Community Collaboratives

FRANCES D. BUTTERFOSS
MICHELLE C. KEGLER

Coalitions are *structured, multiyear* collaborations that are *composed of diverse organizations, factions, or constituencies who agree to work together to achieve a common goal* (Feighery & Rogers, 1990). A coalition is action oriented and focuses on reducing or preventing a community problem by analyzing the issue, identifying and implementing solutions, and creating social change (Butterfoss & Kegler, 2002; Butterfoss et al., 1993).

Coalitions develop when different sectors of the community, state, or nation join to create opportunities that will benefit all their partners in achieving mutual goals. *Community coalitions* operate in neighborhoods, towns, cities, or counties and usually serve a defined location that is recognized by residents as representing and serving them (Clarke et al., 2006). Its members reflect the diversity and wisdom of that community, at both grassroots and "grasstops" (professional) levels (Butterfoss et al., 1993). These members have direct experience with the social/health problem of interest, either through their professional roles or through their lived experience, and are actively engaged in decisionmaking and problem-solving. Community coalitions often collaborate with state and regional coalitions when they recognize the need to disseminate information and strategies widely. The terms *coalitions* and *partnerships* are used interchangeably, but partnerships may assume a more business-like arrangement and involve as few as two partners. Coalition size varies, and its members may be individuals, organizations, or groups. However, if a coalition is composed solely of individuals, then it should be classified as an organization or network.

Over the past thirty-five years, thousands of coalitions anchored by government or community-based organizations have been created to support community-based, health-related activities across the United States. For example, coalitions of health-related agencies, schools, and community-based groups have formed to prevent alcohol, tobacco, and other drug abuse and promote healthy weight and physical activity among youth. Advocates for environmental issues, such as asthma and lead-contamination, have rallied to highlight their issue or enable favorable policy and legislation. Civic and faith-based groups developed coalitions to ensure adequate housing for the elderly and health insurance for low-income populations. The best of these coalitions are vehicles that bring people together, expand available resources, focus on a problem of community concern, and achieve better results than any single group or agency could have achieved alone (Butterfoss & Kegler, 2002).

Coalitions, however, are not a panacea. Although they are usually built from unselfish motives to improve communities, coalitions may still experience difficulties that are common to many types of organizations, as well as some that are unique to collaborative efforts (Dowling et al., 2000; Wolff, 2010). Promised resources may not materialize, conflicting interests may prevent the coalition from having its desired effect in the community, and recognition for accomplishments may be slow in coming. Because it involves a long-term investment of time and resources, a coalition should not be built if a simpler, less complex structure will get the job done or if the community does not embrace this approach.

Clearly, communities are committed to the *practice* of building coalitions to improve health, but we must continue to build and refine the *theories* that ground our *practice*. Community Coalition Action Theory (CCAT), complete with constructs and propositions, has been developed to increase our understanding of how community coalitions actually work (Butterfoss & Kegler, 2009). Before this model is presented in detail, the rationale for and benefits of collaboration will be highlighted.

Coalitions and Collaboration

Collaboration begins when a perceived need exists and two or more organizations anticipate deriving a benefit that depends on mutual action toward common goals (Gray, 2000). These organizations often enter into a formal, sustained commitment to mutual relationships and goals, jointly developed structures, shared responsibility, mutual authority and accountability, and shared resources and rewards. When real community collaboration exists, coalitions address community health concerns while empowering or developing capacity in those communities (Butterfoss, 2007).

The overarching benefits that coalitions provide are improved trust and communication among agencies and organizations, as evidenced by increased networking, information sharing, and access to ideas, materials, and resources. This may help coalitions to more effectively engage their priority populations. In turn, community members are more likely to support and use public programs and services when they have input into setting priorities and tailoring programs and services to local needs and circumstances. Open and transparent communication that is facilitated through community coalitions may also increase public awareness of relevant policy/legislative issues and provide better evaluation of the impact of coalition strategies (Jackson & Maddy, 2001). Finally, coalition membership may lead to increased resident participation and leadership, skills, resources, social/interorganizational networks, sense of community, community power, and successful community problem solving (Kegler et al., 2007, 2009; Kegler & Swan, 2011, 2012). The benefits of community coalition approaches are widely accepted by government agencies and foundations, and, as a result, many prevention initiatives over the past three decades have required the formation of community coalitions as a condition of funding. The next section describes the theory, constructs, and assumptions developed to further our understanding of community coalitions.

Community Coalition Action Theory (CCAT)

The literature is rich with case studies, evaluation/research findings, and conceptual frameworks to explain how coalitions function and how they are instrumental in creating community change. CCAT attempts to synthesize and provide an overarching framework for what is known about coalitions both empirically and from years of collective experiences (Butterfoss & Kegler, 2009). The theoretical underpinnings of CCAT, which are articulated in "practice-proven propositions," draw from a rich volume of prior work in community development, participation and empowerment, interorganizational relationships, and social capital (Butterfoss & Kegler, 2002; Kawachi et al., 2008; Kreuter & Lezin, 2002; Minkler & Wallerstein, 2012; Putnam, 2000; Wendel et al., 2009).

CCAT has been described in detail elsewhere (Butterfoss & Kegler, 2002; Butterfoss & Kegler, 2009); the definitions of constructs are listed in table 18.1 and its propositions in table 18.2. According to the model, coalitions progress through stages from formation to institutionalization, with frequent loops back to earlier stages as new issues arise or as planning cycles are repeated (Proposition 1). Although researchers have presented various series of stages, we suggest three: formation, maintenance, and institutionalization (Butterfoss & Kegler, 2009). The next sections describe these stages of coalition development and associated tasks, as well as factors that influence success at each stage (Proposition 2). Each of these stages is influenced by community context, including the sociopolitical climate, norms and values, geography, and history of collaboration or race relations that surround collaborative efforts (Proposition 3). Reputation of the convening agency and history of past collaborations can affect who will join a coalition and who will share resources, geography can shape assessment methods, community values can influence the types of intervention strategies prioritized, and historical economic or racial divides can affect who participates in coalition activities (Kegler et al., 2011).

Coalition Formation (Propositions 4–14)

Coalitions typically form when a lead agency or convener group responds to an opportunity, such as new funding, a threat such as the closing of a rural hospital,

TABLE 18.1

Constructs, Community Coalition Action Theory

Constructs	Definition
Stages of development	Specific stages or phases that a coalition progresses through from formation to implementation to maintenance to institutionalization. Coalitions may recycle through stages more than once or as new members are recruited, plans are renewed, and/or new issues are added.
Community context	Specific factors in the community that may enhance or inhibit coalition function and influence how the coalition moves through its stages of development. These factors include history of collaboration, politics, social capital, trust between community sectors and organizations, geography, and community readiness.
Lead agency/ convener group	Organization that responds to an opportunity, threat, or mandate by agreeing to convene the coalition; provides technical assistance, financial or material support; lends its credibility and reputation to the coalition; and provides valuable networks/contacts.
Coalition membership	Core group of people who represent diverse interest groups, agencies, organizations, and institutions and are committed to resolving health or social issues by becoming coalition members.
Processes	Means by which business is conducted in the coalition setting by developing clear processes that facilitate staff and member communication, problem solving, decisionmaking, conflict management, orientation, training, planning, evaluation, and resource allocation. These processes help create a positive organizational climate in which the benefits of participation outweigh the costs.
Leadership and staffing	Volunteer leaders and paid staff with the interpersonal and organizational skills to facilitate the collaborative process and improve coalition functioning.
Structures	Formalized organizational arrangement, rules, roles, and procedures that are developed in a coalition to maximize its effectiveness. These include vision and mission statements, goals and objectives, an organizational chart, steering committee and work groups, job descriptions, and meeting schedules.

(continued)

Table 18.1. (continued)

Constructs	Definition
Member engagement	Satisfaction, commitment, and participation of members in the work of the coalition.
Pooled member and external resources	Resources that are contributed or elicited as in-kind contributions, grants, donations, fund raisers, or dues from member organizations or external sources that ensure effective coalition assessment, planning, and implementation of strategies.
Collaborative synergy	Mechanism through which coalitions gain a collaborative advantage through engaging diverse members and pooling of member, community, and external resources.
Assessment and planning	Comprehensive assessment and planning activities that make successful implementation of effective strategies more likely.
Implementation of strategies	Strategic actions that the coalition implements across multiple ecological levels that make changes in community policies, practices, and environments more likely.
Community change outcomes	Measurable changes in community policies, practices, and environments that may increase community capacity and improve health or social outcomes.
Health/social outcomes	Measurable changes in health status and social conditions of a community that are the ultimate indicators of coalition effectiveness.
Community capacity	Characteristics of communities that affect their ability to identify, mobilize, and address social and public health problems. Participating in a coalition may enhance these characteristics, which include citizen participation and leadership, skills, resources, social and interorganizational networks, sense of community, and power.

Source: Butterfoss and Kegler (2009).

or a mandate from higher levels of administration, such as the state or federal government for local agencies, or regional or national headquarters for other types of organizations. Community-based organizations, health departments or other local government units, educational institutions, or local hospitals may serve as conveners, depending on the project and its required financial accountability systems. The lead agency initiates coalition formation by recruiting a core group of community leaders and providing initial support for the coalition. Some community

TABLE 18.2

Constructs and Related Propositions, Community Coalition Action Theory

Constructs	Propositions
Stages of development	1. Coalitions develop in specific stages and recycle through them as new members are recruited, plans are renewed, and/or new issues are added.
	2. At each stage, specific factors enhance coalition function and progression to the next stage.
Community context	3. Coalitions are heavily influenced by contextual factors in the community throughout all stages of development.
Lead agency/ convener group	4. Coalitions form when a lead agency or convener responds to an opportunity, threat, or mandate.
	5. Coalition formation is more likely when the lead agency or convener provides technical assistance, financial or material support, credibility, and valuable networks/contacts.
	6. Coalition formation is likely to be more successful when the lead agency or convener enlists community gatekeepers to help develop credibility and trust with others in the community.
Coalition membership	7. Coalition formation usually begins by recruiting a core group of people who are committed to resolving the health or social issue.
	8. More effective coalitions result when the core group expands to include a broad constituency of participants who represent diverse interest groups and organizations.
Processes	9. Open and frequent communication among staff and members helps make collaborative synergy more likely through member engagement and pooling of resources.
	10. Shared and formalized decisionmaking helps make collaborative synergy more likely through member engagement and pooling of resources.
	11. Conflict management helps make collaborative synergy more likely through member engagement and pooling of resources.

(continued)

Table 18.2. (continued)

Constructs	Propositions
Leadership and staffing	12. Strong leadership from a team of staff and members improves coalition functioning and makes collaborative synergy more likely through member engagement and pooling of resources.
	13. Paid staff make collaborative synergy more likely through member engagement and pooling of resources.
Structures	14. Formalized rules, roles, structures, and procedures improve collaborative functioning and make collaborative synergy more likely through member engagement and pooling of resources.
Member engagement	15. Satisfied and committed members will participate more fully in the work of the coalition.
Pooled member and external resources	16. Synergistic pooling of member and external resources prompts comprehensive assessment, planning, and implementation of strategies.
Assessment and planning	17. Successful implementation of effective strategies is more likely when comprehensive assessment and planning occur.
Implementation of strategies	18. Coalitions are more likely to create change in community policies, practices, and environments when they direct interventions at multiple levels.
Community change outcomes	19. Coalitions that are able to change community policies, practices, and environments are more likely to increase capacity and improve health/social outcomes.
Health/social outcomes	20. The ultimate indicator of coalition effectiveness is improvement in health and social outcomes.
Community capacity	21. By participating in successful coalitions, community members and organizations develop capacity and build social capital that can be applied to other health and social issues and makes coalition sustainability more likely.

Source: Butterfoss and Kegler (2009).

groups may not have 501(c)(3) status and, therefore, have difficulties accepting grant funds, which often support coalition formation. One model that has worked in some smaller communities is for a regional organization to serve as the fiscal sponsor, while another more local organization takes responsibility for coalition-building and strategic aspects of an initiative. Research on coalitions suggests that coalitions often evolve from other pre-existing coalitions and networks (Butterfoss, Gilmore, et al., 2006), which may accelerate their development. On the other hand, new initiatives can inherit past agendas, old ways of thinking, and grievances and conflicts that may limit coalition effectiveness (Kadushin et al., 2005). Composition of the core group affects its ability to engage a broad spectrum of the community (Kegler et al., 2010). Communities are often divided, sometimes by social class or race/ethnicity, values and ideology, or features of the geography, such as waterways that congest bridges, tunnels, and roads. According to CCAT, the core group must recruit those committed to the prioritized issue and a broad constituency of diverse groups and organizations, including community gatekeepers and residents who have lived experience with the issue. With increased attention to health equity, engagement of residents directly affected by the priority issue is especially critical and should occur early in coalition formation to facilitate equitable processes and power sharing (Wolff et al., 2017). This pooling of diverse views, perspectives, and resources is the hallmark of a coalition approach and enables them to address problems in ways that a single agency could not achieve on its own. Effective coalitions are deliberate in recruiting diverse members with specific expertise, constituencies, perspectives, backgrounds, and sectors.

Another important task in the formation stage of coalition development is the selection of staff and leadership. Effective coalition leadership requires a collection of qualities and skills that are typically not found in one individual, but rather in a team of committed leaders. Coalitions are labor intensive in terms of cultivating and maintaining relationships and ensuring smooth and efficient group processes. Insufficient or poor leadership can lead to coalition failure through endless meetings with no real substance or infrequent meetings with no progress between meetings. Empirical research on coalitions shows a consistent relationship between leader competence and member satisfaction. Research also demonstrates relationships between staff competence and member satisfaction, member benefits, participation, action plan quality, resource mobilization, implementation of planned activities, and perceived accomplishments (Florin et al., 2000; Kegler & Swan, 2011; Kegler et al., 2005).

Coalition leaders and staff organize the structures through which coalitions accomplish their work and are responsible for coalition processes, such as communication and decisionmaking that keep members satisfied and committed to coalition efforts. Practically speaking, coalitions accomplish much of their day-to-day work in small groups. Therefore, managing group processes, such as decisionmaking, communication, and conflict management, is critical (Butterfoss, LaChance, et al., 2006; Florin et al., 2000; Kegler & Swan, 2011; Kegler et al., 2005).

CCAT asserts that more formal coalitions are better able to engage members, pool resources, and assess and plan well. Formalization is the degree to which rules, roles, and procedures are precisely defined. Examples of formal structures include committees, written memorandums of understanding, bylaws, policy and procedures manuals; clearly defined roles; mission statements, goals, and objectives; and regular reorientation to the mission, goals, roles, and procedures of collaboration (Butterfoss, 2007). Formal structures often result in the routinization or persistent implementation of the coalition's operations. The more routinized operations become, the more likely it is that they will be sustained. Some coalitions, especially those with a high proportion of grassroots residents, may view formalization as inconsistent with local culture. The external trappings of formalization may not be essential (e.g., bylaws, Robert's Rules of Order), but the underlying advantages of clarity of mission, continuity between meetings, and transparent processes are usually essential to success.

Coalition Maintenance and Implementation (Propositions 15–20)

Following coalition formation, coalitions must plan, select, and implement actions to address their priority issues. The maintenance stage involves sustaining member involvement and creating collaborative synergy toward this end. At this point in a coalition's life cycle, members have been recruited, structures and processes are in place, and ideally, members are enthused about their upcoming collaborative work. Members are the *lifeblood* of a coalition—they set its vision, course, and outcomes. Importantly, when both grassroots and professional residents are actively engaged (Wolff et al., 2017), members represent the *authentic voices* of the community. Capable and well-connected coalition members are sought after, recruited, trained, and valued. Member engagement is best defined as the process by which members are empowered and develop a sense of belonging to the coalition (Butterfoss & Kegler, 2009). Positive engagement is evidenced by commitment to the mission and goals of the coalition, high levels of participation both in and outside of coalition meetings and activities, and satisfaction with the work of the coalition (Butterfoss & Kegler, 2009). Engaging members over time is more likely when the benefits of membership outweigh the costs and when members experience a positive coalition environment (Butterfoss, 2007).

Success in this stage depends on the mobilization and pooling of member and external resources. To foster member engagement, coalitions should review their roster annually and ask for continued commitment. However, members often participate in coalitions with varying levels of intensity—they may be core members who assume leadership roles or those who seek networking opportunities. Members rarely stay active throughout the coalition's life and may experience burnout if they do. Having different categories of membership provides flexibility that allows members to move into and out of activities depending on competing loyalties or demands from home or work. Being attentive to barriers to engagement (e.g., days and times of meetings, childcare, translation), especially for those who cannot attend as part of their paid positions, is critically important in efforts to implement equity-oriented processes (Wolff et al., 2017). Categories of members for community coalitions include (Butterfoss, 2007) the following:

- *Active members*—involved in the work of the coalition, attend most meetings/events, serve on work groups, assume leadership roles, recruit members, and help with fundraising.
- *Less-active members*—lend their name and credibility to coalition efforts, publicly promote its work, and provide valuable connections to key organizations or populations, even if they only attend occasional coalition meetings or events. These members include community leaders, administrators, school officials, politicians, or religious leaders.
- *Inactive members*—networkers or those who want to stay informed and receive mailings but rarely attend meetings. They may be asked to do specific tasks or become active later.
- *Shared members*—more than one individual is selected by their organization to alternately attend meetings and share responsibilities. The downside of this arrangement is that valuable time is spent in "catching members up" and they often are unprepared to make decisions.

Coalition maintenance also entails the ongoing pooling of resources and mobilization of talents and diverse approaches to problem solving. When human and material resources are relatively scarce, collaboration is a necessary and logical strategy for addressing community problems, such as health inequities. Disparities and inequities in health have multiple causes and consequences that require complex solutions from multiple disciplines, organizations, and perspectives. In some communities, health and human services organizations are limited in addressing such issues due to fragmented services, unequal access to resources, and an emphasis on service delivery over changes in policies, systems, and environments. By sharing their human and material resources, finances, and time, coalitions provide a multifaceted approach that can reverse the declining trend in civic engagement and re-engage organizations and interested residents to address local problems (Wolff, 2010).

Members are a coalition's greatest asset—they bring energy, knowledge, skills, expertise, perspectives, connections, and tangible resources to the table. The power to combine the perspectives, resources, and skills of a group of individuals and organizations has been termed *synergy* (Lasker et al., 2001). This pooling of resources ensures more effective assessment, planning, and implementation of comprehensive strategies that give coalitions unique advantages over less collaborative problem-solving approaches (Lasker et al., 2001). Both internal and external partners can provide meeting facilities, mailing lists, referrals, loans or donations, equipment, supplies, cosponsorship of events, and valuable community connections (Braithwaite et al., 2000).

Effective coalitions have leaders that promote productive interactions among diverse members and make good use of their participants' in-kind resources, financial resources, and time (Lasker et al., 2001). High levels of synergy result from collaborative administration and management and the ability of coalitions to obtain enough nonfinancial resources from their participants (e.g., skills, information, connections, and endorsements). In short, the synergy that is created from collaborative work results in greater accomplishments than each group working on its own could ever achieve (Lasker et al., 2001).

Coalitions achieve their goals by pooling resources, combined with assessing a situation and selecting actions that target the most critical determinants of a problem. Once a coalition is formed and has its structures and processes in place, one of its first priorities is often to conduct a community assessment. Community assessment is the process of understanding a community in terms of its strengths, needs, constituencies, history and politics, leadership structure, and related factors that affect community problem solving (Bartholomew et al., 2016; see also chapter 10). Assessment also involves identifying a priority health issue or social issue, determining who it affects disproportionately, and assessing its behavioral and environmental determinants using a socioecological lens. Critical reflection on root causes of persistent inequities, including structural racism and other social determinants of health, has heightened urgency with recent events of police violence and COVID-19. According to CCAT, coalitions that conduct comprehensive community assessments are better positioned to select and implement strategies that will make a difference.

The coalition relies on resources from members and external sources to design culturally appropriate, creative, and comprehensive strategies and to identify and adapt evidence-based interventions or best practices that are appropriate for the local context and have the greatest chance of leading to the desired health or social outcomes. Adaptations of interventions that have been previously evaluated (evidence-based) or are commonly accepted as best practices increase the likelihood that interventions will result in community change, and ultimately, desired health and social outcomes. Newly developed or untested strategies may also be valuable, of course, but warrant evaluation to ensure movement toward desired goals. Most researchers and practitioners agree that effective health promotion efforts require change at multiple levels, including environmental and policy change. Using best practices or evidence-based interventions should minimize a past tendency of coalitions to focus on building community awareness. While a focus on quick wins may help to maintain member interest, it is unlikely to lead to more valued outcomes (Kreuter et al., 2000).

Successful implementation depends on numerous factors, such as sufficient acquisition of resources, completion of tasks on schedule, fidelity to the planned strategies, engaged coalition members, and supportive organizational and community environments. Assuming the strategies link logically to planned outcomes, the likelihood of achieving these outcomes depends on the extent to which the strategies are implemented and reach the priority populations. Additionally, implementation of strategies must be of sufficient duration and intensity to have an effect. If these strategies are effective, shorter-term outcomes, such as changes in individual knowledge, beliefs, self-efficacy, behavior, and public support for policy change occur, as well as changes in community systems, policies, practices, and environments. These intermediate changes should lead to long-term outcomes, such as reductions in morbidity and mortality or substantive progress toward other social goals.

Institutionalization: Planning for Sustainability (Proposition 21)

Finally, in the *institutionalization stage*, successful strategies lead to outcomes. If resources have been adequately mobilized and strategies effectively address an ongoing need, coalition strategies may become institutionalized as part of a long-term coalition or be adopted by other community organizations. The coalition itself may or may not be institutionalized in a community. Most communities currently face a tough environment with limited and shorter funding cycles, increased competition for resources, and economic downturns. Sustainability is often misunderstood as only involving sustained funding, since when the funding ends, so does the commitment. However, sustainability does not depend on one strategy, policy, or approach, but instead requires developing community understanding and leadership to embed new solutions in institutions; literally, *institution*alizing polices and organizational practices within community norms. With this understanding of sustainability, even if funding and efforts diminish, health has been embedded and lasting change remains (Batan et al., 2012).

Despite their critical role in promoting health and preventing disease, many coalitions are unable to sustain their efforts long enough to change policies, systems, and environments. In order to create and build momentum to maintain community-wide change, coalitions must fulfill their missions and be effectively managed and governed. Sustainable coalitions (1) develop strong, experienced leaders; (2) have broad, deep organizational and community ties; (3) coordinate efforts; (4) implement interventions based on best practices; and (5) allow adequate time for sustainability planning (Feinberg et al., 2008; Nelson et al., 2007). Sustainability planning should begin early and continue throughout the life of the coalition. A sustained coalition will be more likely to attract varied funding sources and establish credibility among its constituency and policymakers (Centers for Disease Control and Prevention, 2008).

Besides developing coalitions and partnerships, sustainability involves initiating a groundswell of community strategies that create change at the local level and assembling a wide range of disciplines to work with communities to improve their health. Sustainability can be considered from short- and long-term perspectives (Centers for Disease Control and Prevention, 2011). *Short-term sustainability* deals with tasks that must be done to keep a strategy in place long enough to achieve its objectives. It means having buy-in and support from key decisionmakers and community volunteers; having enough leadership and funding, and clear communications; and putting procedures in place to monitor results and modify strategies that are not working. *Long-term sustainability* is more proactive and future oriented. It means (1) having a long-term plan for assuring the viability of an organization or a community-led initiative that manages several policy, systems, and environmental change strategies; (2) developing a diverse funding portfolio, collaborative leaders, and marketing/branding strategies; and (3) ensuring that the community, its organizations, and strategies are ready to respond to changes in the environment.

Both maintenance and institutionalization stages of coalition development have the potential to increase community capacity to solve problems, and community capacity, in turn, can be viewed as a sustainable outcome. Progress in ameliorating one community problem can potentially increase the capacity of local organizations to apply these skills and resources to addressing additional issues that resonate with the community.

Future of Coalition Approaches

Coalitions are excellent vehicles for consensus building and active involvement of diverse organizations and constituencies in addressing community issue(s). They enable communities to build capacity and to intervene using a social ecological approach, which helps to ensure that needs are met and interventions are culturally sensitive. Community engagement through coalitions also facilitates ownership, which, in turn, is thought to increase the chances of successful institutionalization into the community (Butterfoss, 2007). Future research efforts should focus on what coalitions contribute to community-based strategies above and beyond more traditional approaches (Berkowitz, 2001; Butterfoss et al., 2001; Lasker et al., 2001). For example, do coalitions develop more innovative strategies due to the pooling of expertise and resources? Do they reach previously untapped community assets? Are they better able to implement certain interventions than traditional public health and social service agencies, such as policy or media advocacy for social change? What are the long-term benefits and unintended positive outcomes for communities? How should coalitions be structured to ensure equity-oriented processes that meaningfully address social determinants of health, such as racism (Wolff et al., 2017).

Community coalitions, like other community-level initiatives, are challenged to document long-term outcomes and to quantitatively attribute resulting changes to the initiative (Ellen et al., 2015; Florin et al., 2000; Gabriel, 2000; Kegler et al., 2020; Woods et al., 2015), although a few studies have done so (Feinberg et al., 2010; Flewelling & Hanley, 2016; Plescia et al., 2008). In contrast, the contributions of coalitions to community changes, such as programs, policies, systems, and environments that support health have been documented in a large number of studies (Brownson et al., 2012; Cheadle et al., 2010, 2018; Collie-Akers et al., 2013; Kegler et al., 2008, 2020; Kowalczyk et al., 2017; Sanchez et al., 2015). By strengthening the theoretical base and developing a model of action for community coalitions, this overall area of scientific inquiry will be advanced. Researchers and evaluators have used the CCAT model to field test our assumptions and deepen our understanding of which coalition characteristics and interactions are most likely to fuel goal attainment (Flood et al., 2015; Klushman et al., 2006; Miller et al., 2017; Reed et al., 2014; Wolfe et al., 2020). In one of the more in-depth applications of CCAT, researchers interviewed over 300 key informants to characterize how coalition factors and community context, as articulated by CCAT, influenced the ability of fourteen Connect-to-Protect Coalitions to reduce youth risk for HIV through structural change (Ellen et al., 2015; Miller et al., 2017; Reed et al., 2014). This study found general support for CCAT propositions, but it also sparked additional conversation about the challenges of designing studies that capture the impact of improved policies, systems, and environments on health (Ellen et al., 2015; Woods et al., 2015). Equally as important, practitioners, the front-line coalition pioneers, will determine whether this model continues to be useful in increasing local support and capacity for further coalition development.

Questions for Further Discussion

1. How does community context influence how you develop an appropriate structure and operating procedures for a community coalition?
2. What are some situations in which a community coalition would be the best approach for community mobilization? In what types of situations might a different approach be more appropriate?

Acknowledgments

Portions of this chapter were adapted from Butterfoss, F. D., & Kegler, M. C. (2009). Community Coalition Action Theory. In R. DiClemente, L. Crosby, & M. C. Kegler (Eds.), *Emerging Theories in Health Promotion Practice and Research* (2nd ed, pp. 237–276). Jossey-Bass/Wiley. Reprinted with permission of authors and John Wiley and Sons.

REFERENCES

Bartholomew, L., Markham, C., Ruiter, R., Fernandez, M., Kok, G., & Parcel, G. (2016). *Planning Health Promotion Programs: An Intervention Mapping Approach* (4th ed.). Jossey-Bass.
Batan, M., Jaffe, A., Butterfoss, F. D., & LaPier, T. (2012). *A Sustainability Planning Guide for Healthy Communities.* CDC Division of Adult and Community Health, Healthy Communities

Program. https://www.cdc.gov/nccdphp/dch/programs/healthycommunitiesprogram/pdf/sustainability_guide.pdf.

Berkowitz, B. (2001). Studying the outcomes of community-based coalitions. *Am J Community Psychol, 29*(2), 213–228.

Braithwaite, R., Taylor, S., & Austin, J. (2000). *Building Health Coalitions in the Black Community.* Sage.

Brownson, R., Brennan, L., Evenson, K., & Leviton, L. (2012). Lessons from a mixed-methods approach to evaluating Active Living by Design. *Am J Prev Med, 43*(5, suppl 4), S271–S280.

Butterfoss, F., Cashman, S., Foster-Fishman, P., & Kegler, M. (2001). Roundtable discussion of Berkowitz's paper. *Am J Community Psychol, 29*(2), 229–240.

Butterfoss, F., Goodman, R., & Wandersman, A. (1993). Community coalitions for prevention and health promotion. *Health Educ Res, 8*(3), 315–330.

Butterfoss, F. D. (2007). *Coalitions and Partnerships for Community Health.* Jossey-Bass.

Butterfoss, F. D., Gilmore, L. A., Krieger, J. W., LaChance, L. L., Lara, M., Meurer, J. R., Nichols, E. A., Orians, C. E., Peterson, J. W., Rose, S. W., & Rosenthal, M. P. (2006). From formation to action: How Allies against asthma coalitions are getting the job done. *Health Promot Pract, 7*(2_suppl), 34S–43S.

Butterfoss, F. D., & Kegler, M. C. (2002). Toward a comprehensive understanding of community coalitions: Moving from practice to theory. In R. DiClemente, L. Crosby, & M. C. Kegler (Eds.), *Emerging Theories in Health Promotion Practice and Research* (pp. 157–193). Jossey-Bass.

Butterfoss, F. D., & Kegler, M. C. (2009). The Community Coalition Action Theory. In R. J. DiClemente, R. A. Crosby, and M. C. Kegler (Eds.), *Emerging Theories in Health Promotion Practice and Research* (2nd ed., pp. 237–276). Jossey-Bass.

Butterfoss, F. D., LaChance, L. L., & Orians, C. E. (2006). Building allies coalitions: Why formation matters. *Health Promot Pract, 7*(2_suppl), 23S–33S.

Centers for Disease Control and Prevention (CDC). (2008). *Best Practices Users Guide: Coalitions; State and Community Interventions.* US Department of Health and Human Services, National Center for Chronic Disease Prevention and Health Promotion, Office on Smoking and Health. http://www.ct.gov/sustinet/lib/sustinet/referencelibrary/tobacco/cdcuser_guide.pdf.

Centers for Disease Control and Prevention (CDC). (2011). *A Sustainability Planning Guide for Healthy Communities.* Division of Community Health. National Center for Chronic Disease Prevention and Health Promotion. http://www.cdc.gov/nccdphp/dch/programs/healthycommunitiesprogram/pdf/sustainability_guide.pdf.

Cheadle, A., Atiedu, A., Rauzon, S., Schwartz, P., Keene, L., Davoudi, M., Spring, R., Molina, M., Lee, L., Boyle, K., & Williamson, D. (2018). A community-level initiative to prevent obesity: Results from Kaiser Permanente's Healthy Eating Active Living Zones Initiative in California. *Am J Prev Med, 54*, S150–S159.

Cheadle, A., Egger, R., LoGerfo, J. P., Schwartz, S., & Harris, J. R. (2010). Promoting sustainable community change in support of older adult physical activity: Evaluation findings from the Southeast Seattle Senior Physical Activity Network (SESPAN). *J Urban Health, 87*(1), 67–75.

Clarke, N. M., Doctor, L. J., Friedman, A. R., Lachance, L. L., Houle, C. R., Geng, X., & Grisso, J. A. (2006). Community coalitions to control chronic disease: Allies against asthma as a model and case study. *Health Promot Pract, 7*(2_suppl), 14S–22S.

Collie-Akers, V. L., Fawcett, S. B., & Schultz, J. A. (2013). Measuring progress of collaborative action in a community health effort. *Rev Panam Salud Publica, 34*, 422–428.

Dowling, J., O'Donnell, H. J., & Wellington Consulting Group. (2000). *A Development Manual for Asthma Coalitions.* The CHEST Foundation & the American College of Chest Physicians.

Ellen, J. M., Greenberg, L., Willard, N., Korelitz, J., Kapogiannis, B. G., Monte, D., Boyer, C. B., Harper, G. W., Henry-Reid, L. M., Friedman, L. B., & Gonin, R. (2015). Evaluation of the effect of human immunodeficiency virus-related structural interventions: The connect to protect project. *JAMA Pediatrics, 169*(3), 256–263.

Feighery, E., & Rogers, T. (1990). *Building and Maintaining Effective Coalitions.* Health Promotion Resource Center, Stanford Center for Research in Disease Prevention.

Feinberg, M. E., Bontempo, D. E., & Greenberg, M. T. (2008). Predictors and level of sustainability of community prevention coalitions. *Am J Prev Med, 34*(6), 495–501.

Feinberg, M. E., Jones, D., Greenberg, M. T., Osgood, D. W., & Bontempo, D. (2010). Effects of the Communities That Care model in Pennsylvania on change in adolescent risk and problem behaviors. *Prev Sci, 11*(2), 163–171.

Flewelling, R., & Hanley, S. M. (2016). Assessing community coalition capacity and its association with underage drinking prevention effectiveness in the context of the SPF SIG. *Prev Sci, 17*(7), 830–840.

Flood, J., Minkler, M., Lavery, S. H., Estrada, J., & Falbe, J. (2015). The collective impact model and its potential for health promotion: Overview and case study of a healthy retail initiative in Dan Francisco. *Health Educ Behav, 42*(5), 654–668.

Florin, P., Mitchell, R., Stevenson, J., & Klein, I. (2000). Predicting intermediate outcomes for prevention coalitions: A developmental perspective. *Eval Program Plan, 23*(3), 341–346.

Gabriel, R. (2000). Methodological challenges in evaluating community partnerships and coalitions: Still crazy after all these years. *J Community Psychol, 28*(3), 339–352.

Gray, B. (2000). Assessing inter-organizational collaboration: Multiple conceptions and multiple methods. In D. Faulkner & M. de Rand (Eds.), *Cooperative Strategy: Economic, Business and Organizational Issues* (pp. 243–260). Oxford University Press.

Jackson, D., & Maddy, W. (2001). Introduction to coalitions. Ohio State University Fact Sheet CDFS-1. Ohio Center for Action on Coalitions. https://ohioline.osu.edu/factsheet/CDFS-1.

Kadushin, C., Lindholm, M., Ryan, D., Brodsky, A., & Saxe, L. (2005). Why it is so difficult to form effective community coalitions. *City and Community, 4*(3), 255–275.

Kawachi, I., Subramanian, S. V., & Kim, D. (2008). *Social Capital and Health.* Springer.

Kegler, M., Norton, B., & Aronson, B. (2007). Skill improvement among coalition members in the California Healthy Cities and Communities Program. *Health Educ Res, 22*(3), 450–457.

Kegler, M., Norton, B., & Aronson, R. (2008). Achieving organizational change: Findings from case studies of 20 California Healthy Cities and Communities coalitions. *Health Promot Int, 23*(2), 109–118.

Kegler, M., Painter, J., Twiss, J., Aronson, R., & Norton, B. (2009). Evaluation findings on community participation in the California Healthy Cities and Communities Program. *Health Promot Int, 24*(4), 300–310.

Kegler, M., Rigler, J., & Honeycutt, S. (2010). How does community context influence coalitions in the formation stage? A multiple case study based on the Community Coalition Action Theory. *BMC Public Health, 10,* 90.

Kegler, M., Rigler, J., & Honeycutt, S. (2011). The role of community context in planning and implementing community-based health promotion projects. *Eval Program Plann, 34*(3), 246–253.

Kegler, M., & Swan, D. (2011). An initial attempt at operationalizing and testing the Community Coalition Action Theory. *Health Educ Behav, 38*(3), 261–270.

Kegler, M., & Swan, D. (2012). Advancing coalition theory: The effect of coalition factors on community capacity mediated by member engagement. *Health Educ Res, 27*(4), 572–584.

Kegler, M. C., Halpin, S. N., & Butterfoss, F. D. (2020). Evaluation methods commonly used to assess effectiveness of community coalitions in public health: Results from a scoping review. *New Dir Eval, 2020*(165), 139–157.

Kegler, M. C., Williams, C. W., Cassell, C. M., Santelli, J., Kegler, S. R., Montgomery, S. B., Bell, M. L., Martinez, Y. G., Klein, J. D., Mulhall, P., & Will, J. A. (2005). Mobilizing communities for teen pregnancy prevention: Associations between coalition characteristics and perceived accomplishments. *J Adolesc Health, 37*(3_suppl), S31–S41.

Kluhsman, B., Bencivenga, M., Ward, A., Lehman, E., & Lengerich, E. (2006). Initiatives of 11 rural Appalachian cancer coalitions in Pennsylvania and New York. *Prev Chronic Dis, 3*(4). Serial online. https://www.cdc.gov/pcd/issues/2006/oct/06_0045.htm.

Kowalczyk, S., Randolph, S. M., & Oravecz, L. (2017). Community coalitions' gender-aware policy and systems changes to improve the health of women and girls. *Women's Health Issues, 27*(suppl 1), S6–S13.

Kreuter, M., & Lezin, N. (2002). Social capital theory: Implications for community-based health promotion. In R. DiClemente, L. Crosby, & M. C. Kegler (Eds.), *Emerging Theories in Health Promotion Practice and Research* (pp. 228–254). Jossey-Bass.

Kreuter, M., Lezin, N., & Young, L. (2000). Evaluating community-based collaborative mechanisms: Implications for practitioners. *Health Promot Pract, 1*(1), 49–63.

Lasker, R., Weiss, E., & Miller, R. (2001). Partnership synergy: A practical framework for studying and strengthening the collaborative advantage. *Millbank Q, 79*(2), 179–205.

Miller, R. L., Reed, S. J., Chiaramonte, D., Strzyzykowski, T., Spring, H., Acevedo-Polakovich, I. D., Chutuape, K., Cooper-Walker, B., Boyer, C. B., & Ellen, J. M. (2017). Structural and community change outcomes of the Connect-to-Protect Coalitions: Trials and triumphs securing adolescent access to HIV prevention, testing, and medical care. *Am J Community Psychol, 60*(1–2), 199–214.

Minkler, M., & Wallerstein, N. (2012). Improving health through community organization and community building: A health education perspective. In M. Minkler (Ed.), *Community Organizing and Community Building for Health and Welfare* (3rd ed., pp. 37–58). Rutgers University Press.

Nelson, D. E., Reynolds, J. H., Luke, D. A., Mueller, N. B., Eischen, M. H., Jordan, J., Lancaster, R. B., Marcus, S. E., & Vallone, D. (2007). Successfully maintaining program funding during trying times: Lessons learned from tobacco control programs in five states. *J Public Health Manag Pract, 13*(6), 612–620.

Plescia, M., Herrick, H., & Chavis, L. (2008). Improving health behaviors in an African American community: The Charlotte racial and ethnic approaches to community health project. *Am J Public Health, 98*(9), 1678–1684.

Putnam, R. (2000). *Bowling Alone: The Collapse and Revival of American Community.* Simon and Schuster.

Reed, S. J., Miller, R. L., Francisco, V. T., & Adolescent Medical Trials Network for HIV/AIDS Interventions. (2014). The influence of community context on how coalitions achieve HIV-preventive structural change. *Health Educ Behav, 41*(1), 100–107.

Sanchez, V., Andrews, M. L., Carrillo, C., & Hale, R. (2015). New Mexico community health councils: Documenting contributions to systems changes. *Prog Community Health Partnersh, 9*(4), 471–481.

Wendel, M., Burdine, J., McLeroy, K., Alaniz, A., Norton, B., & Felix, M. (2009). Community capacity: Theory and application. In R. DiClemente, L. Crosby, & M. C. Kegler (Eds.), *Emerging Theories in Health Promotion Practice & Research* (2nd ed., pp. 277–302). Jossey-Bass.

Wolfe, S. M., Long, P. D., & Brown, K. K. (2020). Using a principles-focused evaluation approach to evaluate coalitions and collaboratives working toward equity and social justice. In A. W. Price, K. K. Brown, & S. M. Wolfe (Eds.), Special Issue: Evaluating Community Coalitions and Collaboratives. *New Dir Eval, 165*, 45–65.

Wolff, T. (2010). *The Power of Collaborative Solutions: Six Principles and Effective Tools for Building Healthy Communities.* Jossey-Bass.

Wolff, T., Minkler, M., Wolfe, S. M., Berkowitz, B., Bowen, L., Butterfoss, F. D., Christens, B. D., Francisco, V. T., Himmelman, A. T., & Lee, K. S. (2017). Collaborating for equity and justice: Moving beyond collective impact. *Nonprofit Q, 9*, 42–53.

Woods, W. J., Pollack, L. M., & Binson, D. (2015). The broad approach of a structural intervention study and the lack of effect detection: Target population and sampling issues. *JAMA Pediatr, 169*(8), 790.

19

Addressing Food Insecurity and Tobacco Control through a Neighborhood Coalition

Applying Community Coalition Action Theory and Principles for Collaborating for Equity and Justice

PATRICIA WAKIMOTO

SUSANA HENNESSEY LAVERY

MEREDITH MINKLER

JESSICA ESTRADA

Even before the COVID-19 pandemic threw millions of Americans out of work and left one-third of households with children food insecure, one in seven Americans suffered from food insecurity, which is defined as having "limited or uncertain access to adequate food" (Coleman-Jensen et al., 2020). However, as Farley and Sykes (2015) note, for many low-resource communities, the problem is not lack of access to food per se, but lack of access to *healthy* food. In densely populated neighborhoods, food insecurity intersects with an overabundance of advertising, display, and availability of tobacco and alcohol in the local retail environment (Minkler, Falbe et al., 2018, p. 294). Under-resourced communities frequently lack a single full-service grocery store but have numerous small corner stores that are heavily stocked with processed foods, sugary beverages, cigarettes, and liquor. These small stores are often owned by immigrants or other residents of color who have modest incomes and lack the funds and infrastructure to maintain fresh produce and other healthy foods. A small business owner is commonly offered attractive incentives by large conglomerates to stock their tobacco or other products and display their product advertising (Laska et al., 2018). Neighborhoods in which these small stores operate have elevated rates of morbidity and premature mortality, linked in part to poor diets, smoking, heavy drinking, and other unhealthy behaviors that are often a response to stressors of life in low-resource environments (Hagan & Rubin, 2013; Kaplan et al., 2015).

Here, we describe an established coalition in San Francisco, California, and its efforts to study and address the challenges of food insecurity and tobacco saturation in its neighborhood and citywide. Our case study is the Tenderloin Healthy Corner Store Coalition, a community-driven and led coalition between residents and local community-based organizations (CBOs), agencies, the San Francisco Department of Public Health (SFDPH), and university partners. This coalition played a leadership role to make the case for and develop, implement, and monitor interventions on the community and municipal policy levels. We explore its formation and evolution from 2011 to the present, using the conceptual framework of Butterfoss and Kegler (2009; chapter 18) known as Community Coalition Action Theory (CCAT). While many other conceptual models exist (Christens & Inzeo, 2015; Kegler et al., 2020), CCAT is the most rigorously developed, and advantages include its strong, overarching theoretical framework and practice-proven propositions to guide assessment of coalition stages, processes, and outcomes. In addition, following Wolfe et al.'s recommendation that a "principles-focused evaluation approach" be employed when assessing equity-oriented coalitions (2020, p. 45), our case study also incorporates many of the principles of Collaborating for Equity and Justice (CEJ) (Wolff et al., 2017; chapter 1; box 1.1) as an alternative to more-constraining, top-down models.

Case Study: The Tenderloin Healthy Corner Store Coalition

Background and Overview

The Tenderloin is one of San Francisco's most diverse and vibrant neighborhoods, but it is also its poorest, with a poverty rate of 25 percent versus 11 percent citywide (San Francisco Planning Department, 2018). It has one of the city's highest tobacco and alcohol outlet densities and correspondingly elevated rates of tobacco use and alcoholism. Together with deep racial and social inequities and chronic stressors associated with life in poor neighborhoods, these forces compound health risks for residents, who had some of San Francisco's highest rates of acute and chronic diseases (San Francisco Health Improvement Partnership, 2016), even prior to the pandemic.

When the Tenderloin Healthy Corner Store Coalition (hereafter the Coalition) began, its forty-five-block area lacked a full-service grocery store but had seventy-one small corner stores. The small stores stocked primarily prepackaged and heavily processed foods, sugary beverages, tobacco, and alcohol, creating an environment that the local health department saw as significantly contributing to the neighborhood's high rates of heart disease, cancer, and premature death (San Francisco Department of Public Health, 2012). But the Tenderloin also has a long history of activism; it was the site of the first major protest for transgender rights in the 1960s (Grant, 2010), and successfully advocated against unlawful evictions and lack of building compliance with the Americans with Disabilities Act. Consistent with this tradition, the Tenderloin took on the problem of pervasive food insecurity and tobacco saturation and quickly engaged a broad cross sector of supporters.

The Coalition defined as its mission a commitment to improve the community's access to healthy, affordable food and reduce the prevalence of tobacco and alcohol advertising and availability in local corner stores. It sought to change the food and tobacco landscape by focusing on its many small stores, and it employed a multipronged approach that included regular coalition and policy meetings, community events, merchant education and outreach, hiring and training of local "food justice leaders," and advocating for and conducting research. Its contributions on the community and policy levels included gathering and using "data and stories" (chapter 10) to engage the public and policymakers, and helping to craft, pass, implement, and monitor a municipal ordinance creating the Healthy Retail SF (HRSF) program. HRSF incentivized local merchants to shift to a healthy retail business model (www.healthyretailsf.org). In addition to creating and sustaining a strong community-led coalition, it played a significant role in the citywide healthy retail program, through which nine corner stores (six located in the Tenderloin) have formally converted to healthy retail to date. Most of the other stores that participated in the Coalition's annual and detailed store assessment also showed measurable improvements, in part out of a desire to remain competitive and respond to customers' desires and, in some cases, to be better positioned to apply for participation in the program (Minkler et al., 2019). Despite notable challenges, the Coalition developed strengths over time that enabled it to expand and include two other food-insecure neighborhoods, thereby increasing its impact fighting for access to some of life's most basic needs in under-resourced communities.

Formation Stage

Butterfoss and Kegler (2009) presented a series of CCAT propositions that are discussed in detail in chapter 18 and presented in table 18.2. Sample propositions and their relevance to the Tenderloin Coalition case study also are presented in table 19.1. CCAT's fourth proposition, for example, states that *Coalitions form when a lead agency or group responds to an opportunity, threat, or mandate.* For the Tenderloin Coalition, the catalyst was a Google map of the neighborhood's stores made in 2011 by youth from the Vietnamese Youth Development Center (VYDC), with training and funding assistance from the SFDPH Tobacco Free Program and incorporating its Community Action Model (CAM) (Hennessey Lavery, 2005). The five-step model helps communities identify and name their issues, critically analyze root causes, and develop needed skills and resources to "plan, implement and evaluate health-related actions and policies" (p. 611). The youth's Google map showed thirty-five of the neighborhood's approximately seventy corner stores and used the image of an apple, half an apple, or a rotten apple core to capture each store's aggregate rating based on items such as the presence of fresh produce, signs forbidding smoking—and ashtrays! Creation of a literal map provided the youth and their agency both a powerful visual and a starting point for action (table 19.1).

Consistent with CCAT's seventh proposition, *recruiting a core group of committed people* early on, the VYDC shared the apple map with several CBOs and agencies. This prompted follow-up group meetings and a larger community meeting hosted by the VYDC and attended by roughly sixty residents and agency representatives

TABLE 19.1

**Sample CCAT Propositions and Application to the Tenderloin
Healthy Corner Store Coalition**

Proposition	*Example*
4. Coalitions form when a lead agency or convener responds to an opportunity, threat, or mandate.	Vietnamese youths' Google Map showing poor healthy food access and heavy tobacco marketing in local corner stores sparked interest in action. Their agency took the lead in hosting meetings with others, resulting in an agreement to formalize as a coalition.
3. Coalitions are heavily influenced by contextual factors in the community through all stages.	Low-resource and heavily disinvested neighborhoods meant no single agency had the resources to serve as lead, necessitating co-leadership. But a neighborhood history of activism for social justice and a supportive health department (SFDPH) helped the Coalition take hold and succeed. When the COVID-19 pandemic hit, with its outsized impact on the Tenderloin, some Coalition staff and key supporters had to pivot to mitigation efforts and addressing impacts, including large increases in homelessness. Uneven internet access resulted in lower Coalition meeting attendance, but plans were made for a postpandemic resumption of in-person work, including a new store conversion in fall 2021 and more in 2022.
6. Coalition formation is more successful when community gatekeepers are enlisted to help develop credibility and trust with others in the community.	Coalition co-leads hired four residents trusted by merchants and residents alike to serve as Food Justice Leaders (FJLs) and gatekeepers to both. Their role in community and merchant education, store assessments, and other research, plus advocacy for new policies, proved critical to success, and when more funding became available, their number was doubled.
7. Coalition formation usually begins by recruiting a core group of people who are committed to resolving a health or social issue.	Despite their different foci, a core group of agencies initially recruited by the Vietnamese Youth Development Center (VNDC) agreed that healthy food access was "a social justice issue" and that they would work together to address it. Many other agencies in and beyond the neighborhood soon joined, along with local residents.
10. Shared and formalized decisionmaking helps make collaborative synergy more likely.	To accommodate varied levels of education and experience in decisionmaking bodies, a simple majority-rules procedure was employed. All members had equal say at monthly community meetings and on the policy committee, increasing

(continued)

Table 19.1. (continued)

Proposition	Example
	buy-in and belief that the Coalition was more likely to succeed in getting change than any one partner could on its own.
15. Satisfied and committed members will participate more fully in the work of the coalition.	Holding meetings in a familiar community setting, providing refreshments and icebreakers, and including time for participants to share and discuss new issues and upcoming events helped keep members coming back. Democratizing procedures from the formation through institutionalization stages, with opportunities for members to participate at every level from researching issues to helping in store conversions to work on policy development and advocacy, proved satisfying to members who were, in turn, even more committed to their Coalition work.
17. Successful implementation of effective strategies is more likely when comprehensive assessment and planning occur.	Detailed observational assessment of roughly two-thirds of all neighborhood corner stores biannually; education and assistance to merchants interested in possible conversion to healthy retail; use of assessment data in store selection; and detailed planning process with merchants, SFDPH, architects, and Coalition members helped ensure that the stores selected for conversion had the best possible chance for success.
19. Coalitions that are able to change community policies, practices, and environments are more likely to increase capacity and improve health/ social outcomes.	The Coalition's key role in helping secure passage of the SF Healthy Retail ordinance and in implementation and monitoring of the HRSF program, plus merchant and resident education, store conversions, and work on additional policy issues (e.g., soda tax), helped increase community capacity and the building of a healthier community. Measurable increases in selling space for healthy products and decreased space for tobacco in the majority of local stores, plus substantially increased sales of healthy foods, plus some decrease in tobacco sales in intervention stores, may have been *indirect* indicators of improved health outcomes for some patrons. Increased role of Coalition leaders, members, and FJLs in other capacities (e.g., on a citywide advisory group or helping on other policy issues) helped build both community and Coalition capacity.

Column I sources: Butterfoss and Kegler (2009) and chapter 18.

who were enthusiastic about forming a coalition. As a founding member commented, "We had various topics for [discussion] but converting the corner stores from something negative into having a positive influence . . . had the greatest support" (Flood et al., 2015, p. 660). Thus, the Coalition's early mission was to improve access to healthy food and decrease tobacco and other unhealthy influences in the neighborhood by using the network of corner stores as a resource.

The Coalition's formation benefited from two committed CBOs, the VYDC and the nonprofit Tenderloin Neighborhood Development Corporation (TNDC), which volunteered to serve as its cochairs. Ideally, a coalition benefits from a single lead agency, but in low-resource communities, there may not be a single organization with the wherewithal to do this singlehandedly. CCAT's third proposition applies, emphasizing that *coalitions are heavily influenced by contextual factors in the community throughout all stages of development* (Butterfoss & Kegler, 2009, p. 244). In the context of the Tenderloin, a low-resource and heavily disinvested neighborhood, having two committed CBOs sharing leadership and providing sufficient support for the first several years proved to be a solution that worked well (table 19.1). In fact, most members participating in an early in-depth qualitative study named this leadership approach and the cochairs' strong working relationship as major contributors to the Coalition's early success (Flood et al., 2015). In addition to the co-leads and the SFDPH, organizational membership grew to include the Tenderloin Community Benefit District; the Central City SRO (single-room occupancy) Collaborative; the Alleviating Atypical-Antipsychotic Induced Metabolic Syndrome (AAIMS) project; the National Council on Alcoholism, Bay Area; the South East Food Access (SEFA) Food Guardians Project; and the Asian Pacific Islander Wellness Center, among others. Although coalitions are traditionally made up of organizations and groups of which individuals serve in a representative capacity, in the Tenderloin's Coalition the majority of members were neighborhood residents. Some were affiliated with groups like the AAIMS project, but most joined simply because of their personal commitment to the Coalition's mission. Finally, individual members from outside the neighborhood included several University of California, San Francisco, Medical School students; a UC Berkeley School of Public Health faculty member with long ties to the neighborhood; and four graduate community organizing students, one of whom lived in the Tenderloin.

In chapter 18, Butterfoss and Kegler note that "Members are the *lifeblood* of a coalition—they set its vision, course, and outcomes. Importantly, when both grassroots and professional residents are actively engaged (Wolff et al., 2017), members represent the *authentic voices* of the community." This key proposition is reflected in the Coalition's community-driven and community-led nature and the fact that many residents regularly attended monthly meetings and participated in decision-making. Also salient, however, are CCAT's ninth proposition, stressing that *open and frequent communication among staff and members helps make collaborative synergy more likely,* and the tenth proposition, stressing *the importance of shared and formalized decisionmaking* (Butterfoss & Kegler 2009; chapter 18). Holding meetings in a popular community location, on the same day and time each month, paying attention to the four most important words in community work—"refreshments will be served"—and using simple majority rules decisionmaking were keys to getting a strong turnout and helping community residents see that their opinion mattered (table 19.1). The above aspects of Coalition functioning also are illustrative of the second CEJ principle, which recognized that for real power and empowerment, *community stakeholders should be a driving force from the very beginning* (Wolff et al., 2017; box 1.1).

CCAT's sixth proposition states that *coalition formation is more likely to be successful when the lead agency or convener enlists community gatekeepers to help develop credibility and trust with others in the community* (Butterfoss & Kegler, 2009, p. 244). Crucial to the Coalition's mission was the early hiring and training of four residents, who already had strong relationships with residents and merchants, as Food Justice Leaders (FJLs). The idea was in part based on the Bayview neighborhood's Food Guardian model from the SEFA coalition (Breckwich Vásquez et al., 2007; Hennessey Lavery et al., 2005). Tenderloin's FJLs were in the 20s to 60s age range, received a living wage (albeit, working only part time), and after six weeks of training, they conducted much of the Coalition's community-driven research and community education, with technical assistance from Coalition staff, SFDPH, and later university partners. The centrality of their roles, along with those of the cochairs, was in keeping with the CEJ's second and third principles, *recognizing and building resident power* and *having community stakeholders in key leadership positions* (Wolfe et al., 2017, 2020; box 1.1). The FJLs' role in community-engaged research also reflected the CEJ's fifth principle, which puts a premium on work that "shows what works, acknowledge[s] the complexities" and helps in evaluation (Wolfe et al., 2020, p. 47; chapter 1; box 1.1).

Early in its formation stage, the Coalition benefited from the interest of a critical external partner who became an early influential ally. A city supervisor, for whom the Google "apple map" prompted an eye-opening Tenderloin visit and walking tour, publicly commented, "A lot of the stores are covered in cigarette and alcohol ads, or junk food and junk drink ads. . . . *I've really come to see food access as a civil rights issue*" (Minkler et al., 2019, p. 852). The Coalition took advantage of the growing interest of policymakers in sponsoring a healthy retail measure, and, together with Bayview neighborhood counterparts, Coalition members actively involved additional policy allies, interested merchants, the SFDPH, and an architectural design firm (Sutti & Associates) that specialized in corner store redesigns to work out many of the details and more effectively make the case for the new measure.

The Coalition's early strategies also involved collection and use of data to further assess the neighborhood foodscape, consistent with CCAT's seventeenth proposition, emphasizing the importance of *comprehensive assessment and planning* (tables 18.2 and 19.1). A 2012 survey of 640 residents was conducted in several languages and revealed that each month, roughly half spent nearly half of their grocery money outside the neighborhood to purchase staples (fresh fruit, vegetables, meats, dairy, and grains) that were not available locally, were of poor quality, or sold at higher prices. Extrapolating to the Tenderloin as a whole, the TNDC calculated a potential loss of roughly $11 million annually from the revenue base of a neighborhood that could ill afford it (Minkler, Estrada et al., 2018). This informative example illustrates Hagan and Rubin's (2013) point that substantial economic development impacts of improving healthy food access in low-resource communities may be just as important as their nutritional and public health value.

The survey finding that roughly 80 percent of survey respondents reported that they *would* buy healthy food locally if available and affordable and the earlier Google "apple map" findings were highlighted in a December 2012 Coalition and VYDC press conference. The media coverage included voices of youth on public radio and prompted a city policymaker to remark that "the fact that local people provided numbers and facts from work on-the-ground made a difference," thus recognizing that any proposed policy measure needs support from the community (Minkler, Falbe et al., 2018).

To help assess changes in the local environments over time, FJLs conducted a critical baseline assessment for fifty-six of the neighborhood's corner stores in early 2013. They used SFDPH's Corner Store Standards for Health and Sustainability Tool (http://www.healthyretailsf.org/tenderloin-shopping-guide), which their Bayview counterparts had piloted (Minkler et al., 2019). Aggregate findings on items like availability of low-fat dairy and the amount of shelf space allocated to tobacco were translated into a star rating from 1 (worst) to 4 (best). Forty-three stores (77 percent) received composite ratings of 1–2 (poor–fair), 12 (28 percent) received a score of 3 (good), and a single store rated a 4 (Minkler, Falbe et al., 2018). FJLs held private meetings with each store owner to discuss their scores, share feedback packets, and discuss strategies for improvement. This early and continuing assessment and evaluation work was congruent with CCAT's sixteenth proposition, that *successful implementation of effective strategies is more likely when comprehensive assessment and planning occur* (Butterfoss & Kegler, 2009; p. 245; table 19.1). At the same time, the CEJ's sixth principle, *construct core functions . . . based on equity and justice*, is a reminder to ensure that the Coalition and its community be deeply involved in, and benefit from, such work. Based on FJLs' assessment findings, a colorful Shopping Guide (http://www.healthyretailsf.org/tenderloin-shopping-guide), which included photos of each store, its star rating, and healthy highlights (e.g., having fresh produce and acceptance of food stamps), was translated into four languages and distributed at a community meeting attended by over 150 residents. The meeting also highlighted healthy foods made of locally sourced ingredients, two city policymakers who presented a new healthy retail ordinance they hoped to sponsor, and opportunities for residents to offer their own ideas. The outreach benefited the broader community and helped the Coalition gain visibility and new members (Staples, 2016; chapter 12; appendix 8).

Coalition actions during its formative stage illustrated several CCAT propositions and CEJ principles. It *pooled member and external resources*, including funding and in-kind support from the co-led organizations and SFDPH and a small foundation grant. The funding covered most staff, research, and programmatic needs, but it was not optimal to address some important challenges. There was strong resident engagement with a membership that consisted mostly of people of color and with members who identified as LGBTQ, disabled, and immigrants, among others. However, the Tenderloin's extraordinary diversity also meant that a subset of community members did not engage due to linguistic or cultural barriers. The Coalition tried to provide flyers to advertise special events in Arabic, Vietnamese, and other local languages and make an annual Shopping Guide available in multiple languages, but linguistic inclusion of all residents remained a challenge.

Maintenance Stage

The second stage in the Coalition's life cycle successfully reflected CCAT's emphasis on *high levels of participation both in and outside of coalition meetings and activities* (Butterfoss & Kegler, 2009). Maintaining meeting size (typically twenty to thirty individuals) and the increasingly diverse audience was critical, as was growing collaborations to include key stakeholders beyond the Coalition. In addition to the previously mentioned Sutti & Associates CEO, and faculty and staff with UC Berkeley's School of Public Health, added members included staff from SFDPH's Feeling Good project and members of the Youth Leadership Institute. Finally, a postdoctoral scholar in public health nutrition joined the Coalition at this stage and quickly became a critical addition in assisting the FJLs with data analysis.

The striking diversity of the Coalition's membership along multiple axes could have led to frequent tensions and conflicts. Fortunately, the cochairs fostered respectful participation and dealt with the few conflicts that arose in timely and effective ways, such that their skills were widely recognized as important contributions to success (Flood et al., 2015). These leadership approaches are in line with CCAT's tenth and eleventh propositions' emphases, respectively, on *formalized decisionmaking* and effective *conflict management making collaborative synergy more likely*. The fact that many Coalition members had previously worked together or were currently working together in other capacities (e.g., on a safer streets project and advocating for affordable housing) contributed to trust building that extended to their Coalition work. The belief among the largely White, professional, and highly educated Coalition members from outside the Tenderloin, that the lived experience and wisdom of resident members should hold sway in issue selection, strategizing, and decisionmaking was reflective of bedrock community organizing and community building practice, particularly in work with often marginalized communities (cf. Minkler et al., 2019; Sen, 2003; Staples, 2016; chapters 5, 12, 13). Such beliefs and actions also reflect a seventh CEJ principle added to the original six (Wolff et al., 2017) for its centrality to equity-focused community building and organizing. As discussed in chapter 1 and box 1.1, this last principle stresses the need for *embodying cultural humility* through "a lifelong commitment to self-evaluation and critique, redressing power imbalances . . . and to developing mutually beneficial and non-paternalistic partnerships with communities on behalf of individuals and defined populations" (Tervalon & Murray-García, 1998, p. 123). But it also emphasizes the need to *continue to strive for more cultural competence*, not as something outsiders can ever hope to achieve, but as part of an unending learning process (Greene-Moton & Minkler, 2020). Continued attention to CCAT's ninth proposition of *open and frequent communication* and to the model's overall promotion of diverse membership and power sharing in decisionmaking are critical for this work.

Despite the Coalition's achievements during its maintenance stage and its ability to positively address CCAT and CEJ components, it encountered challenges. Insufficient funding limited staff hours and number of FJLs, whose workload escalated during this crucial stage. Personnel turnover was challenging, particularly among the FJLs, whose part-time status and requirements for selection (e.g., strong pre-existing relationships with merchants and residents) sometimes led to periods of even leaner staffing. Fiscal constraints also limited multilingual community outreach such that the Coalition began holding community events with translation typically available only in Spanish, if at all. Finally, active engagement of merchants to provide updates about new programs and feedback sessions following store assessments was difficult. Eighty percent were immigrants, and many worked long hours, typically six days a week, with minimal time available beyond accommodating brief in-store meetings (McDaniel et al., 2018).

In contrast, a hallmark of the maintenance stage was increased engagement of key players who shared the Coalition's goals. The Coalition increased its work with policymakers interested in sponsoring a healthy retail measure, and met with them, a few interested merchants, the Coalition's Bayview counterpart, the SFDPH, and Sutti & Associates about healthy retail legislation. Coalition members helped draft a municipal ordinance, and iterations were shared with stakeholders (e.g., the Arab American Grocers Association, which represented 450 corner stores in the city and whose input and buy-in would be critical for success). Heavy engagement in policy work at this stage, concurrently with its work on the community and corner store levels, was in keeping with Wolff et al.'s (2017) fourth CEJ principle calling for a *focus on policy, systems and structural change*. It also reflected CCAT's twentieth proposition and emphasized that *coalitions are more likely to create change in community policies, practices, and environments when they direct interventions at multiple levels* (Butterfoss & Kegler, 2009, p. 245; table 19.1).

On the policy level, the Coalition played a key role in working with SFDPH, the Office of Economic and Workforce Development, merchants, and other partners to iron out the details of the proposed healthy retail ordinance (Minkler, Estrada et al., 2018). The final proposed program would provide technical assistance with redesigns and other benefits for selected stores, which, in turn, committed to changes that would meet the legislation's definition of a healthy retailer. The definition included devoting more than or equal to 35 percent of selling space to produce and other healthy foods and less than or equal to 20 percent to alcohol and tobacco combined, removing specific amounts of cigarette and alcohol ads and paying minimum wage (San Francisco Department of Public Health, 2013). Plans for ensuring accountability, monitoring, and evaluation were also included in the draft measure, each with significant roles for the Coalition. Implementation planning involved the FJLs collecting point-of-sale data and completing biweekly report cards with each store, and continued use of SFDPH's corner store assessment tool in HRSF stores and those not participating in the program. This allowed assessment of changes in the intervention stores and in neighborhood healthy retail trends over time. The continued engagement in data analysis of Coalition coleads, the SFDPH, and a university nutrition postdoctoral researcher also helped convince decisionmakers of program accountability.

The Coalition's major investments recognize the importance of proposition 16, *continued comprehensive assessment and planning for effective implementation of strategies* (Butterfoss and Kegler, 2009). Those investments helped to secure passage of the HRSF measure and plan for its effective implementation and ongoing assessment. In late summer and early fall 2013, Coalition leaders and members attended meetings with key city stakeholders to provide testimony in hearings of a subcommittee and the full board of supervisors to advocate for passage of the ordinance. Those efforts and others helped contribute to an important policy win, when the HRSF ordinance was unanimously passed by the board on October 9, 2013, and signed by the mayor. Reflecting back on the Coalition's role in this process, a city supervisor commented that "The Coalition was extremely influential in drafting, refining, and then passing the healthy retailer ordinance. . . . They held meetings with [and testified before] the Land Use Committee and the full board. They brought members in to educate the legislators. They had very clear ideas in working with our staff to develop the HRSF Ordinance."

Before HRSF became a reality, the Coalition and its SFDPH and TNDC partners secured staffing and funding for technical assistance and equipment that would enable the conversion of a pilot store to healthy retail. Two store owners came to the Coalition to make their case for selection, and the CEO of the store redesign firm presented his feasibility analysis for each. Members discussed preferences and concerns (e.g., resident safety in relation to the stores and owners' motivations) with the Coalition, then selected one store for the first redesign (Flood et al., 2015). The store selection decisions were made by the full Coalition, not simply by its leaders or policy committee, in keeping with the CEJ's sixth principle that core functions be based on equity and justice and *build membership, ownership, and leadership* (Wolff et al., 2017; box 1.1). But it also underscores the Coalition leaders' and partners' embodying of a seventh principle, not in the original CEJ but added for this book (chapter 1): *emphasizing cultural humility and cultural competence* (Greene-Moton & Minkler, 2020; box 1.1). Cultural humility in particular was captured in the Coalition's continuous recognition that the lived experience of local resident members should outweigh the opinions of "outside experts" in making such decisions.

Institutionalization Stage

CCAT's third stage is characterized by the recognition that "sustainability does not depend on one strategy, policy, or approach, but instead requires developing community understanding and leadership to embed new solutions in institutions—literally institutionalizing policies and organizational practices within communities" (chapter 18). In this stage, short- and longer-term developments occurred to help institutionalize the Coalition and several of its core strategies (e.g., annual corner store assessments and conversions, new store launches, and community events, some with up to 400 participants) and help contribute to positive intermediate outcomes.

Short-term institutionalization was aided by a three-year grant secured by a university partner, with two-thirds of the funding subcontracted to the Coalition. In keeping with the CEJ's third principle, *work to build resident leadership and power* (Wolff et al., 2017; box 1.1), the grant funding permitted doubling the number of FJLs and increased salary support for a Coalition chair. This contributed to the Coalition's ability to operate for the first time with a single lead organization (TNDC).

The increased number of FJLs was helpful in institutionalizing key Coalition strategies, including the labor- and time-intensive corner store assessments. The HRSF went into effect in 2014, and with the benefit of the FJLs' 2013 baseline assessments, changes in the annual ratings could be assessed for 67 percent and 91 percent of all Tenderloin corner stores, for 2013–2015 and 2017, respectively. As hypothesized, store ratings revealed a ripple effect, through which a steadily increasing number of stores received more positive ratings on healthy retail, despite the great majority not participating in the HRSF program. The number of stores receiving just one to two stars thus dropped markedly from 77 percent in 2013 to 49 percent in 2017 (Minkler et al., 2019). Equally important, monthly point-of-sale data collected by the FJLs for the first four HRSF stores with complete data from baseline through their first year in the program were promising. They showed a 35 percent increase in produce units sold in all four stores and an average 35 percent drop in tobacco sales for three of the four, with the fourth showing no change in the percent of sales from tobacco, albeit with an absolute increase in the number of units sold (Minkler et al., 2019). We share these findings to illustrate CCAT's twenty-first principle, that *coalitions that are able to change community environments, policies and practices are more likely to increase capacity and improve health and social outcomes* (table 18.2). These encouraging findings suggested positive initial impacts of HRSF on intervention store sales (ideally translating into healthier customer consumption patterns) and changes in the overall neighborhood environment from a healthy retail perspective. Further, the FJLs' increased skills in areas including data analysis and public speaking, the large increase in the number of stores moving toward healthy retail, and the contributions of a community coalition and municipal healthy retail policy to support and document these changes illustrate growth in community capacity. In addition to assessing outcomes of change strategies and the policies, programs, and practices to which they contribute, effective coalitions are aided by critical self-reflection and assessment of their strengths and weaknesses, their evolution and new directions moving forward (chapter 21; appendixes 10, 11, 12).

In 2014, a multimethod evaluation of the Coalition and its functioning was led by two university members, with follow-up in 2017, partly in collaboration with an eight-member participatory evaluation (PE) subcommittee. Composed mainly of residents, the subcommittee's activities included learning about and interpreting data from blinded transcribed interviews, and leading and participating in focus groups and other processes. Resident participation added to the richness of the overall evaluation by offering data interpretation grounded in their own lived experience and deep understanding of the community (Flood et al., 2015). In line with both CEJ and CCAT components, PE subcommittee members developed new skills, with some reporting increased confidence in leading small groups and other areas that could contribute to their own ongoing and future development and Coalition functioning.

Funded by a local foundation grant, the Coalition's first annual daylong retreat was held in 2014, enabling this busy and still underfunded organization to step back, focus on its process, undertake strategic planning (appendix 11), and discuss its successes and difficulties and future challenges and opportunities.

Numerous Coalition and Coalition-led events also occurred during the institutionalization stage, including the launch of the pilot converted corner store in early 2014, which was timed to coincide with a neighborhood Sunday Streets celebration. It was followed by the selection, redesign, and launch of five additional Tenderloin healthy retail stores in 2014, 2015, and 2017, with an existing healthy retail store also receiving a second round of funding for higher tier healthy retail upgrades. Each store reopening was followed by a large community celebration with attendance that reflected FJLs' and other Coalition members' increasing effectiveness in mobilizing the community, aided by an increased budget for materials in multiple languages.

Engagement of the Coalition on the municipal policy level and beyond also increased during the institutionalization stage. Policymakers' appreciation of the Coalition's continued role in the implementation of HRSF, and particularly in data collection, monitoring, and evaluation, led to an initial annual city allocation of $50,000 to the Coalition, and to three of its members being invited to serve on the city's HRSF advisory committee, which met quarterly in city hall. When momentum was needed for a statewide healthy corner stores initiative and a proposed city soda tax (which would add a two cent per ounce distributor tax to sugar-sweetened beverages and use the money for improving the public's health; appendix 11), city supervisors and other key stakeholders sought the Coalition's help recognizing its increasingly helpful role in changing food, beverage, and tobacco environments in San Francisco. In the words of one supervisor, "I included [the Coalition] in other

efforts like the 'healthy stores, healthy communities' initiative, which is now operating at the statewide level. . . . They also were very helpful on the soda tax now on
the November [2014] ballot. They've been instrumental in bringing their base out,
in other communities and in linking junk food and junk drinks with alcohol and
tobacco."

Continued appreciation of the Coalition's contributions to HRSF and related
healthy retail efforts also translated into increased fiscal and other support. The
Coalition received permanent project status within its lead agency, TNDC, midway
through the institutionalization stage, and with it regular funding for the director, support for FJLs, and other fiscal and technical assistance. With the passage of
a more modest one cent soda tax initiative on the second try in 2016, new revenue
totaling $11.6 million was generated in FY 2019/2020 (Ettman, 2020; appendix 11)
with $1,150,000 of this allocated to food access. Fully $1 million of this amount went
to healthy food vouchers through the city's SF Eats Program (https://eatsfvoucher
.org), with which the Coalition had long collaborated, and which provides numerous organizations with "veggie vouchers" and the like for distribution to people
who are food insecure. All HRSF stores accept these vouchers, as do many other
corner stores in neighborhoods like the Tenderloin, so a substantial increase in
healthy food stocking and consumer purchasing in these stores is anticipated in
this and future years. The HRSF received $150,000 from the soda tax, plus an addi-
tional $50,000 from the Office of Economic and Workforce Development. Of this
total, $50,000 was allocated to the Coalition for that first year in recognition of its
vital role in the program, with anticipated further funding in the years ahead.

In addition to the Coalition's and HRSF's growth and achievements, numerous examples of growth in individual capacity and leadership were also observed.
Perhaps most strikingly, a young leader of the VYDC who had participated in the
SFDPH's CAM training and helped develop the original Google "apple map," went
on to co-lead the Coalition, then served with the Tobacco Free Program at SFDPH,
and later, as co-director of the HRSF program. Despite such impressive examples
of individual and organizational capacity building contributing to the Coalition's
successful institutionalization, its core strategies, and the HRSF program, however,
Butterfoss & Kegler's (2009) reminder of the continued powerful *influence of "contextual factors throughout all stages of [coalition] development"* (p. 244) remains critical, particularly given escalating environmental challenges.

A growing neighborhood concern that was accelerated during the Coalition's
institutionalization stage was the increasing loss of Tenderloin corner stores due
to skyrocketing rents in this rapidly gentrifying neighborhood. The number of corner stores dropped from seventy-one in 2013 to fifty-seven in 2017, and many merchants reported fears about being priced out, with 2017 rents that were typically
$5,000 per month (and $10,000 per month for two bordering the downtown area)
(McDaniel et al., 2018). Some merchants feared that successful ballot measures,
including a $2/pack increase in the cost of a pack of cigarettes, the soda tax, and a
proposed ban on flavored tobacco products, would hurt their businesses to the

point that they might need to close (Chávez, et al., 2019). Finally, some Coalition members worried that HRSF may inadvertently contribute to gentrification. As San Francisco rents have continued to go through the roof, young professionals looking for more affordable housing have been increasingly attracted to the Tenderloin, and the appealing improvements in HRSF stores might be an added inducement, further contributing to the displacement of lower-income residents. In response to such concerns, the Coalition began participating in affordable housing meetings and hearings and helping in efforts to convert a 5,000-square-foot lot into 140 affordable housing units with healthy retail stores, restaurants, and a communal kitchen (Minkler et al., 2019).

As suggested in the twenty-first and final CCAT proposition, *By participating in successful coalitions, community members and organizations develop capacity and build social capital that can be applied to other health and social issues and make coalition sustainability more likely* (table 18.2). The Coalition's work to address affordable housing is a good example of this proposition at work as is its rapid response to the greatest challenge the neighborhood has faced, the COVID-19 pandemic.

Soon after the Coalition's 2019 expansion to include two other food insecure neighborhoods, the pandemic hit, with its disproportionate toll on neighborhoods comprising predominantly low-income people of color, older, and disabled people with underlying health problems. The Tenderloin was especially hard hit; as the home to almost 4,000 homeless people in 2019, or half the city's total (https://cmtldata.org/data/homeless-residents), it experienced a dramatic increase in the number of unhoused people living on its already crowded sidewalks. At the time of this writing, Tenderloin's COVID-19 case rate, at 381/10,000, was well over twice the city rate of 167/10,000 (https://data.sfgov.org/stories/s/San-Francisco-COVID-19-Data-and-Reports/fjki-2fab/#), and the HRSF co-director (Estrada), who formerly had continued her active involvement with the Coalition, had been redeployed to work full time on the SFDPH COVID-19 response. The Coalition holds its monthly meetings online, and nearly all of its work in the community is on hold. Still, the Coalition continues to find innovative and important ways to help the community through this extraordinary time. FJLs remain engaged in food security advocacy work, including helping bring in a Tenderloin pop-up pantry, securing budget funds for home meal delivery services, and working on a newsletter, *Food Justice News*, to keep residents, agencies, and allies apprised of new developments and opportunities.

As a reminder of the essential services they provide in food insecure neighborhoods, none of the Tenderloin corner stores have closed due to COVID-19. And Eat SF food vouchers, now in far greater supply due to soda tax funding, provide a critical lifeline for many residents of this and other food insecure neighborhoods in one of the nation's most affluent cities. Finally, while no new store conversions took place in 2019 or 2020, a new one is planned for fall 2021, and three more for 2022—an important sign of hope for a Coalition whose primary focus remains addressing food insecurity, one of the foremost issues for residents of this and other low-resource communities in the city and well beyond.

Discussion

The Tenderloin Healthy Corner Store Coalition is one of the thousands of action-focused community coalitions that have emerged over the past forty years in response to a wide range of health and social concerns (Rockler et al., 2019; Wolfe et al., 2020; Wolff et al., 2017). It is also among a growing number of such coalitions focused specifically on issues of food justice and changing the food and tobacco landscape in local communities (Broad, 2017; Butler et al., 2014; Hagan & Rubin, 2013; Silver et al., 2017; https://www.convenience.org/Topics/Foodservice/Healthy-Options/National-Corner-Store-Network). The first such intervention in tribally owned stores also merits attention. Jernigan et al.'s study (2019) used a cluster controlled design and measured changes in customer purchases before and after the intervention, rather than relying on store sales and observational assessments. While our case study focused predominantly on the role of a community coalition and explored changes to which it contributed on the levels of the corner store and municipal policy, a range of measurement tools are available for more detailed study of intervention effects on purchasing behavior and store environments (Glanz et al., 2016; Jernigan et al., 2019). Tools and resources, such as PolicyLink's *Healthy Stores for Healthy Communities* https://healthystoreshealthycommunity.com/ and ChangeLab Solutions' *Healthy Retail: A Set of Tools for Policy and Partnerships* (https://www.changelabsolutions.org/product/healthy-retail-set-tools-policy-partnership) can also help coalitions and partnerships interested in working for healthy retail on the community and policy levels.

We used Butterfoss and Kegler's *Community Coalition Action Theory* toward a comprehensive understanding of our case study coalition, from its formation through its institutionalization stages, and into the uncharted waters of the pandemic. CCAT proved effective for the first eight years of the Tenderloin Healthy Corner Store Coalition because of the emphasis on the importance of community context (from deep poverty and disinvestment, to a long history of local activism, to the potential asset of a network of corner stores, to gentrification and the pandemic). So, too, did the theory's emphasis on strong community leadership, a broad and diverse membership, and the centrality of community gatekeepers (in this case, Food Justice Leaders), all of whom shared the Coalition's commitment to healthy food access as a civil rights issue.

We explored the Coalition following CCAT's three stages. The model's first proposition reminds us that coalitions "recycle through these stages as new members are recruited, plans are renewed, and new issues are added" (table 18.2; Butterfoss & Kegler, 2009, p. 244). When the Coalition was early in its formation stage, the opportunity to partner with a city supervisor and others in helping craft a health retail municipal ordinance came into play and was too good to pass up. Prioritizing that work above other tasks traditionally associated with the formation stage was a potentially risky yet important step for the Coalition. Being involved in this policy work from the ground up contributed to the Coalition's visibility and power in the fight for food justice (Staples, 2016; chapter 12), and later to its institutionalization with permanent organizational and city funding. Of even greater importance was the opportunity provided for the Coalition to work further upstream on a policy measure that could improve healthy food access for residents in multiple food insecure San Francisco neighborhoods (Freudenberg et al., 2015; Iton & Ross, 2017: Plough & Gandhi, 2019), an ability that takes on even greater importance during the pandemic.

Many of CCAT's propositions are complemented by Wolff et al.'s (2017; box 1.1) principles of CEJ, which provided a secondary conceptual grounding for this analysis. The CEJ's third and sixth principles, *[Working] to build resident leadership and power* and developing equity and justice-based facilitating structures that *build member ownership and leadership*, dovetailed with CCAT propositions on power sharing but took it a step further. With its substantial resident majority membership and commitment to majority rules in all decision making—including which stores were selected to become healthy retailers—the Coalition well modeled the building of high-level resident leadership and power. Similarly, the key role of FJLs in much of the Coalition's research both amplified its commitment to community leadership and illustrated its extension into a realm typically under the control of academically trained experts. In retrospect, the Coalition's success and substantial contributions on the community and policy levels may be attributed in large part to the deep commitment of its leaders, members, and partners. Early and continuing roles of the VYDC and the TNDC as co-leads, and then as continued supporters and participants, and of the FJLs, as both community gatekeepers and leaders of the Coalition's community-driven research, were of critical importance. So, too, is the key role of the SFDPH, which, from the onset, shared the Coalition's belief that access to healthy food and a healthier neighborhood environment should be a right and not a privilege (Iton & Ross, 2017; Pastor et al., 2018). The health department's commitment to equity; its role in providing technical support, fiscal, and other resources at every stage of the Coalition's process; and its commitment to ensuring that community members drive the process, were consistent with best practices in the early CAM (Hennessey Lavery et al., 2005), as well as CCAT and the CEJ.

As this book goes to press, the disproportionate toll the pandemic has already taken in the Tenderloin has caused the Coalition to temporarily pause its highly effective on-the-ground strategy of outreach and engagement. Its ability to pivot to new forms of advocacy and engagement bodes well for the communities it serves and for the survival and growth of this impressive community coalition in a postpandemic world. Further, and like countless other coalitions and collaboratives working to address community-identified health and social concerns, the Tenderloin Healthy Corner Store Coalition provides a good example of how community groups, with the support of public health agencies and other partners, can play a leadership role in promoting community- and policy-level change for health equity and social justice. Both Community Coalition Action Theory (Butterfoss & Kegler, 2009; chapter 18) and the principles of Collaborating for Equity and Justice (Wolff et al., 2017; chapter 1) proved valuable tools in better understanding and assessing this work.

Questions for Further Discussion

1. Focus on a coalition familiar to you and apply CCAT's propositions in each of the constructs: Stages of Development, Lead Agency/Convener Group, Coalition Membership, Processes and Leadership, and Staffing (see table 18.2). Discuss the value of applying the framework to an ongoing project and the plans for its future.

2. Discuss the Principles for Collaborating for Equity and Justice (CEJ; see box 1.1) and their application in the two case studies of the Transgender Economic Equity Coalition and Seattle Urban Native Nonprofits (SUNN) presented in chapter 9.

REFERENCES

Breckwich Vásquez, V., Lanza, D., Hennessey Lavery, S., Facente, S., Halpin, H. A., & Minkler, M. (2007). Addressing food security through public policy action in a community-based participatory research partnership. *Health Promot Pract, 8*(4), 342–349.

Broad, G. M. (2017). After the White House garden: Food justice in the age of Trump. *J Food Law & Policy, 13*, 33.

Butler, K. M., Begley, K., Riker, C., Gokun, Y., Anderson, D., Adkins, S., Record, R., & Hahn, E. J. (2014). Smoke-free coalition cohesiveness in rural tobacco-growing communities. *J Community Health, 39*(3), 592–598.

Butterfoss, F. D., & Kegler, M. C. (2009). The Community Coalition Action Theory. In R. J. DiClemente, R. A. Crosby, and M. C. Kegler (Eds.), *Emerging Theories in Health Promotion Practice and Research* (2nd ed., pp. 237–276). Jossey-Bass.

Chávez, G., Minkler, M., McDaniel, P. A., Estrada, J., Thayer, R., & Falbe, J. (2019). Retailers' perspectives on selling tobacco in a low-income San Francisco neighborhood after California's $2 tobacco tax increase. *Tob Control, 28*(6), 657–662.

Christens, B. D., & Inzeo, P. T. (2015). Widening the view: Situating collective impact among frameworks for community-led change. *Community Dev, 46*(4), 420–435.

Coleman-Jensen, A., Rabbitt, M. P., Gregory, C. A., & Singh, A. (2020). *Household Food Security in the United States in 2019.* ERR-275. U.S. Department of Agriculture, Economic Research Service.

Ettman, K. (2020, September 27). $30 million in soda tax revenue: What will it fund in San Francisco and Oakland? SPUR. https://www.spur.org/news/2019-09-27/30-million-soda-tax-revenue-what-will-it-fund-san-francisco-and-oakland.

Farley, T. A., & Sykes, R. (2015, March 21). See no junk food, buy no junk food. *New York Times.* https://www.nytimes.com/2015/03/21/opinion/see-no-junk-buy-no-junk.html.

Flood, J., Minkler, M., Hennessey Lavery, S., Estrada, J., & Falbe, J. (2015). The Collective Impact Model and its potential for health promotion: Overview and case study of a healthy retail initiative in San Francisco. *Health Educ Behav, 42*(5), 654–668.

Freudenberg, N., Franzosa, E., Chisholm, J., & Libman, K. (2015). New approaches for moving upstream: How state and local health departments can transform practice to reduce health inequalities. *Health Educ Behav, 42*(1_suppl), 46S–56S.

Glanz, K., Johnson, L., Yaroch, A. L., Phillips, M., Ayala, G. X., & Davis, E. L. (2016). Measures of retail food store environments and sales: Review and implications for healthy eating initiatives. *J Nutr Educ Behav, 48*(4), 280–288.

Grant, J. M. (2010). *Outing Age: Public Policy Issues Affecting Lesbian, Gay, Bisexual and Transgender Elders.* National Gay and Lesbian Task Force.

Greene-Moton, E., & Minkler, M. (2020). Cultural competence or cultural humility? Moving beyond the debate. *Health Promot Pract, 21*(1), 142–145.

Hagan, E., & Rubin, V. (2013). *Economic and Community Development Outcomes of Healthy Food Retail.* PolicyLink.

Hennessey Lavery, S., Smith, M. L., Esparza, A. A., Hrushow, A., Moore, M., & Reed, D. F. (2005). The community action model: A community-driven model designed to address disparities in health. *Am J Public Health, 95*(4), 611–616.

Iton, A., & Ross, R. K. (2017). Understanding how health happens: Your zip code is more important than your genetic code. In R. Callahan & D. Bhattacharya (Eds.), *Public Health Leadership* (pp. 83–99). Routledge.

Jernigan, V. B. B., Salvatore, A. L., Williams, M., Wetherill, M., Taniguchi, T., Jacob, T., Cannady, T., Grammar, M., Standridge, J., Fox, J., Owens, J. T., Spiegel, J., Love, C., Teague, T., & Noonan, C. (2019). A healthy retail intervention in Native American convenience stores: The THRIVE community-based participatory research study. *Am J Public Health, 109*(1), 132–139.

Kaplan, R. M., Spittel, M. L., & David, D. H. (2015). *Population Health: Behavioral and Social Science Insights.* AHRQ Publication No. 15-0002. Agency for Healthcare Research and Quality and Office of Behavioral and Social Science Research. National Institutes of Health.

Kegler, M. C., Halpin, S. N., & Butterfoss, F. D. (2020). Evaluation methods commonly used to assess effectiveness of community coalitions in public health: Results from a scoping review. *New Dir Eval, 2020*(165), 139–157.

Laska, M. N., Sindberg, L. S., Ayala, G. X., D'Angelo, H., Horton, L. A., Ribisl, K. M., Kharmats, A., Olson, C., & Gittelsohn, J. (2018). Agreements between small food store retailers and their suppliers: Incentivizing unhealthy foods and beverages in four urban settings. *Food Policy, 79*, 324–330.

McDaniel, P. A., Minkler, M., Juachon, L., Thayer, R., Estrada, J., & Falbe, J. (2018). Merchant attitudes toward a healthy food retailer incentive program in a low-income San Francisco neighborhood. *Int Q Community Health Educ, 38*(4), 207–215.

Minkler, M., Estrada, J., Dyer, S., Hennessey Lavery, S., Wakimoto, P., & Falbe, J. (2019). Healthy retail as a strategy for improving food security and the built environment in San Francisco. *Am J Public Health, 109*(suppl 2), S137–S140.

Minkler, M., Estrada, J., Thayer, R., Juachon, L., Wakimoto, P., & Falbe, J. (2018). Bringing healthy retail to urban "food swamps": A case study of CBPR-informed policy and neighborhood change in San Francisco. *J Urban Health, 95*(6), 850–858.

Minkler, M., Falbe, J., Hennessey Lavery, S., Estrada, J., & Thayer, R. (2018). Improving food security and tobacco control through policy-focused CBPR. In N. Wallerstein, B. Duran, J. G. Oetzel, & M. Minkler (Eds.), *Community-Based Participatory Research for Health: Advancing Social and Health Equity* (3rd ed., pp. 293–304). Jossey-Bass.

Pastor, M., Terriquez, V., & Lin, M. (2018). How community organizing promotes health equity, and how health equity affects organizing. *Health Aff, 37*(3), 358–363.

Plough, A. L., & Gandhi, P. (2019). Promoting social justice through public health practice. In B. S. Levy & H. L. McStowe (Eds.), *Social Injustice and Public Health* (3rd ed., pp. 481–494). Oxford University Press.

Rockler, B. E., Procter, S. B., Contreras, D., Gold, A., Keim, A., Mobley, A. R., Oscarson, R., Peters, P., Remig, V., & Smathers, C. (2019). Communities partnering with researchers: An evaluation of coalition function in a community-engaged research approach. *Prog Community Health Partnersh, 13*(1), 105–114.

San Francisco Department of Public Health. (2012). Community health status assessment: City and county of San Francisco. https://www.sfdph.org/dph/files/chip/CommunityHealthSta tusAssessment.pdf.

San Francisco Department of Public Health. (2013, June 18). Healthy Food Retailer Incentives Program. Ordinance no. 193-13. City and County of San Francisco. https://sfgov.legistar .com/View.ashx?M=F&ID=2623379&GUID=929A0821-4749-4CA2-BB1F-42AFC4FB0107.

San Francisco Health Improvement Partnership. (2016). *San Francisco Community Health Needs Assessment 2016*. Appendices. https://www.sfdph.org/dph/hc/HCAgen/HCAgen2016/May% 2017/2016CHNA-2.pdf.

San Francisco Planning Department. (2018). *San Francisco Neighborhoods: Socio-Economic Profiles*. https://default.sfplanning.org/publications_reports/SF_NGBD_SocioEconomic_Pro files/2012-2016_ACS_Profile_Neighborhoods_Final.pdf.

Sen, R. (2003). *Stir it Up: Lessons in Community Organizing and Advocacy*. Jossey-Bass.

Silver, M., Bediako, A., Capers, T., Kirac, A., & Freudenberg N. (2017). Creating integrated strategies for increasing access to healthy affordable food in urban communities: A case study of intersecting food initiatives. *J Urban Health, 94*(4), 482–493.

Staples, L. (2016). *Roots to Power: A Manual for Grassroots Organizing* (3rd ed.). Praeger.

Tervalon, M., & Murray-García, J. (1998). Cultural humility vs. cultural competence: A critical distinction in defining physician training outcomes in medical education. *J Health Care Poor Underserved, 9*(2), 117–125.

Wolfe, S. M., Long, P. D., & Brown, K. K. (2020). Using a principles-focused evaluation approach to evaluate coalitions and collaboratives working toward equity and social justice. In A. W. Price, K. K. Brown, & S. M. Wolfe (Eds.), Special Issue: Evaluating Community Coalitions and Collaboratives. *New Dir Eval, 165*, 45–65.

Wolff, T., Minkler, M., Wolfe, S. M., Berkowitz, B., Bowen, L., Butterfoss, F. D., Christens, B. D., Francisco, V. T., Himmelman, A. T., & Lee, K. S. (2017). Collaborating for equity and justice: Moving beyond collective impact. *Nonprofit Q, 9*, 42–53.

20

Funding for Community Organizing

Tips for Raising Money While Promoting
New Thinking in the Funding Environment

R. DAVID REBANAL

Community organizing is a labor of love. Its ultimate success is rooted in a community's greatest natural resource—the power of its people to build a collective voice for change. Yet despite growing evidence of the importance of community organizing for addressing health and social disparities through an equity lens (Pastor et al., 2018), community organizing work often goes unpaid or underfunded. Further, and while seeking funding to support and sustain organizing efforts often is critical to their effective functioning, those charged with fundraising frequently see it as a necessary but unwanted task that detracts from the "real work" of their grassroots group or organization on the ground. In other cases, seeking funding for such efforts through mainstream sources may be seen as posing significant challenges to the core principles and values of transforming systems of injustice and oppression.

Such views are compounded by the fact that traditionally, funding for public health, social work, and related fields has been structured to support direct services, where grantees can report the number of clients screened for high blood pressure, for example, or the number of residents who attend a community education workshop. Yet, as suggested above, the growing emphasis on health equity and social justice in fields like public health and social work has led more funders to appreciate the need for supporting community organizing in this work (Iton & Ross, 2017; Minkler et al., 2019; Pastor et al., 2018; Plough & Gandhi, 2019; Wolff et al., 2017).

After briefly reviewing the roots of the traditional lack of much philanthropic support for community organizing in the United States, I highlight contemporary developments and movements that have helped shine a spotlight on, and increased public support for, community organizing as an important vehicle for change. Most of the chapter then provides tips and strategies for community organizers to increase fundraising success from institutional funders and individual donors, while also leveraging greater and wider financial support for this work.

Community Organizing and Philanthropy:
Historical Roots and Contemporary Climate

Historically, community organizing has rarely been supported by the field of philanthropy, and was often not recognized as a desirable funding strategy to achieve a philanthropy's mission and goals. This can be attributed, in part, to how institutional philanthropy was established. Since the inception of the Revenue Act of 1913, the field of philanthropy was formalized as a means to minimize the taxable income of wealthy individuals, leading to the creation of a new classification of tax-exempt organizations serving the public interest, commonly referred to as nonprofits. This early history also laid the groundwork for the evolution of the modern-day dependency of most nonprofit organizations on the charity of philanthropists. Subsequently, the Tax Reform Act of 1969 limited how philanthropic funds could be used by prohibiting certain types of foundations from lobbying and discouraging funders from supporting activities perceived as contentious (Suárez, 2012). Institutions receiving, or hoping to receive, philanthropic funding thus could only be as radical or progressive as their funders (Corwin, 2020).

Raising funds for organizing work, however, can also be a tool for community building through programs historically important in fields like social work and public health (Iton & Ross, 2017; Sen, 2020). More importantly, we are currently living in a critical time in our history, in which building grassroots power for social change, and for racial and health equity, is needed, and supported, more than ever (Kramer, 2020; Pastor et al., 2018). While community building and civic engagement programs are seen as "safer" investments by many funders, it is important to distinguish these activities from community organizing, if we hope to lift up the latter. One primary way that community organizing differs from more traditional efforts to build community and increase civic engagement is that rather than focusing primarily on programs or activities, organizing focuses more on leadership development, relationship building, and culture change. Instead of asking people to participate in projects or initiatives *designed by others*, organizing provides the opportunity for people to *develop their own analyses and promote their own decisions* by building individual and collective capacity for study, reflection, deliberation, decisionmaking, and action (https://www.ncrp.org/publication/funding-community -organizing-changing-lives; Doby, 2008).

An important issue for community organizers to reflect on is how we can harness the growing public awareness that community organizers are at the forefront of championing progress in this country and use it to leverage increased funding for community organizing. The contemporary landscape presents numerous examples of the centrality of organizers' roles, from growing a worldwide movement for Black lives, to continuing to fight for immigrant and Indigenous people's rights, climate justice, and food security. Within this context, many philanthropies, like the Robert Wood Johnson Foundation, The California Endowment, the W.K. Kellogg Foundation, and the Seattle Foundation (chapter 9) have already deepened their support for community organizing that not only brings about fundamental systemic changes but is also centered around equity and healing (Iton & Ross, 2017; Jimenez et al., 2019; Plough & Gandhi, 2019). Community organizers are in a good position to encourage other funders to move—or move more strongly—in this direction (Minkler et al., 2019; Pastor et al., 2018; Wolff et al., 2017). Although I have focused so far primarily on philanthropic foundations, the secret to success for coalitions, nonprofits, and other groups that emphasize community organizing is to have a diversified funding strategy (Fyall, 2016). I turn now to some of the approaches and tactics that may be helpful in doing so.

Identifying Potential Funding Partners

More likely than not, your group or organization's plan for fundraising need not start from ground zero. As organizers, you likely value strategy, relationships, and action, which are also valuable in fundraising (Staples, 2016; chapter 12). One place to initiate your search is with the very individuals and institutions who have been your past supporters. These donors and funders are already invested in your organization and work. You may want to generate a database of donors and funders, noting their mission, goals, and strategies, in addition to their funding priorities. Further, funding entities who may not have supported you in the recent past may have had a change in leadership or launched a new strategic plan, in which you may be well positioned as a funding partner to fulfill a shared goal.

Individual Donors

In addition to funding institutions like foundations, discussed in a later section, do not discount individual donors for fundraising support; indeed, many development directors and foundation program officers suggest that grassroots and other groups start by seeking such donors. Individual giving is, by far, the most common form of support, with most reports about nonprofit fundraising consistently citing the statistic that over 70 percent of all donations are from individuals (Fritz, 2019). While over 90 percent of high-net-worth households give to charity, most individual donors would not be considered as such. For these less wealthy individuals, most of their donations (32 percent) go to churches or other faith-based organizations, followed by education (16 percent) and human services (12 percent) (https://nonprofitssource.com/online-giving-statistics/). Yet, even if your group is not affiliated with a local or large-scale faith-based organizing network (e.g., the Gamaliel Foundation, PICO National Network (now Faith in Action and ISAIAH, chapter 5), that still leaves plenty of small individual donor funding available to organizers who can make a strong case on issues that matter to ordinary people.

Further, community organizers working to address issues like climate change or reducing racial/ethnic disparities in access to good quality education, may find that their issues and grassroots groups also appeal to some of those in the highest income brackets. Such interest and largess, of course, can vary dramatically with major fluctuations in the stock market, and events like the coronavirus pandemic, which understandably resulted in a major shifting of support to direct services (Sen, 2020). When two of the world's richest people, Bill Gates and Warren Buffett, launched the "Giving Pledge" in 2010 asking billionaires to give 50 percent of their wealth to charitable organizations in their lifetime (https://givingpledge.org/About .aspx), these individuals were applauded. More recently, some younger tech millionaires and billionaires have begun their own "giving circles," enlisting their friends and colleagues in that sector to pay it forward (Culwell & Grant, 2016). Despite their good intentions, however, many of these efforts have also drawn criticism as a "missed opportunity." Some reports, for example, have suggested that these initiatives have only helped to grow their donors' wealth, or have invested in things like large performing arts centers at elite universities. In this way, they have typically failed to change the funding landscape by investing in efforts that fight social problems, in part to steer clear of challenging the wealthy and elite (https://www.npr.org/2018/08/29/642688220/generous-giving-or-phony-philan thropy-a-critique-of-well-meaning-winners).

Finding individual donors, of course, should not be limited to searching for wealthy patrons. Consider who attends your events, who "likes" your social media posts, who volunteers for your organization, and who has expressed an appreciation for the work you do or has been personally affected by your work. Utilize alumni from any programs in the community you host, as well as past staff and board members who may be connected to potential donors. Board members are often expected to assist in fundraising efforts and can frequently enlist friends and family members as well. Generating a list of individual donors not only demonstrates an appreciation for your work, it may also help convince new foundations to fund your organization; list of donors provides evidence of an influential and important base of support. Finally, offering to list individual donors on your organization's website may be an inducement to those who would appreciate this tangible show of appreciation, as well as to foundations and other funders who look for signs of a diversified funding strategy in making their funding decisions.

Corporate Donors

Another source of funding is corporations, which often have a philanthropic or public relations entity to sponsor events or provide grants or in-kind support to nonprofit organizations in the community, with a special commitment to communities in which they are headquartered or have plants. Although there is considerable variation by corporation, some provide core operating support, and those that do, typically have a less detailed and complex application process for foundation or government entities. According to the Foundation Center (http://data.foundation center.org; http://foundationcenter.org/gainknowledge/research/keyfacts2014/foun dation-focus.html), in 2015 (the most recent year for which data were available), there were more than 2,400 corporate foundations in the United States, with total corporate giving amounting to $5.5 billion annually. Their grants are often smaller than those of foundations and can fluctuate with the economy. While priorities may be less transparent and can often be driven by their executives or by an employee advisory group, corporations are often motivated by positive public relations. This may be particularly true for those wishing to show that they care about the very areas in which their products may be harmful. Gas and oil companies (e.g., Chevron) have for decades made donations to environmental groups, using mottos like "We Care." Although corporate funding may be relatively easy in cases like this, it may also raise substantial ethical challenges (chapter 8). Further, and even if the identity of a potentially embarrassing corporate sponsor is anonymous, it is useful to apply what was labeled years ago "the publicity test of ethics" (Minkler, 1994) before making your decision. Simply put, this involves asking what the consequences might be if the identity of a corporate sponsor becomes known (chapter 8).

When potential conflicts of interest with corporate sponsorships are not an issue, however, it is good to start by considering the ways in which partnering with a corporation may leverage funding from other sources. Community organizers may broaden a partnership with a corporate sponsor, for example, by asking for a staff member to help plan or host a fundraising event, or asking whether the group can use the sponsor's space for an event. Corporations may even be willing to donate furniture, computers, or advertising services for fundraising or campaign efforts.

Again, however, you may need to consider potential conflicts of interest, or how accepting funds or in-kind support from a corporation may affect your core base of support or compromise your mission. (chapters 8, 12). In the former regard, for example, an organization working to address social and economic factors driving childhood obesity disparities in communities of color made the difficult decision to reject funds from a soda company that required pouring rights at all events and branding on their equipment (chapter 8). In the latter regard (accepting corporate donations that conflict with your group's main goals), organizing scholar and activist Lee Staples (2016; chapter 12) warns of the danger of "mission creep" when we accept corporate donations (or apply for grants) that are a poor match for our group's real area of interest, and then must move outside our core mission to satisfy this new funder.

Foundation Funding

Foundations are often thought of as a natural partner for funding community organizing, and several foundations, particularly those committed to social justice and social change, have helped support community organizing in deep ways that have influenced other foundations to follow their lead (Iton & Ross, 2017; Pastor et al., 2018). Further, as more and more foundations have adopted goals to address the root causes of health inequities and the social determinants of health (Easterling & McDuffee, 2018; Iton & Ross, 2017; Plough & Gandhi, 2019), such funding opportunities have broadened as well.

Several foundations have led the way in this regard, including the W.K. Kellogg Foundation, Annie E. Casey Foundation, and The California Endowment, to name a few. More recently, moreover, the nation's largest health philanthropic funder, the Robert Wood Johnson Foundation, funded four leading grassroots base–building organizations to conduct regional multiday convenings with nearly 140 community organizers around the United States. The Foundation's goal was to learn about community organizing strategies that might be useful in its efforts to build a broad Culture of Health in which everyone in our nation "has a fair and just opportunity to live the healthiest life possible" (Plough & Gandhi, 2019). These convenings, and the poignant and powerful messages and recommendations from participants (Minkler et al., 2019), led to new community organizing funding programs at the Foundation, including greater incorporation of the organizing strategies learned in its Culture of Health efforts.

The California Endowment's Building Healthy Communities ten-year, $1 billion comprehensive community initiative launched in 2010 funded community organizers as an intentional mechanism to achieve its vision of health and equity. Their roles included working to advance statewide policy, helping change oppressive narratives (e.g., around health and racial equity) and supporting the transformation of fourteen California communities with high rates of health inequities into places where all people and neighborhoods can achieve optimal health (Ito et al., 2018; https://s26107.pcdn.co/wp-content/uploads/TCE_Pivot_to_Power_FULL-RE PORT_FINAL.pdf). In addition, several regional, state, and "conversion foundations" (created when nonprofit hospitals become for profit) have been early adopters in funding community-organizing efforts to address health inequities. In addition to The California Endowment, these include, among others, the Colorado Health Foundation, McKenzie River, the Neighborhood Funders Group, the Northwest Health Foundation, and the California Wellness Foundation.

An important, perhaps obvious, caveat that bears repeating about seeking funding from foundations is the saying, "If you've seen one foundation, you've seen one foundation." That is, there are several hundred private foundations that range from small, family foundations to large corporate foundations, some with billions in total endowments. In 2015, there were over 86,000 private foundations and charitable trusts registered in the United States, categorized as *operating foundations* (run their own programs and may give grants), *non-operating foundations* (primarily give grants), *family foundations* (funds come primarily from one family), and *community foundations* (raise funds from the community) (http://data .foundationcenter.org/). Finally, and in addition to varying in focus and processes for receiving grants, foundations may be geographically defined (only fund in a particular region), population defined, mission driven, responsive only, or invitation only.

The obvious starting point to identifying foundation partners is to search the internet for foundations that closely align with your work and issues. In addition to a foundation's website, there are online directories and foundation affiliate groups to help identify existing organizations and funders. These range from particular interest areas (e.g., the *Activist's Guide to Religious Funders*, *Grantmakers in*

Health, and *Funders for Justice*), to particular population groups (e.g., *Funders for LGBTQ Issues* and *Grantmakers for Girls of Color*) to state or regional directories (e.g., the *Guide to California Foundations* and *St. Paul and Minnesota Foundations*) to national sites and resources (e.g., *Taproot*, the *Foundation Center*, the *Chronicle of Philanthropy*, and the *National Committee for Responsive Philanthropy*). Finally, using networks and word of mouth can usually produce more detailed and intimate portraits of a funder's priorities and practices.

Finally, an additional consideration for fundraising for community organizing is to set up a giving circle, a form of participatory philanthropy in which individuals come together and pool their dollars, decide together where to give the money (and other resources such as volunteer time), and collectively learn about and invest in their community and philanthropy. Giving circles are becoming popular as a form of more democratic philanthropy, particularly in communities that remain relatively invisible and lack resources such as professional grant writers and development specialists. A recent study about the impact of giving circles found that "members of giving circles are more strategic about their philanthropy, reach beyond their family for philanthropic advice, and engage in conversation about charitable giving with more knowledgeable sources" (Carboni & Elkenberry, 2018; https://scholarworks.iupui.edu/bitstream/handle/1805/17743/giving-circle-membership18.pdf). Giving circles may require a fiscal sponsor to leverage administrative costs and may involve additional startup costs, including time and consultation fees, before generating funds. The Council on Foundations' Community Foundation Locator (www.cof.org/locator) can help identify community foundations in your area to help identify fiscal sponsors too.

Table 20.1 summarizes and identifies other considerations with regard to fundraising for community organizing efforts. While this table does not discuss all other fundraising strategies (such as membership fees and government grants), an overarching consideration to keep in mind is that regardless of the source of funds, all funding comes with strings and demands, rules and expectations, whether explicit or implicit. All funding affects organizational mission, culture, goals, and tactics; thus, organizers are advised not to rely heavily on a single type of funding for organizing. The fact that almost two-thirds of the funding for grassroots groups and community-based organizations, as well as other nonprofits, comes from foundations may be problematic in times of mounting need in poor communities and declining financial health of the nonprofit sector, particularly during a severe recession (Fisher, 2016). Further, many foundations prefer not to give to a particular organization over multiple funding cycles, underscoring again the importance of a diversified funding strategy.

Building Relationships

While there are several guides to nonprofit fundraising, one truth tends to be constant in almost all of them and may be one of the most important takeaways,

TABLE 20.1

Sources of Giving and Pros and Cons for Consideration

Funding Source	Advantages/Considerations	Disadvantages/Considerations
Corporations	Give core support	Tend to be small donations
	Often just need persuasive letter of request and tax ID proof	With recessions, gifts may be less
	Give in areas where they have plants or offices	Potential for image problem (publicity test of ethics)
	Broaden ways for partnerships with corporations (e.g., use of space, donated computers, services)	Potential conflict of interest (e.g., beer company early sponsorship of Mothers Against Drunk Driving)
		Often motivated by public relationships to "look good" (e.g., gas and oil companies to environmental causes)
Foundations	Easy to find out (usually online) their interest areas and grant size	Tend to want new deliverables rather than give core support
	Increasingly support community building, empowerment	Many lose substantial portions of their corpus during recessions and dramatic market fluctuations
	Many support nonprofits in their locale. States have "conversion foundations" (e.g., California Endowment, Colorado Trust) that in accordance with tax status must fund health-related issues, and most define health broadly	Increasingly want evidence-based outcomes over short periods
		Typically can't be counted on for repeat support over many years
	Donor-advised funds can help funding institutions broaden strategies, including community-led organizing	May be conflict averse or prefer to remain "neutral" on controversial or political issues
		Paradigm shift for many from knowledge-driven change to community-driven and -oriented change

(continued)

Table 20.1. (continued)

Funding Source	Advantages/Considerations	Disadvantages/Considerations
Individual donors	A primary source of giving; 75 percent of Americans give even during recessions	Most give small gifts and less during recessions, though this can change with Giving Pledge, One Percent Foundation, and other group-giving by the very wealthy
	Nearly 73 percent of all charitable gifts annually from individuals (albeit with most traditionally going to churches, temples and other faith-based organizations)	
	Tend to give to same causes repeatedly	Individual donor campaign via direct mail or phone calls are labor intensive, though social media and online fundraising tools help
	Other donors, especially foundations, like to see individual donor campaigns	Know your age group! Millennials most likely respond to text requests; 45 percent of Gen Xers respond to crowdsourcing; 49 percent of baby boomers enroll in a monthly giving program
	Donors may also volunteer to help in other ways	
Giving circles	More of a participatory, democratic model	May need a fiscal sponsor
	Facilitates co-learning among community members and networks about issues and responsive philanthropy	May need more time for initial fundraising and may incur startup costs
	May attract additional funding	
	Can be a more strategic approach for fundraising and grant making	

Source: Developed by Meredith Minkler with thanks to Kim Klein, Chris Coombe, R. David Rebanal, and members of the California Senior Leaders Alliance. For more information, see Charitable Giving Statistics, Trends & Data: The Ultimate List of Charitable Giving Statistics for 2018, https://nonprofitssource.com/online-giving-statistics/.

particularly for community organizers: building relationships with a wide variety of donors and funders is paramount to success. Seeking potential partnerships and strengthening individual relationships with potential or existing funders can often be encouraged by collectively thinking about strategies to gain monetary support. The process of fundraising can likewise be an opportunity to clarify your organization or coalition's goals. Although I focus this section primarily on gaining fiscal and other resources from philanthropic institutions like foundations, many of the lessons shared can be applied to building relationships with individual donors and corporations as well.

So how do you approach foundations for funding community organizing and other endeavors that are not typical direct-service projects, and thus may be more challenging to fund? First, there are relatively few health-specific funders in the United States. Furthermore, those that are health focused adopt a wide variety of themes, ranging from oral health, substance abuse, prenatal care, safety net clinics, to rural health, electronic health records, obesity prevention, school-based health centers, reducing health disparities, HIV/AIDS prevention, continuing medical education, and many more. Health-focused funders can feel overwhelmed because health outcomes take decades to change and because funders can't begin to support all the health programs to the degree they would like. Cultivating and soliciting these funders will help develop a more diverse and sustainable funding base for your organizations.

Building strong funder relationships is like building many other relationships with power imbalances—they require work. Do not be shy about calling staff at private foundations and trusts—that is why they are there. Unlike potential individual donors with no funding deadlines or funding parameters, foundation staff often have limitations around deadlines, award amounts, and the types of activities they can support. In addition, foundation program officers care about not only how well their grantees succeed in meeting their respective grant objectives but also how the portfolio of grantees helps the foundation successfully achieve its goals and objectives. Indeed, put yourself in a foundation program officer's shoes, and imagine how you and your group's expertise may contribute to the foundation's programmatic success. Ask yourselves, too, what additional information would likely be most helpful to the program officer assessing your proposal in this regard. Finally, consider how foundation staff can contribute to your program beyond just funding now or in the future, for example, as a convener, a thought leader, or an advocate. Keep in mind that foundation staff look forward to meeting community leaders like community organizers, and they often get ideas for upcoming programs that may directly benefit your work and organization. In addition, foundation staff, particularly if they are local and community foundations, get credit for having a finger on the pulse of community leaders' concerns.

Before approaching foundation staff or anyone else for grants or donations, be sure to prepare as follows:

- Do your homework. This is your first step in the cultivation process. Take the time to research your prospect before you call. This will save you time, and it demonstrates to the program staff that you are considerate of their time. Read the foundation's funding priorities on their website to confirm that your project is a good fit for the fund.

    Try to determine the following: their giving interests, their typical grant range, the key personnel, whether they accept unsolicited proposals, and the approximate length of time between receipt of proposal and when the award will be granted.
- Have specific questions. Define what you want to get out of the conversation before you make the call or email. What questions do you have *that cannot be answered by their website, annual report, or other printed materials?*
- Determine next steps. What would you like the next step to be with this foundation?
- Hone your pitch. While you may wish to speak about the nuances and successes of your program, be prepared to get to the point succinctly, whether it is an "elevator speech" or a five-minute presentation. In addition to minimizing technical jargon, be prepared to give easy-to-understand definitions for common community organizer terms, such as "direct action," "leader," "strategic planning," "power analysis," "base-building," "cutting an issue," and "turnout."

In addition to easy-to-understand definitions, the work of Andy Goodman and others may help with honing your pitch. Andy was previously a television writer and now applies the time-tested concepts and themes that have made novels, movies, and television series successful to helping nonprofits be more effective in building support for their programs. He calls it "Story Telling as Best Practice." He usually starts his workshops by telling a story familiar to us all in language that, unfortunately, most health and social service organizations use in their proposals and presentations. In one of his workshops, he read the following. See if you can guess which story is being described.

> An at-risk youth from a blended family in the farm belt is rendered unconscious during an extreme weather event. When she awakens, she undertakes a long, hazardous journey in which she is aided by an assortment of variously-challenged adults while also being pursued by a person of color, green in this case. Upon reaching her destination, she learns that her journey was all a dream and wakes up in her own bed with a newfound appreciation of the importance of family and community. (from https://www.thegoodmancenter.com)

All right, perhaps your story wouldn't be quite that bland, but storytelling in the public interest sector is often flatter than the Wicked Witch of the East. In their devotion to data, though necessary and compelling in their own right, many professionals have forgotten how to tell a compelling story, even when they have plenty to tell. None of us would choose to tell the story of the Wizard of Oz in such jargon. Yet that is precisely what too many of us do when we tell the story of the work we do. And that is a problem, because stories help engage audiences, making them more receptive to the facts. In addition to incorporating stories, here are several other lessons about cultivating relationships with funders that are worthy of note:

- Contact a foundation program officer *before* submitting an application to discuss your project and confirm its applicability for the fund.
- If your project involves a collaborative relationship, make sure you have actually met with the collaborative partner(s) and, better yet, that you have firmly established what each partner will commit to the project. It is also a good idea to submit a brief support letter from your potential partners, and some funders insist on seeing one.
- Few things frustrate a program officer more than when she provides advice as to what components should be in a competitive proposal, and the grant-seeker ignores it. *If you seek such advice, be prepared to use it.*
- Site visits can be productive, but they do not make sense for every type of project or organization. Typically, site visits are worthwhile if you have something to show or demonstrate that cannot be conveyed over the phone (potentially a conference call) or via the written word. In the case of community organizing, program officers may enjoy seeing a group of committed partners coming together for a common cause so they can put a spirit and faces behind the names in an application. For example, during a site visit of community organizers doing environmental justice work, a program officer remembers seeing maps, photos, and people coming in and out of the office, and the energy and sense of importance helped convince the funder about the potential impact of the organizers' work.
- Lastly, do not overlook the role of practices commonly referred to as the art of stewarding relationships, which often comes naturally to community organizers. There is no exact playbook for doing so but in general, these principles can inform any acts of stewardship:
  - People appreciate being thanked (an immediate email afterward is sufficient, but following up with a short handwritten note, however antiquated it seems, is often still appreciated by a potential funder).
  - Keep your funders informed of your successes, progress, and unanticipated challenges. You may also want to alert them to an upcoming community event that your group is hosting and invite them (or another staff member or intern) to attend. Depending on the cause and the funder, they may even want to say a few words.
  - Share the human stories of what your program means to your community.
  - Be honest about problems you encounter, and ask for advice if you need it.

- Ask your committed funder if they would write a letter on your behalf, if you are pursuing other funding (and offer to send bullet points to make it easy).

These sound like no-brainers. Acknowledging the support that funders gave you and sharing with them what you've accomplished with your last grant are the first steps toward cultivating the next proposal, and growing the field of community organizing within the funding world. The hallmarks of community organizing are public relationships, personal transformation and social change through the power of people. Successful connections with donors are much the same and are worth your time and energy to build and maintain (Dorfman & Fine, 2009; chapter 24).

Conveying and Evaluating Impact

Communicating the impact of community organizing work and why your work matters is critical to fundraising. Oftentimes, this requires providing compelling stories and various examples of the impacts your work has had, and will continue to have, in your community. This is where knowing your audience is important. While some funders value numbers and bottom lines, such as the numbers of people affected by a newly passed piece of legislation or its economic implications, others may prefer firsthand accounts of how your work has changed people's lives. While many organizers want to emphasize the number of people who turn out to an event, or the stories of power-building and new connections, some funders, especially those who are new to funding community organizing, may view these as the means to a greater end. For them, an articulation of "bigger picture" contributions (e.g., to help address a systemic problem, or how a health issue has been improved) may be of particular interest. Be careful in your use of language though: it is usually safer and more accurate to talk about your group's *contribution* to outcomes, rather than to suggest *attribution* (Minkler, 2010). Some community organizers who have built relationships with funders have observed that over time, many who began supporting organizing because of the issues addressed later grow to value the work in its own right and become less driven by issues and more by the process of building grassroots power (Dorfman & Fine, 2009).

It is worth acknowledging again that there are health and social justice foundations that have been supportive of community organizing for years or even decades, and through their shared lessons and knowledge, they have inspired others to adopt community organizing strategies in their grantmaking (Csuti & Barley, 2016; Robinson & Mathew, 2018). In addition to the foregoing examples, others bear special mention. Key among these is the Charles Stewart Mott Foundation, which has been funding community organizing for over three decades as a means to alleviate poverty and promote civic engagement. An assessment (Doby, 2008) of their community organizing support identified several tangible successes, the following among them:

- Gamaliel leaders in Wisconsin negotiated agreements with sixteen banks that resulted in $700 million in loans to 7,000 homeowners and helped gain funding for drug rehab programs as a result of a "treatment instead of prison" campaign.
- PICO (now known as Faith in Action) affiliates in California successfully expanded the State Children's Health Insurance Program, along with access to health insurance for uninsured adults, and gained an investment of $42 million to improve the infrastructure of health clinics.

In another example, the Colorado Trust launched its health-equity advocacy strategy in 2014, which aims to establish a field of advocates who can "promote policy changes addressing social, economic and environmental determinants of health," by funding a cohort of eighteen direct-service, community organizing, and policy advocacy organizations, and shared their lessons learned in a paper entitled "Toward Health Equity in Colorado: Progress and Lessons Learned in Health Equity Advocacy Field-Building" (Inouye et al., 2017; https://www.healthaffairs.org/doi/full/10.1377/hlthaff.2018.0088). Although these examples are on a scale far greater than most of us can expect to see in our work with typically much smaller groups and organizations, they are important as a collective "north star" in suggesting what equity-focused community organizing can help accomplish, particularly as the importance of this work is increasingly appreciated by funders, policymakers, and the general public alike.

Concluding Thoughts

In writing this chapter, it was not my intent to suggest that philanthropy and the private sector could, or should, substitute for large-scale public financing and its accompanying accountability necessary for a more equitable society and the fundamental and systematic changes needed to achieve it. Instead, and toward the end of helping move a sometimes reluctant government further in this direction, I sought to provide some practical tips, potential pitfalls and inspiring examples to those of us working as organizers in helping make change happen. Building on earlier chapters about the hows and whys of doing community building and organizing, I focused on the financial realities—how to successfully bring in the funding and other support needed for community organizing to reach its goals. I argued for the importance of viewing the work of gaining donations and grants as not a necessary aside, but rather as a key part of your efforts to grow community and networks that build grassroots power for health equity and social change.

The examples shared in this chapter, and countless others, reflect the growth and sophistication of community organizing and the growing appreciation of this work by funders and other partners concerned with health and social equity (Minkler et al., 2019; Pastor et al., 2018). Further, and even as we emerge from a global pandemic and economic downturn with heightened discourse about how these and other crises have perpetuated racial and socioeconomic inequities, we have seen both philanthropy and grassroots community organizers mobilize to meet the urgent needs of communities. We saw community organizers pivot from their social change focus to include a far greater focus on mutual aid and direct service in support of their communities (Sen, 2020; chapter 6). We saw foundations increasing their unrestricted spending and flexible administration to support the most affected communities and the organizations that work with them (https://www.cof.org/news/call-action-philanthropys-commitment-during-covid-19). Finally, we saw more urgent calls to action to recognize and support the field of community organizing for health and social justice. All of these may be among the most important lessons learned from this unprecedented time.

Questions for Further Discussion

1. This chapter shares the saying that "if you know one foundation, you know one foundation." Given that there are some 85,000 philanthropic foundations in the United States, and that you'll be lucky to get a call or email response from a program officer at a foundation to which you hope to apply for a grant, what are some of the things you should research and know about the foundation before making contact to ensure that (1) you are reaching out to an appropriate funder, and (2) they will be impressed with the extent to which you have "done your homework?"

2. Many community organizers and progressive nonprofits are reluctant to apply for corporate donations or gifts from wealthy individual donors, which they believe could tarnish the image of their organization. Yet foundations typically want to see a diversified funding strategy that doesn't rely solely on foundation funding as they make their own decision about whether to fund your group. What might be some ways you and members of your organization could find out about corporations or "big money" individual donors who might be interested in funding you and that would not cause concerns about conflicts of interest or "tainted money"? And apart from pleasing foundation funders, what are some of the advantages of seeking and receiving money from corporations or large individual donors?

REFERENCES

Carboni, J. L., & Elkenberry, A. (2018). Giving Circle membership: How collective giving impacts donors. Executive Summary. Collective Giving Research Group. https://scholarworks.iupui.edu/bitstream/handle/1805/17743/giving-circle-membership18.pdf.

Corwin, A. (2020). *Resonance: A Framework for Philanthropic Transformation*. Report, Justice Funders. http://justicefunders.org/resonance/.

Csuti, N., & Barley, G. (2016). Disrupting a foundation to put communities first in Colorado philanthropy. *Found Rev, 8*(4), 9.

Culwell, A. C., & Grant, H. M. (2016). The giving code: Silicon Valley nonprofits and philanthropy. Open Impact LLC. http://baiii.org/wp-content/uploads/2018/08/The-Giving-Code_-Silicon-Valley-Nonprofits-and-Philanthropy-Full-Summary-Authored-by-Alexa-Cortes-Culwell-and-Heather-McLeod-Grant-Open-Imapct.pdf.

Doby, C. (2008). Funding community organizing, changing lives. National Committee for Responsive Philanthropy. https://www.ncrp.org/publication/funding-community-organizing-changing-lives.

Dorfman, A., & Fine, M. (2009). Seizing the moment: Frank advice for community organizers who want to raise more money. National Committee for Responsible Philanthropy and the Linchpin Campaign Center for Community Change. https://www.ncrp.org/wp-content/uploads/2016/11/seizingthemoment.pdf.

Easterling, D., & McDuffee, L. (2018, March 14). Finding leverage over the social determinants of health: Insights from a study of 33 health conversion foundations. Wake Forest School of Medicine. https://www.gih.org/files/FileDownloads/Easterling%20%20McDuffee-Finding%20Leverage%20over%20SDOH.pdf.

Fisher, R. (2016, March 23). Government-funded organizing? *Shelterforce: The Original Voice of Community Development.* https://shelterforce.org/2016/03/23/government-funded_organizing/.

Fritz, J. (2019, September 19). How nonprofits generate revenue streams. The Balance. https://www.thebalancesmb.com/where-do-nonprofits-get-their-revenue-2502011.

Fyall, R. (2016). The power of nonprofits: Mechanisms for nonprofit policy influence. *Public Admin Rev, 76*(6), 938–948.

Inouye, T. E., Estrella, R., & Ravinda, L. (2017). Toward health equity in Colorado: Progress and lessons learned in health equity advocacy field-building. Colorado Trust. https://www.coloradotrust.org/sites/default/files/hea_phase_2_external_paper_final_08.23.17_0.pdf.

Ito, J., Pastor, M., Lin, M., & Lopez, M. (2018). A pivot to power: Lessons from the California Endowment's Building Healthy Communities about place, health and philanthropy. USC Dornsife Program for Environmental and Regional Equity. https://s26107.pcdn.co/wp-content/uploads/TCE_Pivot_to_Power_FULL-REPORT_FINAL.pdf.

Iton, A., & Ross, R. K. (2017). Understanding how health happens: Your zip code is more important than your genetic code. In R. Callahan and D. Bhattacharya (Eds.), *Public Health Leadership* (pp. 83–99). Routledge.

Jimenez, E., Tokunaga, J., & Wolin, J. (2019, November). Scan of the field of healing centered organizing: lessons learned. The Aspen Institute Forum for Community Solutions. https://aspencommunitysolutions.org/wp-content/uploads/2020/01/Healing-Centered-Paper.pdf.

Kramer, M. (2020, June 4). The 10 commitments companies must make to advance racial justice. *Harvard Business Review.* https://hbr.org/2020/06/the-10-commitments-companies-must-make-to-advance-racial-justice.

Minkler, M. (1994). Challenges for health promotion in the 1990s: Social inequities, empowerment, negative consequences, and the common good. *Am J Health Promot, 8*(6), 403–413.

Minkler, M. (2010). Linking science and policy through community-based participatory research to eliminate health disparities. *Am J Public Health, 100* (suppl_1), S81–S87.

Minkler, M., Rebanal, R. D., Pearce, R., & Acosta, M. (2019). Growing equity and health equity in perilous times: Lessons from community organizers. *Health Educ Behav, 46* (1_suppl), 9S–18S.

Pastor, M., Terriquez, V., & Lin, M. (2018). How community organizing promotes health equity, and how health equity affects organizing. *Health Affairs, 37*(3), 358–363.

Plough, A., & Gandhi, P. (2019). Promoting social justice through public health practice. In B. S. Levy (Ed.), *Social Injustice and Public Health* (3rd ed., pp. 481–494). Oxford University Press.

Robinson, N., & Mathew, A. (2018). Examining the role of social justice grantmaking on child-care advocacy and community organizing among women of color. *Soc Work Soc Online, 16*(1). https://www.socwork.net/sws/article/view/540/1066.

Sen, R. (2020, July 1). Why today's social revolutions include kale, medical care, and help with the rent. Zócalo Public Square. https://www.zocalopublicsquare.org/2020/07/01/mutual -aid-societies-self-determination-pandemic-community-organizing/ideas/essay/.

Staples, L. (2016). *Roots to Power: A Manual for Grassroots Organizing* (3rd ed.). Praeger.

Suárez, D. F. (2012). Grant making as advocacy: The emergence of social justice philanthropy. *Nonprofit Manag Leadersh, 22*(3), 259–280.

Wolff, T., Minkler, M., Wolfe, S. M., Berkowitz, B., Bowen, L., Butterfoss, F. D., Christens, B. D., Francisco, V. T., Himmelman, A. T., & Lee, K. S. (2017). Collaborating for equity and justice: Moving beyond collective impact. *Nonprofit Q, 9*, 42–53.

21

Participatory Approaches to Evaluating Community Building and Organizing for Community and Social Change

CHRIS M. COOMBE
PATRICIA WAKIMOTO
ZACHARY ROWE

Evaluation can play a critical role in strengthening community organizing and community building efforts to effect change. In recent years, funders and government decisionmakers have increasingly focused on evidence-based practice, accountability, and measurable outcomes to prove program success. However, community organizing and community building emphasize power, empowerment, collaboration, participation, community competence, and equity as essential to achieving the long-term aim of changing the conditions that contribute to health and well-being (Chávez et al., 2010). While communities see such capacity building as an important outcome, the impact on health can be elusive to evaluation, and the focus on measuring narrow health indicators may not capture longer-term effects on community health and equity (Wallerstein et al., 2011).

The result has been a tension in which community practitioners feel that evaluation is too often imposed externally without considering the unique resources, capacity, or context of their community, and they fear that evaluation will result in loss of funding if decisionmakers deem them unsuccessful (Judd et al., 2001). Further, many organizations lack the skills, knowledge, and resources needed to conduct standard, objective outcome evaluation. Faced with insufficient resources to address complex and intransigent health and social problems, community practitioners are often reluctant to spend scarce funds on an external evaluator to assess the value and worth of their work in a process they perceive to be proving, rather than contributing to improving, the work.

Over the past several decades, these challenges, combined with the expansion of comprehensive community initiatives, coalitions, and community-based participatory research (CBPR), have led to the development and widespread acceptance of collaborative and empowering methods and approaches to evaluation (Fetterman et al., 2017; Springett & Wallerstein, 2008; Wolfe et al., 2020). Central among these approaches is participatory evaluation, which emphasizes partnerships and engages those who have a stake in the project, program, or initiative in all aspects of evaluation design and implementation. Importantly for community organizing and community building, findings are communicated as they emerge so they can be used to solve problems and adjust course. Participatory evaluation also differs from more conventional evaluation by rethinking who owns and controls the process of creating, interpreting, and applying knowledge and to what end. In the emancipatory stream of participatory evaluation, both the process and the products of evaluation are used to transform power relations and promote social action and change (Cousins et al., 2016; Wiggins et al., 2018).

In this chapter, we examine how participatory approaches to evaluation can be used to assess the merit and effectiveness of community organizing and build organizational and community capacity for social change. First, we briefly describe some limitations of conventional evaluation and establish the rationale for a more participatory approach. Next, we describe the theoretical foundation of participatory approaches to evaluation, including its roots in participatory research traditions from several disciplines. We suggest a practical framework that draws on recent and innovative work in participatory evaluation and incorporates participatory approaches at each step of the evaluation process. Finally, we discuss benefits and challenges and consider next steps for community organizers who seek ways to transform their existing approaches to enhance effectiveness and build power.

In the context of the economic, political, and public health crises of our times, and of rapidly growing movements that demand equity and highlight the leadership of youth, people of color, and communities most affected by inequities, the importance of participatory approaches to evaluation has never been clearer. As discussed in chapter 16, dramatic innovations in the rapidity and reach of communication and data sharing, particularly in the online universe, offer a wealth of new tools and approaches that can facilitate the democratization of evaluation and the community capacity building it can facilitate.

Limitations of Conventional Evaluation: Rationale for a Participatory Approach

Participatory approaches to evaluation arose in response to the limitations of conventional program evaluation, and to questions of what knowledge is, who creates it, how, and to what end. The traditional and still predominant approach is rooted in the positivist paradigm of the medical and natural sciences, which views knowledge as an objective reality that can be discovered by impartial observers, using quantitative experimental design as the gold standard. While this is a powerful research model, there are important limitations to its usefulness in evaluating community organizing and community building endeavors.

First, community initiatives and community organizing often involve complex systems change that requires intervention at multiple levels, making it difficult to determine impacts and causal relationships. Community efforts are dynamic and continually evolving to respond to rapidly changing environments. As a result, strategies, targets, and indicators change throughout the project, making summative evaluation unpredictable and limited in adaptability to adjust the program as needed (Patton, 2019). Funder requirements to focus on predetermined quantifiable measures of success may shift priorities to more short-term and easily measured individual behaviors or risk factors instead of empowerment, capacity building, and systems change. When program success is judged by narrowly focused indicators, health problems may be perceived as being caused by individuals, rather than broader social determinants of health, which are more complex, interrelated, and difficult to link to individual health outcomes. In addition, limiting evaluation to simply whether a program is working does not address questions of how, for whom, and under what circumstances, thereby limiting the usefulness of the evaluation (Wolff et al., 2017).

Second, positivist notions of objectivity and expert knowledge will define which types of evidence are valuable and who controls the development of knowledge. For instance, it could be an external expert evaluator who determines what is to be studied, by what methods, and what conclusions may be drawn from the findings. Those directly involved in the program may be considered biased, and, although they may be consulted, the evaluator in the role of impartial observer is regarded as having the expertise, insight, and objectivity for interpreting the meaning of the data.

Notably, evaluations of researcher-centered investigations can be flawed by theory that is rooted in the perceptions, biases, and agendas of the external observer. The outside evaluator may be asking the wrong questions or misinterpreting the results, resulting in an evaluation that may miss the mark or be invalid. In contrast, a constructivist research paradigm is based on the notion that objectivity may be gained through deep involvement in and reflection about the setting rather than through detachment from the setting. As Whyte (1991) famously noted, "Science is not achieved by distancing oneself from the world; as generations of scientists know, the greatest conceptual and methodological challenge comes from engagement with the world" (p. 21).

A research approach that relies on the separate and hierarchical relationship between evaluator and community has the limitation that it fosters dependence and reinforces power imbalances. Participants are in effect dependent on the outside agent for interpretation of the reality of their experience. Decisionmaking as well as knowledge and skills needed for conducting evaluation remain with the evaluator and external to the organization's own process of planning and development. This is counter to the fundamental principles and strategies for promoting health that were captured in the Ottawa Charter for Health Promotion (World Health Organization, 1986) as community empowerment, ownership, and control of the organization's own endeavors and destinies.

A final limitation is that traditional evaluation results may not be applied or as useful as they might be when missing an important aim of evaluation. Stoecker

(2012) refers to the externally driven, summative evaluation as the comprehensive final exam model of evaluation, in which evaluation threatens to expose weaknesses and failures once the project is completed. However, evaluators often have information and insights that could inform program implementation and build organizational capacity throughout the project, but are constrained by role expectations or lack of training in these areas. When reflection and analysis are conducted externally and separate from organizational planning and action, rather than as necessary, sequential steps in an integrated, collaborative decisionmaking process, programs and strategies may be less likely to benefit from evaluation.

Participatory evaluation was developed to address some of these limitations. Community and other stakeholder engagement in the evaluation process is now widely accepted and indeed expected by many practitioners, evaluators, and funders of community health promotion efforts (Springett, 2017). Participatory and traditional approaches to evaluation are not mutually exclusive, and elements of both can provide a more complete assessment. Participatory evaluation has the potential to build a dynamic community of transformative learning, thereby contributing to the empowerment and capacity of disenfranchised communities to bring about change. In the words of the turn-of-the century social reformer Jane Addams (1907), "We slowly learn that life consists of processes as well as results, and that failure may come quite as easily from ignoring the adequacy of one's method as from selfish or ignoble aims" (http://womenshistory.about.com/od/quotes/a/jane _addams.htm).

What Is Participatory Evaluation?

Participatory evaluation is a collaborative approach to evaluation in which those who are involved in the work contribute to understanding it and improving it (Fetterman et al., 2017). It is the systematic assessment of the value and progress of an effort by stakeholders, in a cyclical process of investigation, education, and action (Fetterman et al., 2015; Springett & Wallerstein, 2008).

Participatory evaluation is not new. It arose from several research traditions aimed at legitimizing community members' experiential knowledge, acknowledging the role of values in research, empowering community members, democratizing research inquiry, enhancing the relevance of evaluation data for communities, and applying knowledge for bringing about social change. These traditions include Lewin's (1946) action research and Freire's popular education (chapter 5); feminist research (Frisby et al., 2009; Maguire, 1987); decolonizing methodologies (Smith, 2012); and CBPR traditions (Cargo & Mercer, 2008; Israel et al., 2013; Wallerstein & Duran, 2018).

Participatory approaches to assessing community health and social welfare programs, including empowerment evaluation (Fetterman et al., 2015; Wandersman, 2015) and theory-based evaluation (Weiss & Connell, 1995), gained momentum during the late 1980s and have been applied in varying degrees to a wide range of health promotion programs, coalitions, and CBPR partnerships (Israel et al., 2013; Wiggins et al., 2018; Zeigler et al., 2019), community initiatives (Lachance & Kowalski-Dobson, 2018), policy change capacity building (Coombe et al., 2017), youth participatory research (Ozer & Piatt, 2018; Richards-Schuster & Elliott, 2019), and community organizing and mobilization (Fawcett et al., 2015). It has been suggested that participatory evaluation has emerged in two main streams distinguished primarily by function. The pragmatic stream emphasizes program improvement as the principle aim of participatory approaches. The transformative or emancipatory stream is based on an explicit ideological commitment to reallocating power and promoting social change (Shulha et al., 2016). While the streams are not mutually exclusive, the latter is most consistent with community organizing and community building for health and therefore is the focus of this chapter.

A set of guiding principles forms the basis for transformative participatory evaluation (Shulha et al., 2016):

- Participation and ownership by the community
- Collaborative, co-learning process in which all participants are equitably engaged in and responsible for the evaluation
- Application of findings to promote action and change on multiple levels
- Transformation of power relationships by empowering and building capacity of local community and changing systems

In a spirit of collaborative inquiry and action, community members and outside evaluators work hand in hand on a more equal footing than in traditional evaluation (Fetterman et al., 2017). Local participants are at the center of defining the agenda, determining what issues are investigated and what questions are asked, gathering and making meaning of data, and applying it to change (Sen, 2003; Staples, 2016). As members of the community, local investigators often have experiences and contextualized knowledge that can help shape the inquiry, interpret results, and enhance the capacity of external evaluators (Wiggins et al., 2018). External evaluation facilitators are resources, allies, coaches, and advocates, working in partnership to enhance the capacity of local participants to perform credible evaluation while co-learning from the community. As results emerge, evaluators actively support community planning, organizational development, and action to improve the current organizing effort and work toward broader social change. Professional and academic partners can further apply their expertise and connections to help translate findings into policy or funding opportunities (Springett, 2017). Optimally, both local and external participants are transformed in the process—skills and understanding are deepened, the balance of power shifts, and stronger ties, energy, and commitment are generated (Sánchez et al., 2011; Wiggins et al., 2018).

Like other forms of CBPR, participatory evaluation links knowing and doing through a cyclical process of investigation, education, and action (Wallerstein & Duran, 2018; Wiggins et al., 2018). Using a formative approach that can adapt the effort in response to changing conditions, insights are applied to the program or organizing effort to improve effectiveness. Scarce resources can be targeted or redirected to strategies that work best. More information is gathered on the results of the actions. Going beyond formative and summative approaches (Patton, 2019), this process of critical reflection becomes self-generating and builds capacity of communities for future problem solving, planning, action, and assessment. In this way, both the process and the findings of participatory evaluation build community competence.

A Framework for Using Participatory Evaluation

Participatory evaluation is not a specific methodology, but an approach to evaluation based on a set of key principles that guide evaluation design, process, and methods (Fetterman et al., 2017; Shulha et al., 2016). The evaluation process itself is intended to transform participants and empower communities as co-creators of knowledge, while results are translated into actions, systems, and policies at multiple levels (Wallerstein & Duran, 2018; Wiggins et al., 2018).

As with any evaluation, determining whether, how, and to what degree to use participatory evaluation depends on the history of collaboration among partners, skills and resources available, the evaluation question, and the mission of the coalition or community organizing effort. How participatory an evaluation is can vary along a continuum on key dimensions and may differ at various stages in the evaluation; however, decisionmaking remains a joint responsibility throughout the process, as community control and ownership are defining elements of transformative participatory evaluation.

Participatory evaluation has become more widely adopted in community initiatives and coalitions, resulting in well-documented measures, indicators, and methods, as described by Fawcett et al. (2015), Lachance & Kowalski-Dobson (2018), and Wiggins et al. (2018). In addition, multiple frameworks have been developed that lay out key steps in participatory evaluation (Scarinci et al., 2017; Springett & Wallerstein, 2008).

The following eight-step process of participatory evaluation by Coombe (2012) draws from key elements of several frameworks (Fetterman et al., 2017; Springett & Wallerstein, 2008). Represented as steps in figure 21.1, transformational participatory evaluation is a cyclical, iterative process of learning from the past, applying new understandings to the future, and cycling back through processes as needed (Wiggins et al., 2018).

Step 1: Identify the Purpose and Commit to Participatory Evaluation

Those groups and organizations with a vested interest in the organizing effort jointly identify the purpose and objectives of the evaluation, decide whether to commit to a participatory approach, and determine the extent and type of participation by relevant groups. Once committed, participants establish guiding principles and

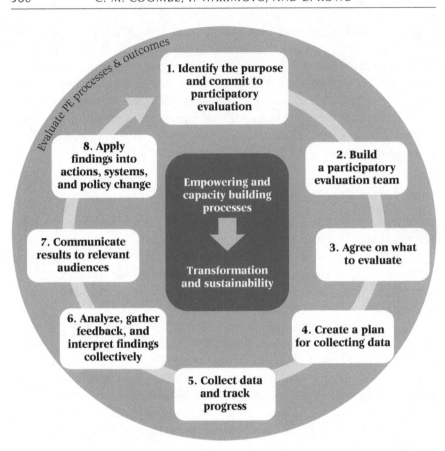

FIGURE 21.1 Transformational Participatory Evaluation.
Source: Wiggins et al. (2018).

processes that foster equitable participation at all steps toward transformative and sustainable change (Fetterman et al., 2017; Israel et al., 2018).

Step 2: Build a Participatory Evaluation Team

Collaborative partnerships require a shared commitment to equity and adequate time to establish and maintain relationships, build trust, and develop processes to understand differences and resolve conflicts. Four key tasks lay the groundwork that is critical to success.

1. *Core team members.* Determining who will be formally involved includes identifying the level and nature of participation expected and what personal and institutional resources each partner brings to the table. Guiding principles and operating norms, such as how decisions are made, can help address power differentials to foster equitable participation.
2. *Roles and multiple mechanisms for participation.* Identifying roles and strategies for substantive participation is important to ensure an equitable, high-quality

evaluation that builds on the assets and strengths within the team. Community members are often involved in data collection, evaluators typically play facilitation and training roles, and all partners are engaged in interpreting, applying, and disseminating evaluation findings. Further, levels of participation may vary over time or in response to changing conditions.

3. *Capacity building.* As noted earlier, the roles of evaluator and community member differ significantly from those in traditional evaluation, and co-learning and capacity building are integral to the process. Enhanced skills and knowledge need to be addressed throughout. For example, external evaluators and funders must gain a deep understanding of the community's historical and current context (Israel et al., 2018; Morelli & Mataira, 2010). Community members may seek enhanced knowledge of research methods.

4. *Relationships with constituencies.* Participants should engage their broader constituencies early on to build trust and ownership of the evaluation process beyond the core team, inspire confidence and vision, address concerns, and build a culture of transformative evaluation and learning.

Step 3: Agree on What to Evaluate

In transformative participatory evaluation, the community decides what is to be evaluated and how. If the initiative's assumptions, goals, and targets of change were clearly spelled out using a participatory process, the evaluation team reviews and adjusts what was proposed or, if needed, makes explicit the community's implicit theory underlying the effort (Weiss & Connell, 1995). Objectives and evaluation criteria emerge from jointly exploring what results are desired and how participants will know if progress is being made (see box 21.1 for sample questions).

BOX 21.1

Sample Questions for Facilitating a Participatory Process to Determine What to Evaluate

What results would we like to see?

How would we know if we achieved them?

What level of change is desirable or acceptable?

How will we know if we are making progress?

What changes (intermediate outcomes) could serve as benchmarks or early markers of movement toward our goals?

How will we assess our participatory process in accordance with our guiding principles?

What facilitators or obstacles might contribute to the results?

How will we account for the effects of environmental conditions outside our control?

While health promotion programs often focus on individual behaviors and health outcomes, community organizing and community building efforts aim for change at multiple levels that may be difficult to specify or that may emerge during the process (Springett, 2017). Including indicators of health-promoting environments, systems, or policies provides evidence of intermediate changes that may lead to longer-term goals (Minkler et al., 2018; chapter 19). In addition to program-specific outcomes, transformational process-related outcomes and impacts to evaluate include participation (Rifkin, 2014), collaboration (Greenwald & Zukoski, 2018; Israel et al., 2020), empowerment and community control (Cyril et al., 2016; appendix 12), community competence or capacity (Coombe et al., 2017; Eng & Parker, 1994), equity (Kastelic et al., 2018; Ward et al., 2018), and sustainability (Quinn et al., 2018). Many frameworks, tools, and methods for collaboratively determining what to evaluate, including multilevel indicators and measures (box 21.2; chapters 10, 11), are now widely available.

Step 4: Create a Plan for Collecting Data

The participatory evaluation team collaboratively develops an evaluation design and methodology that integrates qualitative and quantitative methods for monitoring progress and assessing change. The plan needs to be feasible and make the best use of community resources, such as existing tracking methods, data collection by other projects, and new technologies, while ensuring that results are valid and methods are free enough from bias to be credible to interested audiences. If needed, the evaluation team and other community members can be trained in data-collection methods, such as interviewing, focus groups, or community mapping, thus enhancing capacity and sustainability (chapters 10, 11; appendix 2). Participatory group processes from popular education and CBPR may be particularly useful in equitably engaging diverse stakeholders in developing a plan that values and integrates multiple ways of knowing and is appropriate to the community context.

In the last decade, many innovative participatory assessment and data collection techniques have been developed, including the use of digital technologies and media, that can expand the community's ability to create and use knowledge (chapter 16). Publicly available monitoring, documentation, and data-collection systems may be adapted to local contexts. A sample of these resources is shown in box 21.2.

Step 5: Collect Data and Track Progress

Participatory evaluation involves community members in documenting the organizing effort and its effects. Systems for recording activities and events as they unfold should be jointly developed with those who will be using them to enhance sustainability. Consolidating data collection questions and tools with those of others doing similar research, such as adding questions to an existing survey, can maximize resources, strengthen links between projects, and build ongoing community data capacity (chapter 15). The use of online and digital technologies that integrate data collection and sharing with community organizing and movement building

BOX 21.2
Sample Resources for Evaluating Community and Related Work

The Asset-Based Community Development Institute (cofounded by John Kretzmann and John McKnight, chapter 11) was the catalyst for a growing movement that considers local assets as the primary building blocks of sustainable community development. Resources on Asset-Based Community Development (ABCD), advocacy, community building, strategic planning, and other relevant topics. https://resources.depaul.edu/abcd-institute/Pages/default.aspx.

BetterEvaluation is a global collaboration aimed at improving evaluation practice and theory through cocreation, curation, and sharing information, with frameworks and toolkits that include measures, indicators, and methods for participatory evaluation. https://www.betterevaluation.org.

BOLDERADVOCACY, a program of Alliance for Justice, has resources for effective advocacy, evaluating the ability to organize and tools for effective advocacy. https://bolderadvocacy.org/community-organizing/core-components-of-community-organizing-evaluation/.

The Center for Evaluation Innovation works with foundation leaders and other evaluators to advance evaluation and learning practice in philanthropy. https://www.evaluationinnovation.org/.

Corburn, Ruiz Asari, and Kirschenbaum provide suggestions for numerous web-based tools supporting community mapping projects (appendix 2).

Engage for Equity is a partnered website hosted by the Center for Participatory Research with tools and resources that lay out a step-by-step approach for using the collective reflection and evaluation to strengthen our partnering practices. https://engageforequity.org.

Evaluating Community Programs and Initiatives. KU Work Group for Community Health and Development. 2010. Chapters 36–39. From the Community Tool Box, https://ctb.ku.edu/en/table-of-contents/evaluate/evaluation.

Foster, C. C., & Louie, J. (2010). Grassroots action and learning for social change: Evaluating community organizing. Center for Evaluation Innovation. This publication provides a framework that includes sample benchmarks and data collection methods for the core components of community organizing. https://www.evaluationinnovation.org/wp-content/uploads/2010/03/Foster-Louie-Brief.pdf.

Human Impact Partners (HIP) works in partnerships across strategies of capacity building, advocacy, organizing, and policy-driven research (chapter 10). HIP has products and resources covering their strategies, including A Health Impact Assessment Toolkit (appendix 4, Community Health Indicators). https://humanimpact.org/products-resources/; https://humanimpact.org/hipprojects/a-health-impact-assessment-toolkit-a-handbook-to-conducting-hia/.

PolicyLink's approach, *Lifting Up What Works*, is core to all initiatives to advance policies that enable everyone to participate in an equitable economy, live in a community of opportunity, and thrive in a just society. Through its partnership with Equity Research Institute and the National Equity Atlas, resources have been developed providing data, research, and reports to promote racial equity. https://www.policylink.org/resources-tools/tools; https://www.policylink.org/our-work/economy/national-equity-atlas (table 10.1).

The W.K. Kellogg Foundation's website offers a collection of resources including a logic model development guide. https://www.wkkf.org/resource-directory; https://www.wkkf.org/resource-directory/resources/2004/01/logic-model-development-guide.

exploded during the concurrent social justice movements and global pandemic. This provides enormous opportunities and challenges for participatory evaluation to ensure that data collection is rapid, timely, and rigorous (chapter 16).

Step 6: Analyze, Gather Feedback, and Interpret Findings Collectively

Making sense of the data is a collaborative effort that combines technical expertise, experiential knowledge, and deep understanding of the community. The evaluation facilitator and staff organize and integrate different types of data into a common body of information to gather feedback to the group for discussion and interpretation. Using facilitated group processes, participants interpret meaning, check validity, and identify gaps or connections between data. The aim is to reach consensus on findings and set the stage for moving from knowledge to action at multiple levels, using an equity lens toward social justice. Numerous examples of processes that engage communities in data feedback and interpretation can be found in CBPR and popular education, including a study among Chinatown restaurant workers (chapter 15), community health workers in Nicaragua (Wiggins et al., 2018), and an environmental health community action plan (Schulz et al., 2011; appendix 2).

Step 7: Communicate Results to Relevant Audiences

Participatory evaluation is well aligned with a formative approach that communicates findings to key constituencies as information emerges rather than waiting for a final product. Sharing achievements as they occur and framing findings in terms of community strengths rather than deficits energizes the community and builds trust and commitment. Using evaluation findings to engage participants and the larger community can enhance community building and garner support from prospective funders, new constituencies, and neighboring communities.

Teamwork and mutual learning are critical to combine expertise of professional evaluators in compiling and presenting research data with community evaluators' expertise in communicating with diverse constituencies in understandable and meaningful ways. Creative media, such as video, theater, art, posters, websites, and social media, using community expertise, may communicate more effectively than reports and presentations (chapters 16, 17). Conveying project outcomes to interested parties outside the community contributes to other organizing efforts, expands networks, and sets the agenda for future research and action.

Step 8: Apply Findings into Actions, Systems, and Policy Change

Evaluation findings must be acted upon to be useful to the community. Using the lessons learned, the group can strengthen or expand organizing efforts, institutionalize changes, and plan future actions (Springett, 2017). Valuable information about how the process worked in relation to outcomes may lead the project to redefine objectives, adjust strategies, redirect scarce resources, modify methods, and strengthen collaborative structures. Community efforts for transformative change focus on applying findings for collective power, equity, systems change, and policy advocacy (Coombe et al., 2017; Minkler et al., 2012; Wallerstein et al., 2020). Participatory evaluators can take a more active role in supporting community efforts to effect social change by using their expertise and connections in the philanthropic and policy arenas.

Participatory evaluation is a process of learning, creating knowledge, and building relationships that is an important outcome in and of itself (Roe et al., 2005; Springett, 2017). This requires facilitation and organizational development skills on the part of evaluation facilitators to help the project strengthen its leadership and structure, integrate evaluation into ongoing operations, and seek out new funding resources. There is a growing body of scholarship and practice on evaluating partnership and capacity building as both process and outcomes of community initiatives and coalitions. However, there are fewer published accounts of evaluation of community organizing per se (Fawcett et al., 2015; Foster & Louie, 2010), which may not be evaluated and reported separately from broader initiatives. A notable exception is youth organizing as part of youth participatory action research and evaluation, known as YPAR (Ozer & Piatt, 2018; Richards-Schuster & Elliott, 2019), in which many useful indicators and measures have been developed. There are frameworks, methods, and tools for conducting participatory evaluation and CBPR that are accessible online, especially in sources like the Community Tool Box (https://ctb.ku.edu/en), and can be adapted for community organizing efforts (Israel et al., 2020). Several are listed in box 21.2.

Benefits of Participatory Approaches to Evaluation

As described earlier, participatory evaluation has the potential to advance the field of evaluation and increase its effectiveness. First, it can help overcome resistance to and suspicion of evaluation, demystify the process, and institutionalize evaluation methods within communities (Cousins & Whitmore, 1998; Springett, 2017). When the community shares ownership of goals, process, and skills, evaluation becomes an integral part of organizing for change. Being responsible for evaluation can also push an organization to examine its assumptions and make implicit theory explicit, thus contributing to the development of local theory.

Second, participatory evaluation is well aligned with mixed methods approaches that integrate qualitative and quantitative methods to maximize strengths and overcome weaknesses of each approach (Creswell & Clark, 2017; Lucero et al., 2018). For example, since community organizing and health initiatives are complex and involve multiple factors, quantitative data can inform the extent of accomplishments while qualitative information can increase understanding of which factors contribute to the functioning of the organizing effort and in what ways.

Third, such evaluation can adapt, evolve, and invent evaluation methods, indicators, and instruments. Community participation in evaluation can be a rich source of innovation in methods development. For example, collaborative efforts often lead to unanticipated outcomes that were not specified in the program design and evaluation and can be difficult to identify. Participatory qualitative data-collection processes for capturing such outcomes include photovoice and digital storytelling (Catalani & Minkler, 2010; Sonke, et al., 2019; chapter 17), methods that use stories to identify program impacts through an iterative process of selecting powerful images or events, deliberating on their meaning and value, and engaging in group dialogue to identify implications for action.

Fourth, participatory evaluation can enhance the ability of communities to do systematic data collection (Cousins & Chouinard, 2012; Springett, 2017; Wallerstein et al., 2018). Participatory evaluation can provide an incentive for local organizations to maintain their records in easy to access formats so that records data can be pulled together to create a community database. Community members of the evaluation team can gather new data of their own to give clout and credibility to advocacy efforts, using methods such as mapping conditions of the physical environment and tools such as phone-based apps and social media (chapter 15; appendix 2).

Fifth, participatory evaluation can creatively link community investigators and outside evaluators in a mutual learning partnership (Goold et al., 2016; Zeigler et al., 2019). Training, facilitation, and technical assistance enable community team members to understand and apply evaluation methods within the field's standards for validity and rigor. The experiential wisdom of community leaders and members can ensure that evaluation questions are important, data-collection methods realistic and culturally relevant, and findings applicable within the local context. Evaluators can help ensure that policymakers and other audiences hear community voices. Funders and institutional participants can gain deeper understanding of the critical role of the macrolevel context in the success of community efforts, influencing allocation of resources.

Challenges of Using Participatory Evaluation

There are philosophical and practical challenges to the evolving practice of participatory evaluation (Israel et al., 2018; Springett, 2017). As noted earlier, participatory evaluation frameworks may conflict with traditional assumptions about objectivity and distance. Charges of bias, conflict of interest, and misuse of data or findings can undermine the credibility of the evaluation, thereby lessening its clout. This may be particularly critical in policy and funding arenas. While a central aim of evaluation is ideally program or initiative improvement, evaluation has never been neutral, and participatory evaluation simply makes explicit the importance of community self-determination and the goal of equity.

Participatory evaluation must meet the field's standards for propriety and accuracy, as well as utility and feasibility (Yarbrough et al., 2010). Evaluators can increase accuracy and propriety by exploring ways to minimize participant bias and including multiple methods, measures, and data sources in the evaluation design. Qualitative researchers have developed strategies for addressing concerns of validity and reliability (Creswell & Clark, 2017; Israel et al., 2018). However, because of the paradigm shift involved, participatory evaluation can be challenging for traditional evaluators. As a process of codiscovery, it models the learning process and is quite fluid. Investigators must continually sample a changing environment and evaluate situations by degrees rather than as absolutes.

A second key challenge is that both professional and community evaluators must develop new skills and understanding for genuine collaboration and power sharing to occur. Outside evaluators must develop or hone their skills in working hands-on with community investigators in areas such as organizational development, program development, grant writing, and advocacy. Community evaluators may need training in evaluation methods to ensure rigor. Group-process skills in communication, collaborative problem solving, negotiation, conflict resolution, and consensus building may not be part of the everyday repertoire of many community members or evaluators and must be learned.

Professional evaluators who are outsiders must be cognizant of the history of the community, structural practices of racial and economic injustice, the local ethnic and political culture, and the aims of the project. They must demonstrate humility and self-reflection and be able to openly address power and resource differences; understand power sharing and collaboration as outcomes as well as processes; talk with, not down to, the community; and commit themselves to eliminating racial injustice and inequity. Above all, diverse players must operate under principles of ongoing trust, mutual learning, collaboration, and respect. Participatory evaluation may contribute to increasing the racial and ethnic diversity of the evaluation field.

A third challenge of participatory evaluation is that it takes a great deal of time, effort, and personal commitment, which can be difficult for both evaluators and community members (Sufian et al., 2011). They may feel that the process is diverting precious resources away from what they consider their real work, whether it involves the evaluation or the community organizing. Ironically, what may seem like an opportunity for capacity building to enthusiastic researchers may seem like yet another unfunded mandate to participants, placing too much responsibility on the community for fixing the problem (Caldwell et al., 2015; Israel et al., 2018). Evaluation must be feasible and practical, balancing the interests of all.

A fourth challenge is that the greatest strength of this approach is also one of its greatest hurdles—being responsive to rapid and unexpected shifts in program design and implementation. Effective community organizing and community building must be flexible, developmental, and responsive to changing local needs and conditions (Staples, 2016; chapters 8, 12). This requires continual collection, description, reflection, and feedback of information about a group, organization, or community in all its complexity (and, not uncommonly, all its chaos). Besides being time consuming, such a process conflicts with conventional notions of scientific rigor in evaluation, which preclude continual tampering with the intervention (Springett, 2017; Wallerstein et al., 2011).

A final challenge for participatory evaluation relates to indicators and measurement. As noted earlier, community organizing, community building, and comprehensive community initiatives typically address complex problems with multiple causes affecting different constituencies in interrelated ways. Participation, collaboration, empowerment, power, and community competence and capacity remain challenging to conceptualize and measure, though there is now a substantial body of work in this area as described earlier. Assessing the impacts of these concepts and constructs on policy and systems change is particularly difficult, in part because such changes often take place over a long period of time. Further, as discussed in chapter 22, contextual factors, and the fact that numerous actors typically play a role in hitting the "policy levers" that can bring about change, make it extremely difficult to tease out the impact of an organizing effort or community-based initiative, let alone the role of constructs like empowerment. Yet, here too, the application of new or refined approaches, such as multimethod case study analysis that includes a participatory evaluation component, may help develop a better understanding of the potential contribution of an organizing effort to a larger policy or systems-level change (Coombe et al., 2017; Minkler, 2010; Yin, 2003).

Conclusion

Participatory evaluation can be a powerful tool for community organizing efforts, coalitions, and community-based initiatives that have empowerment, capacity building, and social change as goals. The evaluation process itself can strengthen participation and ownership, build community competence, and reveal important outcomes that might be overlooked in conventional evaluations.

Particularly in the current socioeconomic, political, cultural, and public health contexts, however, a major strength of participatory evaluation lies in how it pays attention to the real voices of real people, demystifying and democratizing the process of developing knowledge. Working as a team, evaluators and community members learn from each other and increase their abilities to have an impact on conditions affecting the community. Participatory evaluation has the potential for transformation.

Finally, participatory evaluation is both an art and a science, requiring changes in philosophy and practice by professional evaluators, community investigators and practitioners, and funders. It requires new skills, new relationships, deep commitment to equity, and a fair amount of faith. Given the ongoing and current imperative to effectively address deeply entrenched systems of inequity, it is an investment we need to make. Participatory evaluation can make an important contribution to building and sustaining healthy, powerful, and self-determined communities.

Questions for Further Discussion

1. What are the key differences between participatory evaluation and conventional approaches to evaluation?

2. Think about your community and a specific participatory research project. What are the considerations and challenges with using a participatory evaluation process? How might the challenges of participatory evaluation be overcome?

REFERENCES

Caldwell, W. B., Reyes, A. G., Rowe, Z., Weinert, J., & Israel, B. A. (2015). Community partner perspectives on benefits, challenges, facilitating factors, and lessons learned from community-based participatory research partnerships in Detroit. *Prog Community Health Partnersh, 9*(2), 299–311.

Cargo, M., & Mercer, S. L. (2008). The value and challenges of participatory research: Strengthening its practice. *Annu Rev Public Health, 2*(9), 325–350.

Catalani, C., & Minkler, M. (2010). Photovoice: A review of the literature in health and public health. *Health Educ Behav, 37*(3), 424–451.

Chávez, V., Minkler, M., Wallerstein, N., & Spencer, M. S. (2010). Community organizing for health and social justice. In L. Cohen, V. Chávez, & S. Chehimi (Eds.), *Prevention Is Primary: Strategies for Community Well-Being* (2nd ed., pp. 87–112). Jossey-Bass.

Coombe, C. M. (2012). Participatory approaches to evaluating community organizing and coalition building. In M. Minkler (Ed.), *Community Organizing and Community Building for Health and Welfare* (3rd ed., pp. 346–365). Rutgers University Press.

Coombe, C. M., Israel, B. A., Reyes, A., Clement, J., Grant, S., Lichtenstein, R., Schulz, A., & Smith, S. (2017). Strengthening community capacity in Detroit to influence policy change for health equity. *Michigan Journal of Community Service Learning, 23*(2), 101–116.

Cousins, J. B., & Chouinard, J. A. (2012). *Participatory Evaluation Up Close: An Integration of Research-Based Knowledge.* Information Age Publishing.

Cousins, J. B., Shulha, L. M., Whitmore, E., Hudib, H. A., & Gilbert, N. (2016). How do evaluators differentiate successful from less-than-successful experiences with collaborative approaches to evaluation? *Eval Rev, 40*(1), 3–28.

Cousins, J. B., & Whitmore, E. (1998). Framing participatory evaluation. *New Dir Eval, 1998*(80), 5–23.

Creswell, J. W., & Clark, V. L. P. (2017). *Designing and Conducting Mixed Methods Research.* Sage.

Cyril, S., Smith, B. J., & Renzaho, A. M. N. (2016). Systematic review of empowerment measures in health promotion. *Health Promot Int, 31*(4), 809–826.

Eng, E., & Parker, E. (1994). Measuring community competence in the Mississippi Delta. *Health Educ, 21*(2), 199–220.

Fawcett, S. B., Sepers, C. E., Jones, J., Jones, L., & McKain, W. (2015). Participatory evaluation of a community mobilization effort to enroll Wyandotte County, Kansas, residents through the Affordable Care Act. *Am J Public Health, 105*(suppl_3), S433–S437.

Fetterman, D. M., Kaftarian, S., & Wandersman, A. (2015). *Empowerment Evaluation: Knowledge and Tools for Self-Assessment, Evaluation Capacity Building, and Accountability.* Sage.

Fetterman, D. M., Rodríguez-Campos, L., & Zukoski, A. P. (2017). *Collaborative, Participatory, and Empowerment Evaluation: Stakeholder Involvement Approaches.* Guilford Press.

Foster, C. C., & Louie, J. (2010, March). Grassroots action and learning for social change: Evaluating community organizing. Center for Evaluation Innovation. http://www.innonet.org/client_docs/File/center_pubs/evaluating_community_organizing.pdf.

Frisby, W., Maguire, P., & Reid, C. (2009). The F word has everything to do with it: How feminist theories inform action research. *Action Res, 7*(1), 13–29.

Goold, S., Rowe, Z., Calhoun, K., Campbell, T., Danis, M., Hammad, A., Salman, C., Szymecko, L., & Coombe, C. M. (2016). The state as community in community-based participatory research. *Prog Community Health Partnersh, 10*(4), 515–522.

Greenwald, H. P., & Zukoski, A. P. (2018). Assessing collaboration: Alternative measures and issues for evaluation. *Am J Eval, 39*(3), 322–335.

Israel, B. A., Eng, E., Schulz, A. J., & Parker, E. (2013). *Methods for Community-Based Participatory Research for Health.* Jossey-Bass.

Israel, B. A., Lachance, L., Coombe, C. M., Lee, S-Y. D., Jensen, M., Wilson-Powers, E., Mentz, G., Muhammed, M., Rowe, Z., Reyes, A. G., & Brush, B. L. (2020). Measurement approaches to partnership success: Theory and methods for measuring success in long-standing community-based participatory research partnerships. *Prog Community Health Partnersh, 14*(1), 129–140.

Israel, B. A., Schulz, A. J., Parker, E. A., Becker, A. B., Allen, A. J., Guzman, J. R., & Lichtenstein, R. (2018). Critical issues in developing and following CBPR principles. In N. Wallerstein, B. Duran, J. Oetzel, & M. Minkler (Eds.), *Community-Based Participatory Research for Health: Advancing Social and Health Equity* (3rd ed., pp. 31–46). Jossey-Bass.

Judd, J., Frankish, C. J., & Moulton, G. (2001). Setting standards in the evaluation of community-based health promotion programmes—a unifying approach. *Health Promot Int, 16*(4), 367–380.

Kastelic, S. L., Wallerstein, N., Duran, B., & Oetzel, J. G. (2018). Socio-ecological framework for CBPR: Development and testing of a model. In N. Wallerstein, B. Duran, J. Oetzel, & M. Minkler (Eds.), *Community-Based Participatory Research for Health: Advancing Social and Health Equity* (3rd ed., pp. 77–94). Jossey-Bass.

Lachance, L., & Kowalski-Dobson, T. (2018, September). Community-driven efforts to increase equity in communities through policy and systems change: Outcomes and lessons learned from 9 years of food & fitness community partnerships. *Health Promot Prac Special Supplement, 19*(1_suppl), 6S–114S.

Lewin, K. (1946). Action research and minority problems. *J Social Issues, 2,* 34–46.

Lucero, J., Wallerstein, N., Duran, B., Alegria, M., Greene-Moton, E., Israel, B., Kastelic, S., Magarati, M., Oetzel, J., Pearson, C., & Schulz, A. (2018). Development of a mixed methods investigation of process and outcomes of community-based participatory research. *J Mix Methods Res, 12*(1), 55–74.

Maguire, P. (1987). *Doing Participatory Research: A Feminist Approach.* Center for International Education, University of Massachusetts.

Minkler, M. (2010). Linking science and policy through community-based participatory research to study and address health disparities. *Am J Public Health, 100*(suppl_1), S81–S87.

Minkler, M., Estrada, J., Thayer, R., Juachon, L., Wakimoto, P., & Falbe, J. (2018). Bringing healthy retail to urban "food swamps": A case study of CBPR-informed policy and neighborhood change in San Francisco. *J Urban Health, 95*(6), 850–858.

Minkler, M., Garcia, A. P., Rubin, V., & Wallerstein, N. (2012). *Community-Based Participatory Research: A Strategy for Building Healthy Communities and Promoting Health through Policy Change.* PolicyLink.

Morelli, P. T., & Mataira, P. J. (2010). Indigenizing evaluation research: A long-awaited paradigm shift. *J Indigenous Voices Social Work, 1*(2), 1–12.

Ozer, E. J., & Piatt, A. A. (2018). Youth-led participatory action research: Principles, implementation, and diffusion in diverse settings. In N. Wallerstein, B. Duran, J Oetzel, & M. Minkler (Eds.), *Community-Based Participatory Research for Health: Advancing Social and Health Equity* (3rd ed., pp. 95–106). Jossey-Bass.

Patton, M. Q. (2019). Expanding futuring foresight through evaluative thinking. *World Futures Rev, 11*(4), 296–307.

Quinn, M., Kowalski-Dobson, T., & Lachance, L. (2018). Defining and measuring sustainability in the food & fitness initiative. *Health Promot Pract, 19*(1_suppl), 78S–91S.

Richards-Schuster K., & Elliott, S. P. (2019). Practice matrix for involving young people in evaluation: Possibilities and considerations. *Am J Eval, 40*(4), 533–547.

Rifkin, S. B. (2014). Examining the links between community participation and health outcomes: A review of the literature. *Health Policy Plan, 29* (suppl 1), ii98–ii106.

Roe, K. M., Roe, K., Carpenter, C. G., & Sibley, C. B. (2005). Community building through empowering evaluation: A case study of community planning for HIV prevention. In M. Minkler (Ed.), *Community Organizing and Community Building for Health* (2nd ed., pp. 386–402). Rutgers University Press.

Sánchez, V., Carrillo, C., & Wallerstein, N. (2011). From the ground up: Building a participatory evaluation model. *Prog Community Health Partnersh, 5*(1), 45–52.

Scarinci, I. C., Moore, A., Benjamin, R., Vickers, S., Shikany, J., & Fouad, M. (2017). A participatory evaluation framework in the establishment and implementation of transdisciplinary collaborative centers for health disparities research. *Eval Program Plann, 60*, 37–45.

Schulz, A. J., Israel, B. A., Coombe, C. M., Gaines, C., Reyes, A. G., Rowe, Z., Sand, S. L., Strong, L. L., & Weir, S. (2011). A community-based participatory planning process and multilevel intervention design: Toward eliminating cardiovascular health disparities. *Health Promot Pract, 12*(6), 900–911.

Sen, R. (2003). *Stir It Up: Lessons in Community Organizing and Advocacy.* Jossey-Bass.

Shulha, L. M., Whitmore, E., Cousins, J. B., Gilbert, N., & al Hudib, H. (2016). Introducing evidence-based principles to guide collaborative approaches to evaluation: Results of an empirical process. *Am J Eval, 37*(2), 193–215.

Smith, L. T. (2012). *Decolonizing Methodologies: Research and Indigenous Peoples.* Zed Books.

Sonke, J., Golden, T., Francois, S., Hand, J., Chandra, A., Clemmons, L., Fakunle, D., Jackson, M. R., Magsamen, S., Rubin, V., Sams, K., & Springs, S. (2019). *Creating Healthy Communities through Cross-Sector Collaboration* [White paper]. University of Florida Center for Arts in Medicine / ArtPlace America.

Springett, J. (2017). Impact in participatory health research: What can we learn from research on participatory evaluation? *Educ Action Res, 25*(4), 560–574,

Springett, J., & Wallerstein, N. (2008). Issues in participatory evaluation. In M. Minkler & N. Wallerstein (Eds.), *Community-Based Participatory Research for Health* (2nd ed., pp. 263–288). Jossey-Bass.

Staples, L. (2016). *Roots to Power: A Manual for Grassroots Organizing* (3rd ed.). Praeger.

Stoecker, R. (2012). *Research Methods for Community Change: A Project-Based Approach.* Sage.

Sufian, M., Grunbaum, J. A., Akintobi, T. H., Dozier, A., Eder, M., Jones, S., Mullan, S, Weir, C. R., & White-Cooper, S. (2011). Program evaluation and evaluating community engagement. In Clinical and Translational Science Awards Consortium Community Engagement Key Function Committee Task Force on Principles of Community Engagement, *Principles of Community Engagement* (2nd ed., pp. 161–183). NIH Publication No. 11-7782. National Institutes of Health. https://www.atsdr.cdc.gov/communityengagement/pdf/PCE_Report_508_FINAL.pdf.

Wallerstein, N., & Duran, B. (2018). The theoretical, historical and practice roots of CBPR. In N. Wallerstein, B. Duran, J. Oetzel, & M. Minkler (Eds.), *Community-Based Participatory Research for Health: Advancing Social and Health Equity* (3rd ed., pp. 17–29). Jossey-Bass.

Wallerstein, N., Duran, B., Oetzel, J., & Minkler, M. (2018). *Community-Based Participatory Research for Health: Advancing Social and Health Equity* (3rd ed.). Jossey-Bass.

Wallerstein, N., Oetzel, J. G., Sanchez-Youngman, S., Boursaw, B., Dickson, E., Kastelic, S., Koegel, P., Lucero, J. E., Magarati, M., Ortiz, K., & Parker, M. (2020). Engage for equity: A long-term study of community-based participatory research and community-engaged research practices and outcomes. *Health Educ Behav, 47*(3), 380–390.

Wallerstein, N. B., Yen, I. H., & Syme, S. L. (2011). Integration of social epidemiology and community-engaged interventions to improve health equity. *Am J Public Health, 101*(5), 822–830.

Wandersman, A. (2015). *Getting to Outcomes: An Empowerment Evaluation Approach for Capacity Building and Accountability.* Sage.

Ward, M., Schulz, A. J., Israel, B. A., Rice, K., Martenies, S. E., & Markarian, E. (2018). A conceptual framework for evaluating health equity promotion within community-based participatory research partnerships. *Eval Program Plann, 70,* 25–34.

Weiss, C. H., & Connell, J. P. (1995). Nothing as practical as good theory: Exploring theory-based evaluation in comprehensive community initiatives. In J. P. Connell, A. C. Kubisch, L. B. Schorr, & C. H. Weiss, (Eds.), *New Approaches to Evaluating Community Initiatives: Concepts, Methods, and Contexts* (pp. 65–92). Aspen Institute.

Whyte, W. F. (1991). *Participatory Action Research.* Sage.

Wiggins, N., Parajon, L., Coombe, C. M., Duldulao, A., Wang, P., & Rodriguez Garcia, L. (2018). Participatory evaluation as a process of empowerment: Experiences with community health workers in the US and Latin America. In N. Wallerstein, B. Duran, J. Oetzel, & M. Minkler (Eds.), *Community-Based Participatory Research for Health: Advancing Social and Health Equity* (3rd ed., pp. 251–264). Jossey-Bass.

Wolfe, S. M., Long, P. D., & Brown, K. K. (2020). Using a principles-focused evaluation approach to evaluate coalitions and collaboratives working toward equity and social justice. *New Dir Eval, 2020*(165), 45–65.

Wolff, T., Minkler, M., Wolfe, S. M., Berkowitz, B., Bowen, L., Butterfoss, F. D., Christens, B. D., Francisco, V. T., Himmelman, A. T., & Lee, K. S. (2017). Collaborating for equity and justice: Moving beyond collective impact. *Nonprofit Q, 9,* 42–53.

World Health Organization (WHO). (1986). Ottawa Charter for Health Promotion. WHO Europe. http://www.who.int/hpr/NPH/docs/ottawa_charter_hp.pdf.

Yarbrough, D. B., Shulha, L. M., Hopson, R. K., & Caruthers, F. A. (2010). *The Program Evaluation Standards: A Guide for Evaluators and Evaluation Users.* Sage.

Yin, R. (2003). *Case Study Research: Design and Methods* (3rd ed.). Sage.

Zeigler, T., Coombe, C. M., Rowe, Z. E., Clark, S. J., Gronland, C. J., Lee, M., Palacios, A., Reames, T. G., Schott, J., Williams, G. O., & O'Neill, M. S. (2019). Shifting from "community-placed" to "community-based" research to advance health equity: A case study of the Heatwaves, Housing, and Health; Increasing climate resiliency in Detroit (HHH) partnership. *Int J Environ Res, 16*(18), 3310.

PART EIGHT

Influencing Policy through Community Organizing and Media Advocacy

A hallmark of community organizing in fields like public health, social welfare, and urban and regional planning lies in its commitment to action and social change. Although that commitment would appear to make engagement in the policy process a logical one in such fields, many professionals shy away from policy advocacy, deeming it too time consuming and risky. Further, for those employed by government agencies (e.g., a state or local department of public health or human services, or a faculty member at a state-funded university), advocacy on behalf of a particular piece of legislation may be forbidden. Finally, community partners may find the policy process confusing, or work on the policy level simply too abstract, to be a good use of their time.

Viewed differently, however, if we and our community partners shy away from working on the policy level, valuable opportunities for increasing health equity and social justice may be lost (Freudenberg et al., 2015; Iton & Shirmali, 2016).

In the final part of this volume, we turn our attention to the role community organizing can play in helping to promote changes in policy or the broader policy environment. In chapter 22, Lisa Cacari Stone and her colleagues offer an introduction to the policymaking process, emphasizing the importance of using an equity lens and ensuring that communities most burdened by health and social inequities are front and center in the work.

Building on earlier conceptual models of the policymaking process (Kingdon, 2011), including one she and her partners in community-based participatory research developed (Cacari Stone et al., 2014), chapter 22 presents a model for bridging evidence, community organizing, and equity policy, including a look at the key steps involved in this process. Recent experiences of the successful and long-term Los Angeles Collaborative for Environmental Health and Justice (Sadd et al., 2014), in securing the passage and implementation of a "Clean Up, Green Up" ordinance in three heavily polluted and largely Latinx communities, is used to demonstrate the utility of the model in real time (Sadd et al., 2014; Yanez, 2016). The contributions of community members and their partners to both policy change and health equity outcomes are described, as is the need for intentionality in setting and working toward equity policy goals from the very beginning of the process if we are to achieve real and sustainable change.

In chapter 23, Amber Akemi Piatt and her partners then explore how two coalitions, each led by currently and formerly incarcerated people and their families but with the support of allies in fields like public health, used the window of opportunity provided by COVID-19 to advance the struggle to end mass incarceration and similarly broken parts of the criminal legal system. The work of Decarcerate Alameda County is explored using Kingdon's model of the three streams in the policymaking process (getting policymakers' attention, coming up with a feasible and politically attractive policy solution, and then negotiating a policy win (2011; chapter 22). We learn how coalition leaders and allies, including health educators at the nonprofit Human Impact Partners, brought attention to the urgent need for decarceration, helped craft policy solutions, and presented them to decisionmakers, achieving some, though certainly not sufficient, policy wins in the process (Health Instead of Punishment Program Team, 2020; Minkler et al., 2020). The authors then turn to the very different approach of the #DeeperThanWater Coalition in Massachusetts, which made the strategic decision to focus on exposing environmental and other abuses and building broad public momentum for abolishing the criminal legal system and *not* working incrementally within the system to change policy. This chapter concludes with Wayland "X" Coleman's powerful essay as an organizer with #DeeperThanWater, whose insights and experiences behind prison walls, and whose determination to share those realities with those of us outside, capture the importance and urgency of this work as little else can.

Media advocacy was one of several critical strategies in the abolition efforts described in chapter 23, and in the book's final chapter we explore this approach in detail. Popular radio commentator Wes Nisker was fond of saying, "If you don't like the news—go out and make some of your own." For Lori Dorfman and her colleagues at the Berkeley Media Studies Group (BMSG), however, the objective has always been not to *make* the news, but rather to strategically *use* the mass media to promote policy initiatives and ensure that stories are told from a community or public health perspective (Wallack et al., 1999). In chapter 24, Dorfman, Prisila Gonzalez, and Shaddai Martinez Cuestas provide an engaging look at media advocacy, including the many questions that need to be answered as we develop an overall strategy, a message strategy, and an access strategy, before we attempt to get media attention to our issue. They also discuss the importance of careful framing, particularly in fields like public health and social welfare, so that the media's popular *portrait* stories (focused on an individual) are presented instead as *landscape* stories that center how the systemic and structural realities in which individuals are embedded have an impact on their health status and well-being. Whether we are tackling problems like junk food in school lunch programs, deep inequities in the quality and availability of health care, the dearth of affordable housing, gender-based violence, or climate change, the effective use of media advocacy can be a critical tool in helping us reframe local and global problems and how they are presented and viewed. In the process, it can also help in efforts to create both healthier communities and healthy, equity- and justice-focused public policies.

REFERENCES

Cacari Stone, L., Wallerstein, N., Garcia, A., & Minkler, M. (2014). The promise of community-based participatory research for health equity: A conceptual model for bridging evidence with policy. *Am J Public Health, 104*(9), 1615–1623.

Freudenberg, N., Franzosa, E., Chisholm, J., & Libman, K. (2015). New approaches for moving upstream: How state and local health departments can transform practice to reduce health inequalities. *Health Educ Behav, 42*(1_suppl), 46S–56S.

Health Instead of Punishment Program Team. (2020, March 13). Taking action for health, justice, and belonging in the age of COVID-19. Human Impact Partners. https://humanimpact-hip.medium.com/taking-action-for-health-justice-and-belonging-in-the-age-of-covid-19-bb6b84648d98.

Iton, A., & Shrimali, B. P. (2016). Power, politics, and health: A new public health practice targeting the root causes of health equity. *Matern Child Health J, 20*(8), 1753–1758.

Kingdon, J. W. (2011). *Agendas, Alternatives, and Public Policies* (updated 2nd ed.). Longman.

Minkler, M., Griffin, J., & Wakimoto, P. (2020). Seizing the moment: Policy advocacy to end mass incarceration in the time of COVID-19. *Health Educ Behav, 47*(4), 514–518.

Sadd, J., Morello-Frosch, R., Pastor, M., Matsuoka, M., Prichard, M., & Carter, V. (2014). The truth, the whole truth, and nothing but the ground-truth: Methods to advance environmental justice and researcher–community partnerships. *Health Educ Behav, 41*(3), 281–290.

Wallack L., Woodruff, K., Dorfman, L., & Diaz, I. (1999). *News for a Change: An Advocate's Guide to Working with the Media.* Sage.

Yanez, E. (2016, April 20). L.A.'s promising Clean Up, Green Up ordinance. The Prevention Institute. https://www.preventioninstitute.org/blog/las-promising-clean-green-ordinance.

22

Moving the Policy Dial through Equity-Focused Community Organizing

LISA CACARI STONE

MANUEL PASTOR

JOSEPH GRIFFIN

RACHEL MORELLO-FROSCH

MEREDITH MINKLER

In public health, urban and regional planning, social work, and related fields, a hallmark of community organizing lies in its commitment to action and social change. Although such action may take many forms, community organizers have increasingly turned to equity-focused policy change approaches as among the most potent for affecting the health and well-being of communities and beyond.

The rationale for an emphasis on policy in the health field is well documented. Despite a decline in life expectancy of one full year in the first six months of 2020 due to the COVID-19 pandemic, with drops of 2.7 years for Blacks and 1.9 for Hispanics (Arias et al., 2021), substantial increases in life expectancy over the last century have been attributed in large part to environmental and other policy-related changes in sanitation, water supply, food quality, and other areas (Braveman & Gottlieb, 2014). More recently, community organizing in areas ranging from climate change and health care for all, to the Movement for Black Lives, and the rights of women, immigrants, Indigenous persons, the disabled, and LGBTQ people, have helped change policies on the local through the national levels (Brown et al., 2012; Cacari Stone et al., 2014; Minkler et al., 2012; Pastor, 2018). Similarly, policy advocacy to promote tobacco control, healthy food environments, affordable housing, curbing the sale of hand guns and assault rifles, and ending police brutality are among many policy-related efforts that took root in community organizing efforts and grew into regional, national, and sometimes global health and social movements (Freudenberg & Tsui, 2014; Iton & Ross, 2017; Pastor et al., 2009, 2016). On the global level, the Healthy Cities/Healthy Communities movement has focused on broad policy-level changes since its inception and in doing so has been helping communities realize their vision of a healthy place in which to live, work, and play. A movement for

Health in All Policies (Rudolph et al., 2013; World Health Organizaton, 2015) has also increasingly worked to influence how we think about health equity and social justice by broadening our gaze beyond the health and social spheres (chapters 1, 12).

As Blackwell and Colmenar (2000) note, for many community residents, the very concept of "public policy" is "unfamiliar and irrelevant, complicated, inaccessible and confusing" (p. 162). Even those who believe in the importance of changing public policy often feel ineffectual in their ability to influence public sphere decisions affecting their lives. Similarly, professionals in health, social work, community psychology, and related fields who work on the community level may be reluctant to focus on policy-related activities, which are perceived as taking place "out there" (e.g., at state and national levels) and far removed from their day to day community organizing efforts (Minkler & Freudenberg, 2010). Confusion over the extent to which nonprofit organizations can engage in policy advocacy without jeopardizing their funding may be cause for concern, although this fear is often exaggerated and not in line with actual federal or foundation grantee guidelines (US Department of Treasury, 2016; chapters 8, 20).

Despite the challenges faced, however, health professionals, urban planners, social workers and other practitioners and researchers, and their community partners, along with policymakers themselves are increasingly recognizing community organizing approaches and strategies as critical to helping effect equity-focused public policy. Indeed, if community organizing and community building principles are taken seriously, policymaking itself may become a process of community building and organizing, with community members engaged at every step, from selecting and framing the issues to interpreting the data, discussing the options, and working for the adoption and enforcement of the policy changes they wish to see.

We begin this chapter by describing the importance of having an equity lens and closing the "know-do" gap in advancing health equity, particularly toward the end of bringing the lived experiences of communities most burdened by health and social inequities to bear in the policymaking process. Next, we offer a conceptual framework for bridging evidence, community organizing, and equity policy, including a look at the key steps or streams involved in this process. Then, we use the Los Angeles Collaborative for Environmental Health and Justice as a case study to demonstrate the utility of the conceptual model in terms of both processes and outcomes. We conclude by suggesting that to truly achieve equity policy, including high-level community involvement in the process, the very nature of our policies should be reconsidered, such that community building becomes a central consideration in how policies are shaped and what they look like.

Framing a Policy Goal from an Equity Lens

The first step in engaging community-based partnerships in efforts to use evidence and organizing to help change policy is to establish processes through which they can identify and frame policy goals from an equity lens. Going beyond the use of the term "disparities," as the noting of differences, the term "equity" connotes unfair and avoidable conditions. In agreeing on a common language (Burke, 2016), partners should find a shared meaning in ways that support the intent of the collaboration. A deep understanding of the historical context of oppression, power suppression, and their intergenerational impacts on communities should be shared by all partners entering a collaboration. Setting a goal to address privilege and oppression is another avenue for developing an equity lens. It is important to name racism, sexism, homophobia, ableism, xenophobia, and Islamophobia as forces in determining how these social determinants are distributed within a given geography or community. Partners must be committed to ongoing dialogue that expands individual and group learning, enhances communication, and holds the collaborative accountable for these equity competencies. Talking about privilege, oppression, and historical injustices, such as racism and genocide, can be challenging for diverse audiences, yet they are critical to creating a policy goal from an equity lens.

Closing the "Know-Do" Gap in Advancing Health Equity

The use of research by policymakers is less likely to occur without interpersonal connections and close linkages between politicians, academics, and community partnerships. The "social ecology of research use" refers to how research use unfolds through linkages of relationships, organizational settings, and political and policy contexts in which policy decisions are made (Nutley et al., 2007; Tseng et al., 2008). In a landmark report, Prewitt and colleagues (2012) highlight the "uncertain connection" between scientific knowledge, how it is used in public policy, and how it can be more effectively used. The transmission of knowledge from communities and the research worlds to that of policymaking is a complex and challenging endeavor because it involves three distinct cultures (practice, research, and policy). Each embodies a distinct culture that the other two need to learn and adapt to in an atmosphere of mutual respect. Each also needs to feel and understand a common purpose (Shonkoff, 2000). Yet community organizing and community-based participatory research (a partnership approach to research that equitably involves community members, researchers, and other partners throughout the research process) (Israel et al., 2013; Minkler, 2010, 2014) create substantial opportunities for engagement, through which community members or practitioners, researchers, and policy makers acquire, interpret, and use research in policymaking to advance health equity.

Community organizers play a critical role in bridging the "know-do" gap illustrated in table 22.1 by fostering the integration and translation of three types of cultures (science, policy, and community practice) that can be linked to policymaking to reduce social inequities (Cacari Stone, 2016). This involves bringing together the three types of partners to pursue a course of targeted action that transcends deeply rooted, and sometimes self-serving, interests of politicians or scientists and researchers to advance their own agendas or keep political or academic

TABLE 22.1

The "Know-Do" Gap in Advancing Health Equity

How Policymakers Perceive Research	How Researchers Perceive Policy	How Communities and Practitioners Perceive Policy and Research
Lack of timeliness	Decisions based on political preferences and money	Both disconnected from real lived experiences of the persons on whom they are doing research or for whom they are making policy
Politically irrelevant research		
Research for the sake of research	Lack of scientific evidence	
Too much focus on describing and managing the problem	Too much partisanship	
	Manipulation of data to support a political position or agenda	Lack of personal contact among researchers, policymakers, and those most affected by the problem
Lack of applicability to "real-life" solutions	Lack of political will or action	Not enough action

Source: Cacari Stone, L. (2016).

power within their respective circles. It also requires continued attention to the three dimensions of equity policy:

- Committing to distributive justice, or equal protection and fair allocation of burdens and resources and procedural justice or fairness in how the decision-making process takes place
- Recognizing the role of intersectional positions of power and privilege
- Leveraging social policies to ameliorate economic or social disadvantage, such as minimum wage laws, progressive taxation, and statutes barring discrimination in housing or employment based on race, gender or gender identity, disability, or sexual orientation (Cacari Stone, 2016)

Community partnerships rooted in and committed to equity policy can help facilitate the willingness of social scientists, health professionals, and others to engage in the political process with community partners. Ideally too, this grounding in concerns with equity can also increase the willingness of politicians to engage with a set of ideas beyond their political or class interests (Cacari Stone et al., 2014). Greater linkages between research, policy, practice, and community can thus serve to challenge the thinking of policymakers and move them toward different, innovative, and transformative conceptualizations and solutions (Iton & Ross, 2017; Minkler, 2010; Nutley et al., 2007; Pastor, 2018).

Conceptual Model: Bridging Evidence, Community Organizing, and Equity Policy

As an approach to bridging these differences, we adapt a conceptual model that has proved useful in theorizing about and exploring the interplay among civic engagement, political participation, and evidence as it contributes to policy changes to reduce social inequities (Cacari Stone et al., 2014; figure 22.1). Following up on earlier testing of a similar model, we illustrate its utility in the context of a case study of the Los Angeles Collaborative for Environmental Health and Justice (Morello-Frosch et al., 2012; Sadd et al., 2014). As this case study illustrates, the Collaborative and its partners initially sought to change policy at the local level, the arena most accessible to local residents, and at the stage of building an equity-focused agenda with multiple partners and sectors.

Our conceptual model draws, in part, on the stages approaches of Bardach (2000), Kingdon (2011), and Longest (2006). Although using slightly different terminology, each of these encompasses (1) problem definition, (2) creating awareness and setting (or getting on) policymaker agendas, (3) constructing policy alternatives, (4) deciding on the policy to pursue, (5) implementing the policy, and (6) evaluation or modification, or both. Although the models have been criticized by some for oversimplifying complex political processes (Sabatier & Weible, 2014), they contribute practical insights, emphasizing the cyclical and interconnected nature of policymaking. Kingdon's (2011) model may be particularly useful in this regard, grouping the various steps into three broad streams: the *problem stream*, convincing policymakers that a problem exists and getting on the agenda; the *politics stream*, proposing feasible, politically attractive solutions; and the *policy stream*, negotiating the politics to win approval of a proposed measure. Kingdon (2011) further notes that when positive policy developments occur in all three streams, a window of opportunity often opens, increasing the likelihood of success (chapter 15).

In the Bridging Evidence, Community Organizing, & Equity Policy Model, the first oval, "Contexts," refers to both *macro-contextual factors* (e.g., the socio-cultural-economic environments, political leadership and power, public attitudes, and policy trends) and the *micro level context* in which community-engaged research takes place. The latter includes patterns of trust (or distrust) among communities, agencies, and university partners; organizational characteristics; and their capacity for high-quality collaborative research (Cacari Stone et al., 2014).

The second oval, "Community Processes," includes *partnership dynamics* among stakeholders and addresses questions such as, "Are there policymakers who are already committed to the issue?" and "Are there democratic decisionmaking processes in place among partners?" This oval also includes the dynamic interplay between the role of science and evidence and the role of civic engagement and political participation. Such work includes traditional outside expert–driven research and compelling "street science" (Corburn, 2017; appendix 2), in which

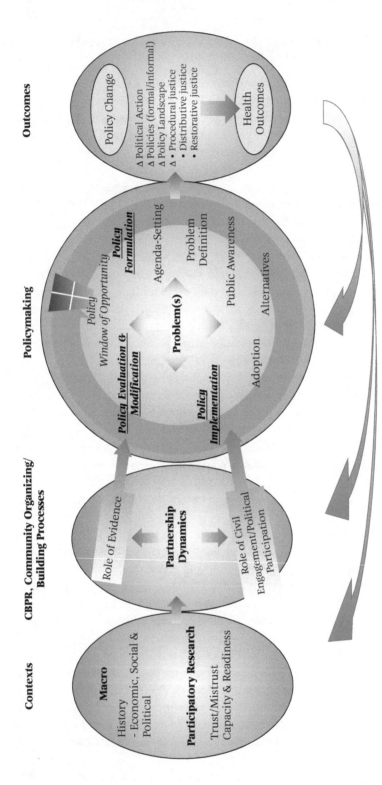

FIGURE 22.1 Conceptual Model for Bridging Evidence, Community Organizing, and Equity Policy.

Reprinted with permission from Cacari Stone L., Wallerstein N., Garcia, P. A., & Minkler, M. (2014). The promise of community-based participatory research for bridging evidence with policy: A conceptual model for bridging evidence with policy. *Am J Public Health, 104*(9), 1615–1623.

community members take the lead in collecting data capturing their often-sophisticated insider understanding of issues affecting their neighborhoods. *Civic engagement* refers to the role of community partners in organizing and advocacy, roles that may be more difficult or restricted for academic or government agency partners, and how community partners can integrate evidence into their organizing strategies. The strategies developed in the "Community Processes" oval influence the policymaking process in a variety of ways.

At the center of the "Policymaking" circle is the problem(s) to be addressed. Surrounding the problem are the stages in which partners may be engaged. Starting at the upper right of the circle, the *policy-formation stage* involves multiple dynamic strategies, which are not necessarily linear. These include agenda-setting, defining and prioritizing the problems within a given political environment, creating awareness of the issue(s) among key policymakers and the public, constructing policy alternatives based on what is timely and feasible, deciding which policies to pursue, and advocating for proposed changes and policy adoption. The last stages typically involve drawing on research findings and community members' stories and experiences. Choices tend to be made when the right combination of conditions, politics (e.g., moods or leadership turnover), and policies (acceptance of ideas by policymakers) converge, creating "policy windows" of opportunity. These windows may open at any stage of the policymaking process (Kingdon, 2011; Longest, 2006).

Finally, the "Outcomes" oval includes policy changes, such as catalyzing political activity (i.e., new leadership, increased civic engagement), formal and informal policies (ordinances, action plans), and changes in the policy landscape. These outcomes, in turn, may increase the likelihood of future policy change and greater opportunity for three forms of justice. The best known of these, *distributive justice*, simply refers to equal protection and fair allocation of burdens and resources. *Procedural justice*, in contrast, refers to fairness in how the decisionmaking process takes place, with marginalized communities getting a seat at the table—and staying at the table, to help shape the decisions that affect their lives and the life of their community (Minkler, 2010). Finally, *restorative justice* speaks to the inclusion of marginalized communities as centric to shaping policy processes that are concerned with balancing power differentials in relationships and healing of trauma due to historical dominant culture abuses in order to achieve equitable social and health outcomes (National Academies of Science, Engineering, and Medicine, 2019).

Illustrating the Model: A Case Study of the Los Angeles Collaborative for Environmental Health and Justice

Background and Overview

Although Los Angeles (LA) has long suffered from some of the nation's poorest air quality, the burden of such pollution is disproportionately borne by low-income communities of color. In such areas, the proximity of freeways, ports, factories, and other pollution sources to both homes and such "sensitive land use receptors" as schools, playgrounds, and senior centers, contribute to the inequitable distribution of asthma, heart disease, and other pollution-related health problems experienced (Morello-Frosch et al., 2001; Sadd et al., 2014).

In 1996, the Los Angeles Collaborative for Environmental Health and Justice (the Collaborative) was created "to study and address community-defined environmental justice issues" in this sprawling region, while also building local capacity by linking research with community organizing and policy advocacy (Morello-Frosch et al., 2012, p. 283). From its roots in another California environmental justice organization (Communities for a Better Environment), the Collaborative operated as a tripartite of community organizers and grassroots groups from across the LA region, university researchers, and funders, beginning with the LA-based Liberty Hill Foundation supporting capacity building and technical assistance to local community-based organizations (Petersen et al., 2006; Sadd et al., 2014).

The Collaborative sought to combine quantitative scientific data with the lived experience and concerns of residents. This led to policy campaigns to change local air district regulations on permissible facility emissions (in one case, reducing the allowable cancer risk for new facilities by 75 percent (https://www.libertyhill.org/campaigns), improving air quality near schools, and reducing diesel truck emissions near ports (Petersen et al., 2006). On a larger scale, the Collaborative's work has been used to support getting the state Environmental Protection Agency (EPA) to consider cumulative rather than simply individual environmental exposures and health impacts in its decisionmaking, and to similarly advocate for changes on the broader municipal and regional levels (Morello-Frosh et al., 2012; Sadd et al., 2014). The research team associated with the Collaborative as well as with other environmental justice organizations across California worked to develop what was called an Environmental Justice Screening Tool that became the precursor to the state's own CalEnviroScreen, a mapping approach that is used to allocate resources to the most environmentally exposed and socially disadvantaged neighborhoods in the state (Sadd et al., 2011).

In the context of this broad arc of work and long history of working together, the Collaborative eventually developed and used a novel ground-truthing method, through which residents, with support from university researchers, collect data about pollution sources and their location in relation to schools and other sensitive land-use areas. Although scientists often rely on government data sets and conduct secondary data analysis on problems such as water and air pollution, the data sets are often dated and badly flawed. Ground-truthing by residents who are familiar with local communities can improve the data set quality and utility by checking their accuracy using area "walk-throughs" with maps or tablets and GIS devices (Minkler, 2014; Sadd et al., 2014; appendix 2). Using this method and their own secondary data analysis, the Collaborative identified LA areas where targeted regulatory strategies might be required to address environmental justice (EJ) concerns, and followed this by organizing and advocacy around the needed specific policy changes (Sadd et al., 2014, p. 282).

The Collaborative's research, organizing, and policy advocacy was described by a variety of stakeholders as a major contributor to the "Clean Up, Green Up" (CUGU) ordinance passed in 2016 and currently being implemented. Through it, green zones have been created in three LA communities (Boyle Heights, Pacoima/ Sun Valley, and Wilmington) that are harshly affected by negative environmental conditions. In these zones, the goal is to reduce pollution, decrease the over-abundance of environmental hazards, and help businesses "clean up and green up" while also creating new jobs (Yanez, 2016; https://cleanupgreenup.wordpress .com).

While the goals have been clear and there was a sense of triumph when the ordinance passed, implementation has been less than stellar. Leaders and residents in Pacoima, for example, report that they are more easily able to get the attention of public agencies when they report problems and "benefit from coordinated inspec-tions, more protective health standards for new and expanded industrial opera-tions, and stronger local public participation" (Binns, 2019). But there are also frustrations that implementation has been stalled, partly by the need to translate broad policy directives into the sort of specific regulations city inspectors need. There are also concerns that the ombudsperson position that was envisioned to better coordinate responses got placed in the city's sanitation department when the original concerns were more about bad zoning and inappropriate uses than accumulated trash.

There is hope that the full potential of the green zone approach will be better realized when the City writes new community plans. In the meanwhile, it is also the case that a policy victory should be judged by its spillovers as well as by its immediate impact. For example, the CUGU campaign induced LA County to cre-ate its own green zone programs in two unincorporated areas, contracting with the research team to update its Environmental Justice Screening Method (http:// planning.lacounty.gov/greenzones/ejsm) and with local EJ organizations in the two communities to do ground-truthing (http://planning.lacounty.gov/greenzones /groundtruthing). The green zone concept also helped inform a "Transformative Climate Communities" program from the state's Strategic Growth Council in which millions of dollars raised by California's cap-and-trade program are reinvested in community-based efforts to reduce both greenhouse gas emissions and local air pollution (https://sgc.ca.gov/programs/tcc/).

Exploring the Collaborative and Its EJ Work within the Conceptual Model

The Collaborative and its environmental justice work in LA well illustrate the util-ity of the Bridging Evidence, Community Organizing and Equity Policy conceptual model.

In the "Contexts" oval, the *macro* context of Boyle Heights, Pacoima/Sun Valley, and Wilmington included decades of disproportionate exposure to air pollution and related health problems with little oversight of the businesses and other sources contributing to these problems (Sadd et al., 2014). The limited political economic clout of the largely Latinx residents, many undocumented and with limited English, may have further limited their capacity (or comfort level) in working for change. On the other hand, LA is a place that has been a center of social movement organizing and this provides a necessary context and infrastructure for communities finding their voice.

On the *micro* level context of *participatory research*, the university and foundation partners' long history of building trust and equitable relationships with the community partners was an important factor facilitating the effective functioning of the partnership. While not without tensions that sometimes occur between academics and activists (Morello-Frosch et al., 2011; Sadd et al., 2014), the Collaborative's centering of community-identified issues, and the readiness of community partners to gain new research skills (e.g., asking the university partners to help them learn how to do air quality monitoring) were important indicators of a favorable micro context vis-à-vis the work. Still, we stress here the long-term nature of the partnership; the researchers were not perceived as being purely transactional because of their long-term commitment, and this is an important lesson for those wanting to replicate these sorts of processes.

In the "Community Organizing / Building Processes" oval, *partnership dynamics* appear at the center, influencing the *role of evidence* and of *civic and community engagement and political participation* in the work. With respect to the role of evidence, the university and foundation partners' clear appreciation of the lived experience and community expertise of the grassroots partners, and the empowering ways in which trainings were conducted for their participation in ground-truthing, spoke to healthy partnership dynamics in this regard. Similarly, community partners expressed appreciation of the substantial time that university scientists devoted to research using detailed EPA and other government data sets, and its importance to creating a strong and equity-focused evidence base (Petersen et al., 2006).

The role of partnership dynamics in both influencing and being influenced by the *role of civic engagement and political participation* was also apparent. As noted above, the long history of collaboration between grassroots groups and organizers, university partners, and foundation funders helped build a dynamic of trust and support that encouraged the engagement of local residents in both an empowering approach to research and civic and political participation, as they shared their findings and lived experience in public settings. Likewise, the commitment of the university partners to improving community health and health equity policy led to their sharing of research findings not only in academic peer-reviewed venues but also with their community partners in local settings to help build support for policy and community change.

The role and assignment of funding were important. The earliest major investor in the Collaborative was The California Endowment, and the initial money was far more focused on organizing groups than on researchers, which helped to establish trust that the research team would be providing support rather than claiming credit. Subsequent support came from the California Wellness Foundation and other funders. But it is important to note that the Collaborative was not the only thing establishing research credibility: the research team also helped facilitate discussions of climate equity and cap-and-trade, designed the precursor to CalEnviroScreen, and helped pilot a similar model in the Bay Area. Being in the mix over years and not just for a short project period was critical. This was important not only for maintaining community trust that outside researchers were committed for the long haul (Israel et al., 2013; chapter 15), but also because the community organizing work involved in building support for new policies can take years. In the case of the CUGU initiative, a full decade of organizing preceded getting to a policy win. The coalition worked hard to meaningfully engage residents and local businesses, which had to feel buy-in (e.g., in helping find potential solutions and mitigation strategies that would help, rather than harm their businesses) if they were to get on board (https://cleanupgreeenup.wordpress.com). Similarly, one may need to wait years to see the results from implementation, and the sort of spillover effects documented above should be included in any full evaluation of the effectiveness of an intervention.

At the center of the "Policymaking" circle are the *problems* around which the policymaking process takes place. Here, the *agenda setting* starting point involved clearly defining the problem around which policy advocacy will take place. In the CUGU campaign, the problem set forth by the Collaborative and other stakeholders was the overconcentration of polluting facilities near homes, schools, senior centers, and other sensitive areas in the three largely Latinx neighborhoods represented by the Collaborative and their disproportionate rates of respiratory and other illnesses associated with poor air quality (Yanez, 2016). The *policy alternative* crafted by the campaign was threefold: reduce local pollution by ensuring existing local businesses comply with the rules, prevent new pollution sources by requiring new industries to meet environmental health standards, and revitalize neighborhoods by concentrating financial and other incentives to help businesses clean up and modernize with new technology while creating new jobs.

To *secure adoption* of the policy proposal, the Collaborative and its partners used their large and diverse, multisector coalition to undertake extensive stakeholder education about the problem and the proposed policy solution, inside and outside city hall (Yanez, 2016). They helped get over 180 organizations from public health to faith-based to local businesses and community groups) to sign on in support of the measure. Collaborative community and academic partners were key among those taking part in community meetings, holding public participation workshops, and being well represented among the over 200 people who presented testimony, including stories and statistics (chapter 10) to help make the case for the measure's passage. Further, and when the CUGU ordinance was unanimously passed by the city council and signed into law by the mayor in April 2016, the Collaborative quickly moved into a follow-up, evaluative and modification role, helping small businesses with compliance and expanding green zone activities by partnering with LA's Department of Water and Power.

The final "Outcomes" oval in our conceptual model lists a range of *policy change dimensions*, from political action and formal and informal policy adoption to changes in the policy landscape to key dimensions of justice (procedural, distributive, and restorative), each of which can then contribute to improved health outcomes. One issue less often considered is implementation, and as noted earlier, this can be especially important. Pastor and colleagues (2016) have drawn a distinction between *winning power* and *wielding power*, between securing a policy victory and developing the administrative and monitoring capacities to ensure that a policy change is also a change in real outcomes. They and others have termed this governing power, and understanding its evolution and deployment is a new frontier for researchers interested in community-engaged collaborations.

The Difficulty of Assessing Contribution to Policy Change

In policy-focused work in which "multiple players are 'hitting' numerous leverage points" (Guthrie at al., 2006, p. 9) and contextual factors are also in play, it can be exceedingly difficult to tease apart a particular partnership's contributions to policy change (Minkler, 2014). Partnerships must consider the role of factors, such as an economic downturn, the opening of a window of opportunity following a media exposé, or the election or appointment of a new policymaker who shares or opposes the partnership's goals (Minkler et al., 2012), as well as the multiple other actors who are actively working for the policy change. Some excellent tools are available for helping evaluate contributions to policy change, among them PolicyLink's Getting Equity Advocacy Results (GEAR) (http://www.pol icylink.org/GEAR and the evaluation section of the Community Tool Box (http://cbt.ku.edu/) (chapter 21). Where time and resources are available, using multi-method case study analysis and triangulating findings can also be useful (Petersen et al., 2006; Yin, 2014).

Finally, and because policy change often takes place over a long period of time, Guthrie et al. (2006) suggested the utility of asking not simply whether policy has changed, but rather, "How did the [partnership's] work improve the policy environment for this issue?" and "How successful was [the partnership] in taking the necessary steps toward policy change?" In the former regard, CUGU would never have passed without the combination of organizing, advocacy, and research. The last part—research—was critical in helping to ground the need in unassailable data, while the first two elements—organizing and advocacy—were essential to changing the political cost-benefit analysis. The challenge has more often been in the boring work of implementation, and this is where researchers and community leaders could team up to build the capacity for more effective monitoring (chapter 15). Finally, in gauging how the policy environment changed, we stress again that the spillover impacts on policy elsewhere have been significant; while the City was a fight, the County essentially adopted the green zones model, brought together researchers and organizers, and is seeking to replicate what the City had initially led on.

Concluding Thoughts

Although efforts to influence policy are messy, time consuming, and fraught with difficulties, they represent critical avenues for improving the public's health and should be considered an important part of the tool kit for community organizers and community builders. By intentionally focusing on the policy level, community-engaged partnerships for research and organizing can help build the evidence base for equity policy, while democratizing knowledge and access, and helping achieve the procedural and restorative, as well as distributive justice dimensions of equity policy.

As illustrated in the case study above, community-based participatory research can improve what Balazs and Morello-Frosch (2013) called the "three R's of Research," its relevance, rigor, and reach. Similarly, it can improve the role of such efforts in the policymaking process, contributing to a stronger evidence base for equity policy, while also enhancing community capacity building and contributing to a more engaged populace. To promote such high-level community involvement, however, the very *nature* of our policies should be reconsidered such that community building becomes a central consideration in how policies are shaped and what they look like. It is only through such reorientation that the oft-repeated phrases "civic engagement, "empowered communities," and, indeed, "community building" itself can reach their full potential, and that "equity policy" in all its dimensions will have the greatest chance of succeeding.

Questions for Further Discussion

1. Balazs and Morello-Frosh (2013) argue that community-engaged research can improve "the three R's of Research"—its relevance, rigor, and reach. Many now agree that involving community members can help ensure that the topic under investigation matters to the community, and that the findings may reach new audiences beyond academics and professionals. But there is still skepticism among some about whether and how community engagement can improve (and indeed, not actually harm) the rigor of the research. Using the case study presented, describe ground-truthing and how this method helped improve the rigor of the science needed to make the case for policy change. How else might ground-truthing be used in other types of research?

2. This chapter illustrates a case example of how community organizing through long-term trusted relationships and various types of evidence supported local policy changes to advance environmental justice at the local level. Reflect on recent political and structural inequities in the United States, such as racism, violence, police brutality, climate justice, family separation and mass deportations, and the disproportionate impacts of COVID-19 on communities of color. Draw from your own experience or that of a community you are familiar with to think about an example of when justice was served (or not served) in policymaking in one of three ways: distributive, procedural, or restorative justice.

REFERENCES

Arias, E., Tejada-Vera, B., & Ahmad, F. (2021, February). *Provisional Life Expectancy Estimates for January through June, 2020*. Vital Statistics Rapid Release Report # 010. https://www.cdc.gov/nchs/data/vsrr/VSRR10-508.pdf.

Balazs, C. L., & Morello-Frosch, R. (2013). The three R's: How community-based research strengthens the relevance, rigor and reach of science. *Environ Justice, 6*(1), 9–16.

Bardach, E. (2000). *A Practical Guide for Policy Analysis: The Eightfold Path to More Effective Problem Solving*. Chatham House.

Binns, C. (2019, March 18). Overcoming an industrial legacy in L.A.'s Pacoima district. NRDC. https://www.nrdc.org/stories/overcoming-industrial-legacy-pacoima-district.

Blackwell, A. G., & Colmenar, R. (2000). Community-building: From local wisdom to public policy. *Public Health Rep, 115*(2–3), 161–166.

Braveman, P., & Gottlieb, L. (2014). The social determinants of health: It's time to consider the causes of the causes. *Public Health Rep, 129*(suppl_2), 19–31.

Brown, P., Morello-Frosch, R., & Zavestoski, S. (2012). *Contested Illnesses: Citizens, Science, and Health Social Movements*. University of California Press.

Burke, N. S. (2016). Get ready for equity. In *Framing the Dialogue on Race and Ethnicity to Advance Health Equity. Proceedings of a Workshop*. National Academies of Science, Engineering, and Medicine. National Academies Press.

Cacari Stone, L. (2016). *Lost in Translation Learning Module: Health Policy, Politics and Social Justice*. College of Population Health, University of New Mexico.

Cacari Stone, L., Wallerstein, N., Garcia, A. P., & Minkler, M. (2014). The promise of community-based participatory research for health equity: A conceptual model for bridging evidence with policy. *Am J Public Health, 104*(9), 1615–1623.

Corburn, J. (2017). Urban place and health equity: Critical issues and practices. *Int J Environ Res, 14*(2), 117.

Freudenberg, N., & Tsui, E. (2014). Evidence, power, and policy change in community-based participatory research. *Am J Public Health, 104*(1), 11–24.

Guthrie, K., Louise, J., & Foster C. C. (2006). *The Challenge of Assessing Policy and Advocacy Activities, Part II: Moving from Theory to Practice*. The California Endowment. http://www.pointk.org/resources/files/challenge_assessing_policy_advocacy2.pdf.

Israel, B. A., Eng, E., Schulz, A. J., & Parker, E. A. (2013). Introduction to methods for CBPR for health. In B. A. Israel, E. Eng, A. J. Schultz, & E. A. Parker (Eds.), *Methods for Community-Based Participatory Research in Public Health* (pp. 3–38). Jossey-Bass.

Iton, A., & Ross, R. K. (2017). Understanding how health happens: Your zip code is more important than your genetic code. In R. Callahan & D. Bhattacharya (Eds.), *Public Health Leadership* (pp. 83–99). Routledge.

Kingdon, J. W. (2011). *Agendas, Alternatives, and Public Policies* (updated 2nd ed.). Longman.

Longest, B. B., Jr. (2006). *Health Policymaking in the United States* (4th ed.). AUPH/Health Administration Press.

Minkler, M. (2010). Linking science and policy through community-based participatory research to study and address health disparities. *Am J Public Health, 100*(suppl_1), S81–S87.

Minkler, M. (2014). Enhancing data quality, relevance, and use through community-based participatory research. In N. Cytron, K. Petit, & G. T. Kingsley (Eds.), *What Counts? Harnessing Data for America's Communities* (pp. 245–259). Federal Reserve Bank of San Francisco and the Urban Institute.

Minkler, M., & Freudenberg, N. (2010). From community-based participatory research to policy change. In H. E. Fitzgerald, C. Burack, & S. D. Seifer (Eds.), *Handbook of Engaged Scholarship: Contemporary Landscapes, Future Directions* (vol. 2, pp. 275–294). Michigan State University Press.

Minkler, M., Garcia, A. P., Rubin, V., & Wallerstein, N. (2012). *Community-Based Participatory Research: A Strategy for Building Healthy Communities and Promoting Health through Policy Change.* PolicyLink.

Morello-Frosch, R., Brown, P., Brody, J., Altman, R., Rudel, R., Zota, A., & Pérez, P. (2011). Experts, ethics, and environmental justice: Communicating and contesting results from personal exposure science. In B. Cohen & G. Ottinger (Eds.), *Environmental Justice and the Transformation of Science and Engineering* (pp. 93–119). MIT Press.

Morello-Frosch, R., Pastor, M., & Sadd, J. (2001). Environmental justice and Southern California's "Riskscape": The distribution of air toxics exposures and health risks among diverse communities. *Urban Aff Rev, 36*(4), 551–578.

Morello-Frosch, R., Pastor, M., Sadd, J., Prichard, M., & Matsuoka, M. (2012). Citizens, science and data judo: Leveraging secondary data analysis to build a community-academic collaborative for environmental justice in Southern California. In B. A. Israel, E. Eng, A. J. Schultz, & E. A. Parker (Eds.), *Methods for Community-Based Participatory Research in Public Health* (2nd ed., pp. 371–394). Jossey-Bass.

National Academies of Science, Engineering, and Medicine (NASEM). (2019). Adopting restorative policies and practices to achieve health equity. In *Achieving Behavioral Health Equity for Children, Families and Communities: Proceedings of a Workshop*. National Academies Press. https://doi.org/10.17226/25347.

Nutley, S. M., Walter, I., & Davies, H. T. O. (2007). *Using Evidence: How Research Can Inform Public Services.* Bristol University Press.

Pastor, M. (2018). *State of Resistance: What California's Dizzying Descent and Remarkable Resurgence Mean for America's Future.* New Press.

Pastor, M., Benner, C., & Matsuoka, M. (2009). *This Could be the Start of Something Big: How Social Movements for Regional Equity Are Reshaping Metropolitan America.* Cornell University Press.

Pastor, M., Ito, J., & Wander, M. (2016). *Changing States: A Framework for Progressive Governance.* USC Program for Environmental and Regional Equity.

Petersen, D., Minkler, M., Vásquez Breckwich, V., & Baden, A. (2006). Community-based participatory research as a tool for policy change: A case study of the Southern California Environmental Justice Collaborative. *Rev Policy Res, 23*(2), 339–354.

Prewitt, K., Schwandt, T. A., & Straf, M. L. (2012). Research on the use of science in policy: A framework. In *Using Science as Evidence in Public Policy* (pp. 53–63). National Academies Press. doi:https://doi.org/10.17226/13460.

Rudolph, L., Caplan, J., Mitchell, C., Ben-Moshe, K., & Dillon, L. (2013). Health in all policies: Improving health through intersectoral collaboration. National Academy of Sciences Perspectives. Discussion Paper. Institute of Medicine of the National Academy of Science.

Sabatier, P. A., & Weible, C. M. (2014). *Theories of the Policy Process.* Westview Press.

Sadd, J., Morello-Frosch, R., Pastor, M., Matsuoka, M., Prichard, M., & Carter, V. (2014). The truth, the whole truth, and nothing but the ground-truth: Methods to advance environmental justice and researcher-community partnerships. *Health Educ Behav, 41*(3), 281–290.

Sadd, J. L., Pastor, M., Morello-Frosch, R., Scoggins, J., & Jesdale, B. (2011). Playing it safe: Assessing cumulative impact and social vulnerability through an environmental justice screening method in the South Coast Air Basin, California. *Int J Environ Res, 8*(5), 1441–1459.

Shonkoff, J. P. (2000). Science, policy and practice: Three cultures in search of a shared mission. *Child Dev, 71*(1), 181–187.

Tseng, V., & the Senior Program Team. (2008). *Studying the Use of Research Evidence in Policy and Practice.* William T. Grant Foundation 2007 Annual Report. William T. Grant Foundation.

U.S. Department of Treasury, Internal Revenue Service. (2016). Schedule C (Form 990 or 990-EZ), Political Campaign and Lobbying Activities. Schedule C (Form 990 or 990-EZ), Political Campaign and Lobbying Activities.

World Health Organization (WHO). (2015). *Health in All Policies: Training Manual.* WHO Press.

Yanez, E. (2016, April 20). L.A.'s promising Clean Up, Green Up ordinance. The Prevention Institute. https://www.preventioninstitute.org/blog/las-promising-clean-green-ordinance.

Yin, R. K. (2014). *Case Study Research: Design and Methods* (5th ed.). Sage.

23

Abolition as a Public Health Intervention

Building Multisector Momentum for Community Care and Criminal Legal System Policy Change

AMBER AKEMI PIATT
CHRISTINE MITCHELL
WAYLAND "X" COLEMAN
MEREDITH MINKLER

Homelessness, unemployment, drug addiction, mental illness, and illiteracy are only a few of the problems that disappear from public view when the human beings contending with them are relegated to cages. Prisons do not disappear social problems, they disappear human beings.

—Angela Davis, 2000

The United States incarcerates more people per capita than any other nation in the world. As of 2020, almost 2.3 million people were incarcerated in more than 1,800 state prisons, 100 federal prisons, 1,700 youth jails, 200 immigration prisons, 3,000 local jails, and 80 Indian Country jails, as well as in military prisons, locked psychiatric hospitals, and prisons in U.S. territories (Sawyer & Wagner, 2020). Furthermore, because structural racism shapes people's access to opportunity, dictates which communities are more heavily policed, and is baked into federal, tribal, state, and local laws that inform what is and is not criminalized, Black, Indigenous, and Latinx people are disproportionately incarcerated. This is particularly true for Black people, who make up 40 percent of the incarcerated population despite representing just 13 percent of U.S. residents (Sawyer & Wagner, 2020).

The health consequences of incarceration have been well documented and include elevated rates of both communicable and chronic conditions, such as tuberculosis, hypertension, and asthma, among people who have been incarcerated (Fazel & Baillargeon, 2011; Gaber & Wright, 2016). To make matters worse, the health impacts of incarceration do not end upon release: for example, one in twelve for-merly incarcerated people is hospitalized for an acute condition within ninety days of release from prison or jail. Furthermore, incarceration actively harms the health and well-being of an incarcerated person's children and family (Mauer et al., 2009). Approximately 10 million children nationwide have had a parent incarcerated at some point in their lives, and this experience of parental incarceration is associ-ated with a wide range of health issues, including HIV/AIDS, high cholesterol, migraines, and depression, during that child's young adulthood (Lee et al., 2013). The harms do not stop there and indeed extend to whole communities; living in neighborhoods with high rates of incarceration puts residents at elevated risk for depression and related illnesses, even if they personally have never been incarcer-ated (Hatzenbuehler & Pachankis, 2016).

Like many downstream harms due to structural inequities in the social deter-minants of health—or "the conditions in which people are born, grow, live, work and age" (Marmot et al., 2012, p. 1)—it does not have to be this way. The criminal legal system—from criminalization to policing to prosecution to incarceration to immigration enforcement to state surveillance—is a set of policy choices. Issues that are handled by the criminal legal system—including but not limited to drug use, theft, and violence—are largely social, political, or economic in nature and could be better addressed through a public health approach. At its best, public health as a field is interested in addressing the root causes of health inequities, investing in positive social determinants of health, and moving toward primary prevention of illness and bodily harm. Given the robust evidence documenting the health and social harms of incarceration—and their severe exacerbation by the COVID-19 pandemic (Gaber & Wright, 2016; Noonan & Ginder, 2015; WHO, 2020)—abolishing the criminal legal system may be seen as a necessary, if not yet commonly accepted, public health solution.

The movement to abolish the criminal legal system is not new. Building on the legacy of slavery abolitionists, criminal legal system abolition is deeply rooted in Black liberation and the lived realities of people who are incarcerated. The Attica Prison uprising in 1971, in which more than half of the 2,200 people incarcerated in the prison rebelled for their political and human rights, was just one of the flash-points in this movement. The efforts of incarcerated revolutionaries and their allies who are not behind bars have caused measurable shifts in both the policy and the narrative spheres. Between 2001 and 2019, thanks in part to such organizing, some important victories were won, including many states directing funds away from new prison construction and toward evidence-based programs and services (deVuono-Powell et al., 2017).

The overlapping emergencies of the COVID-19 pandemic, police violence, and the worst economic crisis since the Great Depression exposed the interconnected-ness of our health and brought wider visibility and attention to the harms of the criminal legal system, in large part due to the mass protests following the police killings of George Floyd, Breonna Taylor, and Tony McDade. They laid bare what criminalized and incarcerated people have long known, and they increased demands for urgent and transformative action. Carceral facilities routinely dominate the list of the largest hot spots for COVID-19 infection and death in the United States and vastly contribute to the community spread of the virus as well (Henry, 2020; Williams & Ivory, 2020; WHO, 2020). In mid-April of 2020, Illinois's Cook County Jail reported approximately 600 people exposed to COVID-19—the largest source of infections in the country—until about a week later, when an Ohio state prison reported 1,828 people, or close to 75 percent of its prison population, testing positive for COVID-19 (Cases Surge, 2020). Alarmingly, an epidemiological modeling study conducted by epidemiologists, academic researchers, and ACLU Analytics projected that without proper precautions, including mass releases from jails, close to 100,000 additional people could die of COVID-19 (American Civil Liberties Union, 2020). In the face of such widespread devastation and imminent risk, many jurisdictions granted significant though insufficient releases from their carceral facilities, with Colorado reducing its jail population by 31 percent and even conservative Kentucky achieving a 28 percent reduction (American Civil Liberties Union, 2020).

Bearing the fruit of decades of powerful community organizing, social movement building, and storytelling, we find ourselves in a new window of opportunity today in the struggle for decarceration and related abolitionist change. The first case study in this chapter describes how Decarcerate Alameda County—a coalition of currently and formerly incarcerated people, public health workers, and community-based organizations (CBOs) advocating to free people from jail, invest in community health, and divest from incarceration and policing in Alameda County, California—used community organizing, policy advocacy, and media strategy. In this case study, we draw, in part, on Kingdon's (2011) model of the policymaking process (chapter 22) as an example of community-driven policy advocacy for decarceration in the time of the COVID-19 pandemic. Consistent with Kingdon's model, we explore the *problem stream*—how coalition members got the need for decarceration on the policymakers' agenda in the wake of a major global event. We then look at the *politics stream*—how advocates crafted solutions and presented them to decisionmakers in partnership with public health allies. Finally, we explore the *policy stream*—during which the coalition worked to have its proposals debated in the public discourse and political arena and ideally win out over the opposition. We further apply Kingdon's (2011) notion of the *policy window of opportunity*, which often opens when there are favorable developments in all three streams of the policy process simultaneously.

We then turn to our second case study, #DeeperThanWater—a coalition of currently and formerly incarcerated organizers, their loved ones, and abolitionist organizations in Massachusetts, which has used the lens of environmental injustice to illustrate the human rights abuses occurring in state prisons. In this second case study, we see a coalition that intentionally does not collaborate with elected officials for policy change. Instead, we observe how #DeeperThanWater focuses on exposing abuses and building broad public momentum for abolishing the criminal legal system. Finally, as far too infrequently included in books of this kind, we hear firsthand in this chapter from an incarcerated organizer with #DeeperThan-Water, whose insights and experiences behind prison walls, and whose determination to share those realities with those of us outside, even at great personal cost, help convey, as little else can, the urgency of the work.

In each case study, we highlight the strategies and tactics employed, the successes and challenges faced, and the implications for public health workers in their personal or professional lives who wish to contribute to efforts for immediate and necessary policy change and for building a mass movement for transformative systems change during the pandemic and in a new postpandemic world.

Decarcerate Alameda County: The Fight for Health Instead of Punishment

I ended up getting quarantined because I tested positive for COVID. While I was there, there were no medical services given. I requested a blanket through my tablet–never given to me. I told them I was really cold. There was no empathy at all for us. We were left to die.

–Angelo Valdez, incarcerated at Santa Rita Jail

For decades, currently and formerly incarcerated leaders and their families have worked tirelessly to shift public opinion and change laws and practices that criminalize people in California. Despite popular state victories, such as Proposition 47 (2014) and Senate Bill 136 (2020), which both reduced the time people have to serve in jails or prisons, realities on the ground remain bleak. Of particular concern in Alameda County, California, is state violence in the infamous Santa Rita Jail, the third-largest jail in the state and the fifth-largest in the country. Class action lawsuits, labor and hunger strikes, and public testimonies from incarcerated people have highlighted abuses ranging from sheriff deputies forcing a pregnant person to give birth alone in solitary confinement, to failing to provide adequate treatment to those in mental health crises, to murdering incarcerated people. Such abuses sit on top of the tragically mundane but devastating impacts of incarceration discussed earlier in the chapter. Despite the vast majority of people inside Santa Rita Jail being pretrial, and thus legally innocent, the county has largely resisted practical alternatives to incarceration, even in the midst of the COVID-19 pandemic.

Health workers and organizations have long participated in community organizing and coalition building efforts with Decarcerate Alameda County, which is led by a steering committee made up of base-building organizations representing people who are most targeted and harmed by the Alameda County Sheriff's Office, including the Ella Baker Center for Human Rights and Causa Justa: Just Cause. While many health workers themselves have experienced abuse from the Alameda County Sheriff's Office firsthand—often for being Black, Indigenous, or people of color—public health organizations in the coalition, including Human Impact Partners (HIP) and the Public Health Justice Collective, have primarily approached the coalition's work through a lens of solidarity and have played a supportive role (Minkler et al., 2020).

Problem Stream: Creating Public Awareness and Getting on the Policymakers' Agenda

The San Francisco Bay Area enjoys a substantial (although shrinking) local news media network, including mainstream and alternative outlets in print, television, radio, and podcast. Problems with the Alameda County Sheriff's Office and Santa Rita Jail were already on local news media's radar, in part because of journalists' relationships with Decarcerate Alameda County organizers. Coalition organizers and community members' prior successes in getting opinion pieces published and bringing local news media out to press conferences and community mobilizations helped prime local news media to broadcast the coalition's demands when the threat of a COVID-19 outbreak in Santa Rita Jail created a new gravity for moving forward.

Decarcerate Alameda County's steering committee carefully crafted the coalition's demands (e.g., releasing incarcerated people, beginning with the most vulnerable to COVID-19; stopping collaboration with ICE; ending money bail). The coalition then worked closely with HIP to ensure relevant public health research was included to help frame the urgency of the issue. Recognizing that the messenger matters, the coalition asked HIP to be out front on this issue and deliver the letter of demands on HIP's letterhead. Understanding the strategic importance of public health leadership for this particular campaign, HIP stepped up and delivered the demands on behalf of the coalition—illustrating the power of partnerships for social justice and public health in action.

Politics Stream: Developing and Presenting Policy Options

In order to increase political pressure on the policymakers and build community power, the coalition's demands were presented in a letter on HIP's letterhead and disseminated widely. Sent on March 17, just one day after the county began to shelter-in-place, the demands included stopping the flow of people into Santa Rita Jail, safely releasing people who are already incarcerated in Santa Rita Jail, meeting the immediate needs of people who remain incarcerated in the jail, and investing in the assets that promote healthier communities. Since multiple government agencies and officials had the power and authority to make the recommended changes, the coalition emailed the letter of demands to many policy targets, including the sheriff's office, the district attorney, superior court, the Northern California Immigration and Customs Enforcement (ICE) office, and the board of supervisors.

In addition to being emailed to key decisionmakers, the March 17 letter was shared widely with the media, and stories quickly appeared in venues including a local radio show popular with county officials (kpfa.org, March 18, 2020) and five local newspapers. Because the coalition could not control how local journalists covered the issue at hand nor whether its policy demands would be accurately captured, sharing its own stories and creating social media content were crucial. The coalition helped shape the public narrative using digital organizing tactics, including tweetstorms, petitions, sign-on letters, and online community forums. Through relationships with litigators working on class action lawsuits inside Santa Rita Jail, and a partnership with the local chapter of the Incarcerated Workers Organizing Committee, the coalition's social media advocacy was able to consistently highlight the current realities and leadership of people who are incarcerated, as well as the families and communities awaiting their release.

Policy Stream: Negotiating the Politics for Policy Wins

In the continuing uncertainty that is life during a pandemic, winning the demands put forward by the coalition continues to unfold, sometimes quickly—and other times agonizingly slowly or not at all. Yet examples of successful local policy changes can be highlighted, thanks to the wide range of the coalition's work, including powerful testimony from currently and formerly incarcerated people, virtual news conferences, and editorials highlighting the public health imperative of the coalition's clear policy demands. This local work happened alongside national uprisings and the creation of new narratives, campaigns, and resources, including a messaging toolkit designed specifically to provide public health arguments for decarceration during the COVID-19 pandemic (Community Justice Exchange & Public Health Awakened, 2020).

Key among the victories achieved during the policy stream negotiations were several steps toward downsizing Santa Rita Jail, culminating in a reduction from roughly 2,650 residents before the outbreak to 1,929 by the second week of April (Altman, 2020; Bay City News Service, 2020). Advocates also successfully pressured the district attorney's office to adopt additional precautions to protect undocumented people during and beyond the pandemic. For example, the county agreed to suspend a policy that requires longer jail or probation periods in exchange for modification of an immigration-neutral plea agreement—a policy that had harmed, solely on the basis of their citizenship status, immigrants who were caught up in the county criminal legal system. The sheriff's office instituted disgracefully insufficient changes, including giving each person three additional ounces of soap per week. These minimal shifts in policy are not nearly enough to address the need and leave in place a larger pattern of negligence in the sheriff's office.

Window of Opportunity

The opening of Kingdon's (2011) policy "window of opportunity" is well illustrated in the strategies and tactics that took place in each stream of the policymaking process to change systems of criminalization and incarceration in Alameda County. The sustained spotlight on jail conditions prior to COVID-19, and the substantial media and public outcry in its wake, contributed to a surge in the *problem stream* that advocates then complemented in the *politics stream* by identifying targets and specific actions each of them could take to address problems in their purview.

Together with the coalition's successes in negotiating wins with policymakers (*policy stream*), these developments opened a window during which some, albeit still grossly inadequate, policy changes were possible to improve the lives of people who have been criminalized and incarcerated in Alameda County (Minkler et al., 2020).

The Long Arc: Small Policy Wins against Unjust Systems and the Opportunity for Building Larger Abolitionist Movements

Abolitionist scholar Ruth Wilson Gilmore (2007) often emphasizes that "abolition is about presence, not absence. It's about building life-affirming institutions." To Decarcerate Alameda County, this includes the presence of health equity in our communities, which must be achieved through robust investments to address the social determinants of health. Sadly, though not uncommonly among county governments in the United States, the Alameda County budget had long been on a trajectory toward more punishment and harm rather than care and wellness. In the decade preceding the onset of the COVID-19 pandemic, the sheriff's office budget grew by $144 million to $443 million annually, representing a 48 percent increase. Over the same time period, the daily jail population actually decreased by 45 percent. In March 2020, during a massive budget crisis brought on by the COVID-19 pandemic and despite the coalition organizing a *unanimously opposed public comment line at the budget hearing*, the Alameda County Board of Supervisors approved a preliminary budget expenditure of an additional $318 million for Santa Rita Jail. This extra funding alone—not the total sheriff's office budget—amounted to nearly three times the county public health department's entire annual operating budget.

Despite this massive campaign loss, what the coalition won may actually be more valuable in the long run. In addition to the handful of small but important policy wins described above, Decarcerate Alameda County has built a growing base of county residents who are eager and ready to build community and organize for the long haul. With renewed energy for abolitionist change brought on by the international uprisings for Black liberation and local mobilizations to defeat the $318 million jail budget increase, coalition membership more than quadrupled in size. Coalition meeting attendance continues to grow each successive week, and new members are meaningfully contributing and plugging into the coalition work, including efforts to oust county officials who do not serve the interests of Black and other communities of color. Ongoing efforts to orient new people to the political landscape of the county and build relationships in a diverse coalition have also included hosting trainings and developing political education resources.

The importance of these local developments cannot be overstated. In mid-June 2020, amid continued nationwide protests over the brutal police killing of George Floyd and other unarmed Black and Brown people, over two-thirds (67 percent) of people in the United States expressed support for the Black Lives Matter movement, and despite a subsequent decline, by mid-September over half (55 percent) still expressed support for the movement (Thomas & Horowitz, 2020).

Public understandings of ways to address the characteristic racism of the criminal legal system, however, remained far less straightforward. Popular reforms—such as equipping police with body cameras, releasing people who are incarcerated on convictions deemed nonviolent, and allowing pregnant incarcerated people to deliver their babies without wearing shackles—do little to address the root causes of incarceration and its long-term health effects (deVuono-Powell et al., 2018). In fact, while they may provide temporary and immediate relief to a lucky few, these reforms may further entrench a system whose intent and purpose is to punish and control people, especially Black and Brown people, not protect community health.

Decarcerate Alameda County's policy agenda challenges the dominant systems, structures, and narratives by unapologetically recognizing all people's humanity and their potential for transformation, healing, and repair. Especially during a deadly viral pandemic, the coalition doubled down on its commitment to seeking safe releases for everyone inside of Santa Rita Jail—without exception—while recognizing that such a demand would mean an uphill battle in both the policy and narrative arenas. This strategic decision elevated the importance of both pursuing traditional media advocacy and generating our own media, primarily through social media platforms (chapter 24). It also underscored the need to reach a critical mass of residents—locally and beyond—who will join together in a movement for transformative change that will abolish the criminal legal system once and for all.

#DeeperThanWater Coalition: Exposing the Toxicity of Prisons

The #DeeperThanWater coalition formed in 2017 after the *Boston Globe* published an article by journalist David Abel on the toxic water at the largest state prison in Massachusetts, MCI-Norfolk. Abel found that 43 percent of water samples taken from the prison from 2011 to 2017 had levels of manganese higher than 0.3 mg/L, the safety threshold of this mineral determined by the Environmental Protection Agency (EPA) (Abel, 2017). Elevated levels of manganese can lead to health impacts, such as tremors, neurological disorders like Parkinson's disease, and diminished verbal function (Mergler, 1999). A 2017 survey developed and disseminated by incarcerated people at the prison found that many identified dry skin, rashes, and gastrointestinal issues as related to the water quality.

The coalition—made up of public health organizers, as well as organizers from Black and Pink Boston, Black Lives Matter Boston, Showing Up for Racial Justice Boston, and Toxics Action Center—is led by formerly and currently incarcerated people and their loved ones (#DeeperThanWater, n.d.). The name arose in response to organizers' realization that although they had come together around the issue of toxic water in prisons, the problems of incarceration go much deeper than water. The coalition holds prison abolition as its primary goal and works to achieve that goal by amplifying the voices of incarcerated organizers and exposing the human rights abuses that occur behind prison walls.

The coalition is most invested in shaping a window of opportunity for abolition by building power amid a growing national mood and movement that demonstrates "All Cages are Connected"—including prisons, jails, and immigration detention centers. In contrast to organizing efforts that focus on policy change, #DeeperThanWater intentionally does not work in collaboration with elected officials, except when making demands that will meet the specific and immediate needs of those who are incarcerated. Instead, the coalition's aim is to focus energy on amplifying the voices of people behind prison walls in order to expose to the general public the human rights abuses that occur in carceral settings. As was witnessed most recently during the COVID-19 pandemic (#DeeperThanWater, n.d.), when public awareness and outrage grow, more pressure is placed on the Department of Corrections, Department of Public Health, and governor's office to be held publicly accountable.

In order to center incarcerated people's voices in media coverage and circumvent the Department of Corrections regulations prohibiting incarcerated people from speaking to press, a core strategy of #DeeperThanWater has been to pass letters, emails, and voice recordings to media and by posting them publicly on Facebook, Twitter, and the coalition's website. Campaigns have earned print coverage in the *Boston Globe* and *The Appeal*, radio coverage on the Massachusetts NPR affiliate and *Democracy Now*, and widespread social media coverage. The coalition even literally amplifies incarcerated people's voices by creating a system through which incarcerated organizers can call in to protests and be amplified over a set of bullhorns. At one protest organized by the coalition during the 2018 National Prison Strike, the only people who spoke were those who were currently or formerly incarcerated or at risk of deportation.

The #DeeperThanWater coalition is a firm believer that there is no victory until all people are free. Until then, it is working to provide for the immediate needs of incarcerated people, when the state fails to provide for those needs. Through mutual aid fundraising, the coalition has raised money to provide clean bottled water for incarcerated people and to provide soap and cleaning supplies (Becker & Jolicoeur, 2018), especially important during COVID-19. Through media advocacy and concentrated base-building, organizers both inside and outside the prison walls have been successful at getting a new water filtration system at MCI-Norfolk and fixed ventilation, including free fans for incarcerated people who could not afford them, at three prisons during the extreme heat of summer 2018 (Crimaldi, 2018). Individual-focused letter-writing and call-in campaigns have been successful at helping people get parole or get out of solitary confinement, and further helped build the case for and winning compassionate release for incarcerated people who are dying. But perhaps the biggest success of the coalition is in building relationships with incarcerated people: through pen pal programs, book clubs, coordinated inside/outside memorials for those who have died behind bars, and word of mouth, the coalition's base grows ever stronger.

As understanding of and support for police and prison abolition reach the mainstream following the 2020 uprisings for Black liberation, and as it becomes clearer than ever that abolition is a public health vision, the window of opportunity is widening to divest completely from the criminal legal system and invest in addressing the social determinants of health. Such transformative change would be fully in keeping with Gilmore's (2007) aforementioned reminder that abolition is in fact about "building life-affirming institutions." #DeeperThanWater holds that the power to bring about this vision lies with the people—those who are incarcerated and those outside the walls.

A Note on State Repression and Structural Barriers to Media Advocacy from Wayland "X" Coleman, Incarcerated #DeeperThanWater Organizer

Prisons are designed to keep incarcerated people separated from the free people of the world. Walls are erected not out of fear of our escape, but out of fear of the public being able to see what's going on inside. The walls are there to block your view and to keep incarcerated people concealed. In addition to blocking public vision, prisons engage—on a normal basis—in abusive and retaliatory repression in order to keep our voices from reaching the public ear.

For years throughout my incarceration, I have sought out ways in which the incarcerated voice could be amplified so that the inhumane and cruel practices within the institutions could be exposed and so that the public could be made aware of our suffering. I have yet to find a way in which to offer my voice and experiences to the world without administrative retaliation and punishment. However, with #DeeperThanWater I have found a team of people in our free society who are willing to help me to speak. For example, in 2017, I was elected by the incarcerated population at MCI-Norfolk prison in Massachusetts by a ballot vote to serve on the institution's Resident Council as the prison's representative of the incarcerated body. The premise of my campaign was centered on the idea that in order to strengthen the Resident Council, it needed to be connected to and supported by people who are free. Over the course of 2016, I wrote and mailed out approximately 300 letters, which yielded twenty-one external resources who committed to receiving a monthly Council report that I offered to draft if I were elected. Once I was elected, I set out to fulfill my promises to the incarcerated community. A month after I was seated as a chairman of the Resident Council—and after several meetings with the prison administration where other executive board members of the Council and myself attempted to address relevant issues within the prison—I drafted my first monthly report and began to mail copies to outside supporters. Included as an attachment to my Council report was a report regarding the contamination of the drinking water. Once my Council package was sent to the *Boston Globe*, reporter David Abel took an interest in the water report and began to investigate. The prison administration grew furious with me for sending information to the media, resulting in me being placed in solitary confinement for a month and administratively removed from my elected position on the Resident Council.

Shortly after my release from solitary confinement, I was able to communicate with David Abel via letter and email. On June 18, 2017, he published a front page article in the *Boston Globe*, exposing the toxic water at MCI-Norfolk. On June 19—the next day—the prison administration retaliated against the entire incarcerated population by calling for a major lockdown and institutional shakedown where they called upon correctional officers from all over Massachusetts to come in and trash everyone's cells. The prison remained on lockdown for a week. Several months later, the institutional strategy of divide and conquer moved the incarcerated population to vote against my reelection, in favor of someone who would be friendlier toward the administration. Though I didn't win re-election, I did win the respect and approval of many free activists who had formed the #DeeperThanWater coalition on the heels of the *Globe*'s article. Once #DeeperThanWater formed, I—for the first time—felt that I had a true support system and a solid platform through which I could work to expose the inhumanities within the prisons.

The kinds of repressions explained above are common within the prison system. Prison administrators are highly reactive toward incarcerated people who attempt to communicate with the world, as if the ability to communicate alone is a threat to the interests of the penal system. In another disciplinary matter, I was unjustly sanctioned for communicating with the world by way of a podcast that my brother had set up as a means for me to share my thoughts, ideas, philosophies, ideologies, and stories of experiences during my incarceration. Through my podcast, "The Prisoner," I was able to communicate over the phone with a live listening audience. This provided a tremendous platform—and opportunity—for me to speak on the world stage and for people to respond by calling in to the broadcast. Once I began to lecture about the institutional racism and White supremacy that are the root of the prison industrial complex, my brother's phone number was administratively restricted, pending an investigation from the commissioner's office. Soon after, I received a disciplinary report for unauthorized communication with the world and was given sanctions of ninety days' loss of phone privileges and sixty days' loss of canteen. My brother's phone number was illegally restricted for more than a year. Today, I sit in solitary confinement solely because of my association with #DeeperThanWater, which has continued to help raise the voices of incarcerated people and stoke the administrative fear of public exposure.

In our modern world, where technology has connected everybody to each other and has provided a platform for all people to amplify their voices without the fear of punitive retaliation, the contemporary existence of an undercaste of people who can be stripped of that voice via state-sanctioned violence should be appalling to everyone. For how can an entire group of people in this day and age be justifiably restricted from personally and socially evolving with the rest of the world? Remember, the walls of the prison are not there to keep incarcerated people from getting

out. They're there to keep you from looking in. The only "crimes" that I have committed are in attempting to reach the public.

Discussion

Right now, we are in a peak cycle. There's tremendous energy out there, directed
against the state. It's not all focused, but it's there, and it's building. Maybe
this will be sufficient to accomplish what we must accomplish over the fairly
short run. We'll see, and we can certainly hope that this is the case. But perhaps not. We must be prepared to wage a long struggle.

–George Jackson, revolutionary leader, assassinated in 1971 by
prison guards during a rebellion inside San Quentin Prison

In this chapter, we have focused primarily on the work of Decarcerate Alameda
County and #DeeperThanWater, two coalitions led by currently and formerly incarcerated people who partner with public health workers and other allies. Rooted in
the current realities and stories of people who are most directly and intimately
threatened by incarceration—and affirmed by growing public health evidence documenting such harms—these coalitions advance meaningful steps toward abolishing the criminal legal system and building in its place systems of community
care.

Public health professionals have been among those working—sometimes
behind the scenes—with grassroots leaders to change policy on a number of critical issues, including incarceration. As we continue to navigate our way through
the acute and chronic crises triggered by COVID-19 and structural oppression, public health workers' skills in interpersonal and mass communication, participatory
research, and monitoring processes and outcomes—as well as our passion for transformative change to the social determinants of health—may help us work as allies
in the fight for a healthier, more just world (Minkler et al., 2020).

When observed through the lens of Kingdon's (2011) policy "window of
opportunity"—the opening created when positive developments simultaneously
occur in the problem, policy, and politics streams—Decarcerate Alameda County
was able to secure small but important wins despite significant challenges in moving the policy dial in the face of both rapidly changing conditions and longer-term
struggles for liberation. The COVID-19 pandemic constituted a window of opportunity in and of itself, as communities facing the worst health inequities forced
policymakers to take action to address the pandemic.

Equally powerful and important is the work of the #DeeperThanWater coalition, which, rather than seeking to influence policymakers for the sake of policy
change, set its sights on amplifying the voices of people behind prison walls to
expose the public to the human rights abuses that happen in prisons, jails, and
detention centers. The coalition holds that such abuses can only be adequately
addressed when prisons are abolished and systems of community care are built

where people's basic human needs for housing, health care, education, employment, food, and more are met.

Finally, and perhaps most important of all, we heard firsthand testimony from one person among the millions behind bars today, as he shared his story, including the punishments he has suffered for sharing it—to understand with vivid clarity why abolition of the criminal legal system must become a reality. Through ongoing organizing and meaningful relationship building with those most harmed by the criminal legal system, we hope the essentiality of decarceration will blossom into a future where a world without policing, prisons, immigration enforcement, or state surveillance is possible.

Questions for Further Discussion

1. As the Decarcerate Alameda County case study illustrates, strong relationships are crucial for community organizing work, especially when public health workers, organizations, or departments need to move nimbly and strategically between being more or less in the spotlight. Can you think of examples when the strength of your relationships, or those of someone you know, had an impact on the ability to do collaborative work effectively? What are concrete ways you can build collective power for a greater good (e.g., in your workplace, in your school, in social justice movements)?

2. The testimony from Wayland "X" Coleman highlights the ways that prisons repress organizing for human rights and try to keep information from getting out from behind prison walls. In order to counteract this, #DeeperThanWater's work hinges on inside/outside organizing with those who are incarcerated and those who are not. What do you imagine are the benefits and challenges of this style of organizing? What institutions are you (or could you imagine being) "inside of" or "outside of" that you could organize using this strategy?

Acknowledgments

First and foremost, we want to thank the countless currently and formerly incarcerated people and their families who are on the frontlines of abolishing the criminal legal system. This includes many movement scholars and elders, some but certainly not all of whom are quoted in this chapter. We continue to learn from you, and our work is only possible because of what you have done before us. We sincerely thank our many community partners in Decarcerate Alameda County and the #DeeperThanWater coalition, including Annie Atwater, Jose Bernal, Adrian Coleman, Kitzia Esteva, Martin Henson, Jaquelyn Jahn, Jessica Kant, John Lindsay-Poland, Tash Nguyen, Norma Orozco, Sofía Owen, Elizabeth Rucker, Rebecca Ruiz, and Danny Thongsy. Thanks are also due to Patricia Wakimoto and Joseph Griffin for their help on a related paper, as well as to the Safe Return Project. Finally, we tip our hats to the many public health workers who have dedicated themselves to ending U.S. incarceration and related injustices made even more severe by the COVID-19 pandemic.

REFERENCES

Abel, D. (2017, June 17). Water at state's largest prison raises concerns. *Boston Globe*. https://www3.bostonglobe.com/metro/2017/06/17/water-state-largest-prison-raises-concerns/xDEkyL3GFwsqag7qvywl3K/story.html?arc404=true.

Altman, L. (2020, April 16). Santa Rita jail confirms more COVID-19 cases. *The Independent*. https://www.independentnews.com/news/santa-rita-jail-confirms-more-covid-19-cases/article_e7b89a0c-7f93-11ea-8017-effa3f2e50e9.html.

American Civil Liberties Union (ACLU). (2020). *COVID-19 Model Finds Nearly 100,000 More Deaths than Current Estimates, Due to Failures to Reduce Jails*. A Partnership between ACLU Analytics Researchers from Washington State University, University of Pennsylvania, and University of Tennessee. https://www.aclu.org/sites/default/files/field_document/aclu_covid19-jail-report_2020-8_1.pdf.

Bay City News Service. (2020, April 9). Activists call for Santa Rita inmates to be released. *San Francisco Chronicle*. https://www.nbcbayarea.com/news/coronavirus/activists-call-for-more-inmates-to-be-released-from-santa-rita-jail/2270286/.

Becker, D., & Jolicoeur, L. (2018, March 30). Drinking water remains a concern at Norfolk prison in Mass. WBUR News. https://www.wbur.org/news/2018/03/30/drinking-water-norfolk-prison.

Cases Surge in an Ohio Prison, making it the top known U.S. hot spot. (2020, April 20). *New York Times*. https://www.nytimes.com/2020/04/20/us/coronavirus-live-news.html#link-4ced1d.

Community Justice Exchange and Public Health Awakened. (2020). Decarceration during COVID-19: A messaging toolkit for campaigns for mass release. https://www.communityjusticeexchange.org/all-resources.

Crimaldi, L. (2018, August 2). Massachusetts cites two prisons for ventilation problems. *Boston Globe*. https://www.bostonglobe.com/metro/2018/08/02/dph-cites-two-prisons-for-ventilation-problems/r9Lezzud BMs4hgFuiPdkpI/story.html.

Davis, A. Y. (2000). Masked racism: Reflections on the prison industrial complex in the USA. [Article reprinted from Colorlines]. *Indigenous Law Bulletin, 4*, 4.

#DeeperThanWater. (n.d.). deeperthanwater.org. https://deeperthanwater.org/2020/03/16/prisons-and-the-pandemic/.

deVuono-Powell, S., Minkler, M., Bissell, E., Walker, T., Vaughn, L., Moore, E., & The Morris Justice Project (2018). Criminal justice reform through participatory action research. In N. Wallerstein, B. Duran, J. G. Oetzel, & M. Minkler (Eds.), *Community-Based Participatory Research for Health: Advancing Social and Health Equity* (pp. 305–320). Jossey-Bass.

Fazel, S., & Baillargeon, J. (2011). The health of prisoners. *Lancet, 377*(9769), 956–965.

Gaber, N., & Wright, A. (2016). Protecting urban health and safety: Balancing care and harm in the era of mass incarceration. *J Urban Health, 93*(1), 68–77.

Gilmore, R. W. (2007). *Golden Gulag: Prisons, Surplus, Crisis, and Opposition in Globalizing California*. University of California Press.

Hatzenbuehler, M. L., & Pachankis, J. E. (2016). Stigma and minority stress as social determinants of health among lesbian, gay, bisexual, and transgender youth: Research evidence and clinical implications. *Pediatr Clin, 63*(6), 985–997.

Henry, B. F. (2020). Social distancing and incarceration: policy and management strategies to reduce COVID-19 transmission and promote health equity through decarceration. *Health Educ Behav, 47*(4), 536–539.

Kingdon, J. W. (2011). *Agendas, Alternatives, and Public Policies* (updated 2nd ed.). Longman.

Lee, R. D., Fang, X., & Luo, F. (2013). The impact of parental incarceration on the physical and mental health of young adults. *Pediatrics, 131*(4), e1188–e1195.

Marmot, M., Allen, J., Bell, R., Bloomer, E., & Goldblatt, P. (2012). WHO European review of social determinants of health and the health divide. *The Lancet, 380*(9846), 1011–1029.

Mauer, M., Nellis, A., & Schirmir, S. (2009). *Incarcerated Parents and Their Children: Trends 1991–2007.* The Sentencing Project.

Mergler, D. (1999). Neurotoxic effects of low-level exposure to manganese in human populations. *Environ Res, 80*(2), 99–102.

Minkler, M., Griffin, J., & Wakimoto, P. (2020). Seizing the moment: Policy advocacy to end mass incarceration in the time of COVID-19. *Health Educ Behav, 47*(4), 514–518.

Noonan, M. E., & Ginder, S. (2015). Understanding mortality in state prison: Do male prisoners have an elevated risk of death? *Justice Res Policy, 16*(1), 65–80.

Sawyer, W., & Wagner, P. (2020, March 24). Mass incarceration: The whole pie 2020. *Prison Policy Initiative.* https://www.prisonpolicy.org/reports/pie2020.html.

Thomas, D., & Horowitz, J. M. (2020, September 16). Support for Black Lives Matter has decreased since June but remains strong among Black Americans. Pew Research Center. https://www.pewresearch.org/fact-tank/2020/09/16/support-for-black-lives-matter-has-decreased-since-june-but-remains-strong-among-black-americans/.

Williams, T., & Ivory, D. (2020, April 8). Chicago's jail is top U.S. hot spot as virus spreads behind bars. *New York Times.* https://www.nytimes.com/2020/04/08/us/coronavirus-cook-county-jail-chicago.html.

World Health Organization (WHO). (2020, March 20). Preparedness, prevention and control of COVID-19 in prisons and other places of detention. Interim guidance. https://www.euro.who.int/__data/assets/pdf_file/0019/434026/Preparedness-prevention-and-control-of-COVID-19-in-prisons.pdf?ua=1.

24

Media Advocacy

A Potent Strategy for Engaging Communities in the Fight for Equitable Public Policy

LORI DORFMAN

PRISILA GONZALEZ

SHADDAI MARTINEZ CUESTAS

The primary tool available to communities for influencing social conditions and creating healthy environments is policy. Policies define the structures and set the rules by which we live. If public health practitioners and community organizers are going to improve social conditions and physical environments in lasting and meaningful ways, they must be involved in policy development and policy advocacy. And being successful in policy advocacy means paying attention to the news.

The reach of the media is intoxicating. In our society, the news media are an important part of our collective narrative, largely determining what issues we collectively think about, how we think about them, and what kinds of alternatives are considered viable. The public and policymakers do not consider issues seriously unless they are visible, and they are not visible unless the media have brought them to light.

Nonprofit organizations, health departments, and community activists are often unhappy with how their issues are presented in the news. Media advocacy addresses this problem. It is an approach to health communication that differs significantly from traditional mass communication approaches (Wallack et al., 1999). Despite the media's enormous reach and potential as a tool for change, public health professionals rarely use mass media to their full advantage. Rather, they tend to use them in their least effective capacity: to convey personal health information to consumers. By contrast, media advocacy harnesses the power of the news to mobilize advocates and apply pressure for policy change. Media advocacy helps people understand the importance and reach of news coverage, the need to participate actively in shaping such coverage, and the methods to do so effectively.

First Comes Strategy

Media advocacy relies on four layers of strategy. The first is the overall strategy, which includes the policy goal and what it will take to enact it. Based on that, advocates develop their media strategy and their message strategy—what they want to say, who will say it, and to whom. After the first three layers of strategy are in place, advocates can determine the best way to attract news attention—the access strategy.

Develop an Overall Strategy

Getting media attention should never be an advocate's first consideration. Before talking to reporters or even determining what to say, public health advocates must know what they want to change in concrete terms, the more specific the better (Dorfman et al., 2005; Themba, 1999). And advocates need to know how to create the change, for example, through legislation, a vote, administrative petition, or some other process (Chapman, 2001; Wallack et al., 1999).

The overall strategy will determine how to approach the problem, and thus also how to approach the media. Media advocates use these five questions to develop their overall strategy:

1. What is the problem or issue? How the problem is defined will determine the solution.
2. What is a solution or policy? Specific solutions are usually incremental since it is impossible to be comprehensive and strategic at the same time. Health problems have complex root causes. Being strategic means selecting the current solution that will support long-term change, understanding it likely will not solve all of the problem all at once.
3. Who has the power to make the necessary change? The target is the person or body that can enact the policy (e.g., legislature, city council, business, school board, principal, mayor, building manager, CEO, etc.).
4. Who must be mobilized to apply the necessary pressure? The secondary targets are the people who care about the issue and who are likely to persuade—or can put pressure on—the target.
5. What are the actions advocates will take to reach and persuade the target? These can be letter-writing campaigns, one-on-one meetings with elected officials, organizing protests, or other tactics.

The evolution of tobacco control illustrates how the answers to these questions will shape strategy. In the 1950s and 1960s, the problem was defined as smoking so the solution was to warn smokers about the danger and help them quit; the targets were smokers or potential smokers. This usually led to actions such as non-controversial education programs about the harms caused by smoking but could include policies like instituting reimbursement for cessation programs in health insurance.

Eventually, tobacco control advocates learned that greater success would come from understanding the problem at a population level and instituting primary prevention. From this perspective, the problem is defined not as smoking but as tobacco. The solutions now are policies that reshape the environment, such as excise taxes, clean indoor air laws, limiting tobacco retail licenses, or banning flavored vaping products. The immediate target is not the smoker but the policymaker, and those who can put public pressure on policymakers. Advocates can take actions like providing testimony in front of elected officials or organizing to put taxes on the ballot.

Develop a Media Strategy

Traditional mass communication strategies focus on delivering a message so people can make better decisions. They assume that what is needed to improve health is to tell individuals what to do, but this approach ignores the systems and policies that surround individuals that have a major impact on their health. Policy, systems, and environmental change require a different approach to mass communication, one that helps people act as citizens to influence policy decisions. Media advocacy's strategic use of mass media in support of community organizing to advance healthy public policies is that approach (Wallack et al., 1993). Instead of conceptualizing the audience as consumers of information or people with a problem, media advocates think of them as active participants in democracy (Chapman & Lupton, 1994). Media advocacy seeks to raise the volume of voices for social change and shape the sound so that it resonates with the social justice values that are the basis of public health (Beauchamp, 1976; Wallack & Lawrence, 2005).

Media advocacy differs from traditional public health campaigns as it seeks to support community organizing with a focus on five strategies:

1. Public health and social problems as issues rooted in inequities in social arrangements rather than on flaws in the individual
2. Changing public policy rather than personal health behavior
3. Reaching and pressuring decisionmakers rather than only those experiencing the problem (the traditional audience of public health communication campaigns)
4. Working with groups to amplify their voices rather than providing individual behavior change messages
5. Having a primary goal of eliminating the power gap rather than just filling the information gap (Dorfman & Wallack, 2012)

Focus on the News

Decades of communications research show that the news media set the agenda for the public, for policymakers, and for other media (Dearing & Everett, 1996; Leskovec et al., 2009; Pew Research Center, 2019). Policymakers see news as a barometer of public concerns. The media accord legitimacy and credibility to the issues they cover. In reflecting the issues of the day, the news media set the agenda by selecting what topics people and policymakers discuss and shape the debate by determining what is not being discussed. Media advocates aim to get their issues covered by the news media at key moments in the policy process (as determined by their overall strategy).

Developing a media strategy means first deciding when the media spotlight would make a difference. Media attention during the budget negotiations or before an important school board vote has a direct impact on the policymaking process. You must also consider which outlets would reach your target audience. To reach a state legislator, advocates might want coverage in the newspaper at the capitol and in the news outlets in the legislator's home district. For a business executive, an advocate might seek coverage on the business pages in the newspapers near company headquarters. To do this well and get the responses from reporters when they pitch stories, media advocates monitor the media and develop relationships with reporters. Monitoring the media is crucial because it helps advocates identify which reporters are interested in their issue and whether the reporting is covering all the aspects they think are important. For example, media advocates can follow specific reporters on social media to learn about which issues they cover. Finally, media advocates decide whether to create news, piggyback on breaking news, write op-eds, post blogs, submit letters, request editorials, use social media, or purchase advertising.

Develop a Message Strategy

A message strategy includes what you will say (the message), whom you will say it to (the target or audience), and who says it (the messenger). A message has three components: a problem statement, a solution, and a values statement. It answers the questions: *What's wrong? Why does it matter?* And, *What should be done?* These questions should look familiar, because the message will be derived from the overall strategy. There might be several correct answers to these questions, so media advocates must be strategic and choose the answers that link to the current status of the overall strategy. Advocates must be able to articulate why this problem and solution matter, which values support this goal, and what will happen if nothing is done. Advocates have to be willing to say who should take responsibility for enacting the solution.

Whatever message advocates develop is going to be heard in a messy, loud media context that is dominated by well-financed campaigns from corporations or other opposition, some with "anti-health" goals that reinforce personal responsibility. Our task is to characterize or frame our issues to reinforce institutional accountability, in a way that supports our policy goal. If we are successful in garnering news coverage, our message can reach our targets while getting the public's attention, which amplifies the pressure on our target.

Framing for Access and Framing for Content

Framing for media advocates includes both what to emphasize to gain the attention of reporters (i.e., framing for access), which may not be what you emphasize once you have their attention (i.e., framing for content). For example, in violence prevention the dominant frame is that acts of violence are inevitable, unpredictable, and thus probably unavoidable. Framing for content means you shape the story to emphasize that violence is predictable and thus can be prevented (at a population level, if not for any given individual). Framing for content is challenging because media advocates often bump up against larger societal frames that can contradict a public health perspective (we devote a special section to framing challenges later in the chapter). But first, to gain access to reporters so you can make your points about violence prevention and connect them to your policy solution, you will have to identify what is newsworthy about the story, now.

Develop an Access Strategy

Advocates can create news by, for example, releasing a report, organizing a demonstration or a protest, or planning an event. Media advocates pay attention to those tenets of newsworthiness that grab journalists' attention: controversy, irony, a local angle, anniversaries and milestones, breakthroughs, populations of interest, and injustice (Wallack et al., 1999). They emphasize what is newsworthy when they pitch stories or frame for access. Then they provide story elements that make it easy for reporters to tell the story. Story elements can be compelling visuals and symbols, concise media bites, authentic voices, and social math that uses comparisons or analogies to make large numbers meaningful.

Then Comes Framing

How should public health advocates answer challenging arguments from opponents? Gun groups argue the best way to prevent gun injury and death is teaching individuals about gun safety. Alcohol companies insist that most people drink responsibly and the companies shouldn't be blamed if some people abuse their products. Junk food purveyors say that it is the parents' responsibility to control what children eat. Car companies say that the key to greater safety on the road is changes in driver behavior (Dorfman et al., 2005).

These are tough arguments to counter. After all, each one is truthful—if incomplete. But each industry argument has a common feature: each frames the debate in terms of a single, widely held, important American value: personal responsibility. Trouble is, when public health battles are framed solely in terms of personal responsibility, audiences can't see how the systems and structures surrounding individuals contribute to their health status. Public health advocates need to "reframe" the message so the landscape around individuals comes into view. When public health advocates make the landscape visible, they make it easier to see why their arguments make sense for public health solutions. With the landscape in view, the need for policy, systems, and environmental change makes sense.

Regardless of how well public health advocates make their case, if the change is significant, it will be contested (if it is not, then you do not need media advocacy!).

Inevitably, environmental changes are more controversial than changes in personal behavior because they generally require a shift in resources or responsibility. How the message is framed can either strengthen support for public health policy or reinforce the opposition.

Typical News Frames Are More Often Portraits than Landscapes

Most news is framed around newsworthy events or actions from individuals. Shanto Iyengar's seminal research showed that nearly 80 percent of television news focused narrowly on incidents, events, or people, what he called "episodic" stories (Iyengar, 1991). Other research has upheld that finding in studies of television (Chávez & Dorfman, 1996; Dorfman et al., 1997) and in print news (Dorfman et al., 2005; Jankowski & Major, 2020; Marvel et al., 2018; McManus & Dorfman, 2002; Woodruff et al., 2003).

In a series of experiments, Iyengar (1991) found that when people watch news stories that lack context viewers focus on the individuals. Without any other information, they tend to attribute responsibility for the problem and its solution to the people portrayed in the story—in other words, they blame the victim. After watching episodic news stories, viewers are more likely to distance themselves from the "victims" portrayed, look to them to work harder to solve their own problem or accept the consequences of their behavior, and gain no insight into the social and political circumstances that contribute to the individual problem.

To counter this dominant episodic news frame, advocates must help reporters do a better job describing the landscape surrounding individuals and events so the context of public health problems becomes visible. Iyengar called these stories "thematic." Thematic stories may engage viewers with a personal story, but they also give them more: background, consequences, and other information that provides context. Iyengar found that viewers who see thematic stories understand that responsibility is shared between individuals and their institutions and are more likely to recognize that government or other institutions have a role in solving the problem.

A simple way to distinguish story types is to think of the difference between a portrait and a landscape. In a news story framed as a portrait, audiences may learn a great deal about an individual or an event, with great drama and emotion. But, it is hard to see what surrounds that individual or what brought the person to that moment in time. A landscape story pulls back the lens to take a broader view. It may include people and events, but it connects them to the larger social and economic forces. News stories framed in such a manner are more likely to evoke solutions that don't focus exclusively on individuals, but also the policies, institutions, and conditions that surround and affect them (Dorfman & Wallack, 2012; Dorfman et al., 2005).

There are economic imperatives in the media business that compel reporters to pursue portraits rather than landscapes. Corporate concentration has forced news outlets to abandon public interest goals to pursue profit in the form of larger audiences. Stories framed as portraits serve that purpose better than landscapes because they are easier stories to tell and presumably attract a larger audience. The framing challenge for public health advocates is to create landscape stories that are as compelling as portraits, which is not easy to do, but crucial.

While landscape stories are harder to tell, it can be done, especially when public health advocates provide the story elements that make it easier for reporters. Tobacco is a terrific example of reframing. First it was thought of as a personal problem of smokers who were addicted. Then it was reframed to be understood as a problem of corporate behavior and government regulation, rather than just the behavior of the smoker. Once advocates emphasized that perspective, and used their role as sources to help journalists tell a new story, the issue was understood differently (see table 24.1).

Make Values Visible

Cognitive linguist George Lakoff describes three conceptual levels for framing messages in the context of public health and other social or political issues (Lakoff, personal communication, June 2004). Level 1 is the expression of overarching values like fairness, responsibility, equality, equity, the core values that motivate media advocates to change the world. Level 2 is the general issue being addressed, like housing, the environment, schools, or health. Level 3 is about the nitty-gritty of those issues, including the policy detail or strategy and tactics for achieving change.

Messages can be generated from any level, but Level 1 is most important, since it is at Level 1 that people connect in the deepest way. According to Lakoff, people's support or rejection of an issue will be largely determined by whether they can identify and connect with the Level 1 value. Values are motivators, and messages for policy change should reinforce and activate values. Messages, therefore, should articulate Level 1 values and not get mired in Level 3 minutiae. Public health advocates must know the Level 3 details—what needs changing and how the change will occur—but those details needn't be prominent in the message. In fact, if Level 3 details crowd out Level 1 values, Lakoff contends that the message will be less effective.

Level 2 categories can be a useful device in reframing an issue, as when violence is cast as a public health issue, or housing is seen as an equity issue.

Table 24.2 provides sample messages that share the same Level 1 value, in this case fairness and equity. The policies used here are examples—at any given time, the specific of the policy may change, depending on the overall strategy. When it does, the values statement may remain consistent, or it too may change.

Evaluation

Advocates can focus immediate evaluation efforts on their process objectives. For example, did the op-ed get published, did the reporter pick up the story we pitched, was the story framed with a landscape perspective? Of course, the ultimate outcome measure for media advocacy is whether or not the desired policy passed. However, disentangling media advocacy's contribution to the policy process from the

TABLE 24.1

Reframing Public Health: Examples from Tobacco, Obesity, Housing, and Sexual Violence

	Tobacco	Obesity	Housing	Sexual violence
Problem	Corporate behavior promotes an addictive deadly product that kills when used as directed	A food industry primed to profit from highly processed foods with minimal nutritional value	Legacy of redlining, predatory lending, lack of government investment in housing as a social good, threat of eviction during a pandemic	Reactive strategies to address the impact of violence, lack of institutional accountability, limited definitions of sexual assault
Responsibility	Belongs to the tobacco industry and those who regulate it	Food manufacturers and marketers and those who regulate them	Local, county, and state officials responsible for zoning, growth policy, and budgets and federal agencies and legislators who lead and fund national housing policy	School and university administrators, leadership in small and large corporations, businesses, nonprofits
Solution	Policies on availability and youth access (e.g., raising the minimum age to 21), excise taxes, secondhand smoke, eliminating flavors, target marketing, and phasing out product sales	Policies on menu labeling, default foods in kids' meals, nutrition standards for school meals, produce incentives for SNAP ("double bucks"), excise taxes on sugary drinks,	Renter protections, mortgage assistance, eviction moratoriums, canceling rent, land trusts	Clear guidelines on role and responsibility for reporting assault, staff training to identify early signs of abuse, sexual harassment policies

(continued)

Table 24.1. (continued)

	Tobacco	Obesity	Housing	Sexual violence
Values	Protect youth, promote health, and hold industry accountable	Promote health, children's development and attention in school, hold industry accountable	Community well-being and diversity, health, interconnection	Protection, safety, caring, education, growth
Story element examples *Visuals,* *Social math,* *Media bites,* *Authentic voices*	A graph that compares the number of tobacco retailers (375,000) in the United States with the number of McDonald's (14,339) or Starbucks stores (11,962) is good social math and a compelling visual (Truth initiative, 2017)	A media bite that encapsulates the problem with junk food marketing during the Olympics: "The Olympic Games should be a beacon of human progress and ability, not a place where poor nutrition is given a halo of gold" (Boseley, 2016)	A quote from a medical professional is an authentic voice and media bite: "Nothing I have in my black bag improves the health of a homeless person . . . other than housing" (Katayama et al., 2019)	Displaying red shoes to represent the number of women lost to violence is a powerful visual to bring attention to the magnitude of violence against women worldwide (Barajas, 2020)

Note: financing for supermarkets in underserved areas, shared use of playgrounds on schoolyards

TABLE 24.2

Policy Examples and Sample Messages

Example	Message
For sugary beverages, with a Level 3 policy goal of limiting their accessibility, the message might be:	We want children to grow up in wholesome environments that foster health. It is not fair that everywhere they turn in this neighborhood sugary drinks are cheap and easy to find, but free drinking water is nowhere to be found. Every family should be able to raise their children in a healthy environment. That's why we're asking the parks district to repair drinking fountains and provide cold drinking water where children play.
For street safety, with a Level 3 policy goal of installing safety crosswalk lights across all neighborhoods of the city, the message might be:	While we have achieved great progress in reducing traffic- related injuries, there are still neighborhoods in our city, primarily in low-income communities of color, with few crosswalks or traffic lights. It is not fair that some of our city residents' lives are protected and others are not. Our city should install reliable crosswalk lighting so pedestrians are safe in every neighborhood.

effects of community organizing or policy advocacy—or other events or secular trends—is challenging, especially because policies can take years, sometimes decades, to enact and implement (Schooler et al., 1996; Stead et al., 2002). Most evidence for media advocacy's success comes from tobacco (Niederdeppe et al., 2007) and alcohol (Harwood et al., 2005; Holder & Treno, 1997; Stewart & Casswell, 1993) policy campaigns, likely because media advocacy was developed first in those fields. Many evaluations are qualitative case studies that describe the process of conducting media advocacy (Dean, 2006; Dorfman et al., 2002; Jernigan & Wright, 1996; Seevak, 1997) and provide a framework for evaluators who want to assess media advocacy in relation to other sorts of health communications. As media advocates expand their practice, we should start to see evaluations of media advocacy practiced in a variety of public health policy arenas.

Conclusions

Media advocacy is in service to community organizing and policy advocacy; it does not stand on its own. That is why one cannot have a media strategy without an overall strategy. Advocates must know what they want, why they want it, and how they are going to get it, all before going to the media.

Media advocacy is one of the few public health interventions that focuses on changing the environment in which people make health decisions. Public health matters are too important to be left to strategies that are at the mercy of media producers who have other priorities. That is one reason why, in public health, we cannot depend on public service advertising, for example.

The focus on policy is critical because usually, although not always, it is the mechanism with which we can improve health environments and health outcomes for the broadest population and address the root causes of inequities. Media advocacy can accelerate and amplify that policy work so we can arrive faster at our goals for safe, healthful environments for everyone.

Questions for Further Discussion

1. Reporters will often try to "put a face" to an issue by talking to a "victim" or a person experiencing the issue you are working on. For example, in covering evictions protections, a reporter may want to interview a landlord or a tenant. This risks keeping the conversation at the individual level and triggering personal responsibility frames. What can you do to ensure that the conversation comes back to the systemic solution you are proposing and the "landscape" frame?
2. Articulating values is key for creating effective messages. And yet, advocates tend to rely solely on data and facts to make their case. What values motivate you to do this work? How can you express those in a message? How can you encourage your advocacy colleagues to articulate their values as well?

Acknowledgments

Adapted from Dorfman, L., & Bakal, M. (2018). Using media advocacy to influence policy. Chapter 13 in R. J. Bensley & J. Brookins-Fisher (Eds.), *Community Health Education Methods: A Practical Guide* (4th ed.). Jones & Bartlett Publishers. The authors thank Katherine Schaff, DrPH, MPH, for her inspiring work on health equity and her contributions to table 24.1.

REFERENCES

Barajas, J. (2020, March 10). This artist's red shoes stand in for all the women lost to violence. *PBS News Hour*. https://www.pbs.org/newshour/arts/this-artists-red-shoes-stand-in-for-all-the-women-lost-to-violence.

Beauchamp, D. E. (1976). Public health as social justice. [Reprinted with permission of the Blue Cross Association.] *Inquiry, 13*(1), 3–14.

Boseley, S. (2016, August 4). Olympics are a carnival of junk food marketing, say campaigners. *The Guardian*. https://www.theguardian.com/lifeandstyle/2016/aug/05/olympics-carnival-junk-food-marketing-campaigners-kelloggs-mcdonalds.

Chapman, S. (2001). Advocacy in public health: Roles and challenges. *Int J Epidemiol, 30*, 1226–1232.

Chapman, S., & Lupton, D. (1994). *The Fight for Public Health: Principles and Practices of Media Advocacy.* British Medical Journal Publishing.

Chávez, V., & Dorfman, L. (1996). Spanish language television news portrayals of youth and violence in California. *Int Q Community Health Educ, 16*(2), 121–138.

Dean, R. (2006, October 1). Issue 16: Moving from head to heart: Using media advocacy to talk about affordable housing. Berkeley Media Studies Group. http://www.bmsg.org/resources /publications/issue-16-moving-from-head-to-heart-using-media-advocacy-to-talk-about -affordable-housing/.

Dearing, J. W., & Everett, R. M. (1996). *Agenda-Setting.* Sage.

Dorfman, L., Ervice, J., and Woodruff, K. (2002, November). *Voices for Change: A Taxonomy of Public Communications Campaigns and Their Evaluation Challenges.* Communications Consortium Media Center. http://www.pointk.org/resources/files/Voices_for_Change .pdf.

Dorfman L., & Wallack, L. (2012). Putting policy into health communication: The role of media advocacy. In R. E. Rice & C. K. Atkin (Eds.), *Public Communication Campaigns* (4th ed., pp. 377–350). Sage.

Dorfman, L., Wallack, L., & Woodruff, K. (2005). More than a message: Framing public health advocacy to change corporate practices. *Health Educ Behav, 32*(4), 320–336.

Dorfman, L., Woodruff, K., Chávez, V., & Wallack, L. (1997). Youth and violence on local television news in California. *Am J Public Health, 87*(8), 1311–1316.

Harwood, E. M., Witson, J. C., Fan, D. P., & Wagenaar, A. C. (2005). Media advocacy and under-age drinking policies: A study of Louisiana news media from 1994 through 2003. *Health Promot Pract, 6*(3), 246–257.

Holder, H. D., & Treno, A. J. (1997). Media advocacy in community prevention: News as a means to advance policy change. *Addiction, 92*, 189–200.

Iyengar, S. (1991). *Is Anyone Responsible?* University of Chicago Press.

Jankowski, S. M., & Major, L. H. (2020). *Health News and Responsibility: How Frames Create Blame.* Peter Lang.

Jernigan, D. H., & Wright, P. A. (1996). Media advocacy: Lessons from community experiences. *J Public Health Policy, 17*(3), 306–330.

Katayama, D., Cruz Guevara, E., & Aguilar, E. (2019, May 29). A prescription your doctor can't write: Housing as health care. KQED News. https://www.kqed.org/news/11750637/a-pre scription-your-doctor-cant-write-housing-as-healthcare.

Lakoff, G., & Morgan, P. (2004, June). Rockridge Institute and University of California, Berke-ley. Personal communication with the authors.

Leskovec, J., Lars, B., & Kleinberg, J. (2009). Meme-tracking and the dynamics of the news cycle. In *Proceedings of the 15th ACM SIGKDD International Conference on Knowledge Discovery and Data Mining* (pp. 497–506). Association for Computing Machinery.

Marvel, D., Mejia, P., Nixon, L., & Dorfman, L. (2018, June 18). Issue 25: More than mass shoot-ings: Gun violence narratives in California news. Berkeley Media Studies Group. http:// www.bmsg.org/resources/publications/gun-suicide-community-domestic-violence -news-narratives-california/.

McManus, J., & Dorfman, L. (2002). Youth violence stories focus on events, not causes. *News-paper Research Journal, 23*(4), 6–20.

Niederdeppe, J., Farrelly, M. C., & Wenter, D. (2007). Media advocacy, tobacco control policy change and teen smoking in Florida. *Tob Control, 16*, 47–52.

Pew Research Center. (2019). *State of the News Media (Project) Digital News Fact Sheets.* Pew Research Center Publications. https://www.journalism.org/fact-sheet/digital-news/.

Schooler, C. S., Sundar, S., & Flora, J. (1996). Effects of the Stanford Five-City Project media advo-cacy program. *Health Educ Behav, 23*, 346–364.

Seevak, A. (1997, December 1). Issue 3: Oakland shows the way: The coalition on alcohol outlet issues and media advocacy as a tool for policy change. Berkeley Media Studies Group. http://www.bmsg.org/resources/publications/issue-3-oakland-shows-the-way-the-coalition-on-alcohol-outlet-issues-and-media-advocacy-as-a-tool-for-policy-change/.

Stead, M., Gerard, H., & Douglas, E. (2002). The challenge of evaluating complex interventions: A framework for evaluating media advocacy. *Health Educ Res, 17*(3), 351–364.

Stewart, L., & Casswell, S. (1993). Media advocacy for alcohol policy support: Results from the New Zealand Community Action Project. *Health Promot Int, 8*(3), 167–175.

Themba, M. (1999). *Making Policy Making Change: How Communities Are Taking the Law into Their Own Hands*. Chardon Press.

Truth Initiative. (2017, September 25). How some local governments are keeping the number of tobacco retailers in check. Truth Initiative. https://truthinitiative.org/research-resources/tobacco-industry-marketing/how-some-local-governments-are-keeping-number-tobacco.

Wallack, L., Dorfman, L., Jernigan, D., & Themba, M. (1993). *Media Advocacy and Public Health: Power for Prevention*. Sage.

Wallack, L., & Lawrence, R. (2005). Talking about public health: Developing America's "second language." *Am J Public Health, 95*(4), 567–570.

Wallack L., Woodruff, K., Dorfman, L., & Diaz, I. (1999). *News for a Change: An Advocate's Guide to Working with the Media*. Sage.

Woodruff, K., Dorfman, L., Berends, V., & Agron, P. (2003). Coverage of childhood nutrition policies in California newspapers. *J Public Health Policy, 24*(2), 150–158.

Appendixes

APPENDIX 1

Challenging Ourselves

Critical Self-Reflection on Power and Privilege

CHERYL A. HYDE

One of the more common, and mistaken, assumptions that community practitioners make is thinking that because they are "fighting the good fight," they do not need to address issues regarding their own power and privilege. Yet engaging in practice under the banner of social justice (or any other "right reason") does not result in an automatic community of shared interests. Nor does it inoculate against the dividends that one might accrue because of race, class, gender, sexual orientation, or other aspect of an individual's cultural identity. Because so much of community practice is relational (chapter 6; appendix 5), I suggest that it is essential for practitioners to engage in some rigorous self-exploration as part of their broader anti-oppression work. In this appendix, I offer one approach to such critical reflection that I have used in teaching and training efforts.

Like many individuals who engage in anti-oppression teaching and practice, I ground much of my thinking in Peggy McIntosh's (1989) classic essay "White Privilege: Unpacking the Invisible Knapsack." By delineating the many ways in which White individuals benefit from usually unrecognized or unacknowledged everyday expectations, rituals, and processes (e.g., "I am never asked to speak for all the people of my racial group" [p. 11]), McIntosh connects the personal with broader structures that promote or protect racism. She then issues a call to action: "A 'white' skin in the United States opens many doors for whites, whether or not we approve of the way dominance has been conferred on us. Individual acts can palliate, but cannot end, these problems. To redesign social systems, we need first to acknowledge their colossal unseen dimensions. The silences and denials surrounding privilege are the key political tool here" (p. 12).

Part of the power of McIntosh's essay is that the reader needs to contend with the cumulative impact that seemingly minor activities can have on the perpetuation of racism. These are microaggressions, and there is considerable evidence that over time, such actions contribute to the racial trauma of people of color (DiAngelo, 2018; Sue & Spanierman, 2020). In demanding that Whites dissect their racial privilege, and then take steps to challenge it, McIntosh provided a foundation for much of the anti-racism and related work that followed (see e.g., Came & Griffith, 2018; DiAngelo, 2018; Hill, 2017; Wise, 2011; chapter 4). Comparable examinations can happen for other privileges based on class, gender, sexual orientation, and so forth; indeed, there are many examples in the literature (for varying approaches, see Adams, 1997; Connell, 2005; Gerschick, 1993; Goodman, 2001; hooks, 2000a, 2000b; Kendi, 2019; Tappan, 2006; Wallerstein, 1999).

While McIntosh's contribution to anti-racism work cannot be underestimated, her approach does, I believe, fall short in four important ways. First, it does not distinguish between how we see our own privilege and how others might perceive or experience our identity. McIntosh is focused on the former, yet those with whom we interact also bring to the encounters an awareness (or not) of privilege as beneficiaries or as those denied such benefits. Second, she is focused on race and racism, which is understandable, but incomplete. Race is not the only attribute that shapes how we negotiate the world. Third, because of this primary focus on race, McIntosh does not capture how different cultural attributes interact and differentially shape privilege. For example, a middle-class White woman and a working-class White woman both hold racial privilege, yet the manifestation of that privilege will present differently because of class. It is important to emphasize the pioneering work of critical race theorists who introduced and developed the concept of intersectionality—the understanding of multiple facets to our identity (Collins, 2019; Crenshaw et al., 1995; Delgado & Stefancic, 2017). And fourth, even though McIntosh notes that "unseen dimensions" support societal structures, she nonetheless neglects the broad, systemic impact of labor market, educational, residential, and other forms of institutionalized racism (Jones, 2000). Fundamentally, hers is an intrapersonal framework for identifying one's White privilege, then understanding how that privilege helps racism endure; this is certainly critical but not sufficient. Grappling with these points, while still employing the essential insights of McIntosh, became the catalyst for the approach that I use.

One Approach to Critical Self-Reflection

Before outlining my approach to a *critical self-reflection* for community practitioners, I want to emphasize, first, that this is a framework that I have found useful as a learner, teacher, trainer, and practitioner. It is not, however, the only model out there, and it is well worth the effort to find a process that both works well and authentically challenges you as a community practitioner. Second, two assessments have been constructed for this appendix (see tables A1.1 and A1.2), but they are adapted from tools that others and I have developed (Burghardt, 2011; Center for Community Health and Development, n.d.; Katz, 1978; McIntosh, 1989). These tools

TABLE A1.1

Cultural Identity Inventory

Cultural Dimensions	Manifestations	Interactions	Domination/ Subordination	Vantage Points
Indicate for each (note any conflict concerning this identifier)	What values, action, or messages are associated with the dimension?	Does the effect of this dimension interact with any other dimension? How so?	If dominant— what privileges do you have? How have you responded? If subordinate— what have you been denied? How have you responded?	How do you understand this aspect of yourself? How do you think or experience the way others see you?
Gender				
Race				
Class				
Sexual Orientation				
Citizenship				
Religion				
Physical/mental ability				
Other?				

Review and reflect on your inventory. Consider these questions:

1. What are your overall reactions to this information (any affirmations, surprises, points of confusion)?

2. Does any dimension stand out as particularly important to your overall cultural identity, and if so, why?

3. What have you learned about yourself? What next steps in this process do you see yourself taking?

work best when individuals push themselves to honestly complete them, then a group debriefing can support further exploration and exchange of ideas.

Step 1: Our Complex Cultural Selves

The first step in this process is to understand the basics of one's culture and the impact on identity. Here, I am referring to the values, attitudes, beliefs, practices,

TABLE A1.2

Assessment: Connecting Cultural Identity to Community Practice

Cultural Dimensions	As Strength/ Asset to My Community Practice	As Challenge/ Concern to My Community Practice	What Do I Need to Continue My Development?
Gender			
Race			
Class			
Sexual orientation			
Citizenship			
Religion			
Physical/mental ability			
Other?			

Note the ways in which the different components of your cultural identity have influenced you as a community practitioner. Specifically, record how that attribute has (1) given you strengths/assets and (2) provided challenges/concerns.

1. Indicate what you need to continue your development (i.e., how can you build on your strengths or address concerns).

2. How does this assessment inform your cognizance of "use of self"?

Source: Adapted from Center for Community Health and Development. (n.d.). Chapter 27, section 2: Building relationships with people from different cultures. University of Kansas. Retrieved from the Community Tool Box, https://ctb.ku .edu/en/table-of-contents/culture/cultural-competence/building-relationships /main. Used with permission from the Work Group for Community Health and Development, University of Kansas.

and rituals that shape who we are and how we act, all of which flow from the various groups of which we are members. The primary cultural dimensions that I focus on are race, gender, citizenship status (in the United States), sexual orientation, class, religion, and physical/mental ability. There may be other dimensions that are important to an understanding of the cultural self (e.g., region of the country or level of education), but I find that these are the significant ones and serve as important springboards to self-awareness.

So, turn to the Cultural Identity Inventory (table A1.1) and consider the first three columns: "cultural dimensions," "manifestations," and "interactions." For each dimension, indicate *what you are* (note any conflicting messages or challenges to this self-identification) and whether there are any important values, messages, or actions associated with that dimension. For example, if you are a lesbian, did you receive messages of acceptance or condemnation? Or if you are a male, were you told that certain emotions, or displays of emotion, were not manly (i.e., unacceptable)? As you start this inventory, you may be able to see how different affiliations influence one another, for example, how messages about being female are shaped by one's religion. You should note these connections as they become evident. What should begin to become apparent is that we are more than just one or two cultural attributes. The foundation of our cultural selves is the complex whole that is generated from these dimensions.

It is also important to understand that the level of influence exerted by these dimensions on one's cultural self may not be the same, and may vary over time. You may even want to note if a particular dimension is exerting a relatively strong (or weak) effect on you, and why. If we imagine these dimensions arrayed in a pie chart, some wedges will be larger than others; and sometime in the future, these wedges could be resized. This is one reason why it is unwise (and even foolish) to assume that you know a person's culture based on just one or two characteristics. What is important to you may not be as significant to another, because that individual is perhaps more concerned with, or influenced by, a different cultural dimension. There is fluidity to the components of one's identity, depending on specific challenges of a given time and place, as well as negotiating daily life.

Step 2: Privilege and Power

Within each of these dimensions there is a dominant and a subordinate group (see table A1.1, column 4). A dominant group is one that *as a group* has access to economic, social, political, and civic privileges. This access is temporal and systemic, and the privileges may be consciously sought or unconsciously acquired. The point is not whether each individual in a given group always (and knowingly) enjoys privilege or even wants it (or asked for it). It is about the *societal group*, which, through its collective activity, turns that privilege over time into societal power. So, in twenty-first-century America, the privileged groups include men, Whites, the middle/upper classes, heterosexuals, citizens, the able-bodied, and Christians. Continuing with the Cultural Identity Inventory, indicate whether you are a member of the dominant or subordinate group for each cultural dimension in column 4.

Individuals who find themselves mostly or exclusively in dominant-status groups are not bad or evil. Rather, by virtue of these group memberships, they have benefited from various societal "perks," whether they asked for them or not. But once such privilege is revealed, these individuals have an obligation to question, challenge, and otherwise act in good faith to work toward the dismantling of a system that generates such disproportionate rewards based on group membership.

The key here is to take action; wallowing in guilt or engaging in excessive hand-wringing does nothing to contribute to anti-oppression work (indeed, such responses just further underscore one's privileges).

Conversely, the individuals who find themselves mostly or exclusively in subordinate-status groups do not have license to claim victimhood and then withdraw from any constructive action. The task for those with less privilege is to understand the injuries, hidden or explicit, that group subordination may have caused (for an excellent analysis of this, see Sennett and Cobb's (1972) classic work *The Hidden Injuries of Class*). How, for example, has one addressed internalized oppression or recognized and healed from racial trauma (Kendi, 2019; Winters, 2020)? Individuals from subordinate-status groups also need to take action against oppressive structure and processes, though their paths to, and strategies for, that action will likely differ from the work that dominant-group individuals undertake.

For most of us, however, it is not a matter of being in either all-dominant or all-subordinate groups. Instead, our cultural identities are composed of a mix. We might have access to racial or gender privilege, yet be in subordinate groups for religion or sexual orientation. To further complicate this understanding, as noted above, not all dimensions have equal "weight" on our overall identity. We should not, however, let this complexity become an excuse for not owning the privilege that we may have. Yes, I may need to contend with a disability or gender or gender identity discrimination, yet I also need to be mindful that as a White professional, I benefit from race and class privilege. Moreover, these societal dividends provide me with some resources with which to address or cope with subordination that results from membership in other groups. It is essential that we push ourselves to understand the implications of this complexity.

Step 3: Understanding Different Vantage Points

A final factor that I consider in this approach to understanding cultural identity focuses on how we see ourselves versus how others perceive us. While it is tempting to think that we have primary or sole control over the making of our cultural identity, we do not. When we interact with, or are simply in the presence of, others, our cultural identity is being shaped by that individual's ideas, beliefs, attitudes, experiences, and so forth. This may not always be fair, but in relationship building, we are always negotiating the perceptions and reactions of others and hopefully in the process can address any misperceptions.

Referring again to the Cultural Identity Inventory, column 5, push yourself to consider your subjective (self-) understanding of each cultural dimension and then the understandings of others. If you are White, how do you view this and how do you experience others viewing that? If you have a disability that is not readily apparent, how do you understand this and how might others (if at all)? The point of this aspect of the inventory is to understand that how you move through life does not necessarily correspond with how others see that journey. What you think might be central to your identity may not even register with someone else. Conversely, what you minimize (such as racial privilege) may be of central import to others. Making the genuine effort to understand how others experience you is critical to relationship building and essential if you want to deconstruct and challenge your own societal privileges.

Step 4: Synthesis and Next Steps

Now comes the difficult work—digesting and then acting on what you have uncovered by virtue of doing this inventory. Consider these three questions: (1) What are your overall reactions to this inventory? (2) Does any dimension stand out as particularly important to your overall cultural identity and why? and (3) What have you learned about yourself and what next steps in this process do you see yourself taking? In other words, the inventory in itself does not constitute anti-oppression work. It is the precursor to anti-oppression work through action. If you have pushed yourself to be honest and reflective thus far, then you have laid a foundation for considering what you need to do. Perhaps education is needed, and if so, how will you go about getting it? Maybe an important relationship needs to be repaired, and if so, how might you take the steps to make amends? Or perhaps the inventory revealed that some skills, such as assertiveness training, are needed. If so, where will you obtain this training? Did you become aware of new potential problems or challenges for other groups, and if so, how might you respond?

It is tempting, and perhaps even human nature, to try to minimize the inventory messages that we don't want to know. It is not easy to think of oneself as "privileged," particularly if we don't ask for it, don't believe we use that privilege to our advantage, or have experienced injustices in other ways. Often, we become more focused on those parts of our identity associated with subordinate-group membership and then don't see the privilege we might have. We also run the risk of becoming paralyzed by building an identity of victimization. Cultural humility, which is built on self-awareness, flexibility, empathy, and openness, is essential; but perhaps most important is understanding that anti-oppression work takes time (Burghardt, 2011; hooks, 2003). Be patient with yourself and others as more authentic relationships are built.

Connecting to Community Practice

Community practitioners would be wise to take a page from the training manual of most clinical social workers, therapists, and counselors who are trained to be cognizant in the "use of self." *Use of self* may be defined as the knowledge and skill sets employed by the practitioner in such a way that she or he becomes an instrument to facilitate change (Heydt & Sherman, 2005). Within the parameters of the therapeutic relationship, the practitioner is able to model and reflect transformative possibilities for the client. Yet this approach is not without its dangers, and considerable self-awareness is necessary if the practitioner wishes to minimize unnecessarily complicated or messy relationships with clients. As part of this training, these practitioners learn to recognize and address the emotions generated in the therapeutic relationship; identify what client/actions might "push buttons"; negotiate expectations of the client, including the maintenance of "appropriate" boundaries; and work through resistance and reluctance. The cultural selves of both practitioner and client significantly affect these dynamics, as cultural variations in seeking help, dealing with authority and power, and building relationships come into play (Heydt & Sherman, 2005; Reupert, 2007). Thus, the *use of self* is actually the *use of the cultural self.*

How does this translate to community practice? The strategic use of self is concerned with relationship building that encourages constructive change, which in many respects is the core of community practice. To be an effective community organizer or other practitioner who can build the relationships necessary for increasing community capacity, that individual needs to understand how his or her cultural identity affects facilitating and sustaining relationships. The assumption is that if one does not acknowledge or address the effect of privilege, then one risks poisoning this critical aspect of practice. Moreover, the ability to build authentic connections rests on how well one understands oneself. Many practitioners want to move quickly to finding commonalities, but the realities of oppression—including the personal side—need to be addressed first (Burghardt, 2011). Time, patience, and humility are essential ingredients in this process.

Building on the insights from the Cultural Identity Inventory, one needs to turn to making connections between that awareness and community practice. For this, another assessment is suggested (see table A1.2). Adapted the Center for Community Health and Development's (n.d.) exercise, the goal is to identify how one's cultural identity helps and hinders one's community practice abilities and then extend these findings by determining what one needs to continue with their development. This information is then linked to an emerging and intentional use of self. By systematically engaging in this self-assessment, one will not only understand how cultural attributes of the practitioner become part of practice (for better or worse), but also begin to think strategically about how to maximize the assets and minimize the concerns.

Concluding Thoughts

Community practitioners are typically concerned with, and adept at analyzing, the power structures and processes that affect their constituencies. In this appendix, I have challenged practitioners to look at a more personal aspect of power—the privileges derived from membership in dominant-status groups. I have argued that one's cultural identity is largely determined by these memberships, and I have highlighted the need for reflecting on the multiple and often intersecting identities we hold (woman, Latinx, middle class, etc.). With a more comprehensive understanding of our cultural identities, including the ways in which the various dimensions can change and be challenged over time, we are better situated to build authentic relationships with constituents and community members. In more fully understanding how we benefit from oppressive systems, we are more likely to find the tools to dismantle the attendant structures and processes. This is a critical aspect of "fighting the good fight" and takes time, patience, and openness to continued learning. In doing so, we forge better bonds with our partners and allies and, ultimately, create better communities for us all.

REFERENCES

Adams, M. (1997). Pedagogical frameworks for social justice education. In M. Adams, L. A. Bell, & P. Griffin (Eds.), *Teaching for Diversity and Social Justice: A Sourcebook* (pp. 30–43). Routledge.

Burghardt, S. (2011). Why can't we all just get along? Building effective coalitions while resolving the not-so-hidden realities of race, gender, sexuality, and class. In S. Burghardt (Ed.), *Macro Practice in Social Work for the 21st Century* (pp. 176–214). Sage.

Came, H., & Griffith, D. (2018). Tackling racism as a "wicked" public health problem: Enabling allies in anti-racism praxis. *Soc Sci Med, 199*, 181–188.

Center for Community Health and Development. (n.d.). Chapter 27, section 2: Building relationships with people from different cultures. University of Kansas. Retrieved from the Community Tool Box, https://ctb.ku.edu/en/table-of-contents/culture/cultural-competence/building-relationships/main.

Collins, P. (2019). *Intersectionality as Critical Social Theory*. Duke University Press.

Connell, R. W. (2005). *Masculinities* (2nd ed.). University of California Press.

Crenshaw, K., Gotanda, N., Peller, G., & Thomas, K. (1995). *Critical Race Theory: The Key Writings That Formed the Movement*. New Press.

Delgado, R., & Stefancic, J. (2017). *Critical Race Theory* (3rd ed.). New York University Press.

DiAngelo, R. (2018). *White Fragility: Why It's So Hard for White People to Talk about Racism*. Beacon Press.

Gerschick, T. (1993). Should and can a white, heterosexual, middle-class man teach students about social inequality and oppression? In D. Schoem, L. Frankel, X. Zuniga, & E. Lewis (Eds.), *Multicultural Teaching in the University* (pp. 200–207). Praeger.

Goodman, D. J. (2001). *Promoting Diversity and Social Justice: Educating People from Privileged Groups*. Sage.

Heydt, M. J., & Sherman, N. E. (2005). Conscious use of self: Tuning the instrument of social work practice with cultural competence. *J Baccalaureate Soc Work, 10*(2), 25–40.

Hill, D. (2017). *White Awake: An Honest Look at What It Means*. InterVarsity Press.

hooks, b. (2000a). *Feminist Theory: From Margin to Center* (2nd ed.). South End Press.

hooks, b. (2000b). *Where We Stand: Class Matters*. Routledge.

hooks, b. (2003). The oppositional gaze: Black female spectators. In Amelia Jones (Ed.), *The Feminism and Visual Culture Reader* (pp. 94–105). Routledge.

Jones, C. P. (2000). Levels of racism: A theoretic framework and a gardener's tale. *Am J Public Health, 90*(8), 1212–1215.

Katz, J. (1978). *White Awareness*. University of Oklahoma Press.

Kendi, I. X. (2019). *How to Be an Antiracist*. One World.

McIntosh, P. (1989, July/August). White privilege: Unpacking the invisible knapsack. *Peace and Freedom*, 10–12. https://psychology.umbc.edu/files/2016/10/White-Privilege_McIntosh-1989.pdf.

Reupert, A. (2007). Social worker's use of self. *Clin Soc Work J, 35*, 107–116.

Sennett, R., & Cobb, J. (1972). *The Hidden Injuries of Class*. W. W. Norton.

Sue, D., & Spanierman, L. (2020). *Microaggressions in Everyday Life*. John Wiley and Sons.

Tappan, M. B. (2006). Reframing internalized oppression and internalized domination: From the psychological to the sociocultural. *Teach Coll Rec, 108*(10), 2115–2144.

Wallerstein, N. (1999). Power between evaluator and community: Research relationships within New Mexico's healthier communities. *Soc Sci Med, 49*, 39–53.

Winters, M. (2020). *Black Fatigue: How Racism Erodes the Mind, Body, and Spirit.* Berrett-Koehler.

Wise, T. (2011). *White Like Me: Reflections on Race from Privileged Son.* Soft Skull Press.

APPENDIX 2

Community Mapping and Digital Technology

Tools for Organizers

JASON CORBURN

MARISA RUIZ ASARI

JOSH KIRSCHENBAUM

Community mapping can answer countless questions about socioeconomic conditions, health, development opportunities, and neighborhood change. Mapping is the visual representation of data by geography or location, linking information to place to support social and economic change on a community level. The process of mapping is a powerful tool for two reasons: (1) it makes place-based patterns much easier to identify and analyze and (2) it provides a visual way of communicating those patterns to a broad audience, quickly and clearly, which can help residents organize as they "see" their place in a new way. The central value of a map is that it helps tell a story about what is happening in our communities. These stories can help bring people into organizing efforts, deepen local understanding of complex issues linking place and health, and support decisionmaking and consensus building by translating place-based knowledge into program design, policy development, organizing, and advocacy. As activists increasingly use web-based mapping platforms and link these to social media and mobile devices, digital maps of places hold the potential to transform community organizing for health equity. But they may also place new demands on activists to be technically knowledgeable and reliant on technology to address the social and political change they seek (Corburn, 2005).

Community Mapping: A Visual Narrative

Community mapping is a vibrant way of telling a neighborhood's story. It can highlight a rich array of community assets, display the concentration of childhood asthma, analyze the relationship between income and location of services, or document rising housing costs and other neighborhood changes over time.

The products of community mapping can take several forms. *Context maps* represent one or a few variables by a broad unit of geography (e.g., income level by census tract). *Display maps* are more complex, illustrating single or multiple variables by smaller units of geography (e.g., the condition of individual properties at the parcel level). *Analytical maps* are the most complex, layering and analyzing multiple variables by various levels of geography. An analytical map might combine income at the census tract level and condition of individual properties at the parcel level and highlight how the two variables relate to each other.

Community maps can be hand drawn or digitally generated. Some web maps are also interactive, allowing participants to analyze data and create other maps based on the locations and kinds of data that interest them. Community practitioners can use a range of technologies, from geographic information systems (GIS) to prepopulated online mapping tools, to create maps and analyze data. As defined by the U.S. Geological Survey (2020), GIS are "computer system(s) that analyze and display geographically referenced information using data that is attached to a location." GIS are not just tools for making maps or visually displaying data; they are used for analyzing many layers of data, allowing users to see information over time.

Two commonly used desktop GIS are QGIS and ArcGIS. QGIS (formerly Quantum GIS) is an open-source GIS, meaning that it can be downloaded and installed free of charge, whereas ArcGIS is license-based paid mapping and analytics software. A number of web-based platforms allow community organizers to more easily create and share maps without investing in expensive and complex GIS software. One of the most widely used and free web-based mapping tools is Google's My Maps (maps .google.com). Using the My Maps feature in Google Maps, organizers and community residents can mark assets and liabilities in their community, share this information easily on the web with others, and allow a number of users to edit or "ground truth" this information over time. This tool, unlike analytically robust but less user-friendly GIS software, allows users to easily add descriptive text into the map, add photos and videos, and embed collaborative maps on other sites. A web-based version of ArcGIS, ArcGIS online, is also a popular tool for creating and sharing interactive maps that require more in-depth analyses traditionally found in a desktop GIS. While highlighting some of the most widely used and helpful tools available at this writing, given the speed of change in internet technology, some of these will likely be replaced in the years ahead. The rationale for and utility of community mapping, aided by digital technology, will likely remain strong, and the reader is encouraged to explore and test promising new programs and approaches as they develop.

How to Use Community Mapping

Community mapping involves six broad steps, some of which can be implemented simultaneously. The process begins and ends with local communities, and each step builds on the information obtained in a previous step.

Step 1: Identify Community Issues and Build a Community Mapping Collaborative

All community mapping efforts start with community-based organizations and residents and their in-depth understanding of community conditions, assets, and problems. Community knowledge is used to identify challenges; set benchmarks, goals, and outcomes; locate opportunities for investment; frame data-gathering efforts; determine the appropriate types of geography and maps; and use maps for community building purposes. By designing and leading the mapping process, community residents and organizations are better positioned to ensure that the maps offer community benefits and accurately reflect community needs. Community leadership also promotes community values in the mapping process and better equips community groups to use the resulting maps for advocacy and organizing purposes.

Step 2: Identify the Audience

Advancing the long-term goals of community mapping often requires tailoring intermediate outputs to specific stakeholders. In some cases, mapping exercises may be intended to strengthen community organizing movements or increase local awareness around an ongoing process. In other cases, spatial data and community maps are presented directly to policymakers, city planning departments, or community leaders and are used in active decisionmaking. Different audiences may also need varying levels of context or key visual and spatial anchor points within a community map to help orient them. For example, local residents may be familiar with more detailed community assets at the neighborhood scale, while others may need recognizable landmarks and more regional context. Thus, identifying who will engage with the outputs of a community mapping exercise can inform decisions about geographic scale, data collection, and the tools best suited for the task.

Step 3: Determine the Appropriate Geography

Community mapping projects can use a variety of geographic units for mapping, ranging from individual parcels to census tracts to entire neighborhoods. Most initiatives will include several different geographies, from parcels or census tracts to cities and counties, which can allow for a range of data inputs and comparisons across space. The smaller the geography the more detailed the data, but also the more time potentially required for collection. One benefit of online mapping tools is that they are not limited by questions of scale; activists can input their data and display at various scales. Decisions about appropriate scale should be driven by research hypotheses, organizing goals, and models of social change. In some cases community mapping may require redefining geographic boundaries or mapping across traditional geographic units to achieve community-defined goals.

Step 4: Collect and Prepare the Data

Community mapping initiatives are only as strong as the data on which the maps are built. Maps that are most useful in a community context will likely consist of information from many sources while also reflecting community members' lived experiences. There are five major data types used in community mapping projects: public statistics, commercial data, administrative data, survey data, and crowd-sourced data.

PUBLIC STATISTICS. Census data are the primary source of public data for community mapping. They can be categorized into five major groups: demographics, socioeconomic characteristics, housing, business and the economy, and transportation. Data.census.gov is particularly useful for creating thematic maps across specific geographic areas and census characteristics.

ADMINISTRATIVE DATA. Administrative data collected by state and local government agencies (such as tax assessors, police departments, city agencies, zoning offices, and school districts) are key inputs for community mapping projects. These data are usually available for small geographic units (smaller than census tracts) and often for parcel-level mapping. Public health data collected by cities and states are increasingly including geographic information that allows for spatial analysis and mapping.

COMMERCIAL DATA. Data are available for sale from companies such as Data-Quick and Dun and Bradstreet and from real estate brokers, and others seeking current data about available properties often use them. This information is expensive, however, so only a few community mapping efforts use this resource.

SURVEY DATA. Many community mapping and GIS projects augment public and administrative data with information that community organizations collect themselves. Such original data collection is the basis of many asset-mapping programs in which community groups and residents map local assets and resources (http://www.abcdinstitute.org/). Data may be collected about assets such as social networks, health, recreation facilities, volunteer opportunities, trees and green spaces, murals, and community gathering sites. They can be gathered by volunteers, including youth, students, and residents. For original data collection to be most useful, data collectors must know why they are collecting the information and how it will be used (chapters 10, 11). Community-gathered information for mapping is increasingly done using widely available technology, such as cell phones and tablets.

CROWDSOURCED DATA. Original data can also be collected through online platforms, such as OpenStreetMap, that allow public contributors to add to an open repository of spatial data. In many cases, this crowdsourced information is then verified by community organizers or residents. This approach can be useful in situations in which physical access to spaces is limited or when data collection is urgent, such as in the case of a natural disaster.

In the cases where a community mapping exercise is generating new data, activists and organizers may consider who will have access to this information and how the newly created dataset could be used by the broader public. Where relevant, community mappers can take necessary steps to de-identify or protect these data as they relate to shared goals and values.

Step 5: Create Maps Using Freely Available Online Tools

As noted, mapping community data requires not only investments in hardware and software but also staff support. For many community groups, developing in-house technological capacity can be cost prohibitive. Therefore, some community organizations develop partnerships with technology or mapping intermediaries, such as universities, to maintain GIS technology.

Because community mapping projects are reliant on expensive technology, low-income and low-wealth communities may need to strengthen their technology infrastructure. Though community groups may not necessarily build and maintain GIS applications, they often require the technological capacity to engage with these systems. Building organizational and community capacity to use desktop or online GIS technology may also have secondary benefits, such as employment or educational opportunities.

Most mapping projects conducted by organizers can start by using existing, web-based tools that are free. We list a few here, but there are many others. The selection of a particular platform should be driven by activists' values and the objectives of the mapping project, not the technology. Some, but not all, of the existing web-based platforms allow for communities to input their own information and customize the maps. Activists should be attentive to how local knowledge and context can be prioritized in the selection of any "off-the-shelf" mapping platform.

- Centers for Disease Control and Prevention (CDC)—Chronic Disease GIS Exchange, https://www.cdc.gov/dhdsp/maps/GISX/index.html
- US Department of Agriculture (USDA)—Food Atlas, https://www.ers.usda.gov /data-products/food-environment-atlas.aspx
- New York City—Health Map, https://a816-healthpsi.nyc.gov/NYCHealthMap
- City of Richmond, California—Transparent Richmond, https://www.transparent richmond.org
- Community Commons—combines hundreds of datasets at multiple scales and includes maps already designed by others, https://www.communitycom mons.org
- Cares Engagement Network—a national data and reporting platform for communities, https://engagmentnetwork.org

- Healthy City—a California-specific online platform that allows activists to access data, create maps, and, working with others, offers the ability for users to "tell their own story" by uploading their own data or multimedia to the system, http://healthycity.org
- Wikimapia—http://wikimapia.org
- Open Street Map—https://www.openstreetmap.org/#map=14/-1.2943/36.8405
- Opportunity Atlas—https://www.opportunityatlas.org
- National Equity Atlas—https://nationalequityatlas.org/about-the-atlas#us

Step 6: Use Maps to Promote Community Building, Organizing, and Neighborhood Investment

The ultimate purpose of community mapping is to improve living conditions through the built environment and community infrastructure, programs, policy advocacy, and research. Effective community groups will use maps as a foundation for campaigns to promote community building and equitable development. In this step of the mapping process, community organizations transform data and spatial analysis into action. Web-based mapping applications offer easy, low-cost mapping opportunities for community organizations that are reluctant or unable to invest in more intensive technologies, such as GIS. As technology has advanced and become increasingly available to community organizations, "citizen science" mapping has become a regular part of campaigns to promote more healthy and equitable communities. Social media platforms, including Facebook, Twitter, and Instagram, allow activists to communicate with spatial information that can be viewed on mobile devices and can help communities quickly turn their data and maps into place-based advocacy tools. The "story" of a community map should be able to concisely answer what is happening in the community, how the map helps confirm what is already known or highlights new information, and what actions need to be taken and by whom.

Like other forms of technology, map making is just one tool and should not be seen as deterministic, and increasingly demands that community organizations be not just consumers, but builders and producers of the next generation of mapping technologies to ensure that they serve community, not just corporate interests.

REFERENCES

Corburn, J. (2005). *Street Science: Community Knowledge and Environmental Health Justice*. MIT Press.
U.S. Geological Survey. (2020). Geographic Information Systems. https://www.usgs.gov/faqs /what-a-geographic-information-system-gis?qt-news_science_products=0#qt-news _science_products.

APPENDIX 3

Action-Oriented Community Diagnosis Procedure

EUGENIA ENG
LYNN BLANCHARD

Editors' note: Eugenia Eng and Lynn Blanchard developed the tool in this appendix over several years, using the term "Action-Oriented Community Diagnosis," which was originally developed by health education leader and scholar Guy Stewart. The tool's emphasis on assessing and contributing to community competence rather than merely identifying needs well illustrates chapters 10 and 11's perspectives on community assessment. Additionally, the broad range of assessment techniques incorporated in this procedure underscores the utility of triangulation (the use of multiple methods) to provide the richest possible database for analysis.

Reprinted from Eng, E., & Blanchard, L. (1990). Action-oriented community diagnosis: A health education tool. *Int Q Community Health Educ, 11*(2), 93–110. Copyright 1991 by the Baywood Publishing Company, Inc., Amityville, N.Y. All rights reserved.

I. Specify the target population and determine its component parts using social and demographic characteristics that may identify commonalities among groups of people.
   A. Race and/or ethnicity
   B. Religion
   C. Income level
   D. Occupation
   E. Age
II. Review secondary data sources, and identify possible subpopulations of interest and geographic locations.
   A. County and townships
   B. Faith-based organizations, schools, and fire districts
   C. Towns
   D. Agency service delivery areas
   E. Industries and other major employers
   F. Transportation arteries and services
   G. Health and other vital statistics

III. Conduct windshield tours of targeted areas, and note daily living conditions, resources, and evidence of problems.
   A. Housing types and conditions
   B. Recreational and commercial facilities
   C. Private and public sector services
   D. Social and civic activities
   E. Identifiable neighborhoods or residential clusters
   F. Condition of roads and distances people must travel
   G. Maintenance of buildings, grounds, and yards
IV. Contact and interview local agency providers serving targeted areas.
   A. What are the communities most in need, and why?
   B. Which communities have histories of meeting their own needs, and how?
   C. What services are being provided by agencies or other organized groups? Which are utilized and which are underutilized?
   D. What, in their opinion, are the major problems still facing communities they serve?
   E. Where do they recommend finding additional information to document needs?
      1. Referrals to other service providers
      2. Referrals to leaders of community organizations
      3. Referrals to informed members of communities
 V. Select a community and contact and interview community informants most frequently cited in provider interviews.
   A. What is the name their community is most commonly known as?
   B. Describe a time when there was a problem in their community that they tried to resolve.
      1. How was the need determined?
      2. How did the community members organize themselves?
      3. Who were the influential people involved?
   C. In their opinion, what are the present needs in their community?
   D. Who would have to be involved to get things done in the community?
   E. What outside services or resources do people in their community know and use to meet their needs?
   F. What other people like themselves who know about their community do they recommend being contacted?
   G. Would they be interested in attending a meeting to find out the results from these interviews? And what do they suggest as times and places to hold such a meeting?
VI. Tabulate the results from the secondary data, provider and community informant interviews, and analyze the degree of convergence among the needs identified.
   A. Determine the extent of agreement/disagreement across the three lists of needs on how each identified need is defined.

    B. Determine the extent of agreement/disagreement across the three lists of need on priority accorded to each identified need.

VII. Present the findings in meetings with community informants interviewed and other influential community members frequently cited by the providers and community informants.

    A. Assess the validity of definitions for each need and redefine them, if necessary, according to how they are manifested in this community.

    B. Determine a priority list of needs according to interest in undertaking a solution.

    C. Select a high-priority need and determine questions that need to be answered such as:

        1. Who suffers from this problem?

        2. When is this problem most prevalent?

        3. How severe are the short- and long-term consequences from this problem?

        4. What are the possible causes of this problem?

        5. What is the range of solutions for reducing or controlling this problem?

        6. What are the available resources and additional resources required for each possible solution?

VIII. Plan the next steps for finding answers to the questions.

APPENDIX 4

Sample Community Health Indicators for Use in Health Impact Assessment

Human Impact Partners

Health Determinants	Connections between Determinants and Health Outcomes	Measurable Indicators
Livelihood		*Rate of unemployment*
▪ Security of employment	▪ Unemployment is a source of chronic stress and low self-esteem and is associated with health adverse behaviors and premature death	▪ % of jobs in the city that provide self-sufficiency income
▪ Adequacy of wages, benefits, and leave		▪ % of jobs that have guaranteed paid sick leave
▪ Job hazards	▪ Income is strongly associated with life expectancy	▪ % of jobs that have health insurance coverage
▪ Job autonomy		
▪ Economic diversity	▪ Sick leave supports timely use of health care	
	▪ Rates of unemployment and poverty are proportional to crime rates	
	▪ Job autonomy predicts reduced mortality from cardiovascular disease	
Housing		
▪ Crowding	▪ Crowded conditions increase risks for infections, respiratory disease, mental health, and fire	▪ % of housing units affordable to household with median income
▪ Affordability		
▪ Design safety		

(continued)

Appendix 4. (continued)

Health Determinants	Connections between Determinants and Health Outcomes	Measurable Indicators
• Location safety • Stable tenure	• Unaffordable rents or mortgages result in trade-offs between housing, food, and medical care; unafford-ability increases stress	• % of households paying more than 30% of income on rent or mortgage payment • % of population homeless in the past year • % of households evicted in past year

Access to Educational Resources

• Quality, proxim-ity, and capacity of schools and childcare • Adult education and training opportunities	• Children commuting long distances to school have less sleep, less exercise, and greater exposure to vehicle pollution • Local community schools can promote parent participation and good educational outcomes • Quality childcare increases childhood educational and job outcomes	• % of residential units within ¼ and ½ mile of public elementary and middle school • % of residential units within ¼ and ½ mile of childcare centers

Transportation

• Access to jobs, goods, services, and educational resources • Active travel • Public transit options • Transport Safety	• Public transit provides access to employment, education, parks, and health care services • Sidewalks and bicycle lanes facilitate physical activity, reducing heart disease, diabetes, obesity, blood pressure, and osteoporosis, symptoms of depression, anxiety, & falls in the elderly • Vehicle speeds are directly proportional to injury severity	• Rate of pedestrian and bicycle injuries per capita per year • % of street miles with dedicated bike paths or lanes, by class • % of population within ½ mile of regional transit and ¼ mile of local public transit stop, by neighborhood

(continued)

Appendix 4. (continued)

Health Determinants	Connections between Determinants and Health Outcomes	Measurable Indicators

Access to Quality Retail Goods and Public Services

• Quality and proximity of financial institutions • Quality and proximity of food resources • Quality and proximity of health services	• Adequate nutrition prevents infectious diseases • Consumption of fruits and vegetables linked to reduced cancer risk • Local financial institutions help families create and maintain wealth • Timely access to primary health services prevents serious hospitalizations • Close proximity to retail goods and services encourages active modes of transport and physical activity	• % of population within ½ mile of a full-service grocery store or fresh produce market • % of population within 30-minute transit or walking commute of a primary care public health facilities • % of population living ½ mile from commercial district with 75% of common public services (post office, public school, public childcare, community park or playground, community garden, library, recreation center, civic spaces, churches, public art, and transit stops) • % of population living ½ mile from a commercial district with 75% of common private services (bank, produce market, convenience store, supermarket, hardware store, cleaner, auto repair, restaurant, farmer's market, café, and private childcare)

(continued)

Appendix 4. (continued)

Health Determinants	Connections between Determinants and Health Outcomes	Measurable Indicators

Access to Parks and Natural Space

- Quality, proximity, capacity, and programming of parks and open spaces

- Regular physical activity reduces risk of developing heart disease, diabetes, osteoporosis, and obesity; reduces blood pressure; relieves symptoms of depression and anxiety; and prevents falls in the elderly

- Access to places for physical activity increases the frequency of physical activity in children and adults

- People who live in greener environments have better physical and mental health

- Trees and green space remove air pollution from the air and mitigate heat island effects

- % of population within ¼ mile of neighborhood or regional park, open space, or publicly accessible shoreline

- % of creeks and shoreline with public access

- % of population within ¼ mile of community recreational facility

- Acres per capita of neighborhood parks

- % of schools meeting state standards for adequate play areas

Environmental Quality

- Pollutants in outdoor and indoor air

- Contaminants in drinking water and recreational water

- Environmental or occupational noise

- Vehicle emissions exacerbate respiratory disease and increase cardiopulmonary mortality

- Indoor aero-allergens cause or exacerbate asthma

- Contaminated water can spread serious infectious disease

- Chronic noise exposure harms sleep, temperament, hearing, and blood pressure

- % of population living within 500 feet of busy roadways

- % of population living a safe distance from industries emitting hazardous pollutants

- % of creeks, watersheds, and shoreline restored or cleaned

- % of population living with outdoors noise level of more than 65 decibels

- % of land area with unutilized industrial or contaminated land

(continued)

Appendix 4. (continued)

Health Determinants	Connections between Determinants and Health Outcomes	Measurable Indicators

Social Cohesion

- Supportive relationships with friends, families, and neighbors
- Participation in social organizations
- Degree and quality of participation in public decisionmaking
- Responsiveness of public agencies to people's needs

- Physical and emotional support buffers stressful situations, supports illness recovery, prevents isolation, contributes to self-esteem, and reduces the risk of early death
- Social contact across ethnic and class groups ensures equitable access to public health and educational services
- Supporting the effective participation of marginalized groups in governance helps ensure achievement of basic human needs (e.g., food, shelter, health services)
- Control of one's life is a major factor in quality of health

- % of voting age population participating in general elections
- % of community involved in community organizations
- % of community professing "trust" of neighbors
- Level of involvement in planning for a development project

Social Exclusion

- Proportion of the population living in relative poverty
- Attitudes toward or stereotypes of minority racial, social, and ethnic groups
- Segregation of residences by race, ethnicity, religion, or class
- Degree of inequalities in income or wealth

- Economic exclusion in segregated neighborhoods limits wealth, which is a buffer against illness and stress
- Residents of low-income and ethnically segregated neighborhoods experience, high rates of teenage childbearing, tuberculosis, cardiovascular disease, and homicide

- Residential segregation by ethnicity
- Residential segregation by household income
- Equality of income distribution
- Diversity of residential uses

(continued)

Appendix 4. (continued)

Health Determinants	Connections between Determinants and Health Outcomes	Measurable Indicators
Community Violence		
• Violent crime • Property crime	• Direct effects of crime include injury and death • Indirect effects of crime include fear, stress, and poor mental health • Fear of violence inhibits walking	• Assault rate per capita • Rates of robbery and burglaries
Environmental Stewardship		
• Protection of water, land, and air resources	• Reducing electricity and natural gas usage results in reduction in climate change and air pollution emissions • Green business practices may reduce occupational and environmental exposures • Exposure and access to natural areas meets an essential human need improving health, well-being, community image, and identity	• Per capita energy use • Per capita water use • Per capita waste generation • % waste diverted from landfill • % of land preserved as natural area • % of facilities that meet green building standards (public and private) • % of businesses meeting or exceeding the county's green business standards

This appendix is extracted from the following source: Human Impact Partners. (2011, February). *A Health Impact Assessment Toolkit: A Handbook to Conducting HIA* (3rd ed.). Oakland, CA: Human Impact Partners.

APPENDIX 5

Skywatchers' Values-Based Methodology and Guidance for Practice

ANNE BLUETHENTHAL
DIERDRE VISSER
NANCY EPSTEIN
CLARA PINSKY

As described in chapter 17, this methodology and guidance was developed interdependently with, and as a core part of, Skywatchers, the principal program of ABD Productions. Skywatchers has been creating multidisciplinary performance work in San Francisco's culturally vibrant but economically challenged Tenderloin neighborhood for more than ten years.

An enduring collaboration between professional artists and residents of the neighborhood's supportive housing, Skywatchers' emergent work is fueled by conversation and relationship building. The values outlined below serve as the guiding principles of a methodology focused on collective creative process over artistic product. Skywatchers' process is their product; their facilitation is about starting a conversation, remaining genuinely engaged in the dialogue, and seeing it through into art.

While this methodology grew out of Skywatchers' community-based art, this practice guidance is useful for anyone considering values-based community-driven work, such as community organizing and community engagement. One cannot overstate the importance outlined in chapter 17 of cultivating curiosity and nourishing trust. By showing up consistently over time and building caring relationships from which flow meaningful, emergent conversations and community-based problem solving, we promote collaboration, raise up personal narratives and the creativity of community members, and situate those within a social change–oriented justice and equity context.

Methodology Value	Practice Guidance
Relational	
We believe	Show up consistently, on time, when you say you will, with an attitude of curiosity and care.
• in "the power of proximity" (Stevenson, 2015).	
• that larger-scale community and structural change begins with bonds formed by intimate, interpersonal exchange.	Show up in the community (even when you don't need anything) being present for important events, gatherings, meetings, etc.
	Spend unstructured time with community members.
Durational	
"Move at the speed of trust" (Brown, 2017).	Be present over an extended period of time.
Show up regularly and consistently over time to demonstrate you are reliable and trustworthy.	Repeat or iterate on activities.
	Plan and allocate resources for unstructured time (times when it seems like "nothing is happening" can be when it's all happening).
Duration allows for building relationships, emergent conversation, and influencing structures.	
	Cultivate critical self-reflection about your presence in the community and build community capacity.
Conversational	
Process-driven conversations allow for strengths, needs, priorities, ideas, and problem solving to emerge directly from community members, who understand that what they say is heard, valued, and considered important.	Begin with dialogue.
	Stay curious and listen, observe, reflect.
	Be patient; wait for the gems to arise.
	Be prepared to let go of preconceived priorities or ideas.
	Listen for the expertise of community members.
Note also that art emerges; that is, words, movement, rhythm, and music can emerge from conversations.	Reflect back to each other what has been heard, seen, and felt; let this lead to art or other creative forms.
Structural	
Grounded in the above, the structural value emphasizes the importance of getting from arts-based organizing to equity-focused systems or policy change:	Situate personal narratives and art-making in a structural justice and equity context.
• working to address socioeconomic inequities and structural racism	Center the expertise of community members with lived experience in the expression of those experiences.
	Cultivate leadership from within the community through an arts-based process.

(continued)

Appendix 5. (continued)

Methodology Value	Practice Guidance
• confronting difficult political issues in humanizing form	Develop relationships broadly in the community.
• building community leadership and power	Consider the integration of creative expression to change hearts, as well as minds.

Source: Bluethenthal, A., Visser, D., Pinsky, C., Epstein, N., & Minkler, M. (2021). Leveraging arts for justice, equity and public health: The Skywatchers program and its implications for community-based health promotion practice and research. *Health Promot Pract, 22*(1_suppl), 91S–100S.

REFERENCES

Brown, A. M. (2017). *Emergent strategy*. AK Press.
Stevenson, B. (2015). *Just Mercy: A Story of Justice and Redemption*. Spiegel & Grau.

APPENDIX 6

Ladder of Community Participation in Public Health

JENNIFER LIFSHAY

MARY ANNE MORGAN

A range of approaches can be used to engage diverse communities around traditional and emerging public health issues. A conceptual framework to help public health leaders plan and evaluate community engagement efforts can be used to stimulate internal dialogue and frame discussions with community partners about how to work effectively to accomplish shared public health goals. Contra Costa Health Services developed a Ladder of Community Participation based on more than ten years of experience with engaging the local community in a range of public health issues. It builds on earlier work in the field (Arnstein, 1969; Chess et al., 1995).

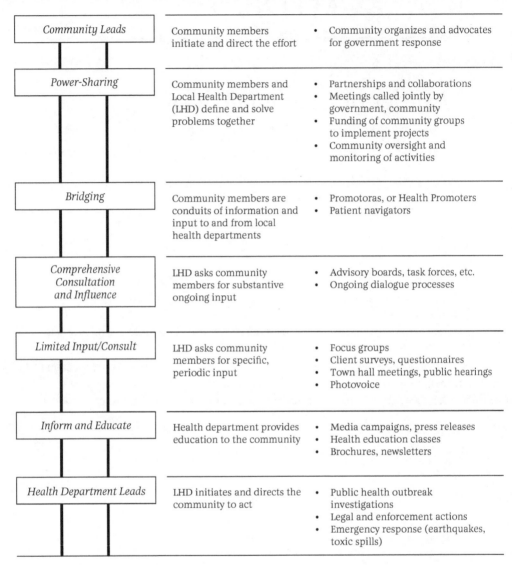

FIGURE A6.1 Ladder of Community Participation in Public Health. Created by Mary Anne Morgan and Jennifer Lifshay.

REFERENCES

Arnstein, S. R. (1969). A ladder of citizen participation. *J Am Inst Plann, 35*(4), 216–224. *Note:* In light of its continued importance, this article was reprinted in the *Journal* in 2019: *85*(1), 24–34.

Chess, C., Hance, B. J., and Sandman, P. M. (1995). *Improving Dialogue with Communities: A Short Guide for Government Risk Communication.* New Jersey Department of Environmental Protection, Division of Science & Research.

Member Assessment of Coalition Process and Outcomes

TOM WOLFF

For each item, please circle the number that best shows your agreement with the statement about that aspect of the coalition.

Vision: Planning, Implementation, Progress

1 = Strongly agree   5 = Strongly disagree

1. The coalition has a clear vision and mission.	1 2 3 4 5
2. There is consistent follow-through on coalition activities.	1 2 3 4 5
3. The coalition has developed targeted action planning for community and systems change.	1 2 3 4 5
4. The coalition effectively reconciles differences among members.	1 2 3 4 5
5. The coalition engages in collaborative problem solving of jointly shared problems, resulting in innovative solutions.	1 2 3 4 5
6. The coalition expands available resources by having partners bring resources to the table or identify others with resources.	1 2 3 4 5

Leadership and Membership

1 = Strongly agree   5 = Strongly disagree

7. The coalition develops and supports leadership.	1 2 3 4 5
8. There are opportunities for coalition members to take leadership roles, and members are willing to take them.	1 2 3 4 5
9. Leadership responsibilities are shared in the coalition.	1 2 3 4 5
10. The coalition has broad and appropriate membership for the issue it is addressing.	1 2 3 4 5
11. The coalition membership is diverse.	1 2 3 4 5
12. Members display commitment and they take on tasks.	1 2 3 4 5

Structure

1 = Strongly agree   5 = Strongly disagree

13. The coalition has regular meeting cycles that members can expect.	1 2 3 4 5
14. The coalition has active workgroups and committees.	1 2 3 4 5
15. Members get agendas for the meetings prior to the meeting and minutes afterward.	1 2 3 4 5
16. The work of the meeting, as outlined in the agenda, gets accomplished.	1 2 3 4 5
17. The coalition has a viable organization structure that functions competently.	1 2 3 4 5

Communication

1 = Strongly agree   5 = Strongly disagree

18. Communication among members of the coalition is effective.	1 2 3 4 5
19. Communication between the coalition and the broader community related to its chosen issues is effective.	1 2 3 4 5
20. Coalition members are listened to and heard.	1 2 3 4 5

Activities

1 = Strongly agree   5 = Strongly disagree

21. Information gets exchanged at coalition meetings.	1 2 3 4 5
22. The coalition advocates for change.	1 2 3 4 5
23. Outcomes are more comprehensive than those achieved without a coalition.	1 2 3 4 5

Outcomes

Open-Ended Question

24. What changes occurred because of the coalition that otherwise would not have occurred?

1 = Strongly agree   5 = Strongly disagree

25. The coalition has been able to achieve its goals and create concrete outcomes.	1 2 3 4 5
26. The coalition is serving as a catalyst for positive change related to the issues it has chosen to work on.	1 2 3 4 5
27. The coalition creates community changes as seen in changes in programs, policies, and practices that enhance people's lives.	1 2 3 4 5
28. The coalition has effected changes in programs, policies, and practices in many sectors and systems in the community related to the issues it has chosen to work on.	1 2 3 4 5

Definitions

Programs can be new or modified interventions, new protocols, and new products, such as educational materials, marketing or branding materials, and new presentations.

Policies can include facility or agency policies, state policies, federal policies, or institutional or agency policies.

For practice changes, consider changes at facilities as well as other institutions and organizations; changes by various practitioners (including physicians, nursing or social work staff members, and facility administrators); changes by government; or changes by individuals affected by the issue.

Open-Ended Question

29. What specific changes in programs, policies, and practices have you seen that were created by the work of this coalition?

Relationships

1 = Strongly agree   5 = Strongly disagree

30. Old or existing partnerships have been enhanced as a result of the coalition.	1 2 3 4 5
31. New relationships have been built with new partners as a result of the coalition.	1 2 3 4 5

Systems Outcomes

1 = Strongly agree   5 = Strongly disagree

32. As a result of the coalition's formation, systems changes have happened.	1 2 3 4 5
33. As a result of the coalition, partners are more collaborative and more cooperative.	1 2 3 4 5
34. The coalition helped the people in the community gain access to more resources both within and outside the coalition in order to reach their goals.	1 2 3 4 5

Benefits from Participation

1 = Strongly agree   5 = Strongly disagree

35. The community and its residents are better off today because of this coalition.	1 2 3 4 5

36. I have benefited from participation in the coalition through
    a. Building relationships with other coalition members
    b. Exchanging information with others—networking
    c. Working with others on issues of importance
    d. Being part of a process that brings about meaningful change

37. My agency has benefited from its participation in the coalition through
    a. Modified programs
    b. Developing new programs
    c. Gaining access to new or more resources
    d. Creating solutions collaboratively with other coalition partners

Collaborating for Equity and Justice

1 = Strongly agree   5 = Strongly disagree

38. The coalition explicitly addresses issues of social and economic injustice and structural racism.	1 2 3 4 5
39. The coalition employs a community development approach in which residents have equal power in determining the coalition's agenda and resource allocation.	1 2 3 4 5
40. The coalition employs community organizing as an intentional strategy and as part of the process and works to build resident leadership and power.	1 2 3 4 5
41. The coalition focuses on policy, systems, and structural change.	1 2 3 4 5

Overall Rating

Open-Ended Questions

42. What changes happened in your own organization as a result of the coalition that would not otherwise have occurred?

43. What happened that surprised you that you did not plan for as an outcome?

44. As a result of the coalition work, what are the three most significant things you have learned?

APPENDIX 8

Issue-Development Worksheet

RINKU SEN

List your criteria for a good issue in order of priority with the most important at the top. Describe how well each issue meets each criterion by giving it a rating from 1 to 5 (with 5 the highest). After comparing the total rankings for the issues, consider the rankings going down the chart. Are the rankings high on your priority criteria? If not, you may not want to pick an issue even though its total ranking is high.

Example Criteria	Example Issue: Living Wage	Your Criteria	Issue 1:	Issue 2:
1. Gives a sense of power, changes conditions, and shifts power relations	Wage hike, right to organize and new constituency of low-wage workers, 5			
2. Worthwhile	Deeply felt, 5, but not widely felt, 1 (small impact)			
	Average: 3			
3. Nondivisive	Small business owners in our cross-class organization don't like it, but everyone else does, 4			
4. Clear demands	Model already written but lots of detail to fight for, 4			
5. Clear target, challenges corporations	City council members, 5			
Average 3.5	All public-sector targets, 2			

(continued)

Appendix 8. (continued)

Example Criteria	Example Issue: Living Wage	Your Criteria	Issue 1:	Issue 2:
6. Easy to understand	Basic idea, yes; complicated clauses, no, 3			
7. Winnable	Not in current city council, 2			
8. Attracts allies	Unions, 5			
9. Reveals race, gender, and economic inequity	Subsidy handle, 5			
10. Clear time frame	Before city council runs again, six months; clear but short time, 3			
11. Leads to other issues	Health care, childcare, affordable housing, environmental protection, 5			
12. Creates new handles	Makes it easier to organize workers, 5			
13. Surfaces discrimination, good data	Requires research to compare, data not easily available, 2			
14. Uses race- and gender-discrimination handles	No, 1			
15. Introduces new or stronger language	Living wage is better wage, but doesn't meet the Self-Sufficiency Standard, 2			
16. Variety of tactics	Research, press, direct action, 4			
Total rankings	56.5			
Criteria placement considerations	Most important criteria are 1–10. Rankings there are between 3 and 5 (except for 7); rankings for 13–16 are generally lower. Do it.			

Source: Sen, R. (2003). *Stir It Up.* Jossey-Bass. Reprinted with permission of the publisher and author.

APPENDIX 9

Choosing Tactics and Framing the Action

Key Questions and Considerations for Getting It Right

MARK S. HOMAN

Selecting the right tactics is critical in helping get to a win on the issue(s) your group is fighting for. The following criteria for tactics selection have stood the test of time and are recommended for consideration in this important part of your group's strategic planning.

Five Criteria for Selection of Tactics

1. It is likely to produce the desired response from the selected target—that is, it will probably work.
2. You and your partners feel confident that you are sufficiently capable of pulling it off—that is, you really think you can do it, know how to, and will.
3. You have sufficient resources—that is, you have enough of what you need to make it work.
4. It builds the organization—that is, it provides leadership opportunities, skill-building opportunities, cohesion, confidence, and so forth, and it attracts attention and new members.
5. It is consistent with your ethics.

Like the care needed in selecting the right tactics, similar thoughtful attention is needed in thinking strategically about the action(s) your group is considering. The following checklist will become so routine that these questions will frame your perspective of any setting for action. Your need to answer these questions will guide everything you do, and your ability to answer them will powerfully increase the likelihood of your success.

A Checklist for Action

- From whom do we want to get a response?
- What responses do we want to get?
- What action or series of actions has the best chance of producing that response?
- Are the members of our organization able and willing to take these actions?
- How do the actions we decide to take lead to the needed development of our organization?
- How do our actions produce immediate gains in a way that helps us achieve our long-term goals?
- Is everything we are doing relevant to the outcomes we want to produce?
- How will we assess the effectiveness of our chosen approach to help refine the next steps we should take?

For a more detailed discussion of these issues, see Homan, M. S. (2016). *Promoting Community Change: Making It Happen in the Real World* (6th ed.). Cengage Learning.

APPENDIX 10

Engaging Coalition and Community Organization Members in a "River of Life" Exercise to Create a Historical Timeline

MAGDALENA AVILA

SHANNON SANCHEZ-YOUNGMAN

REVA HINES

LESLIE GROVER

NINA WALLERSTEIN

In many communities, organizing is a way of life, a way of thinking, and a critical form of consciousness that emanates from being stewards for our communities. Organizing is for many a legacy-based oral history skill set known intuitively through inheritance by seeing, by doing, and by listening. It is founded on the organic intellectualism of rural and urban communities that builds on each succeeding generation. Its many ways of knowing and understanding come from the unique lens of those born within these communities.

Organizing means learning about all the different nuances that bring our communities together. It is about creating a dialogue for collective consciousness and action to understand how each community and its people are unique. It is about building a strength and resilience that comes from antiquity, the history of our ancestors, the present forces, and then the future visionary ability of what can be accomplished by organizing. For many communities of color, organizing is both an intellectual and a spiritual action. The meaning of the action itself is grounded in so many dimensions of thought that it is like a continued seedling of intellectual and spiritual thought emanating from the social, cultural, political, and historical legacy of the people that can advance and protect safe spaces.

Community organizing is also an educational and learned skill set that builds on what many communities intuitively know. Organizing means learning about all the different ways and nuances that bring communities together. There are many different levels of attaining this skill set, and those who master it can sense, feel, and navigate through the endless forces of meaning in their environments.

Organizing is rooted in present-day action to create a realm of possibilities for change that require a deft sense of perspective to understand when one has truly mastered this skill set. From formal academic education, we learn about models of organizing, from Alinsky, Freire, and Gandhi's nonviolence, with Martin Luther King and Cesar Chavez representing a generation of social change from the civil rights movement. Today, current social movements are confronting the roots of systemic change and injustice that stem from a history of social contracts that benefit those in power, mainly White society, which has not had to think beyond its consciousness of benevolence. Initially perceived as fostering a just and equal society, this idea of benevolence has shown its deception, and through its inaction has ushered in a new generation of oppositional consciousness that has always been present but now has broken through like a mega volcano. Western society's foundational social contract anchoring has moved us forward to a breaking point of national rage and patience lost.

As part of organizing approaches, community-based participatory research (CBPR) is as much community based as academically based. It is a bidirectional mode of thinking, which is an equalizer for all research partners regardless of rootedness and orientation. CBPR uses as part of its primary base of engagement a "research tool" known as the River of Life. From a community-based perspective, the River of Life is a metaphor story tool, a story that can only start when the community engages with its different partners. Working with a metaphor and story is a natural form of thinking for many frontline communities. It is a way of "starting from the people," their values, principles, and community history.

The CBPR River of Life metaphor tool brings to the table everyone involved in working with their communities (Sanchez-Youngman & Wallerstein, 2018). It is a lens that helps to magnify collective community scholarship to create change, using thought, action, and engagement. For organizers who serve as social change agents within our communities, the River of Life story metaphor tool brings a people's story to the forefront of the political action, research, and processes for social change. It highlights the many as part of the individual and the one as part of the many. It is as collective as it is singular, honoring history and legacy and highlighting who communities are as a people and the issues that are important to them. It brings real-time relevance to communities' way of thinking, and is rooted in how one's individual lens is immersed and unfolds, shaped by community culture and lived experience.

The beauty of the River of Life is that it has so many different points of entry for the person(s) telling their story, providing a personal entry point so that each person is comfortable and feels safe. It uses water, which is sacred to all life and provides a universal understanding to how we become who we are, shaped by the forces and flow of a river. A major component of the River of Life is the listening skill set. You must listen to the stories in order to pull together the collective oral history that makes up the uniqueness of each community. From the actual stories, you learn the language, the meaning, the context, and the legacy of a people. You put the story maps together, and you bring together the collective consciousness of a community, which is a fundamental principle of community organizing, to start where the people are.

Community-based participatory research has brought forth the River of Life as a key teaching tool and skill-based skill set that utilizes people's stories as organic seedlings for any project to promote community empowerment and health. The River of Life is like taking a brush and painting a picture of the community. It is not just an exercise, but is powerful in its emotional affect and the passion that it brings forth. It is an exercise of voice, of personal and community narrative. As a sacred metaphor, the River of Life grounds people in the water running through their communities that serves to connect us, rather than disconnect us. In many southwestern communities, the River of Life can be the acequias that bring much needed water to our communities so we can grow and thrive; it brings the sustenance of life.

River of Life waters that are vibrant as well as quiet can make change through action that is forthright or also subtle, so that only the native community can see and feel the underground forces that carry and sustain what is important. The River of Life is a crucial lens through which one can understand our own communities more profoundly, as well as a tool that introduces us to different ways of thinking and shapes us to identify the issues that are most important to our lives and our communities.

As an example, Engage for Equity, a CBPR research project located at the University of New Mexico with national partners, has used the River of Life tool in workshops to ground partnerships in their own contexts and beginnings of how they started working together (Parker et al., 2020; Wallerstein et al., 2020). Notably, many CBPR partnerships don't start their Rivers with their funding or their first meeting, but use the opportunity to go back decades or even centuries to the core histories that define their work. From Baton Rouge, Louisiana, a team called "Tale of Two Cities" (from the Robert Wood Johnson Foundation Interdisciplinary Research Leadership Cohort of 2016–2019) started their drawing from the long history of racism in Baton Rouge, going back to the genocide of Native people in 1669 and African American slavery, starting up again with racist housing policy from the 1920s, through civil rights organizing, to how racism continues to impact the lives of its residents (see figure A10.1). They described the genesis of their project in a desire to confront the twelve-year difference in life expectancy between residents of North and South Baton Rouge. Employing qualitative methods, they sought to examine neighborhood and housing conditions and affordability and their impact on health. Looking at housing as a social construct, they used CBPR data to initiate organizing around issues of housing and community resiliency with goals to advocate for community-based policy recommendations around housing and public health. As they created their River of Life with its disturbing history, they also inserted community strengths and values, mobilizing the advocacy they wanted to bring to the state capitol. As they shared their River with other teams, they declared, "in the soul of the river, beautiful things grow in spite of the pollution."

The steps to create a River of Life are listed here. This exercise can take from one and a half to three hours, depending on the depth of sharing and use of the stories for setting the stage for future actions.

Step 1: Each member of the partnership, coalition, or organizing group reflects independently about their community of interest, their advocacy work, and their collective partnership using the metaphor of a river. The goal is to reflect on your origins and journey together as a coalition or partnership. You may ask questions, such as, how and why did you join the partnership or organizing? What is important to know about your community's history and stories? What is important to know about previous advocacy efforts? How and why did you start collectively working together? What have been important events and changes you have seen?

Step 2: Lay out a long sheet of paper (or two flip charts taped together) and other art supplies (markers, crayons, construction paper, glue) so that together you can draw your partnership River of Life. You may also use construction paper to create images, such as hearts to show positive moments or good river flow and boulders or rocks to illustrate obstacles.

Step 3: Draw the River of Life for your partnership or organizing group. Using visual symbols, describe the beginnings, the influences, the obstacles, and the peaceful moments of your work together. Imagine these as key aspects of your advocacy or coalitional work and your collective commitment to community, social, health, and policy change. Begin where you think it is important to start, which may be before your partnership or your specific organizing group started working together, paying close attention to the historical conditions that led to the formation of your coalition.

If it helps, write these instructions on a flipchart:

- Start where you think it is important to start, such as before the partnership or organizing began, historical moments that shaped your coming together, when you received funding, etc.
- Fill in life moments of your partnership and organizing, and key influences that were important motivations for continued involvement in community/advocacy work.
- Draw important or influential stages.
- Draw key tributaries coming in, such as core leaders or activists joining.
- What were factors that facilitated the work?
- What were obstacles that were challenging?
- Where are you headed?

Step 4: Make a historical timeline with dates and months, years (or decades) below the River of Life. Relate important historical and current events within the community, region, state, or nation that might influence what is currently happening in your coalition. How do these conditions influence your collective efforts?

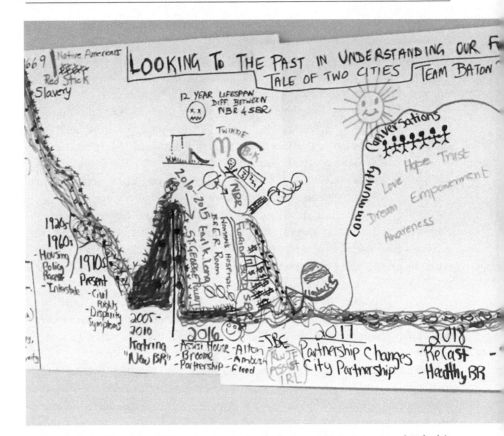

FIGURE A10.1 Tale of Two Cities, created by Reva Hines, Leslie T. Grover, and Valachie Miles, 2019. As explained by the creators of the River of Life shared in this appendix, the state capitol was intentionally drawn on its side, in part to capture that "it is a side step to the policies that affect our communities" and because "often, legislators sidestep work that benefits communities."

Step 5: Stand back and admire your River of Life, and answer the following questions:

- What stood out for you while doing this collective process? (Any general thoughts about what you learned or feelings this exercise raised are helpful).
- What were/are some of the facilitators you identified that were important for your partnership or organizing group?
- What were/are some of the challenges or obstacles you have faced in terms of moving forward in a good way with your partners and fellow organizers?
- Were there important external events that made a difference?
- When do you think you could use the River of Life tool in your own work?

Step 6. If there are multiple teams, partnerships, or organizing groups (or individuals) creating Rivers at the same time, you will need enough time for the

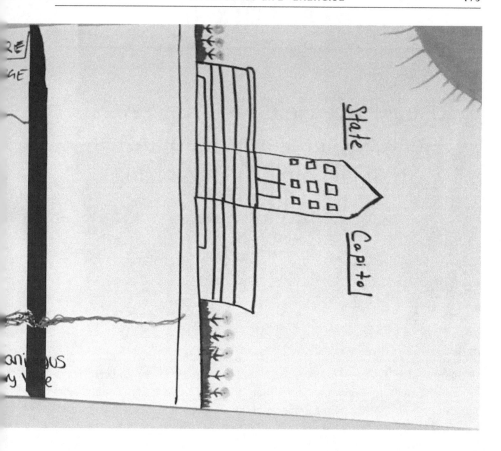

sharing of journeys and discussion of similarities and differences within different contexts and experiences.

REFERENCES

Parker, M., Wallerstein, N., Duran, B., Magarati, M., Burgess, E., Boursaw, B., & Koegel, P. (2020). Engage for equity: Development of community-based participatory research tools. *Health Educ Behav, 47*(3), 359–372.

Sanchez-Youngman, S., & Wallerstein, N. (2018). Partnership River of Life: Creating an historical timeline. In N. Wallerstein, B. Duran, J. Oetzel, & M. Minkler (Eds.), *Community-Based Participatory Research for Health: Advancing Social and Health Equity* (3rd ed., pp. 375–378). Jossey-Bass.

Wallerstein, N., Oetzel, J., Sanchez-Youngman, S., Boursaw, B., Dickson, E., Kastelic, S., Koegel, P., Lucero, J., Magarati, M., Ortiz, K., Parker, M., Peña, J., Richmond, A., & Duran, B. (2020). Engage for equity: A long-term study of community-based participatory research and community engaged research practices and outcomes. *Health Educ Behav, 47*(3), 380–390.

APPENDIX 11

Using Force Field Analysis, SWOT Analysis, and Power Mapping as Strategic Tools in Organizing

MEREDITH MINKLER
ANGELA NI
CHRIS M. COOMBE
JENNIFER FALBE

More than seventy years ago, the German social psychologist Kurt Lewin (1947) developed what he termed "force field analysis" as a tool for understanding dynamic social situations and promoting change (Dubey, 2017). Twenty years later, in the mid-1960s, Albert Humphrey at the Stanford Research Institute developed a related tool, "SWOT analysis," to help professionals in business and other fields examine the strengths, weaknesses, opportunities, and threats that exist relative to their organizations or agencies as a technique for strategic planning (Chermack & Kasshanna, 2007; Gürel & Tat, 2017). Although neither of these tools was designed with fields like public health, social work, or city and regional planning in mind, let alone for community organizers, both have been used effectively in each of these areas and are briefly summarized and illustrated below. In contrast, a third tool, power mapping, has, from the start, been more directly concerned with helping community organizers and others concerned with changing the balance of power around a legislative measure or other change initiative. By identifying "targets" with the power to make change and other players and their stance on a proposed change, as well as their relative power to influence targets, a map is created, which has proven effective in subsequent strategic planning and action for change (Ritas et al., 2008).

This appendix provides an introduction to these methods, with steps and graphics for using them in the context of community organizing and professional practice in fields whose goals increasingly focus on higher-level changes in the organization and policy environments to improve health equity and social justice.

Force Field Analysis

In a classic work, Lewin (1947) argued that social situations exist in a state of "quasi-stationary social equilibria" caused by driving and resisting forces that work in opposition to one another. When the forces are weighted most heavily on the driving side, change is likely to take place. When the resisting or restraining forces are most powerful, however, no change is likely. Strengthening existing driving forces, or adding new ones, helps increase the likelihood of change, as does removing or weakening resisting forces. Of the two, however, the latter is most likely to enable change to occur that is of a more sustained or lasting nature. As Dubey (2017) points out, with its implicit grounding in systems thinking, force field analysis "helps with this complex task of reading the situation in its totality" and understanding what may be needed to change it (p. 700). It can further help health and social change professionals, and community organizers and other grassroots groups, decide when and how to take an action, and when not to act.

Lewin's easy-to-use approach has proved effective in working with adolescents, community advisory boards, grassroots organizations, and health and social service departments to address a wide range of interests and concerns. These range from HIV/AIDS to tobacco control, gender-based violence, and food insecurity. The Minnesota Department of Health (2020), indeed, prominently features force field analysis and simple steps for its use on its department website (https://www.health.state.mn.us/communities/practice/resources/phqitoolbox/forcefield.html).

Finally, and in part *because* it requires a nuanced insider understanding of a situation as experienced by the people concerned about an issue, force field analysis has been a valued tool for community organizers from Saul Alinsky in the 1950s through the present (Dubey, 2017).

To conduct a force field analysis as part of a community organizing effort, draw a diagram as in figure AII.I and follow these simple steps:

1. On a large chalkboard, whiteboard, or large piece of paper or easel pad, write the change being sought in the middle of the page, atop a line running down the paper or board. On one side of the line, have group members list those factors or forces working for the change they want to see. These forces might include, for example, buy-in from the president of the board or other key players, likely positive media attention as a result of the change, and so on.

2. On the other side, list those forces likely to work against a change (e.g., fiscal costs, opposition of a key coalition or other community group, labor-intensive nature of enacting the change).

3. Beneath each force listed, draw an arrow whose thickness is used to illustrate the relative strength of that factor. Group members may, if preferred, use numbers from 1 to 5 to indicate the relative strength of the force under consideration.

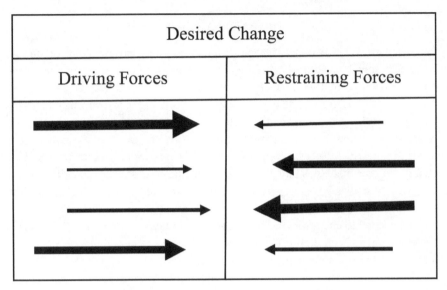

FIGURE A11.1 Sample Model for Conducting a Force Field Analysis.

4. Brainstorm first about which resisting forces can most easily be removed or weakened and how this might occur, having a notetaker keep track of the ideas generated. Remove or change the thickness of the arrows (or change the number assigned to denote weakened strength) to indicate which forces can be weakened or removed through the various tactics discussed.

5. Repeat this process for the driving forces, in this case looking at which forces can be strengthened and what new driving forces might be added to increase the chances of success in achieving the desired change.

6. Decide on "next steps": which strategies will you use in what order, and who will be responsible for follow-up on each of the action steps involved?

SWOT Analysis

Although SWOT analysis is most often used in the field of business as part of corporate strategic planning, it has become a commonly used approach in community-based organizations, and health and social welfare departments and universities, as well as in community organizing (Gürel & Tat, 2017). Also called environmental scanning or situation analysis, SWOT analysis is a process by which participants assess where they are by identifying strengths and weaknesses internal to their organization, and opportunities and threats in the external environment that may influence the effectiveness of potential new directions. Public health professionals in China thus drew on their prior experience with the SARS epidemic, as well as new epidemiological and other data, in a SWOT analysis designed to determine

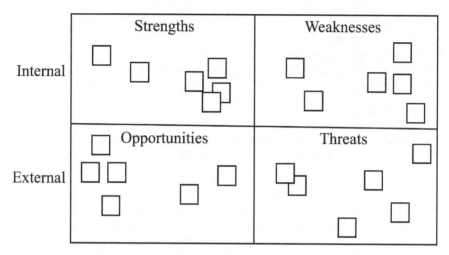

FIGURE A11.2 A Simple SWOT Analysis Schema.

the highest-priority policies for addressing the COVID-19 pandemic (Wang & Wang, 2020). Though not without pitfalls and sometimes misuse (Chermack & Kasshanna, 2007), a strong SWOT analysis can help develop strategies that maximize strengths and take advantage of new opportunities while overcoming weaknesses and avoiding or mitigating threats.

Although there are several ways of conducting a SWOT analysis, one of the most common ways, and one that works well in a community setting, involves the following steps (see figure A11.2):

1. Place four large sheets of paper on the wall or a tabletop, with the papers labeled Strengths, Weaknesses, Opportunities, and Threats.
2. Explain to the group that *Strengths and Weaknesses* refer to factors internal to their organization or agency, and thus ideally within their control; *Opportunities and Threats* refer to forces in the external environment, such as a budget cut or a new and community-friendly mayor or city council, that may have an impact on the organizing issue at hand.
3. Give each participant a set of several blank stick-on notes or other small adhesive papers in each of four colors, using a different color for each of the four categories. Have each participant think of important SWOT factors and write each on individual colored papers, for example, a Strength on yellow, a Weakness on blue, and so forth.
4. Have team members place the colored papers they have filled out on the appropriate large sheets of paper (S, W, O, or T).
5. As a group, look for common themes in each area and cluster items together by moving the colored papers around as needed. Add any new factors that come up and identify urgent or high-priority issues.

6. Stepping back, look across all four areas to identify the strategic or critical issues that emerge from the discussion. A *critical issue* is typically a challenge, dynamic tension, or conflict around which change needs to occur. For example, your environmental justice organization has just received a grant for neighborhood organizing (Strength), but it is already stretched thin by existing work (Weakness). External to the organization, a new toxic waste incinerator is being proposed for siting in a low-resource neighborhood already heavily effected by air pollution and asthma (Threat), and a key planning commission official has been exposed for accepting bribes from the industry backing the incinerator (Opportunity).

7. Look for a "fit" between different forces and your core issue. Prioritize strategic issues by importance and timing, decide what area to focus on, and brainstorm possible scenarios.

There are several variations on the SWOT analysis, including approaches for creating strategic action plans to prioritize issues by available resources, appropriate timelines, and barriers to reaching goals (VeneKlasen & Miller, 2002). A variant of the SWOT analysis created specifically with advocates and organizers in mind was developed by the Berkeley Media Studies Group (BMSG) for use in developing "a coordinated strategy toward policy goals" (Dorfman & Herbert, 2007; chapter 24). Called the ACTION framework for strategic planning, this approach involves group brainstorming around factors that can advance or serve as obstacles to the group's policy goals, the new information or intelligence needed (which might include polls, media monitoring, etc.), and the most important "next steps" to be taken to advance the overall policy goal. The acronym ACTION is used by BMSG to capture the following elements:

Assets and strengths

Challenges, barriers, or liabilities

Threats (external)

Information needs

Opportunities

Next steps

Power Mapping

Long a staple in community organizing, power mapping is of particular use to grassroots groups, coalitions, and partnerships to better understand local or regional policy environments. Best used in small groups of five to seven members, the power-mapping exercise demonstrated here can help identify key organization, community, and individual players; their stance on the issue; and their relative strength and influence (Ritas et al., 2008). It has been used with youth, environmental and social justice organizations and in other settings.

As Falbe et al. (2018) suggest, "policy mapping is particularly useful in cases of "strange bedfellows," for example, when an organization that has historically favored measures promoting public health takes an uncharacteristic opposing stand on a health-promoting measure" (p. 405). This reality was illustrated in one advocacy group's power mapping vis-à-vis a soda tax measure in San Francisco, California, in 2014. The measure would have levied a two-cent-per-ounce tax on the distributors of sugar-sweetened beverages (SSBs), with tax revenues to be earmarked for physical activity and nutrition programs, child dental care, and healthy food and drinks access for those most at risk for chronic diseases. The robust evidence base linking SSBs with diabetes and a host of cardiometabolic health problems (Malik & Hu, 2019) was used by public health professionals and others to make a strong case for the measure. Advocates did their homework and had a good understanding of the measure's key supporters, opponents, and neutral players. They also knew from experience that the immense financial and lobbying resources of the American Beverage Association (ABA) would enable it to spend millions of dollars on defeating the measure—though the advocates couldn't know which targets the ABA would be able to influence (Falbe et al., 2018). Further, power mapping could not explain some of the whys in this situation. For example, did the city's popular mayor remain neutral because of his close ties to the business community? Because at least one city department (Recreation and Parks Department) had in recent years accepted funding from the beverage industry? Or did he have other reasons (e.g., a concern that the measure could penalize smaller merchants or low-income residents)?

Power mapping was more successful in helping advocates understand why other potentially key players stood where they did. For example, when a progressive city supervisor, originally supportive of the soda tax, suddenly became silent on the measure, they "followed the money" and discovered that a progressive LGBTQ group, which was actively campaigning for the supervisor in his bid for higher office, had recently received a substantial donation from the ABA. As Falbe et al. (2018) note, "This infusion of campaign funds, and its apparent influence, led advocates to move the supervisor from 'supporter' to 'opponent' on the power map" (p. 409). Other likely supporters (e.g., the local Department of Public Health) were legally prohibited from taking a stand, while nutrition researchers and other experts from a prominent state-funded university, some of whom had come out in favor of the measure, received emails warning them not to take a stand in their roles as a university researchers, since they, too, were government employees. Finally, the silence of a large, progressive medical organization, as well as other health players whose support could have provided credibility with voters, further hurt the ballot's chances, and it failed to get the two-thirds majority vote required for passage in California of earmarked taxes.

A modified and somewhat weaker soda tax measure was passed in San Francisco two years later, thanks in part to the important lessons learned from the first unsuccessful experience and the successful soda tax experience in nearby Berkeley. For advocates and organizers, however, there were other important take-home messages as well. Key among these was that while power mapping clearly has limitations, "creating and periodically updating a power map that can track support, help explain why an initiative is succeeding or failing, and inform course corrections" can be a valuable tool in better understanding and navigating the political landscape in which we operate (Falbe et al., 2018, p. 409).

To make and use a power map, first select the *specific policy measure* that your group wants to help pass or defeat, for example, a state legislative initiative to increase the smoking age from eighteen to twenty-one, or a city council proposal to ban the shipping of coal from its port.

Then, as a group, do the following:

1. Identify the policy *target(s)*: the individuals and organizations with the power to make a particular change happen.
2. Identify the other *key players* in this situation: the individuals, organizations, or communities that may be affected by the problem or policy or that have the potential to influence the situation. Keep in mind that as change becomes imminent, many people will be drawn into the issue who did not know or care about it before. Try to anticipate whom this will be.
3. On a sheet of paper, write your *policy objective* at the top. Label the left side *supporters*, the middle *undecided* (or divided), and the right side *opposition*. Indicate on this page your *targets* (depicted as circles) and *key players* (squares), according to where they fall along the spectrum. As illustrated in figure AII.3, for visual reference use *larger* squares and circles to indicate more powerful targets and players, or those with more at stake, and *smaller* ones to indicate those who are weaker or less affected by the outcome.

Policy goal of objective _____

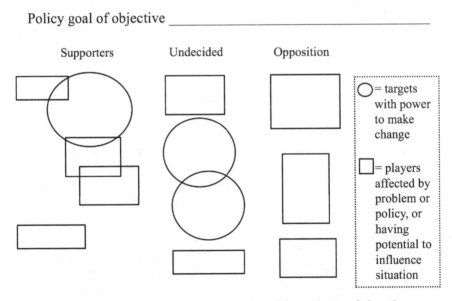

FIGURE AII.3 Creating a Power Map. Source: Adapted from Ritas et al. (2008).

4. In your mapping, remember that many considerations go into decisions about relative power (depicted in the size of the squares or circles), among them the target's or player's *scope* (size), *resources* (staff, money, lobbyists), *skills*, and *access*, as well as *how intensely the issue affects each target or player* (e.g., is it a burning or a tangential issue?). A small group that cares deeply about an issue and has great resources and organization may be more effective than a larger group with few resources or poor organization or one that feels less strongly (Ritas et al., 2008). When possible, allow the circles and squares to overlap where interests overlap. However, because some supporters may share interests with those opposed to your policy, finding areas of (sometimes unspoken) overlap between supporters may not always be possible (Ritas et al., 2008).

5. Particularly important in an election or decision year is to find out what campaign contributions, donations, or perks may have been received in current or recent years and by which player(s) in a position of influence. This step is typically not included in an initial power map and often takes place subsequently because there is usually a time lag between when campaign contributions are made and when they are publicly disclosed. However, when available, campaign contribution information may be useful in updating the map and considering strategic choices. Such information may serve as an important reality check or point of leverage in your group's efforts.

6. Given your current knowledge base, choose the three most important individuals and organizations to influence. Consider the following questions:
   - Is it more important now to strengthen your allies, persuade those who are neutral, or weaken the opposition?
   - Is it time to approach a target or to work with key players?
   - Can we get more information to increase the map's accuracy? If so, where, when, and how?

Conclusion

Whether using force field analysis, SWOT analysis, or such variations as BMSG's ACTION framework, environmental or strategic analyses like these can lay the foundation for generating potential organizing and policy advocacy strategies and providing criteria for making informed planning decisions. Further, and "consistent with health promotion values and trends for evidence-based practice, they provide systematic and multilevel approach(es) to problem assessment, resolution, and social change" (MacDuffie & DePoy, 2004). Finally, and when addressing a problem or creating an exciting new program involves working in the political arena, another strategic analysis tool, power mapping, may also be usefully employed, helping us better understand the political landscape in which we operate. In the challenging world of the present, becoming familiar with, and comfortable using, such tools will help health and social work professionals, urban and regional planners, and community organizers and our community partners, more strategically and effectively address the concerns and goals we have collectively set.

REFERENCES

Chermack, T. J., & Kasshanna, B. K. (2007). The use and misuse of SWOT analysis and implications for HRD professionals. *Human Resource Development International, 10*(4), 383–399.

Dorfman, L., & Herbert, S. (2007). *Communicating for Change / Planning Ahead for Strategic Media Advocacy.* The California Endowment.

Dubey, S. (2017). Force Field Analysis for community organizing. *Proceedings from ICMC 2017: The 4th International Communications Management Conference.* MICA.

Falbe, J., Minkler, M., Dean, R., & Cordeiro, A. J. (2018). Power mapping: A useful tool for understanding the policy environment and its application to a local soda tax initiative. In N. Wallerstein, B. Duran, J. G. Oetzel, & M. Minkler (Eds.), *Community-Based Participatory Research for Health: Advancing Social and Health Equity* (3rd ed., pp. 405–410). Jossey-Bass.

Gürel, E., & Tat, M. (2017). SWOT analysis: A theoretical review. *J Int Soc Res, 10*(51), 994–1006.

Lewin, K. (1947). Quasi-stationary social equilibria and the problem of social change. In T. M. Newcomb & E. L. Hartley (Eds.), *Readings in Social Psychology* (pp. 340–344). Holt, Rinehart & Winston.

MacDuffie, H., & DePoy, E. (2004). Force Field Analysis: A model for promoting adolescents' involvement in their own health care. *Health Promot Pract, 5*, 306–313.

Malik, V. S., & Hu, F. B. (2019). Sugar-sweetened beverages and cardiometabolic health: An update of the evidence. *Nutrients, 11*(8), 1840.

Minnesota Department of Health. (2020). Force Field Analysis. https://www.health.state.mn.us/communities/practice/resources/phqitoolbox/forcefield.html.

Ritas, C., Ni, A., Halpin, H., & Minkler, M. (2008). Using CBPR to promote policy change. In M. Minkler & N. Wallerstein (Eds.), *Community-Based Participatory Research for Health: From Process to Outcomes* (2nd ed., pp. 459–464). Jossey-Bass.

VeneKlasen, L., & Miller, V. (2002). *A New Weave of Power, People, and Politics.* World Neighbors.

Wang, J., & Wang, Z. (2020). Strengths, Weaknesses, Opportunities and Threats (SWOT) analysis of China's prevention and control strategy for the COVID-19 epidemic. *Int J Environ Res, 17*(7), 2235.

APPENDIX 12

Scale for Measuring Perceptions
of Control at the Individual,
Organizational, Neighborhood, and
Beyond-the-Neighborhood Levels

BARBARA A. ISRAEL
AMY J. SCHULZ
EDITH A. PARKER
ADAM B. BECKER

Note *from Barbara Israel*: My colleagues at the University of Michigan and I initially developed the Perceived Control Scale with respondents from Detroit, Michigan, who are primarily of African American or European American descent (Israel et al., 1994; Schulz et al., 1995). The Revised Perceived Control Scale presented here is a revision of this earlier scale and has been tested with African American women living on the east side of Detroit as part of a longitudinal, community-based, participatory research project known as the Eastside Village Health Worker Partnership (Becker et al., 2002, 2005; Schulz et al., 1998, 2003). The scale assesses individual perceptions of control or influence at four levels of analysis—individual, organizational, neighborhood, and beyond the neighborhood. In accordance with our conceptualization of empowerment across all four levels, the intent of the items at the individual level is to assess perceptions of individual influence over decisions that affect the individual's life in general. At the organizational and neighborhood levels, the intent is to assess both perceptions of individual influence within an organizational and neighborhood context and the perceived influence of the organization and neighborhood. Items measuring perceived control beyond the neighborhood level are intended to assess the perceptions of influence of the neighborhood in broader areas, such as the city, state, and national levels (Becker et al. 2002, 2005). Questions measuring perceived control at the organizational level pertain to the organization that respondents identify as being most important to them.

The scale provides a partial measure of empowerment, examining individual perceptions of control or influence at multiple levels. It does not, however, measure the development of conscientization, or critical consciousness (chapters 3, 5, 15), nor does it assess the broader social, political, economic, and cultural contexts that affect empowerment. The scale is further limited in that it does not measure actual control or obtain a collective assessment, at the organizational, neighborhood, or beyond-the-neighborhood levels of perceived or actual control. For these reasons, we strongly suggest that this survey instrument be used in combination with qualitative approaches, such as focus groups, community observations, and in-depth semistructured interviews. Finally, concepts of neighborhood, community, control, and empowerment may differ across cultures and regions, and these differences should be taken into account when the scale is adapted to other areas or population groups.

Despite these limitations, the perceived control indexes presented here have considerable potential use for health educators and other social change professionals engaged in empowerment interventions. See Becker et al. (2002) and Israel et al. (1994) for a more detailed look at the instrument's conceptual grounding and development, its strengths and limitations, and its applications in the field.

Revised Perceived Control Scale Items:
Multiple Levels of Empowerment Indexes

For the first nine items, the interviewer asked the participants, "For each of the following, please tell me whether you agree strongly, agree somewhat, disagree somewhat, or disagree strongly."

1. I can influence decisions that affect my life.
2. I am satisfied with the amount of influence I have over decisions that affect my life.
3. I can influence decisions that affect my neighborhood.
4. I am satisfied with the amount of influence I have over decisions that affect my neighborhood.
5. By working together with others in my neighborhood, I can influence decisions that affect my neighborhood.
6. My neighborhood has influence over things that affect my life.
7. By working together, people in my neighborhood can influence decisions that affect the neighborhood.
8. People in this neighborhood have connections to people who can influence what happens outside the neighborhood.
9. People in my neighborhood work together to influence decisions at the city, state, or national level.

Participants were asked a number of general questions about organizational membership. For the last five items of the Revised Perceived Control Scale, the interviewer asked the participants, "Thinking about the organization that you identified as most important to you, would you say that you agree strongly, agree somewhat, disagree somewhat, or disagree strongly with the following statements?"

10. I can influence the decisions that this organization makes.
11. This organization has influence over decisions that affect my life.
12. This organization is effective in achieving its goals.
13. This organization can influence decisions that affect the neighborhood or community.
14. I am satisfied with the amount of influence I have over decisions that this organization makes.

Indexes

- Perceived control at the individual level includes items 1 and 2 above (alpha = .61).
- Perceived control at the organizational level includes items 10 through 14 above (alpha = .67).
- Perceived control at the neighborhood level includes items 3 through 7 above (alpha = .77).
- Perceived control beyond the neighborhood level includes items 8 and 9 above (alpha = .64).
- Perceived control at multiple levels includes all fourteen items above (alpha = .77).

The alpha coefficients presented here were generated from the longitudinal survey questionnaire administered as part of the Eastside Village Health Worker Partnership (Becker et al., 2002) and reprinted with the permission of the authors.

REFERENCES

Becker, A. B., Israel, B. A., Schulz, A. J., Parker, E. A., & Klem, L. (2002). Predictors of perceived control among African American women in Detroit: Exploring empowerment as a multilevel construct. *Health Educ Behav, 29*(6), 699–715.

Becker, A. B., Israel, B. A., Schulz, A. J., Parker, E. A., & Klem, L. (2005). Age differences in health effects of stressors and perceived control among urban African American women. *J Urban Health, 82*(1), 122–141.

Israel, B. A., Checkoway, B., Schulz, A., & Zimmerman, M. (1994). Health education and community empowerment: Conceptualizing and measuring perceptions of individual, organizational, and community control. *Health Educ Q, 21*(2), 149–170.

Schulz, A. J., Israel, B. A., Parker, E. A., Lockett, M., Hill, Y. R., & Wills, R. (2003). Engaging women in community based participatory research for health: The East Side Village Health Worker Partnership. In M. Minkler & N. Wallerstein (Eds.), *Community-Based Participatory Research for Health* (pp. 293–315). Jossey-Bass.

Schulz, A. J., Israel, B. A., Zimmerman, M. A., & Checkoway, B. N. (1995). Empowerment as a multi-level construct: Perceived control at the individual, organizational and community levels. *Health Educ Res, 10*(3), 309–327.

Schulz, A. J., Parker, E. A., Israel, B. A., Becker, A. B., Maciak, B. J., & Hollis, R. (1998). Conducting a participatory community-based survey for a community health intervention on Detroit's east side. *J Public Health Manag Pract, 4*, 10–24.

EPILOGUE

This book could not have come at a better time. As we grapple with the intersecting dangers of the times in which we live, and the growing evidence of their widespread and likely long-lasting impacts, Meredith Minkler and Patricia Wakimoto bring us a resource that offers a path and shines a light. The chapters speak of courage, hope, and choices that mattered. They bring our attention to the essential skills and time-honed discipline that moves an issue forward or crafts a message that cuts through the noise. They show us how to "make a way out of no way," how to seize a moment, and how to recognize a lively possibility. This book reminds us of what is possible when we center connection and the goodness of life in our practice and our politics, no matter the storm around us. They make us proud of what people can do together. They call us to action.

As we are reminded in these chapters, community building and community organizing have deep roots and far-reaching branches. As practice, theory, and sensibilities, they are both the natural response and the necessary challenge to strangling power and systemic forces that create, as poet Langston Hughes (2009) so powerfully called it, "this fenced off, narrow space assigned to me." The close to eighty authors, and the people they bring forward in the stories they tell, demonstrate over and over again that there is an art and science to this, with each situation its own combination of timeless struggle and emerging possibility. This is sentient work.

As they shaped this collection, Minkler and Wakimoto drew a throughline across time and place, artfully revealing the interplay of key principles and ethical questions as they are expressed in diverse settings. Turning the prism one more time reveals yet another throughline—dynamic, essential tensions often embedded in community-based work for equity and justice. Three of the most salient are briefly described below.

- *Insiders and outsiders.* As we see in this book, effective organizers learn to move with respectful awareness between being a part of and apart from communities they care about deeply. This can be a strategic choice, with different leverage and resources attached to different insider or outsider designations. In contrast, boundaries can be redrawn as people share experiences—outsiders can earn community trust, insiders can be seen as having moved too far from the center. In community-based work where the stakes are high and power imbalances are real, trust can take years to build and just moments to break. Community identity is and must be reciprocal. Living with this heightened awareness is an essential tension of community building, particularly when that work centers equity, power, and justice.

- *Inner work and outer work.* This book rings with accounts of individuals willing to give extraordinary effort to organizing. That kind of work is visible, action oriented, alive in the world. At its most intense, it can be infused with heady urgency and the riveting thrill of risking and growing in community. "Outer work" is what many good organizers live for. But there is an essential tension here as well, because the most effective community organizers also know that the work is not always outside ourselves and with others, but deep within. "Inner work" is the honest, essential, and iterative process of learning, un-learning, re-learning, and co-learning that deepens our critical consciousness and empathic capacity. It can be frustrating to be driven inward when there is so much to be done outside. It can be humbling, sometimes alarming, to interrogate ourselves and our assumptions, impulses, and past actions. It can be hard to step away, and it can be excruciating to realize—or to be told—that we don't have the skills or the right to do the work the moment calls for. None-theless, attending to the necessary tension between inner and outer work is a hallmark of equity-informed community change.

- *Outrage and hope.* Community organizing and community building are fueled by these passions. At times they diverge, as if located within separate paradigms— one that centers what is and what is wrong versus the other that looks to a far-ther horizon to move toward what could be. This central tension can come between organizers, experienced as strategic, even moral, opposites that threaten the effectiveness of a campaign or a movement. But when held in the same space, this tension can enjoin evidence and imagination, experience and vision like no other. This is the dynamic energy of change.

To see the world with an organizer's gaze is to know and appreciate essential ten-sions and use them with grace. Minkler and Wakimoto give us countless exam-ples of the ways in which communities worked together to "collectively identify their assets and concerns, prioritize and select issues, intentionally build power, and develop and implement action strategies for change" (Minkler et al., 2019, p. 10S). Each example, so vividly drawn, tells the story of a complex process in a particular moment, with concrete gains, inevitable setbacks, and an as yet unknowable con-nection to what comes next.

For many years now, my favorite image of community organizing has been the fire metaphor developed by Quin Hussey (2000). With insight born of decades of community building and community organizing experience, Hussey suggests that the process of community change resembles the natural stages of fire—a spark in just the right ecological context ignites material already present, perhaps unnoticed, which then kindles until it burns with its own unique flame. Where most organizing stories stop with the fire at its most direct and powerful—the law changed, the statue removed—Hussey gives equal time and importance to what happens next, moving through three more stages before the fire dies and the ash becomes deceptively still energy that will nurture the next growth.

We are once again in interesting times. There is quiet while fire rages, denial as power shifts, cowardice and courage among us, exhaustion and mourning, awakening, uncertainty, new resolve, all in the same historical moment. Through exquisitely curated theory, tools, and case studies, Minkler and Wakimoto give us what we need to remember, in the words of Howard Zinn, "times when people behaved magnificently" in large and small ways (1994, p. 208). Our task now is simply to do the same.

Kathleen M. Roe, DrPH, MPH

REFERENCES

Hughes, L. (2009). I look at the world. In C. Wiman (Ed.), *Poetry* (4th ed.). Poetry Foundation.

Hussey, Q. (2000). The Hussey stages of community organizing. Unpublished manuscript. San José State University, San Jose, CA.

Minkler, M., Rebanal, R. D., Pearce, R., & Acosta, M. (2019). Growing equity and health equity in perilous times: Lessons from community organizers. *Health Educ Behav, 46*(1_suppl), 9S–18S.

Zinn, H. (1994). *You Can't Be Neutral on a Moving Train.* Beacon Press.

ACKNOWLEDGMENTS

Any edited book is, above all, a gift to the editors. But when most of the writing occurs during a once-in-a-century pandemic, it is truly a gift without measure. We owe a large debt to the many overcommitted individuals who made this book possible. Ranging in disciplines from public health and medicine to social work and community psychology, to law, philanthropy, and urban and regional planning, to political and social science, they were invited because of their demonstrated commitment to equity-focused community organizing and community building. But they were also selected because of their gifts in telling their stories and sharing the theory, methods, tools, and perspectives that are so central to such work in lively and accessible ways. Each one writes from the heart, and their combination of passion and professionalism has contributed greatly to the final product. Although all the authors gave selflessly, we are particularly indebted to Cheryl Hyde, Nina Wallerstein, Tom Wolff, and Ella Greene-Moton, who helped us envision a new edition that would expand its lens still farther in its addressing of the "isms" and the centrality of critical self-reflection on power and privilege in our work. Meredith's deepest thanks are also due Kathleen M. Roe, who not only agreed to write the epilogue, but whose ever-present support as a dear friend, sounding board, and sage adviser both on the book and on sometimes heartbreaking personal matters has been a gift beyond compare.

A book of this size, scope, and complexity requires extraordinary attention to detail, follow-up, and editing skills, plus an ability to juggle countless moving parts and deadlines. I had all of these in my longtime friend, collaborator, and right arm, Dr. Patricia Wakimoto, who graciously agreed to serve as coeditor, despite the extraordinary challenges of doing so during the pandemic.

We are deeply grateful to the team at Rutgers University Press, and particularly to our editor, Peter Mickulas, who believed in this project from the very beginning, as well as to Daryl Brower and Brice Hammack. Also, our thanks to John Donohue at Westchester Publishing Services and Diane Ersepke of Miccinello Associates, who helped make this final edition a reality.

Many colleagues, practitioners, and community activists have shared with us and our fellow authors case studies and examples, ethical dilemmas faced in practice, and new ways of conceptualizing and assessing key aspects of community organizing and community building. Although too numerous to mention by name, their contributions are cited throughout the book, and they are deserving of special thanks and recognition.

As Barbara Kingsolver (1990) reminds us in her book *Animal Dreams*, "The very least you can do with your life is to figure out what to hope for. And the most you can do is to live inside that hope. Not admire it from a distance but live right in it, under its roof." Like many of our coauthors, we have been blessed in the choice of careers in public health that place a strong emphasis on the centrality of empowerment, equity, and social justice for health and well-being. As coeditors, we have also been deeply privileged to "live our hope" under the literal roof of the University of California, Berkeley's School of Public Health, under visionary deans like Joyce C. Lashof and Michel Lu, and with colleagues like Denise Herd, Emily Ozer, Amani Allen, Laura Stock, Diane Bush, Mahasin Mujahid, John Schwartzberg, and Colette Auerswald, along with others who are coauthors in these pages. We also express our deep gratitude for the wisdom, wit, and immense contributions to health and social equity of our late colleagues William Satariano and Kirk Smith, who left us far too soon. Thanks in large part to these and other individuals too numerous to mention, and to the School's unparalleled and deeply caring staff, "going to work" has been a source of pleasure and inspiration over more than three decades.

I (Meredith) also have had the privilege of working with and learning from many leaders and social justice activists and scholars who remain sources of immense inspiration in their unstinting efforts to promote health and social equity. In addition to those who have contributed to this book as authors, this list includes Angela Glover Blackwell, Nick Freudenberg, Nancy Krieger, Robert Ross, Arnold Perkins, and the late H. Jack Geiger, Steven P. Wallace, Steve Wing, and Ruth and Victor Sidel.

The fourth edition of this book owes its existence, in part, to my former graduate students at UC Berkeley, and I owe them tremendous gratitude for teaching me far more about community organizing and community building than I could ever have hoped to teach them. Although too numerous to name, many have become treasured friends as well as colleagues, and working with them has been a blessing and an honor.

Many of our other best teachers, however, have been community leaders and members on the front lines working with groups including the Tenderloin Healthy Corner Store Coalition; Richmond's Safe Return Project; the Chinese Progressive Association; Concerned Citizens of Tillery, North Carolina; Mujeras Unitas y Activas; the Gray Panthers; and the Disability Rights Movement. Together, they have deepened our understanding of what committed organizing and community building are all about, while reminding us of the importance of the Indigenous Peoples' and disability rights movement's mantra, "Nothing about us without us."

I (Meredith) also owe great thanks to the former scholars, leadership, staff, and board of the W.K. Kellogg Foundation's Community Health Scholars Program, which trained many leading faculty and community leaders of color, from whom I continue to learn a great deal about community-engaged research and the imperative of undoing policies rooted in systemic racism. Finally, and for more than a decade, I had the privilege of learning from the masters—older activists, predominantly of color and many from LGBTQ and other often marginalized communities, as part of the California Senior Leaders Program and the California Senior Leaders Alliance it created. With their motto, "Don't think outside the box—think outside the warehouse," the Senior Leaders have brought wisdom and lifelong modeling of effective community building, organizing, and policy advocacy. I remain deeply grateful to them; to the project's former directors, Lisa Romero, Marty Martinson, Julia Caplan, Analilia P. Garcia, Jonathan Malagon, and Meena G. Nair; and to the Atlantic Philanthropies, and particularly to Jeff Kim and the California Wellness Foundation for their long belief in and support of this work.

The fourth edition of this book came to fruition thanks in part to the stimulation and support of my family and friends. My parents were lifelong supporters and role models, providing encouragement and love beyond measure, even as their days grew more difficult. A school principal and believer in teaching and celebrating Black history long before it was popular, my late father, Roy Minkler, was my inspiration and shining star, and the greatest teacher I have ever known, both in the public schools and with his own five children. My mother, Frances Minkler, showed in her fifteen-year struggle with Alzheimer's disease the same gifts of love, concern for others, and optimism that characterized her entire life. My late uncle, Donald H. Minkler, was a tremendous role model and a source of pride and love. His long and courageous battle with Alzheimer's, like his lifelong giving as a physician, teacher, and global leader in family planning and women's reproductive rights, touched many lives. My siblings, Donna, Jason, Chris, and Joan, my niece Lauren, my Aunt Betsy, and their families have, each in their own way, contributed to this project's coming to fruition.

Although I did the lion's share of the work on this book in the wee hours to avoid cutting into family and other work time, any project of this type takes a toll. I am grateful above all to my husband, Jerry Peters, for his love, support, patience, outstanding dinners night after night, and for all the big and little things he did to make life easier and somewhat more manageable during times of chaos and uncertainty. My son Jason continues to give the gifts of his over-the-top sense of humor, his resilience, his lifelong concern for those who are bullied or mistreated, and his determination not to give up. Our beloved twin granddaughters, Ana and Aria, and their incredible mom and environmental educator, Liana Labarca, bring great joy and hope for the future. Our dear friend, Rose Marie Springer, and the two amazing young men, Marquis Parks and Paul Peña, who are like sons to us, have each been part of our family for many years and keep me filled with gratitude. Together with my late parents and nephew, my husband, son, siblings, niece, and their families, they have been a constant reminder that real "family values" are embedded, in large part, in the support and love that families, however they are defined, give to and receive from their members.

NOTES ON CONTRIBUTORS

MARISA RUIZ ASARI, MS, BA, is a data visualization designer and developer from Oakland, California. Her work combines data science with graphic design, illustration, mapping, and other visual media to tell stories that move from understanding to action on policies and practices that shape inequality. She currently supports research institutes, community-based organizations, and city governments around the world, working on issues of health equity and social justice. Previously, she was a policy analyst in the Institute of Urban and Regional Development at the University of California, Berkeley, where she supported work including urban gun violence reduction in the Bay Area and community-led planning in Nairobi, Kenya. Marisa received her BA in public health and her MS in urban and regional development from the University of California, Berkeley, and her MS in data visualization from Parsons School of Design in New York.

MAGDALENA AVILA, DrPH, MPH, MSW, is an associate professor and community health educator in the Department of Health, Exercise and Sports Science, College of Education, University of New Mexico. She self-identifies as an activist scholar in community health and community-based participatory research (CBPR), in her partnering with Latinx and other Indigenous communities of color, and in her use of a social justice framework. Her areas of research are environmental health, environmental racism, and community health impact assessments in working with rural and urban communities. She has also expanded her research capacity by incorporating digital story making into her CBPR work with Latinx communities.

NICKIE BAZELL, MPH, is a passionate health advocate and practitioner whose work supports social justice–based organizations that focus on the root causes of health inequities. Bazell has over eighteen years of experience working with nonprofits, health departments, health care organizations, advocacy organizations, and community planning bodies on community health initiatives across the United States. She spent much of this time providing capacity building in HIV prevention and organizational development, most recently serving as director of the National Capacity Building Program at the Asian and Pacific Islander American Health Forum. She currently lives in London and is a public health specialist with a focus on COVID-19 program delivery in the Borough of Sutton. She is a savvy facilitator and coach, and is a master trainer for numerous HIV-prevention interventions and organizational development topics. She received her MPH in health and social behavior from the School of Public Health at the University of California, Berkeley.

LIONEL J. "BO" BEAULIEU, PhD, is professor of rural and regional development in the Department of Agricultural Economics at Purdue University and was director of the Purdue Center for Regional Development from 2013 to 2020. He played a key role in the launch of several innovative national research/outreach programs across the nation, including the Stronger Economies Together program and the Rural Economic Development Initiative, both in partnership with U.S. Department of Agriculture (USDA) Rural Development, as well as the Food Assistance Research Program in collaboration with the USDA Economic Research Service. Since joining Purdue in 2013, he has led the development and implementation of the Hometown Collaboration Initiative, the launch of the Rural Indiana Stats website, and the Rural Opportunity Zones initiative, all in partnership with the Indiana Office of Community and Rural Affairs. He is a past president of both the Rural Sociological Society and the Community Development Society.

ADAM B. BECKER, PhD, MPH, is associate professor of pediatrics and preventive medicine in the Feinberg School of Medicine at Northwestern University. He is also executive director of the Consortium to Lower Obesity in Chicago Children (CLOCC) at Ann and Robert H. Lurie Children's Hospital of Chicago. He has used CBPR to examine and address the impact of stressful community conditions on the health of women raising children, youth violence prevention, and the impact of the social and physical environment on physical activity.

LYNN BLANCHARD, PhD, MPH, is director of the Carolina Center for Public Service at the University of North Carolina at Chapel Hill. She also holds an appointment as clinical associate professor in health behavior in the Gillings School of Global Public Health. Her interests center on public service and how people work together to address issues of shared concern, with a focus on faculty development around community-engaged scholarship. Dr. Blanchard has developed and worked with a wide array of community programs, including those that focused on visioning and priority setting, health improvement, including children with special needs, HIV/AIDS, and community coalitions. In 2016, she was inducted into the National Academy of Community Engagement Scholarship.

ANNE BLUETHENTHAL has been bridging dance and community-engaged art for over three decades. Advancing justice and equity through bold, nuanced performance works that tackle subjects from globalization and climate change to genocide and gender violence, Bluethenthal believes that relationships are the first site of social change. Her ongoing program, Skywatchers, brings artists into durational, collaborative relationships with residents of the San Francisco (SF)

Tenderloin neighborhood, interrogating the poverty industrial complex and positioning community voices in civic discourse through the arts. Her six-year collaboration in El Salvador, ANDARES, has become part of the country's historical memory movement and remains in the repertoire of its National Dance Company. She has received recognition from *Curve* magazine, the *San Francisco Chronicle*, *SF Weekly*, the *San Francisco Bay Guardian*, and *Theatre Rhinoceros*; cofounded the Center for Art and Social Justice; and founded and produced the SF Lesbian and Gay Dance Festival and the Dancing the Mystery series.

FRANCES D. BUTTERFOSS, PhD, MSEd, is a health educator committed to building, sustaining, and evaluating partnerships to promote health and social justice. She is president of Coalitions Work and a professor at Eastern Virginia Medical School. She has founded and directed several coalitions and received research support from many agencies and foundations. She has published widely, and her books, *Coalitions and Partnerships in Community Health* and *Ignite! Getting Your Community Coalitions Fired Up for Change*, are best sellers for academics and practitioners. She is a past president and distinguished fellow of the Society for Public Health Education. She earned her BS in nursing and her MS in education from the University of Pennsylvania, and her doctorate from the Arnold School of Public Health at the University of South Carolina. Dr. Butterfoss is a recognized expert on coalition building and organizational development, with thirty years of experience training and consulting with organizations, coalitions, and communities across America.

LISA CACARI STONE, PhD, is a professor in the College of Population Health at the University of New Mexico. She has dedicated over thirty years of public health leadership to advance health equity for diverse racial, under-resourced, rural, border, Latinx, and immigrant populations. She is the founding director and principal investigator of a Transdisciplinary Research, Equity and Engagement Center, which invests in team science in testing multilevel interventions with scholars and communities of color. As a method for building community-academic capacities for policy change, she launched an "Equity 'n Policy Institute," which trains place-based teams in evidence-informed policymaking. Her collaborative and scholarly portfolio comprises over $26 million in grants from private and public funders and encompasses the macrolevel determinants of health, to the community level, to the interpersonal level. She received her doctorate in health and social policy at The Heller School, Brandeis University, completed postdoctoral training at Harvard's T. H. Chan School of Public Health, and was a fellow with the late senator Ted Kennedy.

HEATHER CAME, PhD, is a seventh-generation Pākehā New Zealander (Tangata Tiriti). She has worked for twenty-eight years in health promotion and public health and has a long involvement in social justice activism. Dr. Came is a founding member and cochair of STIR: Stop Institutional Racism, a fellow of the Health Promotion Forum, and chair of the Auckland University of Technology (AUT) branch of the New Zealand Public Health Association. She embraces life as an activist scholar. She was lead author of *Te Tiriti–Based Practice in Health Promotion* (2017), has prepared evidence for the Waitangi Tribunal claims, and has led shadow reports to various United Nations human rights committees. She is currently co–principal investigator on a Marsden Grant focusing on reimaging anti-racism theory for health professionals. Dr. Came is head of the Department of Public Health within AUT. Her research focuses on critical policy analysis, *te Tiriti o Waitangi*, anti-racism, and institutional racism in the health sector.

CARICIA CATALANI, DrPH, MPH, is a designer, researcher, and public health scientist. Her work focuses on radical, participatory, and even beautiful ways to improve health through digital innovations. Using a human-centered design approach, she has worked on over a hundred health projects in twenty-eight countries. She earned her MPH from Columbia University and her DrPH from the University of California, Berkeley. She is the former director of health for IDEO and current director of product for Pear Therapeutics.

CHARLOTTE CHANG, DrPH, MPH, was coordinator of Research to Practice and Evaluation and associate project scientist at the Labor Occupational Health Program in the School of Public Health at the University of California, Berkeley. Her work has focused on advancing the movement of research into practice in worker health and safety, with a strong interest in the role and processes of research partnerships with workers and community members. Dr. Chang has worked and written on a range of projects involving immigrant worker populations and communities as well as on research to practice lessons learned in construction health and safety. She also recently served on the board of directors of the Chinese Progressive Association and remains an important supporter of its work.

ROXANA CHEN, PhD, MPH, is a social research scientist at Public Health—Seattle & King County and affiliate assistant professor in the School of Public Health at the University of Washington. She has over twenty years of experience in public health practice and evaluation, with a focus on community-based participatory research, chronic disease disparities, social determinants of health, and using mixed methods to evaluate community and population-level interventions. She is currently leading the evaluation of the Communities of Opportunity Initiative.

WAYLAND "X" COLEMAN was born in Birmingham, Alabama, in 1978, the third child of Rosemary and Mack Coleman III. He moved with his family to Worcester, Massachusetts, in 1988 to escape conditions of poverty that they suffered in Birmingham. In 1997, when he was nineteen years old, he was falsely accused and arrested for a shooting incident at a night club. In 1998, Wayland was wrongfully convicted of the shooting by an all-White jury panel and sentenced to serve life without parole. After having been dealt such an unjust blow by the criminal justice institute, he vowed to expose the injustices, racism, and inhumanities that exist within the criminal justice empire, and within the prison industrial complex as a whole. During his time in prison, Wayland has studied law, history, and social movements, among other things, and is dedicated to the eventual abolition of the prison-industrial complex. In 2018, Wayland graduated from Boston University with honors, earning his bachelor's degree. He is a founding member of, and an internal organizer for, the #DeeperThanWater coalition in Massachusetts. He is still appealing his conviction.

CHRIS M. COOMBE, PhD, MPH, is assistant research scientist in Health Behavior and Health Education in the School of Public Health at the University of Michigan and is affiliated with the Detroit Community-Academic Urban Research Center. She has extensive experience developing, implementing, and evaluating collaborative research and community interventions using a community-based participatory research (CBPR) approach. Dr. Coombe designs and conducts capacity-building training programs in CBPR and policy advocacy for community–academic partnerships and coauthored a widely used, web-based training on CBPR. Her participatory evaluation research focuses primarily on equitable research partnerships, and she is currently a co-investigator on a study to develop a validated tool to measure success in long-standing CBPR partnerships. She works collaboratively with community and academic partners in Detroit to examine and address health impacts of inequities in urban environments, to translate research findings into policy, and to advocate for policy and systems change to advance health equity and social justice.

JASON CORBURN, PhD, is a professor of city and regional planning and public health at the University of California, Berkeley. He directs the Institute of Urban & Regional Development and the Center for Global Healthy Cities. He is a global leader in research and action linking urban and environmental planning and population health. His research explores such issues as urban governance and health; place, toxic stress, and health equity; citizen science; urban climate justice; and informal settlements and health. He co-leads urban health projects in Richmond, Sacramento, and Stockton, California; Medellín, Colombia; and Nairobi, Kenya. He has written about and developed projects focused on Health in All Urban Policies; healthy climate change resilience; urban air pollution; urban gun violence reduction; urban greening; and health and slum upgrading and health equity. Professor Corburn chairs the International Science Council, Program in Urban Health and Well-Being, is on the board of the International Society of Urban Health, was named one of the world's "Top 40 Thinkers on Cities" by Routledge, and is a recipient of the United Nations Association Global Citizenship Award. Professor Corburn received his PhD in city/urban, community and regional planning from the Massachusetts Institute of Technology.

LORI DORFMAN, DrPH, MPH, is on the faculty of the School of Public Health at the University of California, Berkeley, and directs the Berkeley Media Studies Group, a project of the Public Health Institute. BMSG works with advocates to build their capacity to use media advocacy so they can focus attention on transforming systems and structures to foster health. She studies media portrayals of health issues, including alcohol, tobacco, food, children's health, health equity, and violence, among others. Her publications are available at bmsg.org.

EUGENIA ENG, DrPH, MPH, is professor of health behavior in the Gillings School of Global Public Health at the University of North Carolina at Chapel Hill, where she codirects the Cancer Health Disparities Postdoctoral Program and the MPH concentration in health equity, social justice, and human rights. She has over thirty years of community-based participatory research (CBPR) experience, including field studies conducted with communities of the U.S. South, sub-Saharan Africa, and Southeast Asia to address socially stigmatizing health problems, such as pesticide poisoning, cancer, sexually transmitted infections, and HIV. Her CBPR projects include the National Cancer Institute–funded Accountability for Cancer Care through Undoing Racism and Equity; the Centers for Disease Control and Prevention–funded Men as Navigators for Health; and the National Heart, Lung, and Blood Institute–funded The Black Church and Cardiovascular Disease: Are We Our Brother's Keeper? In addition to her coedited book, *Methods for Community-Based Participatory Research for Health*, she has over 130 publications on the lay health adviser intervention model, concepts of community competence and natural helping, and community assessment procedures.

NANCY EPSTEIN, RABBI, MPH, MAHL, is professor in the Department of Community Health and Prevention in the Dornsife School of Public Health at Drexel University, where she directs the school's new program in Arts in Public Health. Originally trained as a community health educator at the University of North Carolina at Chapel Hill, she has spanned the boundaries of academia, policy, and community-based practice for more than forty years. Rabbi Epstein is an award-winning Drexel teaching professor and a contributing author to *Why Religion and Spirituality Matter for Public Health* as well as numerous other publications focused on religion, spirituality, arts, social justice, and public health.

JESSICA ESTRADA is a health program coordinator with the San Francisco Department of Public Health (SFDPH)–Community Health Equity & Promotion branch. She currently works with the Department's COVID-19 response team, prior to which she was co-manager and community engagement coordinator of the Healthy Retail SF Program. She also implements work as a team at SFDPH with the San Francisco Tobacco-Free Project. Prior to working at SFDPH, Jessica worked in youth development and prevention programs in Yolo County and with community-based organizations in San Francisco. In 2012, she helped form the Tenderloin

Healthy Corner Store Coalition and served as its co-lead. Jessica has over twelve years of experience in program coordination and development, community organizing, public health advocacy, youth development, outreach, coalition building, and working with unique populations like merchants and resident leaders.

JENNIFER FALBE, ScD, MPH, is assistant professor of nutrition and human development at the University of California, Davis, in the Department of Human Ecology. Dr. Falbe's research focuses on studying programmatic, policy, and environmental interventions to prevent chronic disease and reduce health disparities. She led an evaluation of the nation's first soda tax in Berkeley, California, and is examining other interventions for discouraging consumption of added sugars. Dr. Falbe also has examined community-based participatory research–informed approaches to promoting healthy retail in disadvantaged neighborhoods, primary care nutrition, and physical activity interventions for underserved youth, multisector community interventions to address childhood obesity, and the impact of screen time on adolescent sleep and health.

STEPHANIE A. FARQUHAR, PhD, is clinical professor and associate dean in the School of Public Health at the University of Washington (UW). Her work draws from the principles of community-based participatory research to address issues of social and environmental equity. She teaches core courses in the undergraduate and graduate public health programs at UW. Stephanie completed her PhD at the University of Michigan and a W.K. Kellogg postdoctoral fellowship at the University of North Carolina–Chapel Hill.

PRISILA GONZALEZ, MPH, RN, FNP-C, is a family nurse practitioner at the Indian Health Center of Santa Clara Valley, where she provides care to vulnerable populations. Prior to becoming a nurse practitioner, she worked as a research associate at the Berkeley Media Studies Group, where she helped research how media advocacy could inform policies regarding tobacco, violence prevention, and food marketing to children and communities of color. She received her MPH from the University of California, Berkeley, her BA from Stanford University, and her RN and FNP from the UC San Francisco School of Nursing.

JOSEPH GRIFFIN, DrPH, MPH, is director of peer learning at the Health Alliance for Violence Intervention. His research looks at gun violence as a form of toxic stress and focuses on strategies for community-level healing from the associated trauma. He takes a community-based participatory research approach to his work, which is primarily focused in his hometown of Richmond, California. Joseph is a Health Policy Research Scholar with the Robert Wood Johnson Foundation, where he looks at how research can be used to inform policy that leads to a more equitable society. Prior to his doctoral work, Joseph worked at Youth ALIVE!, a violence prevention organization in Oakland, California, and the Zuckerberg San Francisco

General Hospital. He received his BA, MPH, and DrPH degrees in public health from the University of California, Berkeley.

DEREK M. GRIFFITH, PhD, is a founding co-director of the Racial Justice Institute, founder and director of the Center for Men's Health Equity, and professor of health systems administration and oncology at Georgetown University. He also is a contributor to and editor of *Men's Health Equity: A Handbook* (2019) and *Racism: Science and Tools for the Public Health Professional* (2019). Trained in psychology and public health, Dr. Griffith has published more than 140 articles, and his program of research focuses on pursuing racial, ethnic, and gender equity in health, and addressing racism as a determinant of health. A fellow of the American Academy of Health Behavior, Dr. Griffith's research has been funded by several institutes within the National Institutes of Health, and also by several foundations. He received the Tom Bruce Award from the Community-Based Public Health Caucus of the American Public Health Association, and he was named by the Community of Scholars one of Cell Mentor's 1,000 Inspiring Black Scientists in America.

LESLIE GROVER is president-founder of Assisi House, Inc. She is certified in community storytelling, story exchange facilitation, and narrative medicine. A community-based participatory research expert, she works with graduate students to conduct research, develop community-based research designs, and create community-centered programs in her role as an associate professor of public policy and public administration at Southern University, Baton Rouge. An avid scholar-activist, her work is widely published on issues associated with social justice, health disparities, community polarization, and vulnerable populations.

LORRAINE M. GUTIÉRREZ, Arthur F. Thurnau Professor, has a joint appointment with the School of Social Work and the Department of Psychology, and is associate dean for educational programs in the School of Social Work at the University of Michigan, Ann Arbor. Dr. Gutiérrez is also a faculty associate in Latinx studies at the University. She focuses on multicultural praxis in communities, organizations, and higher education; multicultural education for social work practice; and identifying methods for learning about social justice. She has served as an editor of the *Journal of Community Practice* and the *Journal of Social Work Education* and is the 2020 recipient of the 2020 Career Achievement Award of the Association for Community Organization and Social Action, which honors the lifetime contribution of a person in the field who has made a major contribution to the conceptual definition of community practice.

TREVOR HANCOCK is a public health physician and health promotion consultant. He is professor emeritus in the School of Public Health and Social Policy at the University of Victoria in British Columbia. Much of his past work has been focused on healthy cities and communities, an approach he helped to pioneer. As an advisor to the World Health Organization in Europe, he helped organize the first technical workshop on healthy city indicators in Barcelona in 1987 and has maintained his interest in the subject. In 1999, he coauthored a major review for Health Canada of population health indicators at the community level. His current areas of interest are population health promotion, healthy cities and communities, and health in the Anthropocene. He recently established a local nongovernmental organization to promote dialogue about "One Planet" communities and writes a weekly column on population and public health for the *Times Colonist*, the daily newspaper in Victoria.

SUSANA HENNESSEY LAVERY, MPH, is a retired health educator with the San Francisco Department of Public Health, Community Health Equity and Promotion Branch, where she worked from 1992 to 2018. In that capacity, she designed and implemented comprehensive health promotion plans and codesigned and implemented the Community Action Model for policy development with San Francisco's diverse communities. She played a lead role in the development of healthy retail efforts in San Francisco and was on the staff of the San Francisco Department of Public Health Healthy Retail SF program. She also sat on the steering committee of the Tenderloin Healthy Corner Store Coalition. For over a decade, she participated on the Bay Area committee of Vision y Compromiso, a California statewide community health worker network. Previously, she was the Community Health Education supervisor at La Clinica de La Raza in Oakland, California, for many years. She also participated for many years on statewide, national, and global health equity planning and implementation initiatives. She also is coauthor on numerous professional publications.

REVA HINES, PhD, is the Alphonse Jackson Professor of Political Science at Southern University and A&M College, Baton Rouge, Louisiana. She is an Interdisciplinary Research Leader Cohort I, Alumni. As a fellow, her research explored the links between health and housing in Baton Rouge. She holds certification in narrative therapy and in community storytelling and is keenly interested in utilizing storytelling as a conduit for empowerment and resiliency among marginalized groups in her community. She is the founding president of Red Stick Bras and All Project, a nonprofit organization that provides resources to unhoused women in the Baton Rouge area. She is also a member of various boards and commissions with her most recent appointment by the Louisiana governor as a commission member on Louisiana Women Policy and Research and by the mayor of Baton Rouge as an institutional partner on the Commission of Racial Equity and Inclusion.

MARK S. HOMAN, MSW, LCSW, recently retired from the faculty at Pima Community College, where he was chair of the Social Services Department. He has also taught and lectured in graduate and undergraduate programs at numerous colleges and universities in the United States and abroad. For more than forty years, he has been active in community organization and development work, and he often serves as a consultant to public and private groups working to strengthen communities. Homan is the author of two widely used books, *Promoting Community Change: Making It Happen in the Real World* (6th ed., 2016) and *Rules of the Game: Lessons from the Field of Community Change* (2nd ed., 2018).

CHERYL A. HYDE, PhD, MSW, is associate professor in the School of Social Work at Temple University. Her primary areas of scholarship and teaching are organizational and community capacity building, multicultural education, feminist praxis, social movements and collective action, and socioeconomic class issues. She is a past president of the Association for Community Organization and Social Administration, former editor of the *Journal of Progressive Human Services*, and a member of several social science and social work editorial boards. She also has practice experience in feminist, labor, and anti-oppression movements.

BARBARA A. ISRAEL, DrPH, MPH, is professor of health behavior and health education in the School of Public Health at the University of Michigan. She has published widely and is actively involved in a number of community-based participatory research partnerships examining and addressing areas including the social and physical environmental determinants of health inequities in cardiovascular disease and childhood asthma and capacity building for, and translating research findings into, policy change.

ANTONY B. ITON, MD, JD, MPH, is senior vice president for Healthy Communities at The California Endowment (TCE), the state's largest health foundation. His primary focus is on TCE's ten-year Building Healthy Communities Initiative, which transforms communities into places where children are healthy, safe, and ready to learn. Previously, he was director and county health officer for the Alameda County Public Health Department. Under his leadership, the county launched an innovative plan to improve the health and lifespan of low-income communities by addressing poverty, racism, and discrimination that prevent residents from obtaining quality housing, jobs, health care, and educational opportunities. He recently coauthored *Advocacy for Public Health Policy Change: An Urgent Imperative* with H. Snyder. Dr. Iton is a regular public health lecturer and national conference keynote speaker. He earned his BS in neurophysiology from McGill University, his JD and MPH from the University of California, Berkeley, and his MD from Johns Hopkins University.

WHITNEY JOHNSON is a project manager at Public Health—Seattle & King County, supporting communications and special projects for Communities of Opportunity. Whitney has worked for over ten years in public health research and programs focused on health equity, policy change, and systems of community-based health.

MICHELLE C. KEGLER, DrPH, MPH, is a professor in the Department of Behavioral, Social and Health Education Sciences in the Rollins School of Public Health at Emory University. She directs the Emory Prevention Research Center and the Intervention Development, Dissemination and Implementation shared resource at the Winship Cancer Institute.

JOSH KIRSCHENBAUM, MS, chief operating officer at PolicyLink, enjoys building projects, initiatives, and organizations. As one of PolicyLink's original staff members, Josh works across the programmatic, communications, and operations teams, which allows him to bring comprehensive organizational knowledge to bear on supporting diverse alliances of internal and external teams to deliver on the promise of equity. His broad understanding of PolicyLink programs, funding, and partners enables him to design and launch new initiatives, drive organizational strategy, and chart the future of the institute. Prior to joining PolicyLink, Josh was the director of special projects in the Institute of Urban and Regional Development at the University of California, Berkeley. He received his BA from Brown University and his MS in city and regional planning from the University of California, Berkeley.

JOHN P. KRETZMANN is cofounder and codirector of the Asset-Based Community Development (ABCD) Institute in the Institute for Policy Research at Northwestern University. The ABCD Institute works with community building leaders across North America as well as on five other continents to conduct research, produce materials, and otherwise support community-based efforts to rediscover local capacities and to mobilize citizens' resources to solve problems. The Institute continues to build on stories and strategies for successful community building reported in his popular book *Building Communities from the Inside Out: A Path toward Finding and Mobilizing a Community's Assets* (1997), written with longtime colleague John McKnight. He formerly worked as a community organizer and community development leader in Chicago neighborhoods, and as a consultant to a wide range of neighborhood groups.

RONALD LABONTÉ, PhD, is Distinguished Research Chair in Globalization and Health Equity and professor in the School of Public Health and Epidemiology at the University of Ottawa. For the past twenty-five years, logically following his earlier work on health and community empowerment, his research has focused on the health equity impacts of diverse globalization processes, many of which form the content of his 2019 book, *Health Equity in a Globalizing Era*. He is editor-in-chief of the BioMed Central journal *Globalization and Health*. He is active with the People's Health Movement, a frequent contributor to its flagship publication *Global Health Watch*, and a co-editor of its forthcoming sixth edition. His most recent work focuses on the global governance of infectious disease and antimicrobial resistance, the political economy of tobacco farming in low- and middle-income countries, and the health impacts of "free" trade and investment treaties.

BLISHDA LACET, MPH, MBA, is a program manager at Public Health—Seattle & King County. She leads the Community Partnership—Place-Based and Cultural Community Partnership Strategy for the King County Communities of Opportunity Initiative. As the strategy lead for the COO partnership work, she provides support and resources such as training and technical assistance to these partnerships. Blishda received her BS in social psychology from Tufts University in Medford, Massachusetts, her MPH from Boston University School of Public Health, and her MBA from Babson College, Olin Graduate School of Business in Wellesley, Massachusetts.

PAM TAU LEE, BA, is a retired instructor at City College of San Francisco and a former project director at the Labor Occupational Health Center in the School of Public Health at the University of California, Berkeley. She was also a founding member of both the Chinese Progressive Association, San Francisco (CPA), and the Asian Pacific Environmental Network, and recently served as chair of the board of the CPA. A longtime activist and practitioner of popular education, community organizing, and community-based participatory research, she has made major contributions to improving the working conditions of immigrants and women.

EDITH A. LEWIS, PhD, MS, is emerita professor of social work and women's studies at the University of Michigan, Ann Arbor. Her primary research interests include methods used by women of color to offset personal, familial, community, and professional role strain. This has included involvement in studies identifying strengths within African American women's communities; the intersections of gender and ethnicity in the lives of women of color; outcomes of an intervention project for pregnant, substance-dependent women; multicultural organizational development, isolating the successful methods used by Ghanaian women in community development projects; and the development of the Network Utilization Project intervention to systematically address individual, family, and community concerns. She has taught in the areas of ethnoconsciousness, community and social systems methods, global and feminist practice, and family and group theories and practice. Her other areas of interest include teaching innovations, particularly those that help prepare social work students for practice within diverse national and global communities.

JENNIFER LIFSHAY, MPH, led community health assessment, planning, and evaluation projects for Contra Costa Health Services' Public Health Department for nearly fifteen years. Prior to her work with CCHS she did strategic planning and monitoring and evaluation work with several Bay Area youth development organizations. She received her MPH in behavioral sciences from the University of California, Berkeley, and her MBA from Columbia University.

LAURA A. LINNAN, ScD, is senior associate dean, academic and student affairs, and professor in the Department of Health Behavior at the University of North

Carolina Gillings School of Global Public Health, Chapel Hill. She is also a director of the Carolina Collaborative for Research on Work and Health. She has more than three decades of experience planning, implementing, and evaluating successful multilevel community-based interventions focused on a wide range of chronic disease outcomes among individuals and groups that suffer health disparities. She is particularly focused on promoting healthy equity though individual, organizational, and policy-level intervention strategies. Linnan's community-based participatory research has been in collaboration with key stakeholders in worksites, beauty salons and barbershops, childcare centers, and churches, and she has employed innovative mixed methods to evaluate key processes and outcomes associated with these efforts.

SHAW SAN LIU is the executive director of the Chinese Progressive Association, San Francisco (CPA). During her fourteen years at the CPA, she has led the development of grassroots organizing and leadership development programs with the Tenant Worker Center, which includes services for low-wage Chinese immigrant workers and tenants living in San Francisco's Chinatown. She has also spearheaded campaign and alliance building to advance policy on labor and economic issues in the Bay Area. She cofounded the Progressive Workers Alliance, an alliance of low-wage worker centered in San Francisco, and has extensive experience with labor and community organizing.

SHADDAI MARTINEZ CUESTAS, MPH, is the strategic communication specialist at Berkeley Media Studies Group (BMSG), where she supports advocates in enhancing their media and communication strategies to advance their policy goals. Shaddai received her MPH from the University of California, Berkeley, with an emphasis on health and social behavior. Before joining BMSG she was the HIV services director at Mission Neighborhood Health Center (MNHC), overseeing the HIV care, psychosocial support, and prevention programs serving low-income and Latinx communities in San Francisco. Prior to this role, she filled various direct service and managerial positions at MNHC. Shaddai is originally from Tijuana, Mexico, and is fully bilingual in English and Spanish.

MARTY MARTINSON, DrPH, MPH, is associate professor and department chair in the Department of Public Health at San Francisco State University. Her work explores the uses of critical pedagogies and political economy lenses in public health education. Formerly, she also critically explored the promotion of ideals of healthy aging that privilege productivity and other capitalist values over other ways of being and growing old. She previously directed the California Senior Leaders Program and Alliance, a program that provided support for the community building and advocacy efforts of diverse elders throughout the state. She earned her DrPH and MPH from the University of California, Berkeley, and her MEd in social justice education from the University of Massachusetts, Amherst.

JOHN L. McKNIGHT is founding director (emeritus) of the Community Studies Program in the Institute for Policy Research at Northwestern University, where he is an emeritus professor in both the School of Speech and the School of Education and Social Policy. He has worked with communities across the United States and Canada and is author of *The Careless Society: Community and Its Counterfeits* (1995) and the coauthor of the widely cited workbook *Building Communities from the Inside Out: A Path toward Finding and Mobilizing a Community's Assets* (1997).

MEREDITH MINKLER, DrPH, MPH, is professor emerita in the School of Public Health and a professor in the Graduate School at the University of California, Berkeley, where she was also founding director of the University's Center on Aging. Dr. Minkler continues to work with community and other partners to develop the evidence base for implementing healthy public policy in areas including food security, environmental justice, immigrant worker health and safety, and reforming the racialized and broken criminal legal system. She conducts multimethod case study analyses of short- and long-term contributions of community-engaged research to equitable public policy and building healthy communities. She has published nearly 200 articles and coauthored, edited, or co-edited ten books, including *Community-Based Participatory Research for Health: Advancing Social and Health Equity* with Wallerstein et al. (3rd ed., 2018). She continues to work with universities, government agencies, philanthropic organizations, and grassroots groups in the United States and other countries on community and policy approaches to health and social equity.

CHRISTINE MITCHELL, ScD, is a research associate with the Health Instead of Punishment program at Human Impact Partners, a national nonprofit based in Oakland, California, committed to bringing the power of public health to social justice campaigns and movements. She is an organizer with the Boston-based abolitionist #DeeperThanWater coalition and a coauthor of the American Public Health Association policy statement on law enforcement violence.

RACHEL MORELLO-FROSCH is a professor in the Department of Environmental Science, Policy and Management and the School of Public Health at the University of California, Berkeley. Her research examines structural determinants of community environmental health with a focus on social inequality, psychosocial stress, and how these factors interact with environmental chemical exposures to produce health inequalities. Her work explores this environmental justice question in the context of climate change, air pollution, environmental chemicals, and effects on women's and children's health, often using community-based participatory research methods. In collaboration with communities and scientists, she has developed science-policy tools to assess cumulative impacts of chemical and non-chemical stressors to improve regulatory decisionmaking and advance environmental justice. This includes California's Drinking Water Tool and the Environmental

Justice Screening Method, which served as a foundation for Cal-EPA's CalEnviro-Screen, to identify vulnerable communities that are disproportionately burdened by multiple sources of pollution and social stressors, and require enhanced regulatory attention.

MARY ANNE MORGAN, MPH, has over thirty years of experience working with local health departments, community-based organizations, health advocates, and community leaders to address critical public health issues. She has provided technical assistance, training, and program development to regional public health associations and statewide health department initiatives in areas that include community engagement strategies, chronic disease prevention through policy and systems change, elder abuse, community violence prevention, and social and environmental justice.

ANGELA NI, MPH, has dedicated her career to working with health care systems and companies, foundations, and public entities to improve health and health care in the United States and abroad. She currently manages strategic planning efforts for Kaiser Permanente's (KP) national corporate strategy team. In this role, she facilitates the development of effective strategies and engaging discussions for KP's national and regional leadership, and helps drive alignment on ambitions and more detailed operational planning, implementation, and measurement. Previously, Angela was a manager in the health care strategy practice at Strategy&, the strategy consulting business unit of PricewaterhouseCoopers. Angela received her MPH in health policy and management from the Harvard School of Public Health.

BARACK OBAMA, the forty-fourth president of the United States, previously served as a U.S. senator from Illinois. He also served as director of the Developing Communities Project, an institutionally based community organization on Chicago's far South Side for three years, where his roles included that of community organizer. Obama was a consultant and instructor for the Gamaliel Foundation, an organizing institute working throughout the Midwest. After graduating from Harvard Law School, Obama taught constitutional law at the University of Chicago Law School for twelve years. During this time, he also directed the Illinois Project Vote, which registered 150,000 African Americans in the state. In 1996, he was elected to the Illinois State Senate and gained support for ethics reform and health care laws. Obama was re-elected twice and held the position until he was elected U.S. senator in 2004, then resigned from the Senate in 2008 to serve as President of the United States from 2009 to 2017.

EDITH A. PARKER, DrPH, MPH, is professor and chair of the Department of Community and Behavioral Health in the College of Public Health at the University of Iowa and was previously associate professor in the School of Public Health at the University of Michigan, Ann Arbor. Her research focuses on community-engaged health promotion interventions. She has served as the principal investigator or the co–principal investigator on more than twenty federally funded grants.

SUSAN R. PASSMORE, PhD, is senior scientist and assistant director for community-engaged research with the Collaborative Center for Health Equity in the School of Medicine and Public Health at the University of Wisconsin–Madison. As an anthropologist, Dr. Passmore's scholarly work focuses on the social construction of trust and the practical application of this knowledge to create innovative approaches for building researcher "trustworthiness." In her previous role as assistant director for the University of Maryland Center for Health Equity, Dr. Passmore worked closely with Dr. Stephen Thomas to adapt and re-create much of the community-engaged infrastructure originally established in Pittsburgh to the Washington, DC, metro area, including the Maryland Community Research Advisory Board and the HAIR network of barbershops and beauty salons as well as several other initiatives for community-engaged health promotion.

MANUEL PASTOR, PhD, is a distinguished professor of sociology and American studies and ethnicity at the University of Southern California (USC), where he directs the USC Equity Research Institute. He is the Turpanjian Chair in Civil Society and Social Change and received his PhD in economics from the University of Massachusetts, Amherst. Pastor's research focuses on the economic, environmental, and social conditions facing low-income urban communities—and the social movements seeking to change those realities. His latest book is titled *State of Resistance: What California's Dizzying Descent and Remarkable Resurgence Means for America's Future.*

AMBER AKEMI PIATT, MPH, is the Health Instead of Punishment Program director at Human Impact Partners, a national nonprofit organization focused on transforming the field of public health to center equity and building collective power with social justice movements. She is an experienced advocate and researcher who has collaborated with grassroots groups on successful campaigns to curb U.S. militarism, incarceration, policing, and state violence. She organizes with the Public Health Justice Collective and has served on advisory boards for issues ranging from gender equity to stigma reduction. Her publications have appeared in books, peer-reviewed journals, and local and global media, such as *The Guardian*. She is based in Oakland, California, and is an alumnus of the University of California, Berkeley, School of Public Health; the University of California, Los Angeles; and the Women's Foundation of California's Women's Policy Institute.

CHERI A. PIES, DrPH, MPH is clinical professor emerita in the School of Public Health at the University of California, Berkeley. She served as principal investigator for the Best Babies Zone Initiative, which developed a place-based multisector approach to reducing infant mortality through community-driven transformation. She previously directed the Family, Maternal, and Child Health Programs for Contra Costa Health Services. Her work has included implementing a life course perspective in maternal and child health practice, education, and training; community capacity building; photovoice; women's health and reproductive issues; women and HIV; and parenting support for nontraditional families. Dr. Pies is a pioneer in understanding social determinants of health and the ways in which social and economic disparities and inequities influence birth outcomes and generational health across the life course. In 2018, she received two prestigious honors: the American Public Health Association Section Award for Leadership & Advocacy and the Maternal and Child Health Bureau Champion Award.

CLARA PINSKY, MS, works at the intersection of arts, public health, and urbanism. She formerly served as senior program manager of Skywatchers, an innovative community arts ensemble in San Francisco, and is an assistant choreographer at Forklift Danceworks, a nationally recognized, community-based dance company. She is coauthor of the recent study *Creative Placemaking Finance*, published by the Lindy Institute for Urban Innovation and commissioned by ArtPlace America and The Kresge Foundation. She also is author of "Community Collaborations as Creative Disruptions" in *The Journal of the Texas Arts Education Association*. Clara earned her BA in dance from Wesleyan University and her MS in urban strategy from Drexel University.

R. DAVID REBANAL, DrPH, MPH, is assistant professor of public health in the College of Health and Social Sciences at San Francisco State University (SFSU). His research focuses on building evidence for policy- and population-level interventions focused on structural and social determinants of health inequities. His current research examines the roles of neighborhood features, immigrant political participation, and neighborhood social capital on the mental health of Asian Americans. Dr. Rebanal has nearly two decades of public health experience, including working in public health program development and evaluation. This includes leadership roles in philanthropy, policy advocacy, and community-based participatory research initiatives. Prior to his current appointment, Dr. Rebanal was senior research and evaluation associate at the Health Equity Institute at SFSU, and is currently an affiliate faculty member. Dr. Rebanal received his DrPH with a focus on social epidemiology and community development at the University of California, Berkeley.

KATHLEEN M. ROE, DrPH, MPH, is editor-in-chief of *Health Promotion Practice*, a journal of the Society for Public Health Education dedicated to the art and science of community-based practice for equity and social justice. She also is professor emerita in the Department of Health Science and Recreation at San Jose State University, which she chaired from 2000 to 2012. Deeply interested in the ways in which people experience and become engaged in the issues of their time, she bases her work on principles of inclusion, voice, and agency. Among her many community building and community organizing projects over several decades were long-term community–academic partnerships in the United States and Mexico. Her career was based at San José State University, where she was professor of public health for over thirty years, MPH director for twelve years, and chair of the Department of Health Science and Recreation from 2000 to 2012.

ZACHARY ROWE, BBA, is executive director of Friends of Parkside, a grassroots community-based organization on Detroit's east side that promotes solidarity among Parkside residents, helps build the self-esteem of youth residents, offers educational and employment-related resources to the community, and promotes the health and well-being of residents. Mr. Rowe has been involved with community-based participatory research projects for close to twenty-five years and is a founding member of the Detroit Urban Research Center board. He served as a co–principal investigator on National Institutes of Health and Agency for Healthcare Research and Quality–funded projects.

ALICIA L. SALVATORE, DrPH, MPH, is the director of community-engaged research at the Christiana Care Value Institute. She conducts participatory and partnered research in the community and within health systems to examine and address social, environmental, and organizational determinants of health and health equity. She received her DrPH from the School of Public Health at the University of California Berkeley, her MPH in health behavior from Gillings School of Global Public Health at the University of North Carolina at Chapel Hill, and her BA from Franklin and Marshall College. She completed a National Heart, Lung, and Blood Institute–funded postdoctoral fellowship at the Stanford Prevention Research Center and was an instructor at the Stanford School of Medicine and an associate professor of public health at the University of Oklahoma Health Sciences Center prior to coming home to Delaware.

SHANNON SANCHEZ-YOUNGMAN, PhD, is a research assistant professor and political scientist at the University of New Mexico. Her research focuses on the development and impact of health and social policy on women of color and children in the United States.

AMY J. SCHULZ, PhD, MPH, is professor of health behavior and health education in the School of Public Health at the University of Michigan. She has served as principal investigator for the Healthy Environments Partnership since 2000 and as co–principal investigator for Community Action to Promote Healthy Environments since 2014; both are community-based participatory research partnerships focused on environmental justice and health equity in Detroit. She has authored more than 130 professional publications and has served as principal investigator on eleven federally funded research grants.

RINKU SEN is a writer and a political strategist. She was formerly the executive director of Race Forward and was the publisher of their award-winning news site Colorlines. Under her leadership, Race Forward generated some of the most impactful racial justice successes of recent years, including Drop the I-Word, a campaign for media outlets to stop referring to immigrants as "illegal," resulting in the Associated Press, *USA Today*, the *Los Angeles Times*, and many other outlets changing their practice. She was also the architect of the *Shattered Families* report, which identified the number of kids in foster care whose parents had been deported. Her books *Stir It Up* and *The Accidental American* theorize a model of community organizing that integrates a political analysis of race, gender, class, poverty, sexuality, and other systems.

LEE STAPLES, PhD, MSW, is clinical professor emeritus in the School of Social Work at Boston University. He has been involved in community organizing since 1968 as a street organizer, supervisor, staff director, trainer, consultant, educator, and coach. His organizing has included welfare rights, public and private housing, mental health consumers, childcare, low-wage workers, public health, tax reform, immigrant rights, labor, youth empowerment, and other issues at neighborhood, statewide, and national levels. He has conducted several hundred community organizing training sessions across the United States and internationally (Bosnia, Canada, Croatia, Denmark, Israel, Morocco, Netherlands, Puerto Rico). His research and publications focus on nongovernmental organization development in the Balkans, consumer empowerment in Israel, social capital in Latinx communities, mental health rights, grassroots leadership development, social action groups, immigrant workers' centers, and youth organizing. He has published numerous scholarly articles and is the author of *Roots to Power*, now in its third edition, and coauthor (with Melvin Delgado) of *Youth-Led Community Organizing*.

CELINA SU, PhD, is the Marilyn J. Gittell Chair in Urban Studies and professor of political science at the City University of New York. Her publications include *Streetwise for Book Smarts: Grassroots Organizing and Education Reform in the Bronx* and pieces in the *New York Times Magazine*, *Harper's*, and elsewhere. Her work focuses on everyday struggles for collective governance, centering economic democracy, and racial justice. She has received several distinguished fellowships, including a Berlin Prize. She earned her PhD in urban studies from the Massachusetts Institute of Technology.

MAKANI THEMBA is chief strategist at Higher Ground Change Strategies based in Jackson, Mississippi. A social justice innovator and pioneer in change communications and narrative strategy, she has spent more than twenty years supporting organizations, coalitions, and philanthropic institutions in developing high-impact change initiatives. Higher Ground provides Makani the opportunity to bring her strong sense of history, social justice, and organizing knowledge in support of changemakers seeking to take their work to the next level. Higher Ground helps partners integrate authentic engagement, systems analysis, change communications, and more for powerful, vision-based change. Makani is a highly sought-after public speaker, capacity builder, and trusted facilitator. Previously, she founded and served as executive director of The Praxis Project, a nonprofit organization helping communities use media and policy advocacy to advance health justice. Makani has published numerous articles and case studies on race, class, media, policy advocacy, and public health.

STEPHEN B. THOMAS, PhD, is professor of health policy and management in the School of Public Health and director of the Maryland Center for Health Equity at the University of Maryland in College Park. Over the past three decades, Dr. Thomas has applied his expertise to address a variety of conditions associated with the burdens of race and history, including cardiometabolic diseases, HIV/AIDS, and COVID-19. He is the principal investigator of the Research Center of Excellence on Race, Ethnicity and Disparities Research, funded by the NIH–National Institute on Minority Health and Health Disparities. To achieve health equity for all, he believes we must translate the science of medicine and public health into culturally tailored community-based interventions codesigned with people from the neighborhoods being impacted by everyday racism and structural inequality.

MARÍA ELENA TORRE, PhD, is the founding director of the Public Science Project and faculty member in critical psychology and urban education at the Graduate Center at the City University of New York. A mama of a very cool eleven-year-old, she has written about and been engaged in critical participatory action research nationally and internationally for over twenty years with communities in neighborhoods, schools, prisons, and community-based organizations seeking structural transformation. Coauthor of *The Essentials of Critical Participatory Action Research* and co-editor of *PAR EntreMundos: A Pedagogy of the Americas*, her work looks at how decolonizing methodologies, radical inclusion, and a praxis of solidarity can inform a participatory public science that supports movements for justice.

EVAN VANDOMMELEN-GONZALEZ, DrPH, MPH, is grateful for her community organizing mentors and partners. She is the faculty director for the On-Campus/Online MPH Interdisciplinary Program and core faculty for the DrPH program in the School of Public Health at the University of California, Berkeley. Building on years of community health education and outreach, she coordinated bilingual Spanish/English field efforts for research projects in New York and San Francisco with young people and women in the areas of sexual health, partnership dynamics, social networks, and place-based health. Her current community research experience, teaching, and learning centers on participatory, mixed-methods, action-oriented, and strengths-based approaches to multilevel interventions, including with undocumented and gang-involved youth communities and worker justice projects documenting the impact of workload and chemical exposures on janitor and domestic worker health in California. She received her DrPH from the School of Public Health at UC Berkeley and her MPH from the Mailman School of Public Health at Columbia University.

DIERDRE VISSER is a curator, writer, artist, and woodworker. As Curator of the Arts at the California Institute of Integral Studies in San Francisco and publisher of CHROMA books, she strives to promote pluralism in the arts, to support artists in the creation of new and experimental work, and to foster dynamic and critical dialogues within and across communities that propose integrative approaches to the urgent questions we collectively face. With Laura Mays, Deirdre is coauthoring a forthcoming history of women in woodworking titled *Making a Seat at the Table*. As a community-based artist she works collaboratively with Anne Bluethenthal and the Skywatchers Ensemble in the City's Tenderloin neighborhood. She is an active member of the boards of La Pocha Nostra and ABD Productions.

PATRICIA WAKIMOTO, DrPH, MS, RD, is a researcher in the School of Public Health at the University of California, Berkeley, and in the Nutrition Policy Institute at the University of California, Davis. She has over thirty years of experience in clinical and community health and nutrition fields and special interests in diverse communities. As former codirector of the National Center on Minority Health and Health Disparities Center of Excellence, Translational, and Outreach Core, she worked with the Partners in Research project with Black and Latinx communities in Oakland, California. She previously worked with Southeast Asian Hmong communities in multiyear statewide and national collaboratives with teams from California, Wisconsin, and Minnesota. Recent work includes youth pipeline programs, the Tenderloin Healthy Corner Store Coalition, and school-based interventions focused on nutrition, physical activity, and policy. Dr. Wakimoto has expertise in dietary methodology, program evaluation, program management, and training. She received her DrPH from the University of California, Berkeley School of Public Health, her MS in health and safety administration from Indiana University, and her BS in nutrition and dietetics from Arizona State University.

NINA WALLERSTEIN, DrPH, is distinguished professor of public health, College of Population Health, and director of the Center for Participatory Research at the University of New Mexico (UNM). She has developed community-based participatory research (CBPR) and empowerment, Freire-based interventions for over thirty years, and authored over 170 publications and seven books, including the Freirean *Problem-Posing at Work: A Popular Educator's Guide.* She was UNM's inaugural 2016 Community Engaged Research Lecturer awardee. She has a long-term relationship with New Mexican tribes to support intergenerational, culture-centered family prevention programming and has worked for over a decade with the Healthy Native Community Partnership. She has strengthened the science of CBPR and community-engaged research since 2006. As principal investigator of a National Institute of Nursing Research–funded grant, Engage for Equity, she focuses on promising partnering practices associated with outcomes and partnership evaluation and reflection resources. In collaboration with Latin American colleagues, she produced an empowerment, participatory research, and health promotion curriculum available in Spanish, Portuguese, and English. She also cosponsors UNM's annual summer institute in CBPR for health.

TOM WOLFF is a community psychology practitioner who is committed to issues of social justice and community. He is the founder of Tom Wolff and Associates and is a nationally recognized consultant on coalition building and community development, consulting with individuals, organizations, and communities across North America. His most recent book is *The Power of Collaborative Solutions* (2010). Tom's clients include federal, state, and local government agencies, foundations, hospitals, nonprofit organizations, professional associations, and grassroots groups.

KIRSTEN WYSEN, MHSA, is a policy analyst at Public Health—Seattle & King County. In 2018–2019, she was a policy fellow at the Center for Advanced Study in the Behavioral Sciences at Stanford University. She has worked for twenty-one years in health policy and planning at the Seattle/King County health department, focusing on how basic needs contribute to good health and on racial equity. She served as the policy officer for the department's COVID-19 response in spring 2020. Previously, she was the deputy program manager for the Washington State Basic Health Plan, when it grew from 90,000 enrollees to 220,000. She worked on the implementation of Washington State's 1993 health care reform law and on Medicare and Medicaid payment policies in Washington, DC, and Portland, Maine. She received her BA from Brown University and her MHSA from the University of Michigan School of Public Health.

INDEX